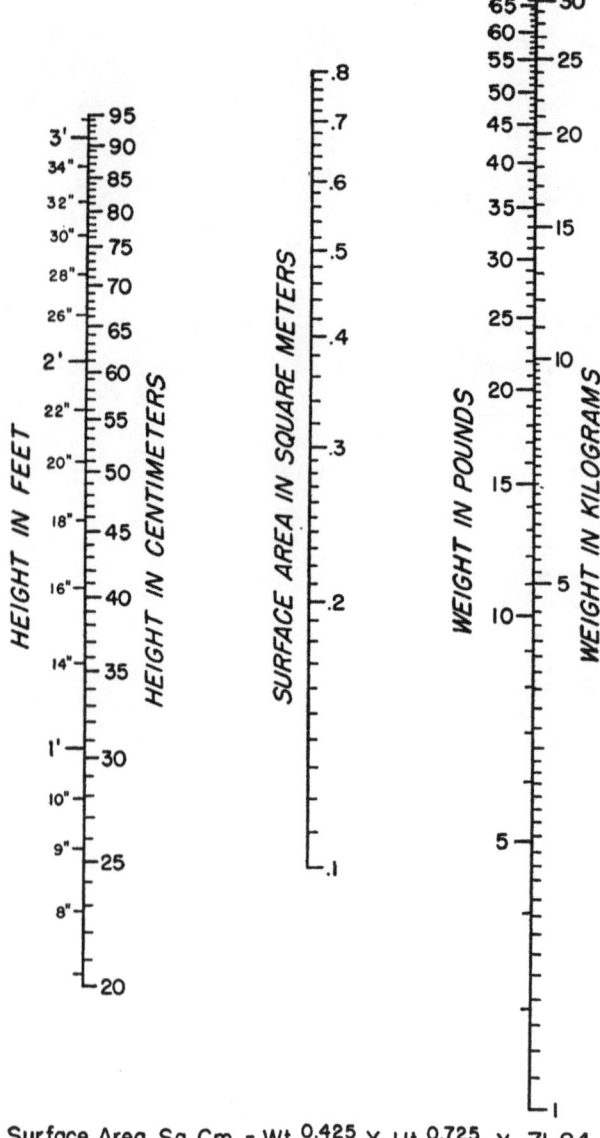

Surface Area, Sq. Cm. = Wt.$^{0.425}$ × Ht.$^{0.725}$ × 71.84

Nomograms estimating surface area from height and body weight. The patient's surface area is found by drawing a straight line between the point representing his weight and the point representing his height. From J. D. Crawford, M. E. Terry, G. M. Rourke, *Pediatrics* 5:783, 1950. See also Figure 1, page 594.

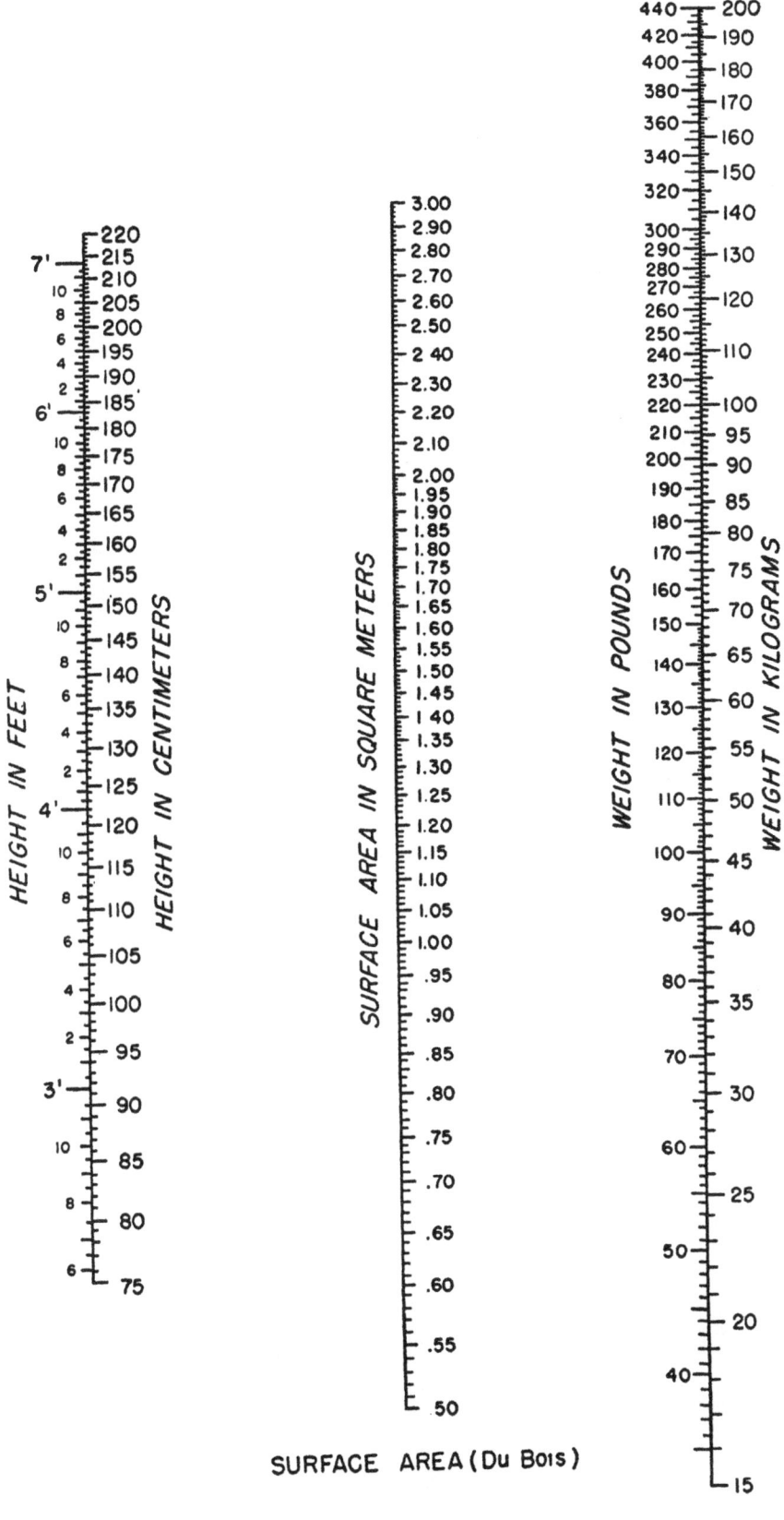

SURFACE AREA (Du Bois)

FUNCTIONAL ENDOCRINOLOGY

FROM BIRTH THROUGH ADOLESCENCE

For approximately a quarter of a century THE COMMONWEALTH FUND, through its Division of Publications, sponsored, edited, produced, and distributed books and pamphlets germane to its purposes and operations as a philanthropic foundation. On July 1, 1951, the Fund entered into an arrangement by which HARVARD UNIVERSITY PRESS became the publisher of Commonwealth Fund books, assuming responsibility for their production and distribution. The Fund continues to sponsor and edit its books, and cooperates with the Press in all phases of manufacture and distribution.

FUNCTIONAL ENDOCRINOLOGY

FROM BIRTH THROUGH ADOLESCENCE

NATHAN B. TALBOT, M.D.
ASSOCIATE PROFESSOR OF PEDIATRICS, HARVARD UNIVERSITY; PHYSICIAN, CHILDREN'S MEDICAL SERVICE, MASSACHUSETTS GENERAL HOSPITAL

EDNA H. SOBEL, M.D.
FORMERLY RESEARCH FELLOW IN PEDIATRICS, HARVARD UNIVERSITY; AT PRESENT INSTRUCTOR IN PEDIATRICS, UNIVERSITY OF CINCINNATI COLLEGE OF MEDICINE; RESEARCH ASSOCIATE, CHILDREN'S HOSPITAL RESEARCH FOUNDATION AND THE FELS RESEARCH INSTITUTE, ANTIOCH COLLEGE

JANET W. McARTHUR, M.D.
INSTRUCTOR IN GYNECOLOGY, HARVARD UNIVERSITY; ASSISTANT PHYSICIAN, MASSACHUSETTS GENERAL HOSPITAL

JOHN D. CRAWFORD, M.D.
INSTRUCTOR IN PEDIATRICS, HARVARD UNIVERSITY; ASSISTANT PHYSICIAN, CHILDREN'S MEDICAL SERVICE, MASSACHUSETTS GENERAL HOSPITAL

PUBLISHED FOR THE COMMONWEALTH FUND

HARVARD UNIVERSITY PRESS
CAMBRIDGE, MASSACHUSETTS
1954

COPYRIGHT, 1952, BY THE COMMONWEALTH FUND

PUBLISHED FOR THE COMMONWEALTH FUND
BY HARVARD UNIVERSITY PRESS
SECOND PRINTING

DISTRIBUTED IN GREAT BRITAIN
BY GEOFFREY CUMBERLEGE
OXFORD UNIVERSITY PRESS
LONDON

PRINTED IN THE UNITED STATES OF AMERICA
BY CASE, LOCKWOOD & BRAINARD

PREFACE

This book is written for practitioners, students and investigators of medicine and surgery who seek practical information concerning (a) the actions of endocrine systems in health and ordinary disease and (b) the management of endocrinopathies as they occur in young people. As much emphasis has been given the former as the latter subjects in the belief that endocrinology encompasses more than the diagnosis and therapy of those gross disorders of glandular function which result in gigantism, dwarfism, Addison's disease, Graves' disease, sexual precocity and the like. The physician may encounter but a handful of patients suffering from these unusual conditions in all his years of practice. Yet he constantly deals with patients whose health or survival depends to no small extent upon the homeostatic efficiency of certain endocrine-controlled systems. Just as we have learned that there is hardly an organ or tissue in the body beyond the influence of endocrine forces, so we are beginning to realize that there is scarcely a disease that is unaccompanied by important homeostatic changes in the functional activity of one or more of the endocrine glands. This book therefore attempts to translate into modern clinical terms the thesis so beautifully expressed by Walter B. Cannon in his classic writings on *The Wisdom of the Body*.

Detailed consideration has been given in separate chapters to all those glands now known to be organs of internal secretion. Certain structures such as the PINEAL BODY and the THYMUS, organs once considered by many to belong to the endocrine family, are not so discussed. It appears that most if not all of the effects once attributed to these structures as endocrine organs can now be explained more satisfactorily by other means. Obesity also is not considered in a separate chapter, though discussion of this condition will be found to occupy a considerable amount of space in the text. This seems a logical decision in view of the fact that the vast majority of obese patients lack any objectively demonstrable endocrine disorder. There is one chapter which we would have included had we felt that there was enough information available to justify it. This chapter might be entitled Neuro-endocrine or Psycho-neuro-endocrine Relations. In the present volume remarks concerning these relations are interspersed through the clinical sections.

In writing this book it has been assumed that the reader may be comparatively unfamiliar with the subject under consideration and with its relation to subjects covered elsewhere in this volume. On this account every effort has been made to build from the ground up and to avoid making statements which are incomprehensible for lack of background information. Toward this end, the initial sections of each chapter are devoted to considerations of the functional dynamics of the particular gland and to indicating by cross references where pertinent related information may be found. It is hoped that the latter will help the reader visualize the highly integrated nature of the endocrine complex. It is hoped also that the reader who gives attention to these basic information sections will find himself equipped with the raw material necessary for independent thinking in clinical areas. Since it is the exception rather than the rule for patients to conform exactly to textbook pictures, this seems a most important objective.

Following these sections on basic considerations, there are in most chapters sections dealing with the practical use of physiologic information in diagnostic tests. In the final clinical sections of each chapter all the foregoing data are brought to bear on the problems presented (a) by patients showing physiologic alterations in endocrine activity secondary to certain non-endocrine diseases and (b) by patients suffering from the various primary endocrinopathies. It will be noted that doses usually are expressed on a per square meter of body surface area basis. Doses thus expressed are applicable to patients of all ages regardless of size. There will be found just inside the covers of the book charts which indicate the approximate surface area of persons of various weights and heights. Incidentally, those unfamiliar with the derivation of such commonly used terms as "milliequivalent," "millimole" and "milliosmole" will find information concerning them in the last pages of the Appendix.

In the foregoing connections, it has been our purpose to make the book as concise, clear and self-sufficient as possible. These goals could be approached only at the price of considerable condensation of facts and of a certain amount of dogmatism. We have been forced to sift available information, to omit much historic, anatomic and histologic information and to present in the main single rather than multiple theses. In doing this we have attempted to review original data and to formulate opinions based on such data rather than simply to restate the ideas and conclusions of others. This method of approach has led us to undertake a number of studies designed to fill gaps in knowledge revealed by

PREFACE   [VII]

review of the literature; this book reports some of these investigations for the first time. For permission to include previously unpublished data we are greatly indebted to certain of our associates, whose names are indicated in the legends of figures representing their work.

In writing this volume we have enjoyed the support and encouragement of many colleagues, particularly Dr. Allan M. Butler, Chief of the Children's Medical Service of the Massachusetts General Hospital. We also take pleasure in expressing our appreciation to the Commonwealth Fund of New York, whose generous aid has made it possible for us to work together as a team both in writing this book and in accumulating much of the information presented herein. In addition we wish to express our thanks to the staff of the Fund's Division of Publications for the many things they have done to improve the quality of this book and to lighten the authors' burden in its making. Finally, we take great pleasure in expressing our appreciation to Mrs. Barbara G. Edwards and Mrs. Ann S. Silin for their devoted assistance in the preparation of the manuscript.

N.B.T.
E.H.S.
J.W.McA.
J.D.C.

November, 1951

CONTENTS

Preface

Chapter I. THE THYROID

BASIC CONSIDERATIONS — 1
  Thyroid Hormone — 1
  Thyroid Hormone Actions — 2
    Cell Metabolism — 2
    Cell Organization — 2
    Body Growth and Maturation — 2
  Relation of Anterior Pituitary and Thyroid Glands — 3
  Effects of Therapy on Thyroid Status — 4
    Athyrotic Individuals — 4
    Normal Persons — 4
  Physiologic Variations in Thyroid Gland Activity (Thyroid Homeostasis) — 5
  Methods of Appraising Thyroid Status — 6
    Basal Metabolic Rate — 6
    Serum Cholesterol in Hypothyroidism — 7
    Hypercarotenemia and Hyperlipemia in Hypothyroidism — 8
    Serum Alkaline Phosphatase in Hypothyroidism — 8
    Epiphyseal Dysgenesis in Childhood Hypothyroidism — 9
    Rate of Skeletal Maturation in Hypothyroidism — 11
    Urinary Creatine Output in Hypothyroidism — 12
    Radio-active Iodine Uptake in Thyroid Disease — 12
    Serum Protein-bound (Thyroid Hormone) Iodine Concentration — 13

CLINICAL CONSIDERATIONS — 14
  Hypothyroidism (Athyrosis, Myxedema, Cretinism) — 14
    Primary Hypothyroidism (Athyrosis) — 15
    Hypothyroidism Secondary to Hypopituitarism (Pituitary Myxedema) — 30
  Hyperthyroidism (Thyrotoxicosis) — 32
  Goiter — 44
    Neonatal Goiter — 44
    Endemic Congenital Goiter — 46
    Adolescent Goiter — 46
    Thyroiditis — 48

REFERENCES — 48

Chapter II. THE PARATHYROIDS

BASIC CONSIDERATIONS — 53
- The Hormone and Its Sites of Action — 53
- Physiology of the Parathyroid Endocrine System — 54
  - Introductory Comments on Renal Excretory Mechanisms — 54
  - The Parathyroids and Phosphorus Metabolism — 62
  - The Parathyroids and Calcium Metabolism — 72
  - Summary Comments on the Probable Nature of Physiologic Factors Influencing Parathyroid Activity — 74
  - Parathyroid Hormone and Bone Catabolism — 75
  - Comparison of the Effects of Vitamin D, Dihydrotachysterol and Parathyroid Extract — 77
  - Relation of the Parathyroids to Other Endocrine Systems — 78

CLINICAL CONSIDERATIONS — 78
- Physiologic Parathyroidism — 78
  - Effect of Variations in Phosphorus Intake — 78
  - Effect of Variations in Calcium Intake — 79
  - Effect of Kidney Disease on Calcium and Phosphorus Metabolism and on Parathyroid Status — 88
- Pathologic Parathyroidism — 102
  - Primary Hypoparathyroidism — 102
  - Primary Hyperparathyroidism — 122

REFERENCES — 129

Chapter III. THE ADRENAL CORTICES

BASIC CONSIDERATIONS — 135
- Chemistry of the Hormones — 135
- Physiologic Actions of the Hormones — 137
  - Electrolyte and Water Hormone (Na-K Hormone) — 137
  - Sugar-Fat-Nitrogen ("S-F-N") Hormones or 11-17-Oxycorticosteroids (11-17-OCS) — 148
  - Normal and Abnormal Adrenocortical Urinary 17-Ketosteroid Precursors (17-KS-Gens)—the So-called Adrenocortical Androgens — 156
  - Factors Controlling Adrenocortical Activity — 158
- Methods of Diagnosis — 163
  - Test 1—the Water Test for Adrenocortical Insufficiency — 163
  - Introductory Comments on Tests 2, 3 and 4 — 163
  - Test 2—the Epinephrine-Eosinophil Test — 168
  - Test 3—the ACTH-Eosinophil and Related Tests — 170
  - Test 4—the Eosinophil Count — 173
  - Test 5—the Twenty-four-Hour Fast — 174
  - Tests 6 and 7—the Insulin and Glucose Tolerance Tests — 175
  - Test 8—Urinary 11-17-Oxycorticosteroid Measurements — 180
  - Tests 9 to 11—Electrolyte Measurements — 185
  - Test 12—the Sweat Test — 189
  - Test 13—Urinary 17-Ketosteroid (17-KS) Measurements — 190

CONTENTS [XI]

CLINICAL CONSIDERATIONS	193
Hypoadrenocorticism	194
Primary Hypoadrenocorticism (Addison's Disease)	195
Overwhelming Sepsis or Other Illness and Acute Hypoadrenocorticism (Waterhouse-Friderichsen Syndrome)	216
Hypoadrenocorticism Secondary to Hypopituitarism (ACTH Lack)	218
Hyperadrenocorticism	223
Adrenocortical Virilism	224
Cushing's Syndrome	235
Adrenocortical Virilism Complicated by Signs Suggestive of Na-K Hormone Lack	245
Abnormal Feminization and Other Changes Due to Adrenocortical Tumor	247
Precocious Adrenarche	247
Therapeutic Hyperadrenocorticism Produced by Means of ACTH or Cortisone	247
REFERENCES	261

Chapter IV. THE ADRENAL MEDULLÆ

BASIC CONSIDERATIONS	271
Origin	271
Adrenomedullary and Related Sympathetic Hormones	271
Control of Adrenomedullary Activity	272
Factors Which Influence Adrenomedullary Activity	272
Actions of Epinephrine and Related Substances	272
Cardiovascular Effects	273
Metabolic Effects	273
Effects on Other Endocrine Glands	275
Anti-Epinephrine or Adrenolytic Substances	275
CLINICAL CONSIDERATIONS	275
Hypoepinephrinism Due to Adrenomedullary Failure	275
Hyperepinephrinism Due to Adrenomedullary Tumor (Pheochromocytoma and Related Tumors)	276
THE PHARMACOLOGY OF EPINEPHRINE	287
USP Preparations	287
Comments on the Therapeutic Use of Epinephrine	287
In Control of Hemorrhage	288
For Congestion of Nasal Mucosa and Conjunctiva	288
For Bronchial Asthma	288
In Miscellaneous Disorders	288
REFERENCES	288

Chapter V. THE OVARIES

BASIC CONSIDERATIONS	291
General Functions of the Ovaries	291
Genetic and Hormonal Influences in Sex Determination	291

Embryology, Anatomy and General Physiology of the Ovaries ... 291
  Embryology ... 291
  Anatomy and General Physiology ... 292
Ovarian Hormones ... 296
  Definitions of "Estrogen" and "Progestin" ... 296
  Estrogen ... 296
  Progesterone ... 300
The Sexual Development of the Child and Adolescent ... 301
  Pseudo-Precocity of the Newborn ... 301
  Genital Status during the Preadolescent and Adolescent Years ... 302
  Appearance of Secondary Sex Characters during Adolescence ... 304
  Hormone Production at Various Ages ... 306
  Correlation between Hormone Production and Sexual Differentiation ... 308
  Summary and Comments ... 309
The Menstrual Cycle ... 309
  Proliferative Phase ... 311
  Secretory Phase ... 311
  Phases of Regression and Menstruation ... 312
Methods of Diagnosis ... 312
  Indices of Estrogen Production ... 312
  Indices of Progesterone Production ... 317
  Indices of Gonadotropin Production ... 319
CLINICAL CONSIDERATIONS ... 320
Types of Sexual Precocity ... 320
  True Precocious Puberty ... 321
  Pseudo-Precocious Puberty ... 329
Types of Sexual Infantilism ... 337
  Primary Hypothalamic Infantilism ... 340
  Primary Pituitary Infantilism ... 341
  Agenesis of the Follicular Elements of the Ovary ... 344
Adolescent Menstrual Disorders ... 345
  Physiologic Considerations ... 345
  Types of Amenorrhea ... 348
  Types of Menorrhagia ... 355
  Dysmenorrhea ... 361
Hermaphroditism ... 365
  Classification ... 365
REFERENCES ... 367

Chapter VI. THE TESTES

BASIC CONSIDERATIONS ... 373
Chemistry of Testicular Hormones ... 373
Physiologic Actions of Testicular Androgens ... 374
  General Metabolic Actions ... 374
  Actions on Various Body Structures ... 375

Contents

Central Nervous System-Pituitary-Gonad Relations	385
Anterior Pituitary–Testicular Relations	385
Timing of Events During Normal Adolescence	392
Methods of Appraising Testicular Status	393
Appraisal of Testicular Androgen Production	393
Appraisal of Testicular Capacity to Produce Androgens	402
Appraisal of Testicular Tubular Status	402
CLINICAL CONSIDERATIONS	408
Isosexual Precocity in Males	408
True Precocious Puberty	408
Pseudo-Precocious Puberty	418
Sexual Infantilism–Hypogonadism with Failure of Sexual Development or Aspermatogenesis	422
Hypothalamic Infantilism	422
Pituitary Infantilism, Primary Type	423
Pituitary Infantilism, Functional Type, Secondary to Athyrosis and Nutritional Deficiencies	430
Testicular Infantilism	431
Clinical Use of Testosterone as a Growth-Promoting Agent	440
Comments on the Use of Testosterone as a Protein Anabolic Agent in Debilitated Patients	441
Comments on Cryptorchidism	442
True Cryptorchidism	442
Pseudo-Cryptorchidism	443
REFERENCES	443

Chapter VII. THE ANTERIOR PITUITARY

BASIC CONSIDERATIONS	449
The Pituitary Growth Hormone (PGH)	451
Chemical Nature	451
Physiologic Actions	451
Methods of Appraising Anterior Pituitary Status	455
CLINICAL CONSIDERATIONS	460
Pathologic Hypopituitarism	461
Primary Organic Hypopituitarism (Simmonds' Disease)	461
Secondary Functional Hypopituitarism	472
Physiologic Hypopituitarism	472
Hypopituitarism Secondary to Primary Athyrosis	473
Hypopituitarism Secondary to Undernutrition (Starvation and Anorexia Nervosa)	473
Note on the Acceleration of Wound-healing by Increasing Caloric Balance	478
Comments on the Selective or Fractional Nature of Hypopituitarism in Certain Patients	480
Pathologic Hyperpituitarism	481

Primary Organic Hyperpituitarism	481
Secondary Functional Hyperpituitarism	484
Physiologic Hyperpituitarism	486
Functional Hyperpituitarism Secondary to Caloric Hypernutrition (Simple Dietary Obesity)	486
Functional Hyperpituitarism with Tall Stature	492
REFERENCES	494

Chapter VIII. THE POSTERIOR PITUITARY

BASIC CONSIDERATIONS	497
Development and Structure of the Posterior Lobe	497
Hormones of the Posterior Lobe	497
Physiology of the Antidiuretic Mechanism	498
Action of the Antidiuretic Hormone on the Kidneys	499
Secondary Effects of Antidiuretic Hormone	510
Control of Posterior Pituitary Activity by the Hypothalamus	511
Factors Which Stimulate the Neurohypophyseal Mechanism	511
Elimination and Inactivation of Antidiuretic Hormone	514
The Role of the Adrenal Cortex in Water Metabolism	516
Summary Remarks on Limits of Control of Water Homeostasis by the Posterior Pituitary	517
CLINICAL CONSIDERATIONS	518
Hypofunction of the Posterior Pituitary	518
Pathologic Posterior Pituitary Hypofunction (Diabetes Insipidus)	520
Functional Deficiency of Antidiuretic Hormone (Psychogenic Polydipsia)	529
Comments on the Water Metabolism of Newborn Infants	530
Non-neurohypophyseal Disturbances Resembling Diabetes Insipidus	531
Nephrogenic Diabetes Insipidus	531
Pannephritis	532
Polyuria and the Adrenocortical Alarm Reaction	534
Hyperfunction of the Posterior Pituitary	534
Pharmacologic Uses of Posterior Pituitary Extract Other Than Those in Diabetes Insipidus	535
REFERENCES	536

Chapter IX. THE PANCREATIC ISLETS

BASIC CONSIDERATIONS	541
The Hormones	541
Action of Insulin	541
Insulin Antagonists	542
Factors Which Influence the Rate of Insulin Production (Blood Glucose Homeostasis by Means of Insulin)	542

CONTENTS [XV]

 Metabolic Effects of Insulin Lack   543
 Metabolic Effects of Insulin Excess   546
 Methods of Estimating Insulin Status   550
  Indications of Insulin Deficiency   550
  Indications of Insulin Excess   552
CLINICAL CONSIDERATIONS   553
 Juvenile "Hypoinsulinism" or Diabetes Mellitus   553
 Hyperinsulinism and Related Conditions Causing Hypoglycemia   577
  Introductory Comments   577
REFERENCES   582

APPENDIX
 Blood, Plasma or Serum Values   587
 Urine Values   589
 Miscellaneous Tests   591
 Units of Measurement   591

INDEX   601

FIGURES

Chapter I. THE THYROID

1. Effect of changes in environmental temperature on thyroid status. — 4
2. Diagrammatic representation of ossification of epiphysis in normal and in hypothyroid subjects. — 10
3. Epiphyseal dysgenesis at the head of the femur in a hypothyroid boy of 10 years. — 11
4. Heights, weights and skeletal ages of untreated hypothyroid infants and children. — 13
5. Cretinism and a large goiter in a girl of 16 years. — 16
6. Hypothyroidism plus goiter. — 17
7. Infantile hypothyroidism in a child of three months. — 18
8. Infantile hypothyroidism in a child of nine months. — 18
9. Juvenile hypothyroidism. — 19
10. Mongolism plus hypothyroidism in an infant. — 24
11. Growth rates of hypothyroid children during the first six months of thyroid therapy plotted against the age at which treatment was instituted. — 26
12. Fingernail change noted in a hypothyroid patient following institution of thyroid hormone therapy. — 27
13. Curves showing the changes in the developmental quotient of six hypothyroid children plotted against the time elapsed after institution of thyroid therapy. — 28
14. Intelligence quotients of hypothyroid children after at least two years of thyroid therapy plotted against the age when hypothyroidism appeared. — 29
15. The relative incidence of the principal symptoms and signs of thyrotoxicosis in 60 children of 7 to 16 years seen in the Thyroid Clinic and Adolescent Endocrine Clinic of the Massachusetts General Hospital over a 10-year period. — 33
16. Moderately severe thyrotoxicosis of approximately three months' duration in a girl of six years. — 34
17. Schematic indication of sites at which iodine and thiouracil are thought to exert their action on the thyroid. — 38
18. Transient congenital goiter in a newborn infant. — 45

19. Diagram of the manner in which large or circular types of goiter may compress structures in the neck.   46

Chapter II. THE PARATHYROIDS

1. Nomogram for the derivation of serum "ionized" calcium concentration from total calcium and total protein concentrations.   55
2. Simplified diagrams of renal tubule reabsorption mechanisms and of the influence of endocrine factors upon them.   57
3. Effect of parathyroid extract on the absolute value for tubular phosphorus reabsorption (TRP) and on the ratio between TRP and glomerular filtrate phosphorus (TRP/GFP).   61
4. The influence of changes in dietary phosphorus intake on intact and parathyroidectomized rats.   63
5. The influence of changes in dietary phosphorus intake on normal human subjects.   64
6. Relations between GFP and the ratio TRP/GFP.   65
7. Effect of dietary phosphorus intake on the size of the parathyroid glands.   67
8. The rapidity of parathyroid adaptative response to phosphorus loading.   69
9. The renal "threshold" for calcium excretion.   71
10. Reciprocal relations between renal tubule calcium and phosphorus reabsorption under conditions of parathyroid extract treatment.   73
11. Relations between renal tubule reabsorption of calcium and phosphorus under conditions of changing dietary phosphorus intake.   74
12. Mechanisms for demineralization of bone by parathyroid hormone.   76
13. Vitamin D resistant rickets in a boy of seven.   83
14. Roentgenographic appearance of osteomalacia.   85
15. Roentgenographic appearance of vitamin D lack rickets.   85
16. Progress of healing in renal rickets.   85
17. Response of an individual with normal kidney function to chloride loading.   92
18. Physical appearance of a 14-year-old girl with loss of renal tubule base economy.   94
19. Roentgenogram of the chest of the patient of Figure 18.   94
20. Urinary losses of calcium and sodium in base-losing nephritis.   96
21. Hyperaminoaciduria with buphthalmos and congenital cataracts in a child of 11 months.   100
22. Monilia albicans of the fingernails in hypoparathyroidism.   106
23. Monilia albicans of the mouth in hypoparathyroidism.   106
24. Response to parathyroid extract in neonatal tetany, pathologic hypoparathyroidism and pseudo-hypoparathyroidism.   109
25. Response to therapy in hypoparathyroidism.   112
26. Pseudo-hypoparathyroidism in twin sisters, aged five years.   113
27. Roentgenograms of the hands in pseudo-hypoparathyroidism.   115
28. Metastatic calcification in pseudo-hypoparathyroidism.   115
29. Electrocardiographic changes in hypocalcemia.   121
30. Skeletal deformities in primary hyperparathyroidism in a girl of 12 years.   124

FIGURES [XIX]

31. Roentgenogram of the knees of the patient in Figure 30, showing diffuse skeletal demineralization. 124

Chapter III. THE ADRENAL CORTICES

1. Diagrammatic representation of probable relations between Na-K hormone and renal excretion of sodium and potassium. 138
2. Effect on the sweat chloride–rate index of various hormones. 139
3. Effect on the sweat chloride–rate index of varying amounts of NaCl in the diet. 140
4. Effect of excess Na-K hormone (DOCA) on body water and electrolyte composition. 141
5. Effect of excess Na-K hormone (DOCA) on the muscle composition of normal dogs receiving ordinary diet or ordinary diet fortified with KCl. 142
6. A focus of necrosis in cardiac muscle caused by intracellular potassium depletion which followed Na-K hormone poisoning. 143
7. Effect of Na-K hormone deficiency on body water and electrolyte composition under conditions of normal or low sodium and normal or high potassium intake. 144
8. Comparison of sodium and potassium losses by a thirsting and fasting normal dog and an adrenalectomized dog whose ACE therapy was discontinued while he was receiving a constant mixed dietary intake. 145
9. Changes in plasma sodium concentration and in extra- and intracellular water occurring during 15 days of thirsting by the normal dog of Figure 8. 146
10. Chart showing the effect of adding to or subtracting from the extracellular compartment a certain amount of NaCl without changing the volume of body water. 147
11. Schematic representation of potential sources of blood glucose and potential routes or mechanisms by which glucose is withdrawn from the circulation. 149
12. Effect of S-F-N hormone on the relative amounts of carbohydrate, fat and protein which are oxidized to provide the organism with energy. 151
13. Urinary 11-17-OCS and 17-KS output by normal individuals of various ages. 154
14. Diagram illustrating the growth in prenatal and postnatal life of a series of structures. 155
15. Microchromatographic fractionation studies of the urinary 17-KS excreted by normal persons and by patients with adrenocortical virilism due to bilateral adrenocortical hyperplasia. 161
16. Excretion of 11-OCS and 17-KS by a patient following extensive burns. 162
17. Diagrammatic representation of factors involved in tests designed to give information concerning capacity for ACTH and 11-17-OCS (S-F-N hormone) production. 166
18. Absolute eosinophil counts on normal subjects of various ages. 167
19. Results obtained by application of the epinephrine-eosinophil test to normal individuals ranging in age between 3 months and 17 years. 169

20. Results obtained by application of epinephrine-eosinophil test to patients with various abnormal conditions. 171
21. Absolute eosinophil counts on patients with various primary endocrinopathies and on sick, convalescent and allergic individuals who were endocrinologically normal. 174
22. Effect of fasting on blood sugar of a normal individual and a patient with 11-17-OCS hormone deficiency. 176
23. Normal insulin tolerance test. 178
24. Insulin tolerance test in adrenocortical insufficiency. 179
25. Glucose tolerance test in a normal person and in a patient with hypoadrenocorticism (i.e., S-F-N hormone lack). 182
26. Glucose tolerance test in a patient with hyperadrenocorticism (i.e., increased S-F-N hormone activity). 183
27. Urinary 11-17-OCS values in patients with various conditions. 184
28. Diagram indicating various possible relations between adrenocortical activity and body needs for adrenocortical hormones, particularly the Na-K and S-F-N types. 193
29. Diagrammatic representation of the chief causes of hypoadrenocorticism. 194
30. Relative incidence of various symptoms and signs of primary hypoadrenocorticism in children. 196
31. Idiopathic Addison's disease in a boy of 14½ years receiving DOCA therapy. 198
32. Roentgenographic demonstration of microcardia in the patient of Figure 31. 198
33. Primary hypoadrenocorticism (Addison's disease), with hypoparathyroidism and moniliasis in a girl of eight years. 200
34. Cardiovascular effects of Na-K hormone (DOCA) intoxication. 207
35. Electrocardiographic tracings in a case of potassium depletion, a normal individual and a case of potassium intoxication. 208
36. Waterhouse-Friderichsen-like syndrome in a boy of 13 years. 217
37. Diagrammatic representation of probable relations between pituitary, thyroid and adrenal status in patients with primary hypopituitarism and in patients with hypopituitarism secondary to hypothyroidism. 220
38. Diagrammatic representation of relations pertaining before and after removal of a unilateral adrenocortical cancer. 221
39. Embryologic development of the urogenital sinus. 226
40. Variations in the type of urogenital sinus seen in female pseudo-hermaphrodites with adrenocortical hyperplasia. 227
41. External genitalia of a pseudo-hermaphrodite with masculinization due to congenital adrenocortical hyperplasia. 228
42. Adrenocortical virilism with pseudo-hermaphroditism due to bilateral adrenocortical hyperplasia in an 11-year-old girl. 230
43. Probable congenital adrenocortical virilism (pseudo-precocious puberty) due to bilateral adrenocortical hyperplasia in a boy of five years. 230
44. Adrenocortical virilism due to bilateral adrenocortical hyperplasia. The patient is shown at 7½ and 11½ years. 232

FIGURES   [XXI]

45. Testicular biopsies on two patients with congenital adrenocortical virilism.   233
46. Height and skeletal ages of three children with congenital adrenocortical virilism due to adrenocortical hyperplasia plotted against chronologic age.   234
47. Cushing's syndrome and masculinization due to adrenocortical carcinoma. The patient is shown at 3½ and 8 months.   236
48. Pseudo-precocious puberty with partial Cushing's syndrome due to adrenocortical carcinoma. The patient is shown at 6½ and 7 years.   238
49. Cushing's syndrome in a girl of 11 years.   240
50. Osteoporosis of the spine due to Cushing's syndrome in the patient of Figure 49.   243
51. Appearance at various ages of a boy with congenital adrenocortical virilism and disturbances in sodium, potassium and chloride metabolism secondary to proved bilateral adrenocortical hyperplasia.   248
52. Hyperplastic adrenocortical cell rest in the testis of the patient of Figure 51.   250
53. "Precocious adrenarche" in a girl of seven years and "precocious gonadarche" in a girl of eight years.   251
54. Transient alleviation of infantile eczema by stress-induced (physiologic) and by ACTH-induced (pathologic) hyperadrenocorticism.   260

Chapter IV. THE ADRENAL MEDULLÆ

1. Effects of sympathetic nerve stimulation.   273
2. Pheochromocytoma in a child of six years.   278

Chapter V. THE OVARIES

1. Schematic diagram of a mammalian ovary showing, in a clockwise direction, the sequence of events in the origin, growth and rupture of the ovarian follicle and the formation and retrogression of a corpus luteum.   293
2. Scale drawings of the fetal, neonatal and infantile uterus showing the transient enlargement of the neonatal uterus produced by maternal estrogens.   303
3. Scale drawings of the uterus and adnexa of the newborn infant and of the girl at puberty.   304
4. Stages in the sexual differentiation of the human breast.   305
5. The urinary excretion of total estrogens in international units by boys and girls of different ages.   306
6. Simplified diagram showing the relations of the hypothalamus, anterior pituitary gland, ovaries and endometrium in the normal sexually mature female during a 28-day menstrual cycle.   310
7. Vaginal smears of childhood and maturity.   314
8. The technique of aspirating vaginal secretion for making smears.   315
9. Graph representing the cytological changes occurring in the vaginal smear during a normal ovulatory cycle.   316
10. Representative basal body temperature records, showing the monophasic curve characteristic of an anovulatory menstrual cycle and the biphasic curve characteristic of an ovulatory cycle.   319

Figures

11. Diagrammatic representation of the relations of the hypothalamus, anterior pituitary gland, gonads and secondary sexual characteristics in the normal child, the normal adult and in patients with sexual precocity of various types. — 323
12. True precocious puberty of the "constitutional" type in a child of 16 months. — 324
13. Typical corpus luteum in a retrogressive phase obtained when an exploratory laparotomy was performed on a patient with "constitutional" precocious puberty at the age of 22 months. — 324
14. Osteitis fibrosa disseminata in a boy of 11 years. — 326
15. Roentgenogram of the left femur of the patient in Figure 14. — 326
16. Roentgenogram of the skull of an 18-year-old patient with osteitis fibrosa disseminata. — 329
17. Osteitis fibrosa disseminata in a child of 3$\frac{9}{12}$ years. — 331
18. True precocious puberty due to an astrocytic hamartoma in the hypothalamus and the floor of the third ventricle, in a child of two years. — 332
19. Pseudo-precocious puberty and abdominal distension due to a huge granulosa cell carcinoma of the left ovary in a girl of seven years. — 332
20. Sagittal section of the brain of the patient in Figure 18. — 333
21. Sagittal section of an ovary of the same patient. — 333
22. Mammoplasia in girls of two, three and four years. — 336
23. Close-up views of the breasts of the three patients shown in Figure 22. — 336
24. Diagrammatic representation of the relations of the hypothalamus, anterior pituitary gland, gonads and secondary sexual characteristics in normal children and adults and in patients with sexual infantilism of various types. — 338
25. Appearance of a girl of 10$\frac{8}{12}$ years who was subjected to a panhysterectomy at the age of three months because of hydrometrocalpas. — 346
26. Sexual infantilism due to agenesis of the follicular elements of the ovary in a girl of 15 years. — 346
27. Gross appearance of the uterus and adnexa in a patient with agenesis of the follicular elements of the ovaries compared with those of a normal newborn child drawn to the same scale. — 347
28. Microscopic appearance of the "ovarian streak" in a patient with agenesis of the follicular elements of the ovary compared with that of a normal newborn infant. — 347
29. Imperforate hymen in a patient of 27 years, showing the bulging due to retained menstrual accumulation of many years. — 349
30. Appearance of a girl of 22 years who began to menstruate at the age of 12 and who had a spontaneous menopause at the age of 17. — 352
31. Vaginal smear of the patient in Figure 30. — 352
32. Microscopic appearance of the ovary in fibrocystic disease. — 353
33. Sample menstrual chart of the type employed at the Massachusetts General Hospital, showing a convenient method for recording menstrual bleeding, endocrine studies and hormone therapy. — 354
34. Simplified diagram showing the relations of the hypothalamus, anterior pituitary gland, ovaries and endometrium in an adolescent girl with moderate ovarian insufficiency resulting in metropathia hemorrhagica. — 357

FIGURES [XXIII]

35. Simplified diagram showing the treatment of metropathia hemorrhagica due to mild ovarian insufficiency and illustrating the "escape phenomenon." 362
36. Simplified diagram showing the relations of the hypothalamus, anterior pituitary and endometrium in an adolescent girl with severe ovarian insufficiency resulting in metropathia hemorrhagica. 363

Chapter VI. THE TESTES

1. Production of positive nitrogen balance, positive potassium balance and transitory hypokalemia by testosterone treatment. 376
2. Effect of 25 mg. of testosterone propionate daily on total urinary nitrogen excretion by subjects receiving various inadequate diets. 378
3. Effect of testosterone on fasting blood sugar concentrations during periods of inadequate dietary intake. 379
4. Effect of testosterone on the urinary acetone-body output of subjects receiving various inadequate diets. 379
5. Diagrammatic representation of the metabolic effects of administered testosterone on a child with progeria. 380
6. Effect of testosterone on the muscular development of a six-year-old boy with progeria. 382
7. Effect of oral methyl testosterone therapy on the growth rates of eight dwarfed children. 383
8. Effect of testosterone on the skeletal maturation of a 12-year-old dwarf. 384
9. Diagrammatic representation of differences between preadolescent and adolescent or adult males. 387
10. Testicular biopsies (testes of the fetal and neonatal periods, infancy, childhood, the prepubertal and pubertal periods, adolescence, maturity and senescence). 388
11. Testicular biopsies from a patient with hypogonadotropic eunuchoidism before and after gonadotropic hormone. 391
12. Diagrammatic representation of the major changes noted during male pubescence. 393
13. Diagrammatic representation of the distribution of boys of various ages among the six classes of masculine development indicated in Figure 12. 394
14. Photographic illustrations of the fact that there may be wide differences in the physiologic age (sexual maturity status) of boys of the same chronologic age. 396
15. Adolescent gynecomastia in three healthy pubescent boys. 397
16. Diagrammatic representation of the chorionic gonadotropin test. 403
17. Complete true precocious puberty in a boy of 2$\frac{9}{12}$ years. 406
18. Testicular biopsy from the patient in Figure 17. 406
19. The family tree of the patient in Figure 17. 407
20. Complete true precocious puberty. The patient is shown at 5 and 13 years of age. 410
21. Testicular biopsies from the patient of Figure 20 before and after the administration of stilbestrol. 412

22. Complete true precocious puberty due to central nervous system lesion in a boy of 10 years. 414
23. Ventriculogram of the patient in Figure 22. 414
24. Incomplete true precocious puberty. The patient is shown at the ages of 1½ and 5½ years. 416
25. Testicular biopsy from the patient in Figure 24. 417
26. Sexual precocity due to a testicular interstitial cell tumor. The patient is shown at 2⁹⁄₁₂, at 3½, and at 4½ years. 421
27. Cross section of the testicular tumor from the patient in Figure 26. 422
28. Diagrammatic representation of the characteristics of panhypogonadism secondary to primary hypopituitarism. 424
29. Diagrammatic representation of primary panhypogonadism. 425
30. Apparent generalized idiopathic pituitary insufficiency with sexual infantilism in a male aged 23. 426
31. Idiopathic testicular atrophy in a boy of 12 years. 432
32. Idiopathic gynecomastia in a boy of 18 years with normal spermatogenesis. 432
33. Appearance of six patients with normal Leydig cells but defective spermatic tubules and increased urinary gonadotropin (FSH) output and gynecomastia. 437
34. Close-up views of the chests of three of the six patients of Figure 33. 438
35. Testicular biopsy from a patient with Klinefelter's syndrome. 439

Chapter VII. THE ANTERIOR PITUITARY

1. Effects of hypophysectomy and of pituitary (growth hormone) extract treatment upon body composition of rats. 453
2. Relations between caloric intake, protein intake and nitrogen balance in a growing child. 456
3. Diagrammatic representation of possible relations between caloric balance and pituitary growth hormone (PGH) production and protoplasmic growth rate. 457
4. Diagrammatic indication of types of change noted in patients with generalized pituitary insufficiency. 458
5. Craniopharyngioma. 460
6. Heights of dwarfed children. 464
7. Weights of various types of dwarfed children. 465
8. Skeletal ages of dwarfed children. 466
9. Idiopathic hypopituitarism in male patients of various ages. 467
10. Functional hypopituitarism secondary to caloric undernutrition with retarded growth and maturation in two physically and mentally healthy girls. 474
11. Growth in height and gain in weight of a child (Figure 10) with nutritional dwarfism before and after hospital admission, when dietary intake was increased. 475
12. Anorexia nervosa in a boy of 14 years. 477
13. Effect of improving caloric balance on wound-healing of a boy with thermal burns of long standing. 479

14. A 15-year-old giant and a normal boy of the same age. 482
15. Gigantism resulting from pituitary adenoma (growth chart of the Hurxthal and Alton giants). 483
16. Physical appearance of two boys of 6 and 18 years suffering from obesity due to overeating. 488
17. Average annual increments in standing height of girls and boys having their maximal growth at the ages of 10½, 12½, 14½ and 17 years, respectively. 493

Chapter VIII. THE POSTERIOR PITUITARY

1. Diagrammatic representation of hypothalamic-neurohypophyseal control of water metabolism. 500
2. Diagrammatic representation of factors regulating facultative water reabsorption. 501
3. Relation of maximum and minimum urine volume to solute load. 502
4. Relation of urine solutes to urine volume in patients with diabetes insipidus and renal disease. 504
5. Renal limitation of maximal urine volume. 506
6. Relation of pitressin dosage to duration of antidiuresis. 507
7. Relation of urine solute excretion to duration of pitressin antidiuresis. 508
8. Effect of antidiuretic hormone on renal solute excretion. 509
9. Metabolic changes in water deprivation in diabetes insipidus. 513
10. Induction of water intoxication. 519
11. Diabetes insipidus due to metastatic pinealoma in a girl of six years. 522
12. Idiopathic diabetes insipidus in a boy of 12 years. 522
13. Water deprivation test in diabetes insipidus. 525
14. Water restriction in psychogenic polydipsia. 526
15. Effects of renal tubule disease on water metabolism. 533

Chapter IX. THE PANCREATIC ISLETS

1. Effect of fasting ketosis and diabetic ketosis on serum electrolyte composition. 547
2. Effect of sudden insulin deprivation on the nitrogen and potassium balances, the urinary glucose excretion, the eosinophil and total white blood cell counts and the corticosteroid excretion of a depancreatized dog. 549
3. Dilatation of the ventricles presumably secondary to repeated insulin reactions in a boy of 7½ years. 559
4. Representation of approximate duration and intensity of action of various types of insulin. 561
5. Diagrammatic representation of certain of the factors to be considered in the management of diabetes mellitus. 562
6. Schematic diagrams showing how under conditions of stress adrenocortical hormones tend to inhibit renal sodium and to facilitate renal potassium excretion. 571

APPENDIX

1. Graph estimating surface area from body weight alone.   594
2. Heights and weights of normal boys.   594
3. Heights and weights of normal girls.   597

End papers. Nomograms estimating surface area from height and body weight.

TABLES

Chapter I. THE THYROID

1. Standard number of calories for girls and boys of specified weight and height. — 7
2. Symptoms of hypothyroidism in approximate order of frequency. — 15
3. Approximate time required for thyroid to effect certain changes in infants and children with primary hypothyroidism. — 25

Chapter II. THE PARATHYROIDS

1. The effect on serum calcium concentration of increases in dietary phosphorus intake without change in dietary calcium intake. — 75
2. The relative effect of vitamin D, dihydrotachysterol (A.T.-10) and parathyroid extract on gastrointestinal calcium absorption and urinary phosphorus excretion. — 77
3. Conditions prompting physiologic (or homeostatic) variations in the parathyroid activity of persons with normal parathyroid glands. — 80
4. Pathologic parathyroidism: characteristics of primary hypoparathyroidism, primary hyperparathyroidism and related conditions. — 81
5. Physiologic hyperparathyroidism in glomerular disease without tubular insufficiency. — 89
6. Distribution of body stores of fixed base. — 93
7. Free base equivalence of commonly used alkaline salts. — 97
8. Clinical manifestations of primary hypoparathyroidism in children and adolescents. — 104
9. Characteristics of conditions resulting in decreased serum ionized calcium. — 108
10. Low calcium diet. — 127

Chapter III. THE ADRENAL CORTICES

1. Apparent effects of normal or abnormal adrenocortical and testicular urinary 17-KS precursors on certain somatic phenomena. — 159
2. Quantitative relations between total urinary 17-ketosteroid output of children with congenital adrenocortical virilisim (due to adrenocortical hyperplasia) and maximum output of normal adult women. — 160

3. Summary of diagnostic methods designed to reveal Na-K, S-F-N and 17-KS-Gens status. 164
4. Low sodium diet used in provocative Tests 10 and 11 (Table 3) for demonstrating adrenocortical Na-K hormone deficiency. 187
5. Representative average results obtained for normal and hypoadrenocortical patients on the second and third days of the low sodium provocative test. 189
6. Urinary 17-ketosteroid excretion in selected conditions. 192
7. Approximate normal minimum parenteral needs per m^2 per day for temporary maintenance of water, electrolyte and caloric balances. 211
8. Approximate losses suffered during acute dehydration in moderately and markedly dehydrated normal persons and in a markedly dehydrated hypoadrenocortical patient. 212
9. Approximate requirements for repair and maintenance of patients with moderate extracellular dehydration due to acute hypoadrenocorticism during the first 24 hours. 213
10. Theoretically expected characteristics of syndromes due to excess production of the various major types of adrenocortical hormone. 222
11. Some manifestations of Cushing's syndrome, adrenocortical virilism, adrenocortical feminism and mixed hyper-hypoadrenocorticism as observed clinically in pure form in children. 225
12. Preliminary grouping of diseases other than ordinary hypoadrenocorticism and hypopituitarism on the basis of response to ACTH and cortisone therapy. 252

Chapter IV. THE ADRENAL MEDULLÆ

1. Responses of effector organs to autonomic nerve impulses. 274
2. Composite listing of various clinical manifestations of hyperepinephrinism which may be observed in patients of all ages. 277
3. Summary of observations on 11 patients with adrenomedullary tumors. 282
4. Eye manifestations of children of Table 3. 284

Chapter V. THE OVARIES

1. The relation between the chronologic ages of 14 girls and the presence of gonadotropic hormone in their urine. 307
2. Clinical characteristics of various types of isosexual precocity in the female. 322
3. Clinical characteristics of various types of sexual infantilism in the female. 339

Chapter VI. THE TESTES

1. Urinary gonadotropins in normal boys. 386
2. The order of appearance of some external changes associated with sexual maturation in boys. 395
3. Representative findings for boys with complete and incomplete true precocious puberty (Table 5, Type I). 398

TABLES [XXIX]

4. Pseudo-precocious puberty in boys due to testicular interstitial cell tumor (primary hyperleydigism). 400
5. Salient characteristics of various types of isosexual precocity in males. 404
6. Salient characteristics of various types of sexual infantilism in males. 405
7. Male eunuchoidism due to selective lack of pituitary gonadotropins with normal testes as evidenced by positive response to chorionic gonadotropin therapy (hypogonadotropic hypogonadism). 430
8. Male eunuchoidism of primary testicular origin with positive urinary gonadotropin assays and failure to respond to chorionic gonadotropin therapy (hypergonadotropic hypogonadism). 434
9. Clinical manifestations of patients with a testicular tubule defect, normal Leydig cells and gynecomastia. 435

Chapter VII. THE ANTERIOR PITUITARY

1. Types of adenohypophyseal hormones. 451
2. Methods of appraising anterior pituitary status, exclusive of general physical examination and of local examinations for pituitary tumor or central nervous system lesion. 459
3. Outline of pituitary conditions and their causes. 461
4. Primary hypopituitarism due to authentic pituitary lesions. 463
5. Causes of short stature. 470
6. Causes of tall stature. 471
7. Pituitary gigantism. 485
8. Fruits classified by carbohydrate content and average composition of common foods. 490

Chapter VIII. THE POSTERIOR PITUITARY

1. Classification and characteristics of several conditions in which polyuria may be the presenting complaint. 520

Chapter IX. THE PANCREATIC ISLETS

1. Approximate composition of body fluid per kg. of body weight and calculated dehydration losses resulting in a 10 per cent decrease in body weight. 545
2. Losses suffered during four days of complete thirsting and fasting by a normal adult weighing 64 kg. 545
3. Losses suffered by a 68-kg. diabetic patient during a 78-hour period of precoma nausea and acidosis following insulin withdrawal plus extrapolated losses for a theoretical day of vomiting and thirsting. 545
4. Differential diagnosis of diabetic coma and insulin reaction. 565
5. Basic parenteral maintenance requirements of a diabetic patient per m² of body surface during the first 24 hours of therapy. 572
6. Repair and maintenance parenteral therapy during the first 24 hours of

treatment for a child of approximately 30 kg., or 1 square meter of body surface. 573
7. Approximate guide to therapy for diabetic coma patients of various sizes during the first 24 hours. 574
8. Composition of solutions suitable for intravenous administration to diabetic coma patients. 574
9. Summary of certain conditions which may be accompanied by hypoglycemia. 579

THE THYROID

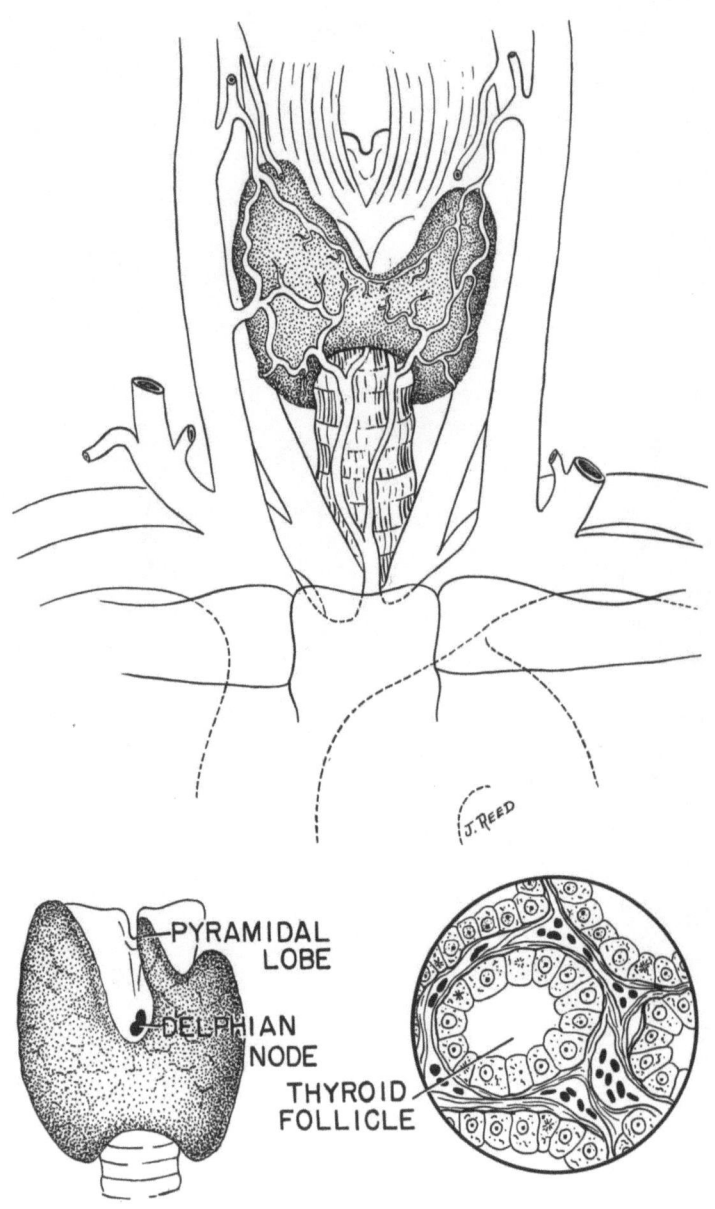

CHAPTER I

THE THYROID

BASIC CONSIDERATIONS

THYROID HORMONE

The thyroid gland creates thyroid hormone from tyrosine and iodine. The fact that tyrosine is not included in lists of so-called essential amino acids suggests that it can be synthesized by the body. The daily requirement of iodine is approximately 75 micrograms. Thyroid hormone is stored in the follicles of the gland as thyroglobulin, an iodine containing protein with a molecular weight of about 675,000. Because of its large molecular size, thyroglobulin is not diffusible into the blood stream. Hence, before it can be liberated as thyroid hormone, it must be digested by a proteolytic enzyme. The gland produces such an enzyme under the influence of pituitary thyrotropic hormone. The exact form in which thyroid hormone circulates in the blood stream is not known. It is linked to the circulating proteins, where it can be measured approximately as serum protein-bound iodine.

$$2I^- \rightarrow I_2 + HO-\!\!\bigcirc\!\!-CH_2CHNH_2COOH \rightarrow HO-\!\!\bigcirc\!\!-CH_2CHNH_2COOH$$

IODIDE IODINE   TYROSINE   DIIODOTYROSINE

- -

$$HO-\!\!\bigcirc\!\!-CH_2CHNH_2COOH + H_2O-\!\!\bigcirc\!\!-CH_2CHNH_2COOH$$

DIIODOTYROSINE   DIIODOTYROSINE

$$\downarrow$$

$$HO-\!\!\bigcirc\!\!-O-\!\!\bigcirc\!\!-CH_2CHNH_2COOH$$

THYROXINE

CHAPTER I:

THYROID HORMONE ACTIONS

The diverse effects of thyroid hormone on the organism will be considered briefly under three arbitrary, but convenient, headings.

Cell Metabolism. Changes in the concentration of circulating thyroid hormone distinctly influences the metabolism of body cells[1]; when thyroid hormone is absent, basal energy production decreases to about 60 per cent of average normal. As the concentration of thyroid hormone in the circulation is increased to normal levels, there is an approximately parallel rise in basal heat production. When the concentration of thyroid in the circulation rises above normal limits, the basal metabolic rate likewise becomes supranormal.

These changes in basal energy metabolism are reflected by corresponding changes in the rate of oxygen consumption, insensible weight and water loss, cardiac output and circulation time. Probably they are also closely related to the changes in appetite, nervous and emotional irritability, peristaltic rate and pulse rate seen in patients with thyroid disease.

Thyroid accelerates the rate of mobilization of nitrogen from muscles under conditions of fasting. As indicated in Figure 37 of Chapter III, thyroid status is an important determinant of adrenocortical hormone requirements.

Cell Organization. When thyroid hormone is absent, certain cellular functions become disorganized. Epiphyseal dysgenesis and myxedema are examples of this type of phenomenon. The former is manifested by spotty and irregular calcification of the developing skeletal epiphyses (see below, page 9). The latter is characterized by the occurrence of a special type of edema due to the formation and accumulation of an abnormal protein in interstitial spaces. Myxedema is not merely the result of a slow rate of cell metabolism, for it persists when the metabolic rate of a hypothyroid individual is elevated to normal or supranormal levels by non-thyroid agents such as dinitrophenol. It can be dissipated only by restoring thyroid status to normal.

Body Growth and Maturation.[2] Thyroid bears both direct and indirect relations to body growth and maturation. The tendency for cells to grow and mature is maximal under conditions of normal thyroid hormone concentration. When the concentration of thyroid hormone in fluids bathing body cells is abnormally low, growth and maturation rates are diminished. But thyroid in excess does not cause growth and development to be accelerated. On the contrary, thyrotoxicosis sometimes results in developmental retardation.

The indirect effects of thyroid on growth and maturation are mediated by the anterior pituitary gland and its hormones. In children and adolescents marked hypothyroidism can lead to an apparent decrease in the production of growth, adrenocorticotropic and gonadotropic hormones by the anterior pituitary (see Chapters III, V and VI). These effects of thyroid insufficiency are manifested clinically by stunted stature, signs of adrenocortical insufficiency and retardation in sex development. Hyperthyroidism has no clearly evident effect upon production of the growth hormone, but it may prompt increased adrenocorticotropic hormone secretion (Chapter III, Figures 27 and 37) and may interfere with the normal cyclic production of gonadotropins in the adolescent and adult female. This results in menstrual disturbances. Thus, thyroid in excess assumes the characteristics of a toxic substance, as is clinically evident in patients with Graves' disease.

Other thyroid hormone actions are considered in the section dealing with methods of diagnosis (page 23).

RELATION OF ANTERIOR PITUITARY AND THYROID GLANDS

The anterior pituitary elaborates a hormone, thyrotropin,* which exerts an important controlling influence over the structure and secretory activity of the thyroid gland. Like other anterior pituitary hormones, thyrotropin is a protein substance. Little is known concerning its exact chemical nature.

In the absence of thyrotropic hormone, the thyroid gland shrinks and becomes inactive. Since the thyroid gland is the chief source of thyroid hormone in the body, thyrotropin lack results in thyroid hormone insufficiency. As pituitary thyrotropic hormone production increases, a roughly parallel increase in thyroid gland size and secretory activity occurs. The concentration of thyroid hormone in the circulation rises correspondingly.

The relation between the anterior pituitary and thyroid glands is reciprocal. As the concentration of thyroid hormone rises above normal, pituitary thyrotropin production is inhibited. This decrease in thyrotropin leads to a decrease in thyroid hormone secretion and hence to a fall in the concentration of thyroid hormone in the blood stream. Conversely, when thyroid hormone concentration becomes abnormally low, there tends to be a compensatory increase in pituitary thyrotropin secretion. This in turn leads to increased thyroid gland activity and consequently to a rise in the concentration of thyroid hormone in the circulation.

While the anterior pituitary occupies this important position in the control of thyroid hormone blood levels, it is not necessarily the master control center. This center may lie in the hypothalamus.

* Alternative name—thyroid-stimulating hormone (TSH).

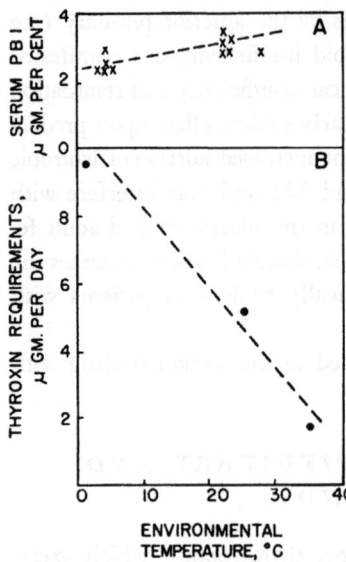

FIGURE I—1. Effect of changes in environmental temperature on thyroid status.

SECTION A: Note that serum protein-bound iodine concentration rises slightly as environmental temperature is increased. The data are derived from observations on normal rats chronically exposed to the environmental temperatures indicated. From C. G. Rand, D. Riggs and N. B. Talbot.

SECTION B: Note that thyroid hormone requirements diminish markedly as environmental temperature is raised. The data are derived from observations on rats treated with thiouracil and various amounts of thyroid hormone. From E. W. Dempsey and B. Astwood, *Endocrinology* 32:509, 1943.

EFFECTS OF THERAPY ON THYROID STATUS

Athyrotic and normal individuals react somewhat differently to thyroid hormone administration.[3] Hence, these two types of person will be considered separately.

Athyrotic Individuals. In the case of athyrotic patients, a constant dose of thyroid must be given orally for about 10 days before the maximum increase in serum thyroid-hormone iodine concentration is attained. It takes from two to four days longer for the maximum rise in basal metabolic rate to occur and several months for all signs of hypothyroidism to disappear. Daily doses of approximately 60 to 90 mg. of USP thyroid per m^2 are required to dispel the symptoms and signs of thyroid deficiency and to raise serum protein-bound (thyroid hormone) iodine concentrations to normal levels; daily doses of more than about 120 mg. per m^2 are apt to cause an abnormal elevation in serum protein-bound iodine values and to result in signs of thyrotoxicosis.

Normal Persons. In contrast to the foregoing, the serum protein-bound iodine values and basal metabolic rates of normal individuals are not easily altered by ordinary therapeutic doses of thyroid hormone. For example, the administration of enough thyroid to eliminate symptoms and signs of hypothyroidism in the hypothyroid patient (60 to 90 mg. of USP thyroid per m^2 per day) usually has no effect on the normal person. In fact, some normal adults have taken as much as 500 to 600 mg. (300 to 450 mg. per m^2) of USP thyroid by mouth daily without showing significant changes in serum protein-bound iodine values or basal metabolic rates and without developing signs of hyperthyroidism. Larger doses usually do cause symptoms and signs of thyrotoxicosis. While detailed studies of a similar nature have not been performed on normal children, clinical observations suggest that they behave like adults in this respect.

The feeding of 90 to 120 mg. of thyroid per m^2 per day to normal persons probably suppresses pituitary thyrotropin production and hence endogenous thyroid hormone secretion. This reaction does not, however, fully explain the normal person's tolerance for thyroid doses greater than 120 mg. per m^2 per day. Since tolerance for such doses is lacking when the thyroid gland is absent, it is presumed that the gland itself is capable of destroying or inactivating limited amounts of unneeded thyroid hormone. These observations find practical application in the management of patients with possible but unproved hypothyroidism (see thyroid therapy test, page 28).

PHYSIOLOGIC VARIATIONS IN THYROID GLAND ACTIVITY (THYROID HOMEOSTASIS)

Clinical and experimental studies indicate that serum protein-bound (thyroid hormone) iodine concentrations normally are maintained at nearly constant values irrespective of environmental circumstances. On the other hand, investigations have revealed that the body may utilize thyroid hormone at widely different rates. For example, there is an inverse relation between environmental temperature and the body's need for thyroid hormone (Figure 1). These changing requirements apparently are met by appropriate changes in thyroid glandular activity.[4]

Functional changes in thyroid activity also are seen in individuals suffering marked caloric undernutrition of the type exemplified by patients with severe anorexia nervosa (see Chapter VII, Figure 12). These patients sometimes show marked lowering of the basal metabolic rate, hypothermia, bradycardia and abnormally low serum protein-bound iodine values.[13b] Such hypometabolism and functional hypothyroidism presumably reflect adaptive changes designed to conserve caloric stores. When the caloric intake is increased to adequate levels, the foregoing adaptive changes disappear spontaneously within one or two weeks.

In these connections it appears physiologically inappropriate to increase the energy metabolism of calorically depleted patients by administering thyroid hormone. This serves only to increase the rate at which body calorie stores are drained. Exhaustion of energy stores results in death.

METHODS OF APPRAISING THYROID STATUS

Basal Metabolic Rate.[1a] This is one of the oldest and best-known indices of thyroid status. It consists of determinations of oxygen consumption under so-called basal conditions of fasting and physical and emotional repose. The actual measurement is carried out for two or three six-minute periods with the aid of an appropriate apparatus. The adult-type apparatus is suitable for use only on children over six or eight years of age; special apparatus, which avoids the use of masks and nose clips, is needed for younger children. Assuming a constant respiratory quotient, the oxygen consumption is multiplied by a conversion factor to give an estimate of calories produced. That is, the measurement is used to estimate basal body energy or heat production. It has become customary to express this value as total (basal) calories per 24 hours even though the actual period of measurement is much shorter.

For this measurement to have any diagnostic meaning in an individual patient it must be compared with average values obtained for normal children of the same sex and height, weight, surface area or protoplasmic mass.[5] Such a comparison can be made with the aid of the standard data which are given in Table 1. For example, if a girl weighing 10 kg. has a total basal heat production of 541 calories, her basal metabolic rate is ±0 per cent. On the other hand, if she should produce only 433 calories, her caloric output would be −20 per cent according to the weight standard. The normal range is commonly considered to be ±15 to ±20 per cent; a small number of normal children will be found to have values outside these limits.

Unfortunately, basal metabolic rates determined respectively according to height, weight, body surface and so forth do not always agree. This is especially true for children who are abnormally fat or thin. It is common experience to compute the basal metabolic rate for an obese child and find that according to the height standard it is about +30 per cent, according to the weight standard approximately −20 per cent and according to a surface area standard somewhere in between these values.[5a] This confusing information is rendered the more difficult to interpret because there is no unqualified reason for choosing one standard in preference to another.

From the foregoing it becomes apparent that the basal metabolic rate determination may be of limited value for defining hypo- or hypermetabolism. Its value as an index of thyroid activity is further reduced by the fact that unknown factors (epinephrine, corticosteroids, androgens, proteins, etc.), as well as thyroid hormone, appear to influence the basal metabolic rate. When an x-factor acts to increase the basal metabolic rate, that of the euthyroid person will tend to rise above normal and that of the hypothyroid patient to reach normal limits.

TABLE I—1. Standard number of calories for girls and boys of specified weight and height. From F. B. Talbot, *Am. J. Dis. Child.* 55:455, 1938.

Wt. (kg.)	Total calories per 24 hr. Girls	Total calories per 24 hr. Boys	Wt. (kg.)	Total calories per 24 hr. Girls	Total calories per 24 hr. Boys	Ht. (cm.)*	Total calories per 24 hr. Girls	Total calories per 24 hr. Boys	Ht. (cm.)*	Total calories per 24 hr. Girls	Total calories per 24 hr. Boys
3.0	136	150	36.0	1,173	1,270	48	134	—	96	709	755
4.0	205	210	38.0	1,207	1,305	50	159	—	98	722	765
5.0	274	270	40.0	1,241	1,340	51	—	160	100	735	785
6.0	336	330	42.0	1,274	1,370	52	186	175	105	770	805
7.0	395	390	44.0	1,306	1,400	54	214	200	110	807	830
8.0	448	445	46.0	1,338	1,430	56	246	225	115	846	875
9.0	496	495	48.0	1,369	1,460	58	278	260	120	894	935
10.0	541	545	50.0	1,399	1,485	60	309	300	125	942	990
11.0	582	590	52.0	1,429	1,505	62	341	315	130	987	1,045
12.0	620	625	54.0	1,458	1,555	64	373	360	135	1,057	1,105
13.0	655	665	56.0	1,487	1,580	66	404	390	140	1,130	1,165
14.0	687	700	58.0	1,516	1,600	68	433	420	145	1,208	1,220
15.0	718	725	60.0	1,544	1,630	70	462	450	150	1,294	1,290
16.0	747	750	62.0	1,572	1,660	72	489	480	155	1,386	1,380
17.0	775	780	64.0	1,599	1,690	74	515	510	160	1,477	1,480
18.0	802	810	66.0	1,626	1,725	76	539	535	165	1,544	1,570
19.0	827	840	68.0	1,653	1,765	78	560	565	170	1,584	1,655
20.0	852	870	70.0	1,679	1,785	80	581	590	175	1,596	1,720
22.0	898	910	72.0	1,705	1,815	82	601	612	180	1,600	1,800
24.0	942	980	74.0	1,731	1,845	84	619	635	190	—	1,900
26.0	984	1,070	76.0	1,756	1,870	86	636	660			
28.0	1,025	1,100	78.0	1,781	1,900	88	652	685			
30.0	1,063	1,140	80.0	1,805	—	90	666	705			
32.0	1,101	1,190	82.0	1,830	—	92	681	725			
34.0	1,137	1,230	84.0	1,855	2,000	94	695	740			

* Since the height standard is based on a normal weight, this can also be called expected weight.

This point is illustrated by the fact that only about two-thirds of the infants and children with authentic hypothyroidism have abnormally low basal metabolic rates according to commonly used standards of metabolism. Conversely, when an x-factor acts to lower the basal metabolic rate, the euthyroid person may have a metabolic rate which is lower than the so-called normal and the hyperthyroid patient may have a metabolic rate which is within normal limits.

Despite these limitations, the basal metabolic rate is useful for following changes in the thyroid status of a given individual. Once the patient's true *basal* metabolic rate has been determined—several measurements on successive days may be needed to train the patient in "basal" behavior and to obtain two or more successive values which agree within a small range—the metabolism measurement serves as a good index of changes in a patient's status under therapy.

Serum Cholesterol in Hypothyroidism.[6] In practically all normal infants and children the concentration of cholesterol in serum or plasma ranges between approximately 110 and 280 mg. per cent. The value obtained in an individual may fluctuate as much as 80 mg. per cent from day to day, but ordinarily is not influenced by the patient's sex, diet or state of nutrition or by a recent meal. The normal values for infants may be slightly lower than those for children over two years of age.

In hypothyroidism, as in certain other conditions such as nephrosis, chronic nephritis, acute obstructive jaundice, diabetes mellitus and xanthomatosis there is a tendency to hypercholesterolemia. The relation between serum cholesterol values and thyroid deficiency varies somewhat with the type of patient.

In adult myxedema patients, hypercholesterolemia is the rule except for those few patients who also are suffering from severe malnutrition or advanced hepatic insufficiency, conditions which tend to cause hypocholesterolemia. The incidence of hypercholesterolemia in the hypothyroid infant or child *who has never received thyroid hormone therapy* is about 30 to 50 per cent. In the remainder of this juvenile group, the serum cholesterol is either within or below normal limits. Thus hypercholesterolemia is not an obligatory accompaniment of either adult or juvenile hypothyroidism.

The administration of thyroid to hypothyroid patients who have hypercholesterolemia causes the cholesterol to fall to normal levels.

When an otherwise healthy hypothyroid infant or child is given desiccated thyroid in adequate doses for eight or more weeks, his metabolic response to the hypothyroid state changes. If thyroid hormone therapy now is discontinued, the patient will usually develop hypercholesterolemia within a period of four months (often within 3 to 10 weeks). Similarly treated infants and children who subsequently prove to be normal do not develop hypercholesterolemia.

In summary—a rise in serum cholesterol to abnormally high values following withdrawal of thyroid therapy or a fall in serum cholesterol from high to normal values after instituting thyroid hormone treatment constitutes good presumptive evidence for a diagnosis of hypothyroidism.

Hypercarotenemia and Hyperlipemia in Hypothyroidism.[7] Hypercarotenemia is a frequent finding in hypothyroid patients. It appears to be due to a loss of hepatic ability to convert carotene to vitamin A. But hypercarotenemia is not diagnostic of hypothyroidism, for it may occur also in such conditions as Cushing's syndrome and liver disease or simply as a result of eating large amounts of foods rich in carotene such as carrots and squash. Hyperlipemia appears to be another consistent finding in childhood hypothyroidism.

Serum Alkaline Phosphatase in Hypothyroidism.[8] During infancy and childhood the serum alkaline phosphatase is normally higher (average 7.5, range 5 to 14 B.U. per cent) than it is in maturity (average about 3, range 1.5 to 4 B.U.

per cent), the values being roughly proportional to the rate of long bone growth. In the case of 80 to 90 per cent of hypothyroid infants and children the serum alkaline phosphatase is abnormally low; following institution of thyroid hormone therapy, it rises to normal in about two months.

In the majority of other conditions where there may be a lowering of the serum alkaline phosphatase (scurvy, severe malnutrition, severe anemia, arthritis, achondroplasia, splenomegaly and abdominal tumors) the differential diagnosis from hypothyroidism is usually easy. Normal values are found in most children with dwarfism due to caloric undernutrition. Normal values are also obtained in mongolism and in primary pituitary dwarfism, diseases which often are mistaken for infantile or juvenile hypothyroidism. These data suggest that the lowering in serum alkaline phosphatase activity seen in athyrosis is not due simply to a decrease in the rate of long bone growth and that it is not a reliable index of osteoblastic activity. It is possible that the low values seen in athyrosis are due in part to disorders in the function of hepatic and other body cells.

An elevation in the serum alkaline phosphatase is the rule in active rickets (either due to vitamin D lack or to renal insufficiency, steatorrhea, etc.). Because rickets is a disease which occurs only with long bone growth and because hypothyroidism results in marked slowing in bone growth, the influence of these two diseases upon the phosphatase is antagonistic. Consequently, when the diseases coexist the alkaline phosphatase is neither as high as in rickets alone (usually > 15 B.U. per cent) nor as low as is usual in uncomplicated hypothyroidism (< 4.5 to 5 B.U. per cent).

Epiphyseal Dysgenesis in Childhood Hypothyroidism.[9] In the absence of thyroid hormone the ossification pattern of skeletal epiphyses may vary from the normal and give rise to fairly characteristic roentgenographic findings.

In considering this condition, it is helpful to review first the normal pattern of epiphyseal ossification (see Figure 2). Before ossification sets in the epiphysis is almost radio-lucent and hence invisible in x-ray films. As the epiphysis matures, a small nucleus of radio-opaque ossification develops near the center of the cartilagenous epiphysis. With passage of time this ossification center grows outward, so that eventually the entire cartilage is evenly calcified and radio-opaque.

When thyroid hormone is lacking, there is a tendency to disorderliness in this ossification process. The resultant condition, epiphyseal dysgenesis, will become evident when calcification occurs. Instead of the normal single center of ossification numerous small foci of calcification are seen (Figure 3). These multiple foci tend to grow slowly, eventually coalescing to form a single center with irregular shape and poorly defined, fluffy margins.

Epiphyseal dysgenesis is not evident in epiphyses which have ossified prior to

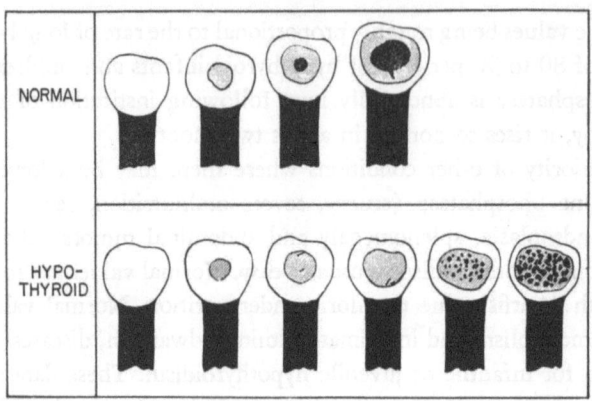

FIGURE I—2. Diagrammatic representation of ossification of epiphysis in normal and in hypothyroid subjects. Shaded areas represent changes which occur in epiphyseal cartilage preparatory to ossification; black areas represent calcification. Under normal conditions calcification develops from a single nucleus in the cartilage which has undergone a preparatory change. In hypothyroidism calcification is delayed by abnormality in the preparatory stage and finally develops from multiple foci scattered over a large area. From L. Wilkins, *Am. J. Dis. Child.* 61:13, 1941.

---

the onset of thyroid deficiency; it may become evident in epiphyses which calcify during the period of hypothyroidism.

Characteristic changes in one or more epiphyses can be found in about 90 per cent of untreated hypothyroid infants and children. In addition, dysgenesis may become apparent in epiphyses which are retarded in development by athyrosis and which calcify after thyroid hormone treatment is started. This is especially so during the first six months following initial treatment; during this period the condition may be missed unless x-ray films are taken at intervals of two or three months.

Epiphyseal dysgenesis may be found in a number of bones, most commonly at the head of the femur and less commonly at both ends of the humerus, ulna, radius, tibia, fibula and navicular and in the vertebral column. When present in the capital epiphysis at the neck of the femur, epiphyseal dysgenesis is often accompanied by coxa vara. This is manifested clinically by a limping gait.

Epiphyseal dysgenesis is to be distinguished particularly from two other bone diseases, osteochondritis deformans juvenilis and chondrodystrophy. Osteochondritis deformans is a degenerative disease in which there are atrophic changes in a previously normal epiphysis. In contrast to epiphyseal dysgenesis, it usually involves but a single epiphysis and is unilateral. Also in contrast to

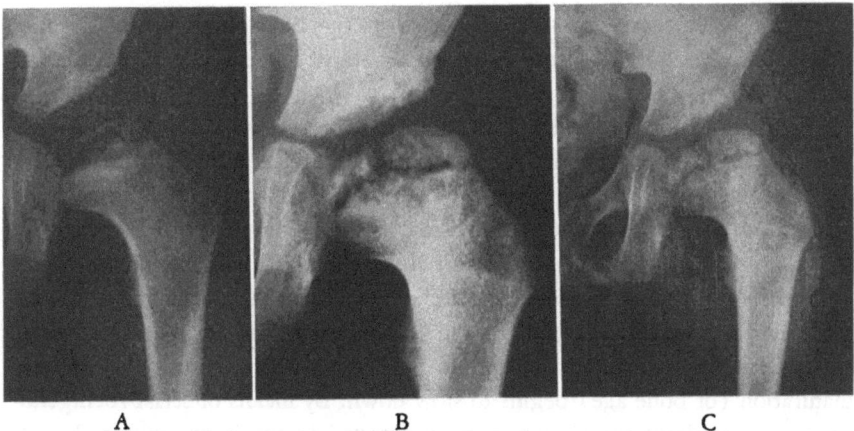

A   B   C

FIGURE I—3. Epiphyseal dysgenesis at the head of the femur in a hypothyroid boy of 10 years. The roentgenogram in Section A was taken prior to starting thyroid hormone treatment. Note the moth-eaten appearance of the epiphysis. In Section B the roentgenogram was obtained after 1½ years of therapy; that in Section C after 2½ years of therapy. Partial healing is indicated by the smooth superior margin of the epiphysis. Fluffy areas of dysgenesis are still evident at the metaphysis.

---

epiphyseal dysgenesis, it is likely to be painful. It occurs most often at the head of the femur and in the navicular of the foot, sites which bear considerable weight. Osteochondritis deformans may occur in hypothyroid as well as euthyroid children. When not associated with thyroid lack, it fails to respond to thyroid hormone treatment. At times it can be distinguished from epiphyseal dysgenesis only with the aid of serial roentgenograms.

Chondrodystrophy is characterized by the grossly abnormal shape of the epiphyses and deformities in the metaphyses and shaft. It resembles epiphyseal dysgenesis only in the occurrence of multiple foci of ossification. In this connection it is noteworthy that a few epiphyses (olecranon, trochlea, patella and os calcis) normally show a few widely scattered but well-defined foci of calcification.

The administration of thyroid hormone to hypothyroid patients causes epiphyseal dysgenesis to heal.

Rate of Skeletal Maturation in Hypothyroidism. The skeletal maturation of hypothyroid infants and children almost always is retarded. A delay in skeletal maturation can be recognized by comparing roentgenograms of the hand and wrist of a patient with normal standards of skeletal maturation such as those prepared in photographic form by Todd and by Flory.[10] The findings obtained are expressed in terms of bone age, which is the chronologic age of average normal children of the same sex showing an equivalent degree of skeletal maturation.

Like their heights and weights, the bone ages of normal children of the same sex show some variation about the average normal for a group. During infancy the bone age may be six months more or less than the actual age. Between the ages of 2 and 12 normal development may deviate from 12 to 18 months, and in adolescence by as much as two years. In dealing with patients of adolescent age it should be remembered that the skeletal maturation of the hand is normally completed in the average girl at 16 and in the average boy at 18 years.

When a previously normal juvenile patient becomes athyrotic, his skeletal maturation (or bone age) begins to slow down. By means of serial roentgenograms the resultant retardation may be detected in the infant within 3 to 6 months and in the older child within 6 to 12 months, periods of time within which a measurable advance in skeletal development normally occurs. The bone age of an infant or child who has been hypothyroid for only a few months may be within normal limits. On the other hand, juvenile patients who have been athyrotic for more than a year or two almost always show definite retardation in skeletal development (Figure 4). In fact, the bone age of a hypothyroid child should serve as an approximate index of the age of onset of this disease.

While bone-age retardation is consistent with thyroid deficiency in children, it is not diagnostic thereof. Essentially equivalent degrees of retardation may be observed in apparently euthyroid children whose growth and maturation have been delayed as a result of such other factors as undernutrition or chronic debilitating illness.

Urinary Creatine Output in Hypothyroidism.[11] It has been shown that the output of creatine in the urine of hypothyroid infants and children is abnormally low and that this disturbance is corrected by thyroid hormone therapy. While of physiologic interest, this phenomenon is not of much practical diagnostic value because of the fact that it is difficult to make accurate 24-hour collections and because creatine output is influenced by diet and other non-thyroid factors.

Radio-active Iodine Uptake in Thyroid Disease.[12] The thyroid gland takes up iodine for the purpose of synthesizing thyroid hormone. By means of radio-active iodine metabolism studies, it is possible to determine what proportion of a standard dose of iodine is trapped in the thyroid gland under normal and abnormal conditions.

When a normal person is fed a small amount of radio-active iodine (100 microcuries of I^{131}), approximately 65 per cent (range 50 to 85 per cent) can be recovered in the urine in 48 hours. Most of the remaining radio-active iodine

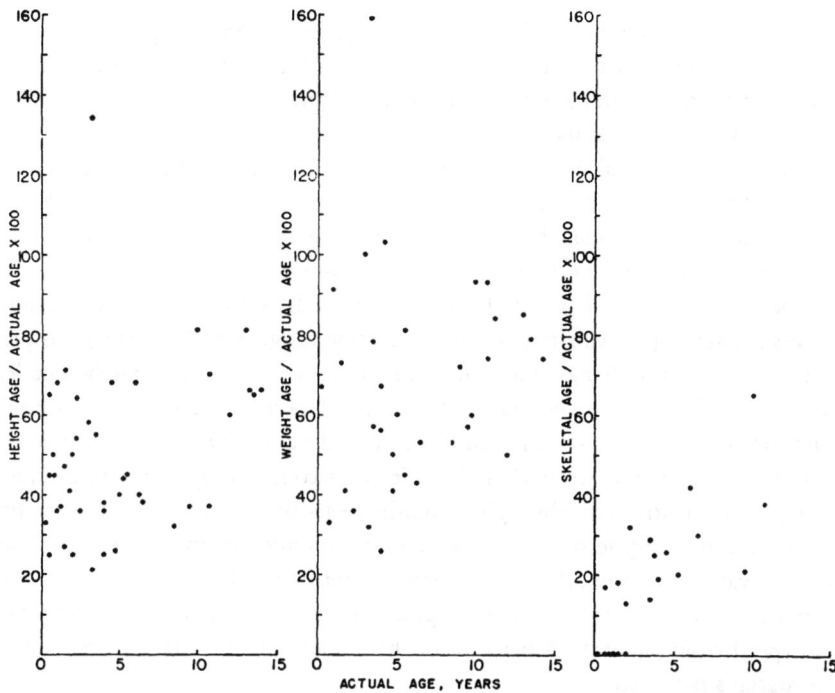

FIGURE I—4. Heights, weights and skeletal ages of untreated hypothyroid infants and children. Measurements are expressed as height age, weight age or skeletal age ÷ by actual age x 100 (ordinate) and are plotted against chronologic age (abscissa). Height age represents the average age of normal children of the same height and sex as the patient. Weight age and skeletal age are similarly estimated. Ratios between 80 and 120 per cent are considered within normal limits.

---

has been taken up by the thyroid gland. When a similar dose is given to an athyrotic patient, 73 to 92 per cent is recovered in the urine within a similar number of hours and none is trapped in the thyroid region. On the other hand, if the radio-active iodine is administered to a thyrotoxic patient, much less (average 19 per cent, range 6 to 32 per cent) appears in the excreta, and much more is taken up by the hyperplastic thyroid gland. The use of this type of measurement for diagnostic purposes is still in the experimental stage.

Serum Protein-bound (Thyroid Hormone) Iodine Concentration.[3, 13] Except in patients who have received organic iodine-containing compounds such as those used for intravenous pyelography and for gall bladder studies, nearly all the protein-bound iodine in the serum is thyroid hormone iodine. Non-precipitable, inorganic iodine in the serum is not related to thyroid hormone concentration. Because protein-bound iodine can be separated from inorganic iodine by suitable treatment of serum or plasma, it is possible to determine the concentration of protein-bound iodine in the blood of patients taking inorganic iodides in food, water or medicines.

The actual chemical determination of serum protein-bound iodine is tedious and exacting, for the quantity of iodine actually measured is minute ($=0.000,06$ mg.). Particular care must be taken to avoid contaminating the patient, physician, equipment or laboratory with substances like tincture of iodine.

The concentration of protein-bound iodine in the serum of normal persons ranges between approximately 4 and 8 (extreme range 3 to 9) micrograms per cent as measured by Riggs' permanganate ashing–starch titration method or its equivalent. With the exception of the neonatal period, there is for practical purposes no age or sex variation in these normal values. During the first week of life values range between 10 and 12, in the second through fifth weeks they average 7.4, in the sixth through eleventh weeks they average 6.9 and in the twelfth through fifty-second week they average 6.3 micrograms per cent.[13c] The average value found in athyrotic patients is approximately 1.3 micrograms per cent, and rarely are the values obtained greater than 2.5 or 3 micrograms per cent. In hyperthyroid patients 95 per cent of the values obtained are greater than 8 micrograms per cent.

While this measurement is not absolutely free from error, it gives more accurate information concerning thyroid status than other available laboratory procedures. The only limitations of any importance are the relatively large amounts of blood required (15 cc. of whole blood), cost of analysis and limited analytic facilities. With more demand and greater experience these limitations will probably be overcome.

CLINICAL CONSIDERATIONS

HYPOTHYROIDISM (ATHYROSIS, MYXEDEMA, CRETINISM)

Thyroid deficiency can develop as a result of (a) primary defects in the thyroid gland, (b) pituitary thyrotropin deficiency and (c) miscellaneous conditions in which production of thyroid hormone is impeded either by lack of raw material (iodine) or by the presence of such agents as thiocyanate, thiourea, thiouracil and the like. Iodine deficiency must be severe to result in clinical hypothyroidism, because the thyroid gland extracts available iodine from the blood stream with great efficiency. Thus it may obtain a minimum essential supply of

TABLE I—2. Symptoms of hypothyroidism in approximate order of frequency.

Onset before 2 yr.: 36 points	Onset after 2 yr.: 11 points
DWARFISM	DWARFISM
SLOWNESS OR APATHY	SLOWNESS OR APATHY
SLOW MOTOR DEVELOPMENT	Easy fatigability
DRY SKIN	DRY SKIN
CONSTIPATION	CONSTIPATION
SLOW TEETHING	Slow teething
POOR APPETITE	POOR APPETITE
LARGE TONGUE	Large tongue
HERNIA	Hernia
Pot belly	Pot belly
	HAIR ABNORMAL
Deep voice	Deep voice
Cold extremities	Cold extremities
Cold sensitivity	COLD SENSITIVITY
Myxedema	MYXEDEMA
Fat pads	Fat pads
Yellow skin	Yellow skin

iodine even under conditions of relative want. When the iodine supply is poor, however, the gland becomes enlarged (goitrous) and hyperplastic. If this state persists for a long time thyroid cells become exhausted with resultant hypothyroidism. Because it has become standard practice to add iodine to table salt in geographical areas of iodine deficiency, hypo-iodinism is becoming a rare cause of hypothyroidism in this country.

Primary Hypothyroidism (Athyrosis). This is the most common type of thyroid insufficiency observed in pediatrics.

ETIOLOGY. In some instances the thyroid gland fails to develop during fetal life (congenital athyrosis). In areas of marked iodine poverty, where pregnant mothers' iodine stores are very poor, the fetal thyroid may develop, but because of iodine want may fail to function at birth. Congenital cretinism results. In many instances there is no satisfactory explanation for the thyroid failure. A rare additional cause of thyroid failure is thyroiditis. Because this is characterized by thyroid gland enlargement, it is considered below under goiter (page 48).

CLINICAL MANIFESTATIONS. Table 2 presents in outline form the more common manifestations of primary hypothyroidism. In this table it is assumed that the hypothyroid state develops and is recognized during infancy, childhood or adolescence. When the condition develops in infancy or childhood, but is not recognized until later life, the symptoms and signs characteristic of the earlier age group persist and become more marked. The symptoms and signs typical of the older age group are likewise present. The following comments and Figures 5 to 9 may serve to clarify the information presented in the table.

Continued on page 20

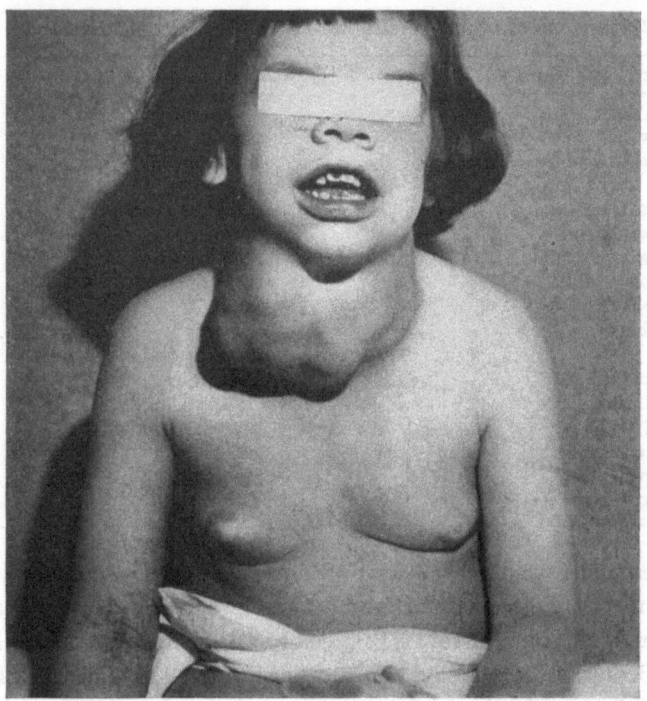

FIGURE I—5. Cretinism and a large goiter in a girl of 16 years. From J. B. Stanbury and A. N. Hedge, *J. Clin. Endocrinol.* 10:1471, 1950.

CASE HISTORY

The cretinous state was not recognized until several months after birth, and treatment thereafter with thyroid was desultory. The goiter was first noticed at the age of seven. The patient was given a tracer dose of radio-active iodine, which was found to accumulate in the thyroid gland within a matter of less than two hours; it then very slowly declined. Administration of thiocyanate 24 hours later was followed by a rapid discharge of the radio-iodine from the gland.

This was interpreted to mean that the thyroid was capable of trapping large amounts of iodide, but was unable to convert it into hormone. Radio-iodine tests of two of the patient's three goitrous siblings produced the same effect; a test of one of three apparently normal siblings showed no discharge after the administration of thiocyanate.

Assay of the excised gland for unbound iodide showed 29.3 micrograms per cent of iodide and 10.4 micrograms per cent of protein-precipitable iodide. The serum protein-bound iodine was 1 microgram per cent.

THE THYROID [17]

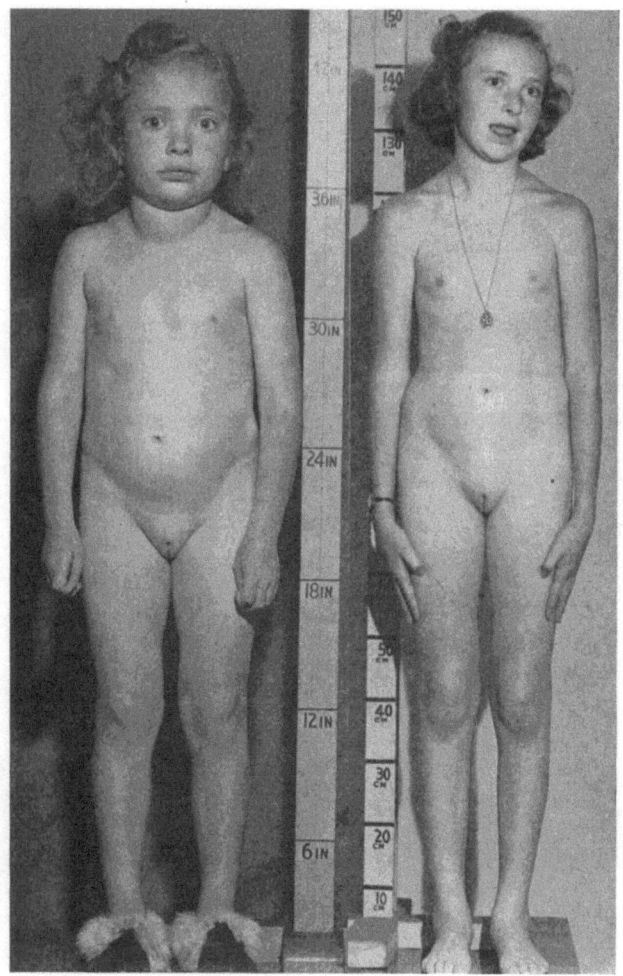

FIGURE I—6. Hypothyroidism plus goiter.
LEFT: The patient at the age of 8 years.
RIGHT: The same patient at the age of 14 years.

CASE HISTORY

The thyroid deficiency probably developed between the ages of one and two. The goiter became noticeable when the child was about five. Iodine medication produced no effect on the goiter or on the hypothyroid manifestations. Thyroid hormone therapy caused both to disappear, but the goiter reappeared within a few months whenever the dose of thyroid was reduced below approximately 100 mg. per m^2 per day. We are indebted to Dr. A. M. Butler for permission to record this case.

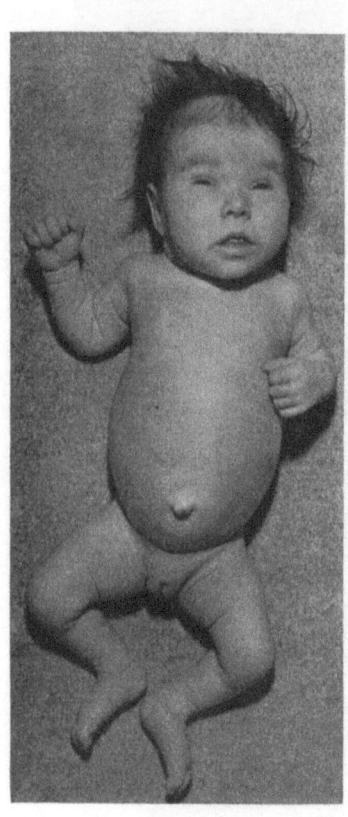 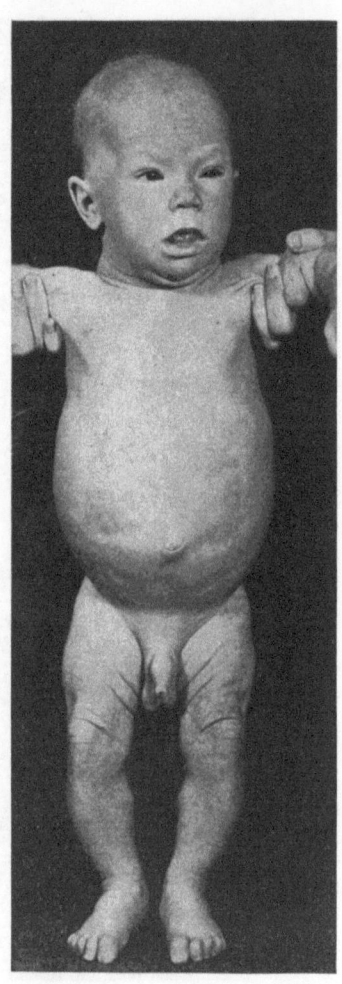

(Left)

FIGURE I—7. Infantile hypothyroidism in a child of three months. Considerable puffiness of the face and body due to myxedema is evident. Note the protrusion of the tongue, pot belly, umbilical hernia and relative shortness of the extremities.

(Right)

FIGURE I—8. Infantile hypothyroidism in a child of nine months. Note the mottling of the skin over the legs, the very protuberant abdomen, the supraclavicular bulges in the neck (so-called fat pads), as well as the porcine facies. Except for the face and tongue, the appearance is one of emaciation rather than myxedema.

We are indebted to Dr. C. A. Janeway for permission to record this case and that in Figure 9 (opposite).

The Thyroid

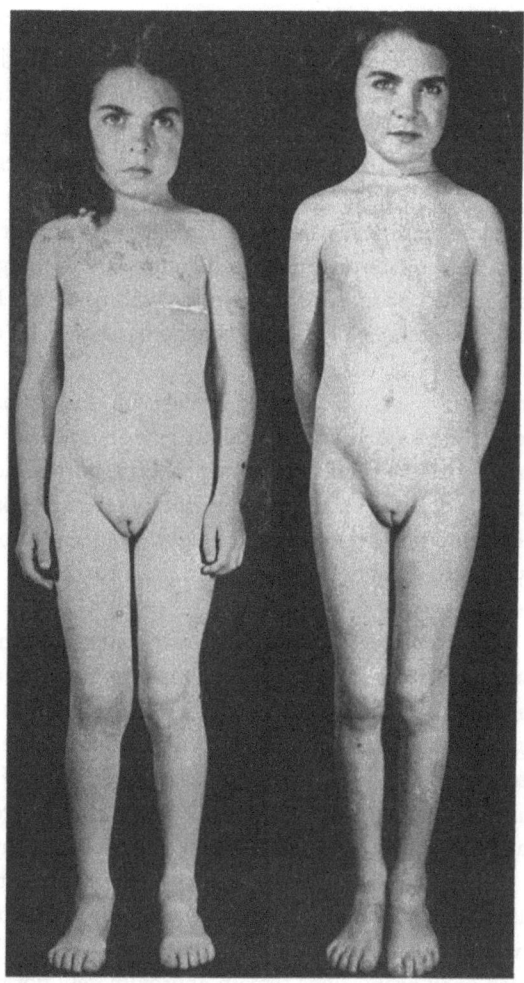

FIGURE I—9. Juvenile hypothyroidism.

LEFT: The patient at 10 years. Insofar as can be estimated, athyrosis developed in this child at the age of two. She had received some thyroid between her fourth and sixth years but none between her sixth and tenth years. Note that body proportions are normal and that there is no pot belly or umbilical hernia. The cheeks have a slight tendency to sag, with the result that the facial expression seems rather "heavy." Light mottling of the skin over the legs is also evident.

RIGHT: The same patient after a year of thyroid hormone treatment. Aside from an increase in stature, the chief change is in the facial expression. The cheeks are rounded and of healthy appearance. The eyes are bright. The figure thus illustrates that, so far as photographic appearances go, patients with juvenile hypothyroidism may show only subtle signs of abnormality.

The thyroid gland. In the majority of patients the gland is small and not readily palpable. On the other hand, in occasional patients the gland is enlarged to inspection and palpation. Under this circumstance its shape and consistency may be of several types. When the goiter has been present for a long time, the gland may be firm and nodular (see Figure 5); when the goiter has developed during childhood and is of only a few years' duration, the lobes and isthmus of the gland are apt to be more or less evenly enlarged, of not more than moderately firm consistency and free from nodules (see Figure 6). If the gland is of hard consistency and contains nodules or if there is swelling of the Delphian node, the possibility of thyroiditis or of thyroid carcinoma should be considered (see also under goiter).

Growth disturbances. As is illustrated in Figure 4, the majority of hypothyroid infants and children are abnormally short when first seen. It is only when thyroid deficiency is of very brief duration or when a normal adult stature has been attained by an adolescent child prior to the onset of hypothyroidism that children with this condition are of normal height. Figure 4 also shows a slight tendency for hypothyroid children to be overweight for height (weight age > height age).

Shortness of the extremities is a normal characteristic of the newborn infant; the lower measurement from the top of the symphysis pubis to the soles of the feet is about one-third of the total body length. During the first year of life the legs normally grow more rapidly than the trunk so that at one year the lower measurement equals about .38 and at two years about 0.41 of the total body length.[14] By stunting long bone as well as trunk growth hypothyroidism prevents this normal change in body proportions. Hence patients with thyroid deficiency dating back to early infancy usually have remarkably short extremities. However, when a patient develops thyroid deficiency after the extremities have grown to equal approximately half the total body length ($\pm$ 8 years), even though growth is retarded body proportions remain approximately normal.

Slow growth of hair as well as of fingernails and toenails is characteristic of thyroid deficiency; it appears from clinical history data that hypothyroid children need fewer hair cuts and fingernail clippings than normal children or than they themselves require after thyroid therapy has been instituted.

The anemia of hypothyroidism is apt to be normochromic and fails to respond to iron or liver but does yield to thyroid therapy. For these reasons the anemia of hypothyroidism is placed under the general heading of slow growth. It is realized that this may be an oversimplification.

Maturation disturbances. Retardation in motor or intellectual development is commonly found in infantile hypothyroidism (see Figures 13 and 14).[15] In older patients, although the rate of cerebration may be slow, the intellect may be normal or superior.

Retardation in skeletal maturation may be recognized in infant hypothyroid patients by a delay in the closure of the cranial fontanelles. In the normal infant digital palpation reveals that the posterior fontanelle is "closed" by the age of 4 months, while the anterior fontanelle usually is "closed" by the age of 18 months. Retardation in skeletal maturation also is evident in roentgenograms of the skeleton.

Delay in the time of eruption of teeth is characteristic of infantile hypothyroidism. Among older hypothyroid children there is also a tendency to delayed shedding of deciduous teeth and eruption of permanent teeth.

Sexual maturation may be markedly slowed (six or more years later than average) in children who develop hypothyroidism at or before the time they reach adolescent age. On the other hand, sexual development usually takes place eventually even if thyroid deficiency persists. When hypothyroidism develops after considerable sexual development has taken place, there may be few if any signs of hypogonadism.

Umbilical hernia and occasionally also diastasis of the rectus muscles may be observed in cases of infantile hypothyroidism. Hernia is not found in children who develop athyrosis after the umbilical opening has closed.

Hypometabolism and allied derangements. These manifestations of thyroid insufficiency are present with considerable regularity in patients of all ages. Of those listed in Table 2, sensitivity to cold weather, cold hands and feet, constipation, easy fatigability and coarse dry skin are the symptoms and signs encountered with greatest regularity.

Poor appetite is most obvious in hypothyroid infants, who often require 30 or more minutes to ingest even a small amount of food. As patients become older, emotional and other factors are apt to overbalance thyroid deficiency as determinants of appetite. In consequence the appetite may not diminish in proportion to the energy metabolism. When this happens the patient develops an excessively positive caloric balance. Because surplus calories are stored as body fat, obesity results.

Sluggish circulation is a frequent clinical finding. In the older patient it is reflected by bradycardia and a tendency to hypotension. In the infant the pulse may not be slow, but poor peripheral circulation is evidenced by mottling of the skin over the abdomen and extremities (see Figure 8). Occasional patients show enlargement of the heart and, in electrocardiograms, low voltage P and T waves.[17]

Hypothermia is common. The oral temperature frequently averages less than

98°F. Patients who are old enough to talk complain of feeling cold under conditions where normal persons are comfortably warm.

The tendency to slowness of motion or lethargy described for athyrotic patients again varies with the age and temperament of the individual. The mothers of athyrotic infants often state that these babies are less vigorous and active than were their normal siblings at the same age, that they are remarkably "good" and placid, that they cry seldom and sleep a great deal. In older patients a tendency to think slowly and easy fatigability may be prominent. Occasionally, juvenile and adolescent patients seem to be suffering from nervous tension.

Slowness of visceral action is almost always evident as constipation. Not infrequently hypothyroid patients give a history of chronic laxative therapy. Presumably as a consequence of poor intestinal and abdominal muscle tone, moderate to marked degrees of potbelly are often seen.

Dryness and coarseness of the skin may give it a sandpapery texture. This may be most noticeable over the trunk.

Metabolic aberrations. The term myxedema is used interchangeably with hypothyroidism by some authors. While it is probably true that hypothyroidism of any severity is always accompanied by myxedema, it also is true that myxedema may be subtle and difficult to detect on clinical examination. In the infant the tongue becomes thick, broad and protuberant (see Figures 7 and 8); occasionally it becomes large enough to obstruct the upper respiratory passages. We know of one instance where macroglossia caused suffocation and sudden death. For unknown reasons, macroglossia is less noticeable in children and adolescents. Hoarseness of the voice, sometimes described as guttural voice, is quite common in hypothyroid patients of all ages. Puffiness of the face may be marked (see Figure 7), or there may be just enough facial edema to cause the cheeks and eyelids to sag a little and give a heavy-jowled appearance. These changes often are more evident in retrospect, after thyroid therapy has caused them to disappear, than they were on first inspection (see Figure 9). "Fat" pads over the clavicles and in the folds of the axillæ are seen occasionally in patients with infantile athyrosis of long duration. They are rarely seen in patients who develop thyroid insufficiency after the age of two.

The skin of hypothyroid patients may have a yellowish color suggestive of jaundice. This is due to an accumulation of carotene in the circulation as a result of inability to convert dietary carotene to vitamin A.[7a] The yellowish tinge is most noticeable on the palms of the hands, soles of the feet, nose and ears. The scleræ are not discolored as they are in jaundice.

Miscellaneous and atypical manifestations. Tonic spasm and rigidity of facial and laryngeal muscles develop in occasional hypothyroid infants and children.

This spasm is intermittent and most apt to occur when the patient cries or becomes excited. The laryngeal spasm may simulate mechanical upper respiratory obstruction. The condition as it is observed in hypothyroid patients bears some resemblance to the disease, myotonia congenita.[16] Both in this disease and in hypothyroidism the urinary creatine output is unusually low. It is presumed that this hypocreatinuria reflects a disturbance in muscle phosphocreatine metabolism. These manifestations disappear with thyroid therapy.

Hypothyroid persons tolerate morphine very poorly.

DIAGNOSIS. Retardation of growth or maturation, constipation, easy fatigability, sensitivity to cool weather and dry coarse skin or the presence of a goiter suggest hypothyroidism as a possible diagnosis. In many instances the manifestations of thyroid lack are so obvious that there is little difficulty in making the diagnosis. In others, however, the signs may be so subtle that the condition must be ruled in or out by application of certain test procedures. Of these the serum protein-bound iodine measurement gives the most direct information. Because the other procedures mentioned in the section on diagnostic methods give only indirect information, they are more difficult to interpret. The thyroid hormone therapy test outlined below is of considerable practical clinical value and can be carried out without laboratory aids.

DIFFERENTIAL DIAGNOSIS. The most common euthyroid conditions to be distinguished from hypothyroidism are those in which there is stunted growth, retarded sexual development, impaired intellectual development, edema or overweight, apparent macroglossia or goiter. For information concerning other causes for dwarfism, retarded sexual development and obesity, see Chapter V, Figure 24, Chapter VI, Table 6, and Chapter VII, Table 5. Goiter in association with thyrotoxicosis is covered in a later section of this chapter. Mental deficiency and macroglossia are discussed briefly below.

The condition most often confused with athyrosis is mongolism or mongolian idiocy.[18] As shown by the patient of Figure 10, the two conditions occasionally coexist. Infants and children with mongolism have a characteristic appearance. The anterior-posterior diameter of the head is short (brachycephalic), and the back of the head is flattened. The eyes slant upwards laterally. The epicanthic folds are prominent. The bridge of the nose is broad and flat. The tongue is long and may protrude between the lips. The ear lobes usually show minor congenital malformations. Signs of congenital heart disease are seen frequently. The extremities are remarkable in two respects. First, they are hypermobile. This can be demonstrated by the ease with which the feet can be placed behind the ears. Second, the fifth digits are frequently abnormally shortened and crooked inward. An unusually deep crease may be found on the soles of the feet between the

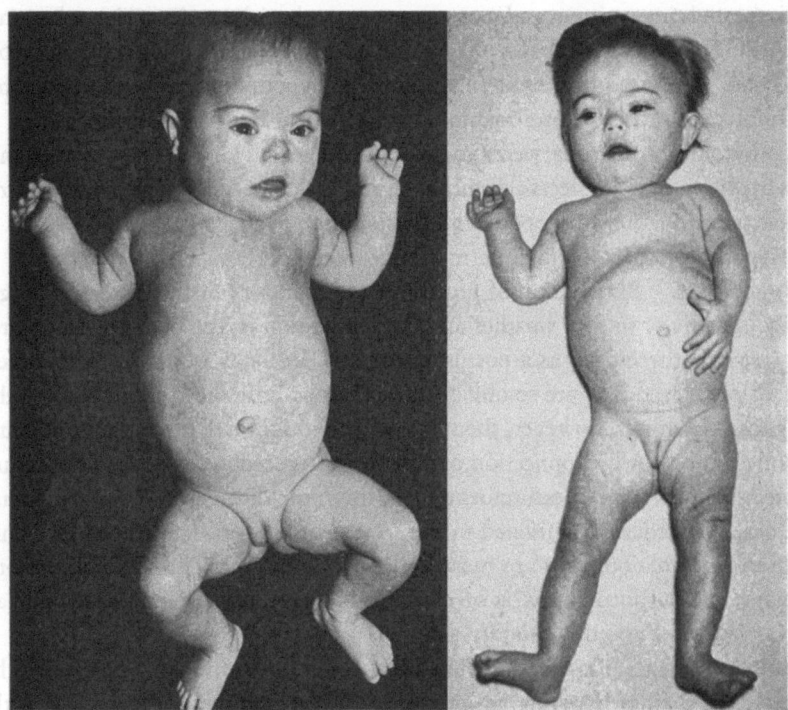

FIGURE I—10. Mongolism plus hypothyroidism in an infant.

LEFT: The patient at 10 months. She was lethargic and constipated and had cold hands and feet. Growth and development had been slow. The photograph shows short extremities, mottled skin, marked epicanthic folds, a thick protruding tongue and a small umbilical hernia. Laboratory studies revealed that her serum protein-bound iodine was 1.88 micrograms per cent; roentgenograms, that her bone age was less than three months.

RIGHT: The same child after five months of thyroid therapy, to which she had a clear response. The features of mongolism now appear without the confusing, superimposed features of hypothyroidism.

---

great and second toes. Finally, mongoloid patients often make facial grimaces.

Most mongolian idiots do not show retarded skeletal maturation, epiphyseal dysgenesis, lowering of the serum alkaline phosphatase or other metabolic signs of marked thyroid lack. However, as illustrated by Figure 10, these two conditions may coexist. Thyroid medication does not eliminate the salient characteristics of mongolism.

True macroglossia can be caused by tumors or congenital malformations. Except for the very rare patient with a thyroglossal duct cyst at the base of the

TABLE I—3. Approximate time required for thyroid to effect certain changes in infants and children with primary hypothyroidism. These data are based on serial observations of 17 patients, of whom 12 were less than two years of age.

Change noted	Time after thyroid therapy started	
	Average, weeks	Range, weeks
1. Body weight loss (average 6 per cent)	2½	1½— 7
2. Increased physical activity	3½	½—11
3. Drop in serum cholesterol	3½	1 — 6
4. Increased appetite	4	1 —11
5. Improved peripheral circulation, skin warmer	5	1 —11
6. Loss of constipation	5½	1 —11
7. Increased growth rate	8	3 —16
8. Disappearance of skin dryness and coarseness	10	4 —20
9. Loss of myxedematous appearance	11	6 —20

tongue, signs of thyroid disease are absent in such individuals. A normal tongue may protrude (pseudo-macroglossia) in an infant with marked hypertrophy of posterior pharyngeal (adenoid) tissue. Moderate edematous enlargement of the tongue also has been observed in one infant with Cushing's syndrome.

TREATMENT. Because of its standardized potency USP thyroid is recommended for the treatment of thyroid deficiency. The daily maintenance dose is between 60 and 90 mg. per m^2 of body surface area irrespective of age or size.

When thyroid is first given, it is to be remembered that the hormone can produce a marked acceleration in body metabolism. Particularly in athyrotic infants, too sudden an acceleration in metabolism can cause trouble in the form of severe diarrhea, vomiting, dehydration, excitement or mania. Such difficulties can be avoided by giving initially one-quarter of the recommended maintenance dose. If no untoward signs develop within two weeks, the dose can be safely increased to half the maintenance dose. If all goes well, three-quarters of the maintenance dose can be started in another two weeks and the full dose about six weeks after treatment is started.

The adequacy of the dose used for maintenance purposes can be judged either by the clinical response (see below) or by measurements of the serum protein-bound iodine concentration. For reasons outlined earlier other laboratory indices of thyroid status are not considered of much value. Ideally the dose used should completely eliminate metabolic signs of thyroid deficiency, but it should not produce signs of toxicity such as hyperactivity, jitteriness, marked tachycardia, chronic weight loss (or failure to gain) or diarrhea. Especially in mentally deficient hypothyroid children, progress and performance are apt to be better with minimal adequate than with maximal adequate maintenance doses. With the

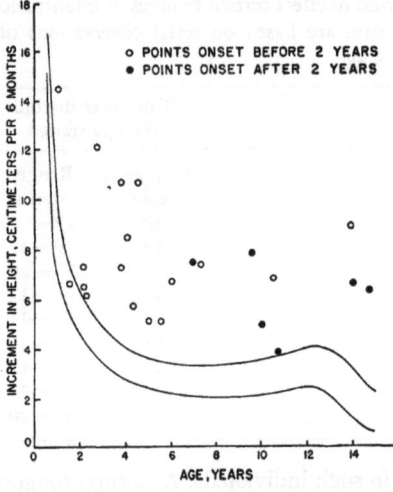

FIGURE I—11. Growth rates of hypothyroid children during the first six months of thyroid therapy (ordinate) plotted against the age at which treatment was instituted (abscissa). The two lines coursing downward from left to right indicate the approximate upper and lower limits of growth rates for normal children at various ages.

larger doses, such patients tend to become easily distractible and difficult to manage. There is little evidence to support the idea that thyroid therapy sufficient to cause mild thyrotoxicosis produces greater progress with respect to intellectual development, body growth or body maturation than do subtoxic adequate doses.

Response to treatment. When a patient has primary hypothyroidism, the response to thyroid hormone therapy is clean cut. Certain of the changes which occur are outlined in Table 3. Most of these changes can be detected within six months after adequate thyroid treatment has been started.

On the average there is a 6 per cent weight loss within two or three weeks. Following this initial loss of weight, there usually is a steady weight gain. Increased activity or liveliness is noted by about four weeks; the patient obviously has more energy. In patients with hypercholesterolemia, the serum cholesterol values fall to normal limits within approximately the same period of time. An increase in appetite may be noted very soon in hypothyroid infants. This is evidenced both by a shortened feeding time and by an increase in the volume of food taken. The serum alkaline phosphatase activity rises from subnormal to normal values on the average in four or five weeks. The temperature of the skin over the extremities becomes appreciably warmer under conditions of cool environmental temperature in about five weeks. When this occurs the tendency to mottling of the skin disappears. Constipation may be eliminated within a few days. On the average this complaint is gone in about five weeks.

It takes a little longer to demonstrate a definite increase in growth rate. This can be documented by measurements of body length. Figure 11 shows that dur-

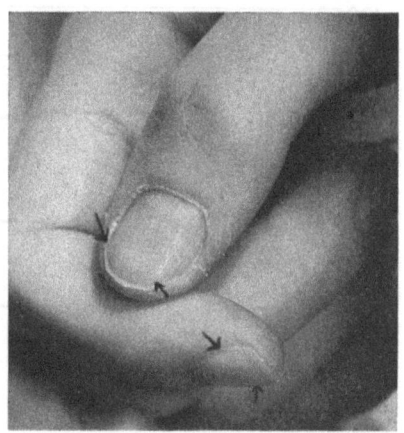

FIGURE I—12. Fingernail change noted in a hypothyroid patient following institution of thyroid hormone therapy. The arrows indicate the crescentic dividing line between the thicker, lighter-colored proximal nail which appeared after thyroid was given and the thinner and slightly darker distal nail produced before thyroid was started.

ing the first six months of adequate thyroid therapy hypothyroid infants and children tend to grow at a greater rate than the expected normal. Regardless of age, an increase in height of at least 5 cm. is to be expected during the first half year of treatment. Thereafter, the growth rate diminishes over the course of about two years to average normal. The diminution cannot be prevented by increasing the thyroid dosage above ordinary maintenance levels. This fact indicates that thyroid hormone is not *per se* a growth hormone.[2] However, it must be present in adequate amounts in order for growth to proceed normally.

When the athyrotic juvenile patient is treated with thyroid hormone, there is a distinct tendency for the rate of skeletal maturation to increase. Ordinarily this increase in maturation rate results in a diminution in the degree of skeletal retardation (i.e., in the difference between actual age and bone age). If thyroid therapy is begun before the age of two, the bone age may reach normal limits within a period of two to four years. In older patients the bone age response to thyroid therapy is more variable; a normal degree of skeletal maturation may not be attained until adolescent development occurs. Very occasionally, following thyroid medication, the bone age advances with remarkable rapidity, surpassing the actual age and even becoming precociously advanced. This unusual phenomenon may be related to heavy thyroid hormone dosage.

A change in skin texture from coarse to fine may take from one to five months of thyroid treatment. An approximately equal amount of time is required for myxedema to disappear completely.

There are a number of other changes which may take place following the institution of thyroid medication to athyrotic patients. Among these, shedding of scalp hair may be striking. When this occurs, it is followed by the regrowth

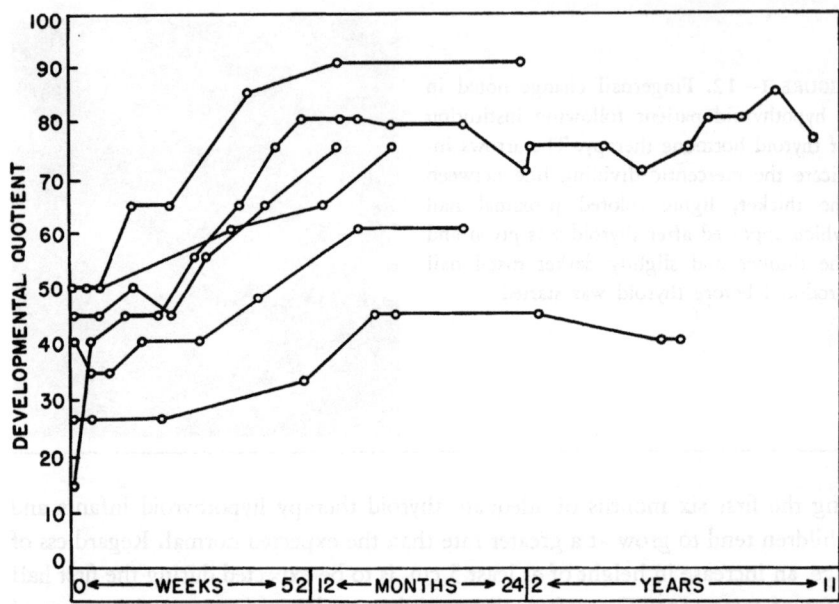

FIGURE I—13. Curves showing the changes in the developmental quotient of six hypothyroid children (ordinate) plotted against the time elapsed after institution of thyroid therapy (abscissa). The developmental quotient is the mental-motor age ÷ by actual age x 100. From A. Gesell, C. S. Amatruda and C. S. Culotta, *Am. J. Dis. Child.* 52:1117, 1936.

of a new and more luxuriant crop. Another phenomenon of interest may occur in the fingernails and toenails. A zone of relatively thick, healthy nail appears near the cuticles. At the junctions of the thicker new nail and the thinner old nail, a semicircular transverse ridge can be made out. As the healthy new nail grows under the influence of thyroid hormone, these ridges move outward at an approximately even pace in all the fingers and toes (see Figure 12).

Another change of great importance may be noted in the intellectual status. As is shown in Figure 13, the intelligence quotient of young, mentally retarded athyrotic patients tends to increase during the first year of thyroid treatment. Thereafter it remains more or less constant. Changes in the intellectual performance of children who are mentally adequate prior to thyroid treatment are in the same direction but less marked.

Therapeutic test with thyroid. Thyroid hormone in ordinary therapeutic doses causes a number of easily recognized changes in hypothyroid infants and children (see preceding section). By contrast, such therapy has no grossly discernible effects on euthyroid persons (see page 4). These facts may be

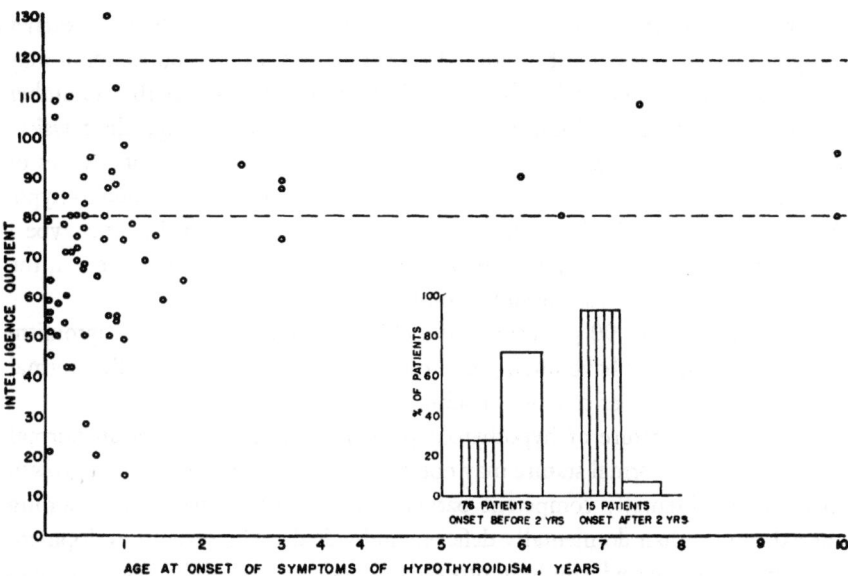

FIGURE I—14. Intelligence quotients (ordinate) of hypothyroid children after at least two years of thyroid therapy plotted against the age when hypothyroidism appeared (abscissa). It is evident that a very large number of children who develop hypothyroidism at an early age have IQ's under 80. The inset summarizes these data with relation to the age of onset; the striped columns represent patients with IQ's of 80 or more; the white columns, patients with IQ's of less than 80.

used to clinical advantage. If a child suspected of hypothyroidism responds in a typical manner to thyroid therapy, it is almost certain that he was deficient in thyroid prior to therapy. On the other hand, if he fails to show clear evidences of benefit after six months of thyroid hormone treatment, it is most unlikely that he has significant hypothyroidism.

There is no danger in giving thyroid hormone for a limited period for therapeutic test purposes except to patients with marked primary pituitary insufficiency or primary adrenocortical insufficiency (see Chapter III, Figure 37, and Chapter VII). Such patients are encountered only very rarely.

PROGNOSIS. This subject has been covered in part above. There it was indicated that the intelligence quotient increases about as much as it ever will during the first year of adequate thyroid therapy. Figure 14 shows that the ultimate intelligence quotient bears some relation to the age of onset of hypothyroidism. Only about 25 per cent of the patients who develop signs of thyroid deficiency before the age of two ever attain an intelligence quotient above

80. It is not known to what extent these statistics could be modified by earlier recognition and treatment of infantile hypothyroidism. In this connection it may be of interest to quote from Tredgold[15 a]: "The general experience that a number of cretins show no mental improvement under treatment, although the physical signs disappear, leads me to think that there are probably two distinct types of cretins. In one type the mental and physical retardation are clearly due to hypothyroidism, and the child becomes normal under treatment. In the other type I am disposed to think that the essential condition is one of primary amentia, the hypothyroidism being a super-added complication."

By contrast, about 90 per cent of the children who develop hypothyroidism after the second year have intelligence quotients above 80 (i.e., in the normal range) and only 10 per cent are of subnormal intelligence.

The ultimate stature of hypothyroid patients is likely to be within normal limits. However, normal stature may not be attained until the adolescent growth spurt occurs. Mentally competent patients have a better chance of attaining normal stature than do mentally deficient individuals. The sexual development of treated hypothyroid children proceeds at average or slightly slower than average rate.

Except in adolescents with mild thyroid deficiency of the type associated with so-called adolescent goiter, most hypothyroid children never cease to need thyroid hormone substitution therapy. To test their need, thyroid treatment may be discontinued for a trial period of observation.

EFFECTS OF THYROID WITHDRAWAL. It is practically impossible to determine whether a patient has a tendency to thyroid deficiency when he is receiving adequate maintenance doses of thyroid hormone. But, as would be expected, hypothyroid patients gradually redevelop most of the cardinal signs of thyroid lack within four months after therapy is discontinued (see Table 2). Among the first changes to be noted are moderate weight gain, loss of pep and tolerance for cold, coolness of the skin and slowing of the pulse. Of particular diagnostic value is the concurrent tendency to develop hypercholesterolemia (see page 8).

If a patient who has been receiving thyroid hormone in full maintenance doses for several months develops these changes when therapy is discontinued, it may be concluded that he is still definitely in need of treatment. If he fails to develop them, therapy should not be resumed until signs of thyroid lack appear.

Hypothyroidism Secondary to Hypopituitarism (Pituitary Myxedema). Patients with a primary defect in the anterior pituitary gland may also be partially or totally deficient with respect to thyrotropic hormone (TSH). This deficiency results in a corresponding lack of thyroid hormone (secondary hypothyroidism). Moreover, since pituitary lesions can cause generalized pituitary insufficiency, adrenocorticotropic hormone (ACTH), gonadotropic hormones (FSH, LH, etc.) and pituitary growth hormone (PGH) deficiency may result. This leads to secondary hypoadrenocorticism, hypogonadism and stunted growth.

A nearly similar condition can develop as a result of primary athyrosis. That is, thyroid hormone lack results in impaired anterior pituitary activity just as it interferes with the economy of other body cells.

These relations create interesting and at times perplexing clinical problems of diagnosis and therapy, for patients with primary panhypopituitarism may present symptoms and signs which are almost indistinguishable from those seen in the primary hypothyroid patient.[19] Certain patients with primary hypopituitarism will have local evidences of a lesion in the region of the sella turcica (see Chapter VII). Such signs aid greatly in distinguishing between these two conditions.

Signs of thyroid deficiency are usually much more subtle in patients with primary pituitary disease than in patients with primary athyrosis. Perhaps this difference is due simply to differences in the degree of hypothyroidism. The concentration of protein-bound iodine in the serum averages lower in patients with primary athyrosis than in patients with hypothyroidism secondary to hypopituitarism.

Whereas such complaints as lethargy, constipation and sensitivity to cold are common in patients with primary athyrosis, they often are minimal or absent in patients with primary hypopituitarism. Moreover, the skin of hypopituitary patients tends to be fine and smooth in texture rather than coarse, sandpapery and dry as in athyrosis.* On the other hand, both types of patients may show abnormally slow growth, abnormally slow skeletal maturation, epiphyseal dysgenesis, retarded sexual development, hypo-17-ketosteroiduria and hypo-11-17-oxysteroiduria. Hypercholesterolemia is a variable finding in both types.

Hypothyroidism due to hypopituitarism can be distinguished from primary athyrosis by observing the effect of thyroid hormone therapy. If the patient is suffering primarily from a lack of thyroid hormone, its administration will result in the changes outlined in the preceding section. The characteristic signs and symptoms of thyroid hormone deficiency disappear and there is a marked increase in growth rate, sexual maturation and 17-ketosteroid excretion. By contrast, while thyroid therapy eliminates signs of hypothyroidism *per se* in the hypopituitary patient, it fails to restore growth rate, sexual development and adrenocortical activity to normal.

* An exception is encountered in patients with marked anorexia nervosa. Such patients may develop functional hypothyroidism of appreciable degree (see above under thyroid homeostasis).

The administration of thyroid hormone to panhypopituitary patients may result in relative hypoadrenocorticism (see Chapter III, Figure 37). This is particularly apt to occur when full therapeutic doses of thyroid hormone are employed. This complication can usually be avoided by beginning with doses of one-tenth to one-quarter of the standard maintenance dose (60 to 90 mg. of USP thyroid per m^2 per day). If the initial substandard dose is well tolerated over a period of two or three weeks, it may be increased stepwise as tolerated until the therapeutic level is reached.

In the latter connections, it is well to ask the parents of patients given thyroid for the first time to report promptly any untoward manifestations such as vomiting, diarrhea, dizziness, marked weakness or the like. On the other hand, one should try not to frighten the family to such an extent that they dare not give any thyroid to their child.

HYPERTHYROIDISM (THYROTOXICOSIS)

Thyrotoxicosis, or Graves' disease, is a widespread disorder in which the muscular, nervous, reticulo-endothelial and lymphatic systems as well as the thyroid, anterior pituitary and eyes may be involved. It is characterized by the presence of a toxic excess of thyroid hormone in the blood stream.

Regardless of age, this condition occurs approximately seven times more frequently in females than in males.[20] The reason for this sex difference is not known. Relatively speaking, hyperthyroidism occurs less often among children than adults. While it occurs but rarely among children under five, it has been reported in infancy. Children are most apt to develop hyperthyroidism at the onset of adolescence (about seven or eight years*) and at about 13 years.

ETIOLOGY. The exact cause of spontaneous thyrotoxicosis is not known. Students of the subject have postulated such factors as (a) hyperthyrotropinism due to hypothalamic disturbances, (b) failure of inactivation of thyrotropic hormone by the thyroid, (c) increased sensitivity of the thyroid to thyrotropic hormone, (d) production of an abnormal thyroid-stimulating hormone and (e) direct neurologic stimulation of the thyroid. There are as yet no reported instances of thyrotoxicosis due to thyroid carcinoma in a child.

CLINICAL MANIFESTATIONS. The onset of juvenile hyperthyroidism varies from insidious on the one hand to abrupt on the other. At times it appears to have been incited by an emotional, infectious or physical trauma.

The outstanding clinical manifestations include thyroid enlargement, eye changes, weight loss despite increased appetite, weakness, irritability, sweating

---

* See Chapter V, page 302, for the definition of "adolescence" as used here.

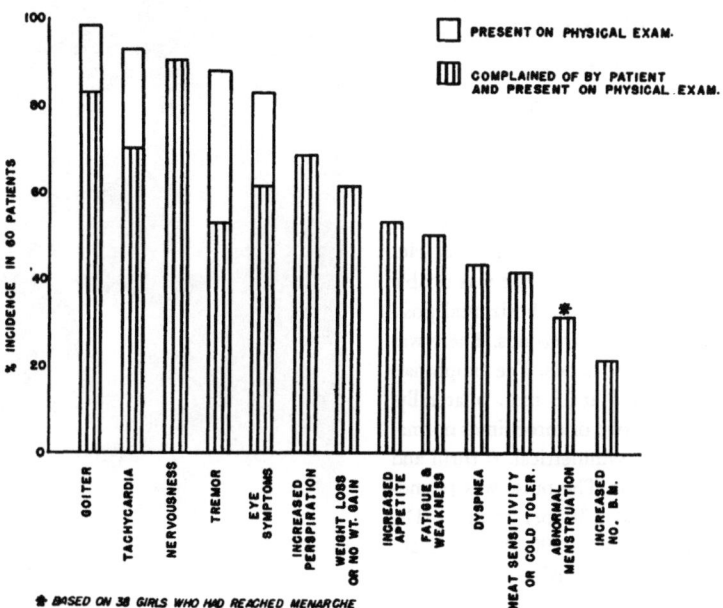

FIGURE I—15. The relative incidence of the principal symptoms and signs of thyrotoxicosis in 60 children of 7 to 16 years seen in the Thyroid Clinic and Adolescent Endocrine Clinic of the Massachusetts General Hospital over a 10-year period. The letters BM in the right-hand legend along the abscissa stand for bowel movements.

and increased sensitivity to heat or tolerance for cold. The pattern of presenting signs varies from patient to patient, especially with respect to the prominence of eye signs. Figure 15 indicates the relative frequency of certain of the manifestations. Brief detailed comments follow.

The thyroid gland is obviously and more or less symmetrically enlarged. Usually it is in its normal position; occasionally it extends downwards. Nodules are very unusual in juvenile hyperthyroid patients. Thrills are noted bilaterally over the superior poles of the thyroid lobes in the majority of thyrotoxic patients. Systolic bruits are present over the lobes and sometimes the isthmus of the toxic goiter. Thyroid thrills and bruits are to be distinguished from thrills and hums occasioned by the passage of blood through the great vessels of the neck.

Possible eye signs are as follows. Lid retraction may result in a widened palpebral fissure and give rise to an overly bright, staring expression (see Figure 16). Lid lag, characterized by a tendency for the upper lid to fall less rapidly

[34]   CHAPTER I:

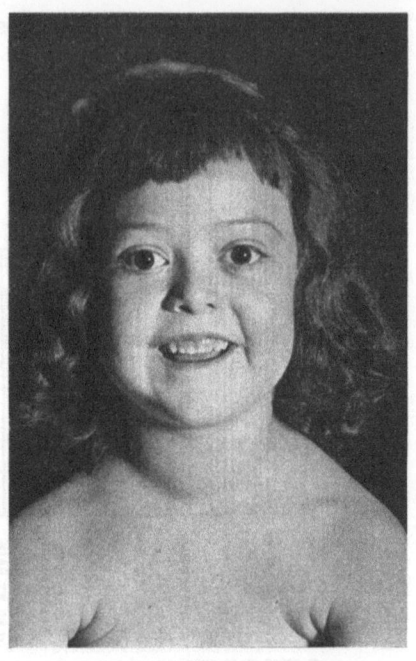

FIGURE 1—16. Moderately severe thyrotoxicosis of approximately three months' duration in a girl of six years.

CASE HISTORY

Protrusion of the eyes, irritability, excessive perspiration and slight elevation of temperature had developed gradually. There was no known precipitating factor. The child had a height age of 5½, weight age of 4½ and bone age of 5$\frac{9}{12}$. Her skin was warm and moist. She was unable to maintain her legs in a horizontal position for longer than 45 seconds. There was a fine tremor of the hands. The exophthalmos was measured at 18 mm. bilaterally. The thyroid was two or three times normal size, smooth and symmetrical. A thrill and bruit were present. The pulse was pounding; the rate was 130 per minute. The blood pressure was 150/90. No other abnormalities were revealed.

---

than the eyeball when it rolls downward, also may be present. This phenomenon is accentuated by fatigue of palpebral muscles. Weakness of extraocular muscles may result in limitation of ocular movements. Swelling of orbital contents may cause forward protrusion of the eyeball. There also may be chemosis of the conjunctivæ. Severe eye changes of the types described for adults[21] are very uncommon in juvenile thyrotoxic patients.

Signs of hypermetabolism and thyrotoxicity. The increase in heat production or caloric output characteristic of the condition leads to a feeling of warmth, increased perspiration and diurnal elevations in body temperature. When there is a compensatory increase in food consumption, no weight loss occurs. However, if the intake of calories is not increased, body weight is apt to diminish. When anorexia, vomiting or diarrhea develops, the large resultant negative caloric balance leads to a rapid loss of weight. This is an ominous sign.

In most hyperthyroid children the resting pulse rate is in excess of 100 beats per minute; in many it is over 120. The heart is not ordinarily enlarged, but it may seem to be so because of the forcefulness of the apical impulse. Frequently there is a diffuse precordial systolic murmur. In addition, a harsh systolic sound, which seems to be "close to the ear" and of scratchy quality, may be heard over the pulmonic area. These signs probably are related to increased cardiac activity and blood flow. Sometimes the pulmonic area signs are accompanied by dilatation of pulmonary vessels, which becomes manifest in roentgenograms of the heart by increased prominence of the pulmonic conus. Though these findings may be quite suggestive of organic heart disease, they tend to disappear after the patient becomes euthyroid. Myocarditis is reported as an occasional complication in severe thyrotoxicosis.

Muscular weakness is sometimes marked. If not obvious, it may be demonstrated by asking the patient to hold the lower legs horizontal while sitting in a chair. Normal persons can maintain them in that position for at least two minutes. Thyrotoxic patients are apt to weaken and allow their legs to fall before that amount of time has elapsed.

Nervous irritability is expressed in a variety of ways such as overactivity, jumpiness, inability to sit still, quickness of reaction, lively tendon reflexes and fine tremors of the tongue and outstretched hands. In addition, there is emotional instability with an inclination to weep at slight provocation. Young patients may become utterly unmanageable.

Abnormalities of menstruation may occur. When hyperthyroidism develops prior to the menarche, there may be a delay in the onset of menstruation. When the disease develops after the menarche, there is a tendency to oligomenorrhea or amenorrhea.

Occasionally the metabolic manifestations of thyroid toxicity suddenly become much intensified. The resultant clinical condition is called *thyroid storm* or *toxic crisis*. It is characterized by the development of weakness, a very rapid pulse, a high fever, either hyperirritability or marked apathy and a tendency to delirium. The patient becomes weak, may become comatose and die in a matter of days.

DIAGNOSIS. The diagnosis of thyrotoxicosis usually presents no problem. It can be confirmed by measurement of the protein-bound iodine in the serum or by observing the patient's response to specific therapy. Very occasionally a diagnosis of thyrotoxicosis is erroneously considered in abnormally anxious but otherwise healthy children.

In rheumatic carditis as in thyrotoxicosis there may be fever, rapid resting pulse, cardiac enlargement, cardiac murmurs and signs of decompensation. While thyrotoxicosis is considered very rarely in the differential diagnosis of rheumatic fever, the reverse is more common. When thyrotoxicosis is controlled, signs of cardiac embarrassment due to thyroid toxicity vanish.

In one five-months-old infant with a cerebral arteriovenous aneurysm, the occurrence of tachycardia, hypertension with wide pulse pressure, cardiac enlargement, failure to gain weight, hyperactivity and exophthalmos was considered strongly suggestive of thyrotoxicosis. This infant's response to thiouracil was not impressive. At post mortem the thyroid gland showed no changes indicative of hyperthyroidism.

Patients with pheochromocytoma may present a clinical picture quite similar to that seen in Graves' disease. Unlike thyrotoxic patients, most of them show changes in the eyegrounds and have cool skin as well as normal serum protein-bound iodine values. This condition is considered in detail in Chapter IV. Other types of goiter are considered in succeeding sections of this chapter.

TREATMENT. Spontaneous hyperthyroidism characteristically shows cyclic fluctuations in severity, and in most patients the disease is self-limited. Both these characteristics and especially the former need to be borne in mind in evaluating therapy and in making predictions. Children are likely to pass through two to four cycles before the disease is burned out. Phases of exacerbation and of remission can last from a few months to several years.

In choosing between the various types of treatment available for juvenile thyrotoxic patients, particular care should be taken to avoid continuing with a form of therapy which makes the child a semi-chronic invalid. In other words, treatment which, after the initial period of recuperation, requires limitation of the child's normal work-and-play activities or frequent visits to the physician is not considered satisfactory. Under this circumstance some more effective form of therapy such as subtotal thyroidectomy is indicated.

Therapeutic agents. Aside from subtotal thyroidectomy, there are three important types of agents which diminish thyroid hormone secretion in patients with spontaneous hyperthyroidism: (a) iodide salts, (b) radio-active iodine and (c) thiouracil and related substances. Current investigations suggest that ACTH also may be of practical value in the management of severe, acute thyrotoxicosis.[22c] Because this type of treatment is in an early experimental phase, it will not be discussed further here.

Decision concerning the proper method of treatment is not always easy. When the disease is mild, little is to be lost by trying iodine first, provided the patient is observed regularly. If the signs of toxicity remain of negligible degree, no other treatment is needed. If, on the other hand, the child's condition is obviously deteriorating and his health and happiness are in jeopardy, thiouracil therapy may be started. Ordinarily, thiouracil will check the disease before it becomes very severe.

By contrast, when it is clear at the outset that a child has severe thyrotoxicosis it usually is best for reasons outlined below to withhold iodine at least pending institution of propyl thiouracil treatment. One is then in a position either to continue with a long course of propyl thiouracil treatment or to perform a subtotal thyroidectomy as soon as the patient can be considered suitably prepared.

There are arguments for and against chronic administration of thiouracil and subtotal thyroidectomy. Present evidence suggests that thiouracil must be continued in juvenile patients for many months and perhaps for several years before a permanent remission in thyrotoxicosis can be looked for.[23 d, g] Moreover, very undesirable side effects are sometimes produced by drugs of this type (see page 41). Subtotal thyroidectomy by an experienced surgeon carries very little risk if the patient has been properly prepared. On the other hand, it must be remembered that operative mishaps and deaths do occur in thyroid as in other types of surgery despite all precautions. While surgery does not guarantee against recurrence of thyrotoxicosis at a later date, residual postoperative thyrotoxicosis becomes a relatively remote possibility after a generous excision has been performed.

No hard and fast rule for decision can be set forth. At the moment we consider skillful surgery to be a more dependable form of therapy than chronic medication with drugs of the thiouracil type. More extensive studies of the end results of thiouracil treatment are needed before its value can be appraised adequately. The same is true for radio-active iodine treatment, which intentionally is receiving scant attention in the present volume.

There follow more detailed comments on the clinical management of thyrotoxic patients and on the use of drugs.

Initial management. Bed rest is indicated in the initial management of a thyrotoxic patient. This alone frequently results in some improvement. The food offered should contain generous amounts of sugar and other carbohydrates, which can easily be used for fuel. Otherwise the diet may conform to the patient's tastes. Because thyrotoxicosis increases the requirements for vitamins, it is well to supplement the diet with concentrates of vitamins A, B complex, C and D. In some cases sedation may be accomplished by iodinization alone (see below). If additional sedation is needed, phenobarbital or chloral hydrate in ordinary doses serves satisfactorily. There is usually no need for administering morphine.

Iodinization. The use of iodides in the therapy of thyrotoxicosis seems paradoxical when it is remembered that iodine is a constituent of thyroid hormone and that iodine lack may lead to thyroid hormone deficiency. Iodine therapy does not, in fact, alter the progress or duration of thyrotoxicosis. It merely puts on the brakes to a certain extent by partially blocking the effects of pituitary thyrotropic hormone (Figure 17).[22 a] The quantity of iodine (as sodium or potassium iodide) needed daily to produce this result is about 6 mg., an amount from 80 to 100 times greater than that needed to prevent iodine-want goiter.

Iodine therapy rarely causes hypothyroidism in thyrotoxic patients and usually

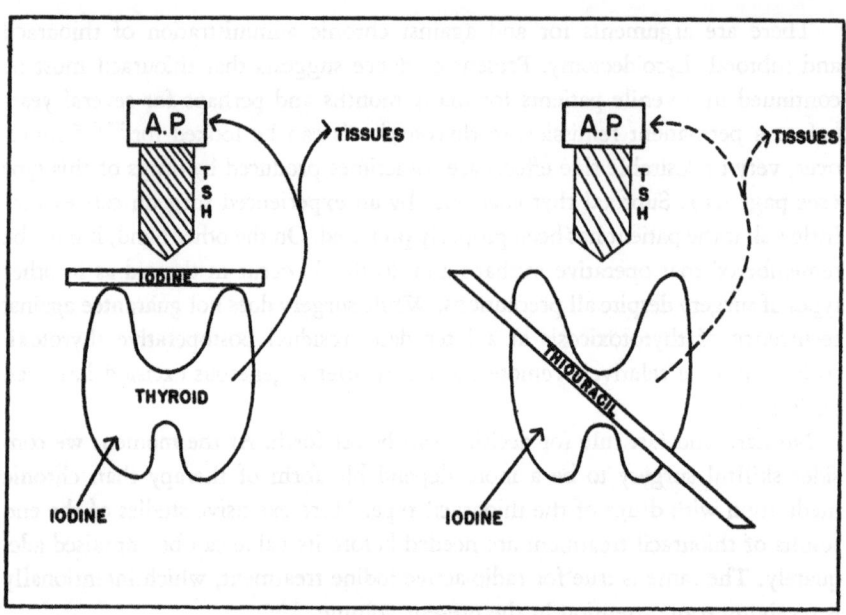

FIGURE I—17. Schematic indication of sites at which iodine and thiouracil are thought to exert their action on the thyroid. Iodine partially inhibits the action of TSH upon the thyroid; thiouracil arrests the synthesis (iodinization) of thyroid hormone.

is without appreciable action in euthyroid persons. It is not known why this is so.

Iodinization can be accomplished by the daily oral administration of 5 minims (0.3 cc.) of a saturated solution of potassium iodide in milk. This gives 230 mg. of iodine, which is greatly in excess of the smallest dose (6 mg.) that will produce maximum benefits. Medication can be withdrawn and reinstituted with undiminished effectiveness. When used as a chronic therapeutic agent, iodine should be continued for six months to a year after all signs of thyrotoxicosis have subsided.

Thyrotoxic patients who have not received appreciable amounts of iodine for several weeks respond to iodinization in a fairly characteristic manner. An appreciable reaction is attained in about 10 days. The thyroid gland usually becomes smaller and of firmer consistency. Thrills and bruits tend to diminish or disappear. The rate and force of the heart and pulse beats diminish. Palpitation disappears as does the sensation of warmth. Nervous excitability and emotional instability subside rapidly. Eye signs are not altered significantly.

As changes in the foregoing symptoms and signs take place, there is a fall in the basal metabolic rate. In adult patients the rate of fall is about 3 or 4 points a day. In children it may be slightly greater. A well-documented* fall of 15 or more points in rate within 12 days is considered a positive response and confirmatory of the diagnosis of thyrotoxicosis. Such a response is obtained in the vast majority of children with Graves' disease. Hence failure to show a comparable rate of fall within the same period suggests either that the patient is not thyrotoxic or that there has been a large intake of iodine in the recent past.

Signs of iodine toxicity are uncommon. A few persons develop an acneiform, pustular rash (but pre-existing acne is not a contra-indication to iodinization). Fever, coryza and salivation may also occur. Such signs sometimes disappear spontaneously within a few days while patients are under iodine therapy. On the other hand, severe, indeed fatal, reactions to iodine have been observed.[22 b] These are apt to be associated with very high fever and edema of the face and respiratory passages. When it appears that iodine medication is responsible for marked toxic manifestations, iodine therapy should be stopped regardless of thyroid status. The patient's thyrotoxicosis will, of course, grow worse. The serious therapeutic problem which thus develops may be combatted by means of the general measures enumerated above (page 37). In addition, a drug of the thiouracil type may be given. This eventually will bring the thyrotoxicosis under control.

Use of radio-active iodine. The therapeutic effect of radio-active iodine is dependent upon the thyroid gland's efficiency as an iodine trap.[24] The gland can increase its iodine concentration over that of the blood by a factor of 10,000. Since radio-active iodine is physiologically indistinguishable from ordinary iodine, it is taken up by the thyroid, where it destroys the thyroid cells by internal irradiation. Such radiation may cause a permanent remission in the thyrotoxicosis. This treatment has been used with success in a number of adult thyrotoxic patients. However, it is not at present recommended for juvenile patients because of the theoretical possibility that the radiation may incite degenerative changes culminating in malignancy after a latent period of 10 to 20 years.

Use of thiouracil drugs. Thiouracil and propyl thiouracil are members of a large group of drugs which depress thyroid function by interfering with the utilization of iodine in the synthesis of thyroid hormone (Figure 17).[23] When given in appropriate amounts they effectively suppress thyroid hormone production by the thyroid glands of hyperthyroid or euthyroid individuals, and when given for a sufficiently long period of time, hypothyroidism results regardless of the original thyroid status.

Thiouracil and related drugs do not prevent secretion of thyroid hormone

* See comments on basal metabolic rate in a previous section of the chapter.

which has already been formed and stored in the gland. Hence, prior medication with large doses of iodine, by saturating the thyroid gland with iodinated hormone, may delay the "antithyroid" effects of such drugs. On the other hand, thiouracil drugs do not block the thyrotropin-inhibiting effect of iodine.

The response to thiouracil treatment is about half as rapid as that described for iodinization. Moreover, in contrast to iodine, thiouracil causes the thyroid gland to develop a softer consistency. Because of this change, the outlines of the gland often become difficult to distinguish with accuracy.

Since thiouracil drugs do not prevent pituitary thyrotropin from causing thyroid gland hyperplasia, enlargement of the gland may take place while they are in effect. In euthyroid subjects thyroid enlargement occurs when the concentration of thyroid hormone in the serum falls below normal; in patients with Graves' disease the same may happen when concentrations fall below thyrotoxic levels. In most patients under thiouracil treatment, it is probable that the gland enlarges somewhat; occasionally it enlarges markedly. Thrills and bruits persist at least for a while.

With one other important exception, the clinical response to thiouracil treatment is similar to that obtained by iodinization. The exception concerns the degrees of decrease in thyroid hormone production. As has been said, iodine does not stop thyroid hormone production. In adequate doses, thiouracil does. Hence, patients receiving thiouracil can be rendered euthyroid or even hypothyroid at will. This means that thiouracil treatment can be used to bring thyrotoxicosis completely under control in preparing patients for subtotal thyroidectomy. The dangers of severe intra- or postoperative reactions are thus appreciably decreased.

The action of thiouracil drugs on thyrotoxicosis depends on continuous administration. Although remission may persist after treatment is discontinued, in juvenile patients especially there is likely to be an exacerbation of the disease within five or six months. The relapse rate—probably 50 to 75 per cent—is very difficult to predict accurately from available data. Further carefully planned studies may modify this estimate. Until the value and safety of chronic therapy with thiouracil drugs has been demonstrated more clearly, their routine use is not recommended.

More is known about thiouracil and propyl thiouracil than about most of the other related drugs. These substances have many characteristics in common and a few distinguishing features which add to the reputation of some and subtract from that of others. They are considered separately below.

Within an hour after a single dose is taken *thiouracil* is rapidly absorbed from the gastrointestinal tract and attains maximum concentrations in the blood stream. The subsequent rates of degradation and excretion are difficult to define. It takes from one to five days to clear the blood and tissues of thiouracil after cessation of therapy.

The initial dose is 350 mg. per m^2 per day. This is divided into three parts and given every eight hours. To maintain an effective concentration of the drug in the thyroid gland for 24 hours, it is essential that a dose of the drug be given at least every eight hours. Accidental omission of one dose or extension of the prescribed eight-hour interval between doses to 10 or 12 hours may permit the concentration of thiouracil to fall below effective levels. Particularly when iodine is being given also, an oversight of this kind may permit the thyroid gland to produce new iodinated hormone. Since thiouracil acts by preventing the formation rather than the discharge of thyroid hormone by the thyroid gland, such an accident may appreciably delay control of thyrotoxicosis by thiouracil therapy.

For chronic maintenance therapy, following a satisfactory initial response, the amount given may be reduced to one-half or one-third of the value mentioned above, and the time interval may be increased to 10 or 12 hours. Signs of hypothyroidism indicate the need for decreasing the dose, while signs of increasing thyrotoxicosis point to a larger dose.

Toxic reactions of various sorts may develop following administration of thiouracil.[23, 25] Agranulocytosis is the major hazard. In approximately 2 per cent of treated patients this develops within eight weeks after starting therapy; occasionally it develops later. Hence it is an ever-present threat. Dose levels do not seem to bear any consistent relation to this toxic reaction. The mortality is appreciable (± 25 per cent). Accordingly, patients receiving thiouracil require careful medical supervision, especially during the first 10 weeks of treatment. Leucocyte and differential cell counts should be taken at weekly intervals. They are also indicated whenever a recipient of the drug develops a fever or sore throat. The presence of agranulocytosis calls for immediate cessation of thiouracil and for the institution of penicillin therapy in full doses intramuscularly.

Leucopenia short of agranulocytosis results in 3 or 4 per cent of cases under treatment. It is characterized by a leucocyte count of less than 1,000 per mm^3, with polymorphonuclear leucocytes comprising between 10 and 50 per cent of the total count. This phenomenon is seen most often after six weeks of therapy. In most instances the withdrawal of thiouracil is followed by recovery within 10 days. Penicillin therapy is indicated in the presence of bacterial infection.

Drug fever is observed in about 5 per cent of treated patients. High drug fevers are an indication for stopping therapy.

Enlargement of submaxillary and salivary glands is seen occasionally. This manifestation may disappear while treatment is continued. Thyroiditis has also been seen. It is apt to be associated with fever, erythema of the overlying skin and discomfort. It is an indication for discontinuing thiouracil.

Other miscellaneous toxic reactions are seen from time to time. They include thrombocytopenia, jaundice, hematuria, maculopapular eruptions, urticaria, neuritis, arthritis and edema of the leg. Generally speaking they are contra-indications to further use of the drug.

With respect to its antithyroid effects, *propyl thiouracil* is similar to thiouracil. However, experience to date indicates that it produces only one-eighth as many toxic reactions. The incidence is about 1.8 per cent. Very few fatalities have occurred as a result of its use in over 1,000 patients. At present propyl thiouracil is therefore considered the drug of choice. The dosage is 120 to 175 mg. per m^2 per day. This is divided into three doses and given every eight hours.

Combined propyl thiouracil and iodine therapy. When these drugs are to be used in combination some consideration should be given to the order in which they are administered.[26] It will be remembered that prior administration of iodine appreciably delays the action of propyl thiouracil. Hence, when prompt control of thyrotoxicosis is important, it is advisable to give propyl thiouracil first and wait for a few hours before giving iodine medication.

When preparing patients with propyl thiouracil for subtotal thyroidectomy, it may be desirable to add iodine to the treatment during the last week before operation. In that interval it will cause the gland to become firmer and less vascular, thus facilitating surgery.

Finally, in treating a patient who has hyperthyroidism of a mild degree, it is reasonable to administer iodine first in order to find out whether the disease can be controlled by the iodinization alone. Should iodine prove inadequate a thiouracil drug may be added as outlined above (page 39).

Preparation for subtotal thyroidectomy. Thyrotoxic patients are poor surgical risks. This is partly because thyroid in excessive concentrations has toxic effects on various systems and organs and partly because thyrotoxic individuals tend to become depleted with respect to calories, protoplasm, hepatic glycogen, minerals and vitamins.[1 b, c; 27] For these reasons it is essential that the patient be rendered euthyroid and be given an opportunity to recuperate before thyroid surgery is undertaken.

Methods for controlling the thyrotoxicosis by medical means are outlined above. The patient may be considered a good candidate for surgery when the pulse and blood pressure have returned to normal, signs of cardiac embarrassment have disappeared, the basal metabolic rate has fallen to a slightly minus value and an appreciable portion of body weight lost during the period of thyrotoxicosis has been regained. He also should have attained a reasonable degree of emotional stability.

Care should be taken to avoid rendering the patient hypothyroid preoperatively, since thyroid deficient patients are intolerant of stress and drugs like morphine.

Detailed comments on anesthesia and surgical procedures are beyond the scope of this book. The importance of engaging a surgeon who is familiar with thyroid problems is clear. Concerning the question of how much thyroid tissue should be removed we have a medical opinion. It is much easier to treat postoperative hypothyroidism than postoperative residual thyrotoxicosis. Therefore extensive rather than limited subtotal resection of thyroid tissue is recommended.

Thiouracil drug and iodine therapy should be discontinued on the day of operation.

When iodine alone has been used preoperatively, fever as high as 103 or 104° F. may develop following subtotal thyroidectomy. The high fever subsides within four days and ordinarily is not associated with a demonstrable infection. With thiouracil preparation, postoperative fever is uncommon. Thyroid storm or toxic crisis is seen occasionally as a complication of thyroid surgery in patients who have been prepared for surgery by means of iodine therapy alone. It has become very uncommon among patients rendered euthyroid with thiouracil drugs.

Surgical complications such as vocal cord palsies due to injury of recurrent laryngeal nerves, infection and edema will not be considered here. Postoperative tetany is considered in Chapter II.

Postoperative supervision. Patients who have had a generous subtotal thyroidectomy stand a good chance of developing mild-to-moderate hypothyroidism within a few weeks. This is considered a desirable postoperative result. The clinical manifestations correspond to those outlined earlier under hypothyroidism. When hypothyroidism develops, thyroid hormone substitution therapy is definitely indicated; often there is little to be lost in starting standard maintenance doses of thyroid soon after the patient has recovered from the operation. Though the need for substitution therapy may disappear with time, thyroid hormone may be continued indefinitely unless signs of thyrotoxicosis supervene. Provided it has been demonstrated that recurrent thyrotoxicosis cannot be alleviated by simply withdrawing thyroid hormone, the method of management is the same as for an initial attack.

GOITER

Enlargement of the thyroid gland is mentioned above both under hypothyroidism and under hyperthyroidism. This section deals with thyroid enlargement not associated with clear clinical signs of either deficient or excessive thyroid hormone production.

Neonatal Goiter.[28] This condition has the following characteristics. At birth the infant is seen to have a horseshoe-shaped enlargement of the lobes and isthmus of the thyroid gland (see Figure 18). The enlargement may be asymmetrical. The gland tends to be of moderately soft consistency and may be slightly nodular. Because the enlarged gland can compress adjacent structures (see Figure 19) serious signs of distress may be present. Upper respiratory obstruction from compression of the trachea leads to dyspnea, intermittent cyanosis, retraction of the intercostal spaces and laryngeal mucous. By interfering with the innervation of the vocal cords, pressure on the laryngeal nerves may aggravate these respiratory difficulties and cause the voice to be hoarse. Dysphagia develops when there is narrowing of the esophagus.

Possibly because of pressure on the great vessels of the neck, there may be striking signs of circulatory embarrassment and marked enlargement of the heart. Protrusion of the eyes may also occur. This seems to be a manifestation of venous hypertension above the thyroid area rather than a sign of thyrotoxicosis. Though objective confirmation by serum protein-bound iodine measurements is lacking, it seems probable that these infants are euthyroid.

The thyroid commences to shrink and the various manifestations of obstruction and compression begin to disappear within a few days. The respirations can return to normal within eight or ten days. Thereafter all remaining symptoms and signs subside gradually. As a rule the infant appears to be perfectly normal within a period of six to twelve months.

Treatment of this complaint is largely symptomatic. Respiratory difficulties may be lessened by letting the head fall back. Oxygen therapy is helpful. If relief from mechanical strangulation by the thyroid must be obtained, subtotal thyroidectomy should be undertaken. Tracheotomy is said to be difficult to perform without killing the patient.

The cause of neonatal goiter is not clear. It appears sometimes to be related to iodine metabolism, for the condition most often occurs in infants born of mothers who have taken large doses of iodine during pregnancy*—asthma being the reason for iodine medication in some instances, tachycardia or thyrotoxicosis

---

* Animal husbandrymen have been aware of this relation between maternal iodine intake and neonatal goiter for some time.[28]

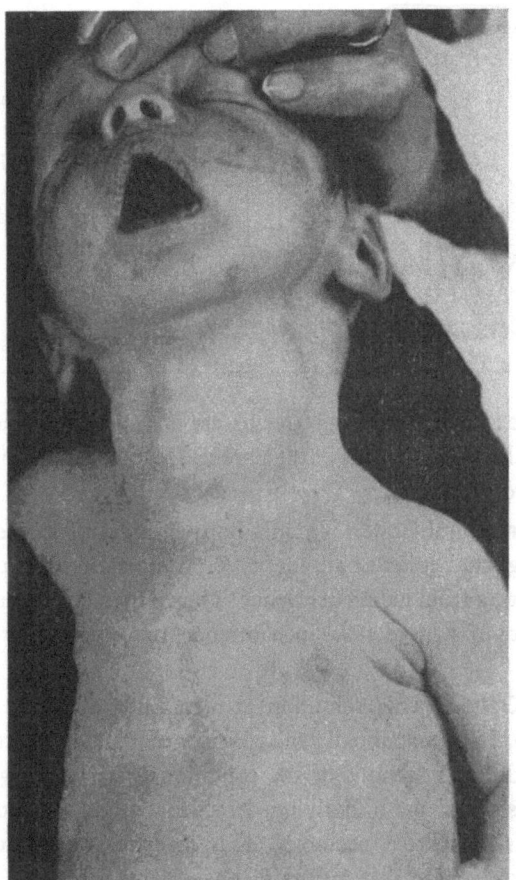

FIGURE I—18. Transient congenital goiter in a newborn infant.

CASE HISTORY

The mother of this baby had been taking from 12 to 40 minims of a saturated solution of potassium iodide daily for three years because of an asthmatic condition. During pregnancy she took 8 minims t.i.d. At birth, the infant was noted to have an enlarged thyroid gland. He suffered one choking and twitching spell, thought possibly to be due to obstruction of the air passages by mucus. There were no evidences of either hypo- or hyperthyroidism. His appearance at the age of one week is indicated in the above photograph. His subsequent course was benign. At the age of one month the thyroid gland seemed a little smaller; at three months it was barely palpable. Growth and development at that time were normal. We are indebted to Dr. A. F. Hardyment of Vancouver, B.C., for the summary and photograph of this case.

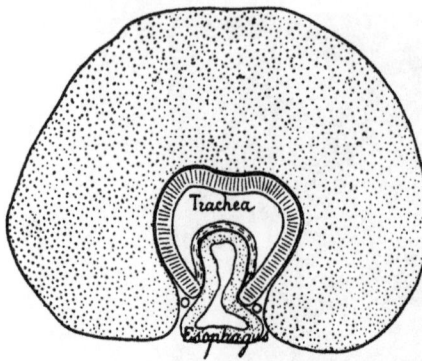

FIGURE I—19. Diagram of the manner in which large or circular types of goiter may compress structures in the neck. From A. Crotti, *Thyroid and Thymus*. Philadelphia, Lea & Febiger, 1938.

in others. There is no evidence that the disease is necessarily related to a primary disturbance in the thyroid status of the parent. Detailed studies on such a patient should be of great interest.

Endemic Congenital Goiter. Infants born in areas of iodine poverty sometimes have congenital goiter of another type. In the majority of cases the mother has goiter resulting from iodine deficiency. The infant's goiter may either subside or grow and attain a large size. Such infants frequently suffer from hypothyroidism.

Adolescent Goiter. This condition is mentioned above in the section on hypothyroidism. It is undoubtedly the commonest malady affecting the thyroid gland. While the pathogenesis of the condition is not entirely clear, the best evidence suggests that the underlying defect is a slight functional inadequacy in the synthesis of thyroid hormone. This inadequacy may follow from the operation of three conceivable factors:

1. Absolute deficiency in iodine intake. Before the widespread use of iodized salt this factor exhibited a striking geographic incidence. Mountainous areas or old glacial areas where the soil had been leached of its iodine were the chief sites of prevalence. Since the brilliant demonstration of Marine that goiters of this type are due to an absolute or relative lack of iodine, and the consequent program of iodine prophylaxis, geographical distinctions have become blurred.
2. Deficient production of thyroid hormone, due to defective absorption of iodine or to interference with thyroid hormone synthesis, in the presence of an adequate iodine intake. The clinical significance of this factor is less easy to gauge, although recent studies employing radio-active iodine have demonstrated that such common foods as rutabagas, peanuts, peaches and strawberries may inhibit the uptake of iodine by the thyroid.[29]

3. Excessive demand for thyroid hormone. It is believed that during adolescence there is a temporary physiologic demand for larger amounts of hormone than the gland has previously been elaborating. A supply of iodine that just suffices for the manufacture of the body's minimum thyroglobulin requirement may become inadequate under these circumstances.

When the iodine store falls below a critical level, the parenchymal cells of the thyroid undergo first hypertrophy, then hyperplasia. These two processes continue until exhaustion or recovery supervenes. Apparently during the hypertrophy stage, an increased quantity of colloid is formed; this is poor in iodine—hence the term colloid goiter. Upon resaturation of the thyroid with iodine, involution of the parenchymá takes place.

Clinically, the patient with adolescent goiter exhibits a diffusely and symmetrically enlarged thyroid which is so soft in consistency that it is difficult to outline. The extent of the thyroid enlargement is ordinarily not great and signs of increased vascularity are uncommon. A few patients having extreme degrees of thyroid enlargement may complain of pressure symptoms, but constitutional symptoms are rare. In occasional cases there may be evidence of mild hypothyroidism. The basal metabolic rate and the serum protein-bound iodine are usually within normal limits, although both may be slightly depressed.

While iodine will exert a curative, as well as prophylactic, effect in a large percentage of cases, desiccated thyroid in a dosage of 60 to 120 mg. per m^2 daily for a period of 12 to 18 months gives good results more uniformly. The dose needed to bring about involution of a goiter may be a little larger than that ordinarily required for elimination of symptoms of thyroid deficiency in athyrotic patients. Thyroid presumably causes the goiter to shrink by suppressing pituitary thyrotropin production and hence by putting the patient's gland at rest.

If thyroid therapy is begun when the disease is in an early stage, the chances of shrinking the gland to normal size are excellent. If treatment is delayed, and the Marine cycle of hypertrophy, hyperplasia, colloid storage and involution is permitted to advance, thyroid medication may still have the capacity to diminish the over-all size of the goiter. However, shrinkage may be uneven, so that nodules which were buried in the substance of the gland before treatment and were therefore not palpable, may stand out like bas-relief. Not only are these nodules unsightly, but in later life they may begin to overfunction and give rise to thyrotoxicosis. Therefore, there is every advantage in treating the condition while it is in an early stage.

Toward the end of adolescence therapy can be stopped and the patient observed for evidences of exacerbation. Usually these will not be seen.

Thyroiditis. Another cause of thyroid gland failure is chronic thyroiditis—a nonspecific inflammatory process leading to atrophy of functioning thyroid tissue. The Hashimoto type, which is seen occasionally in children, is characterized by a diffuse and intense lymphocytic infiltration of the gland, which becomes enlarged and of granular or nodular consistency. The Delphian lymph node often is palpable just above the isthmus in a paramesial position. Other regional lymph nodes also may be felt. As the lesion in the thyroid gland progresses, symptoms due to pressure on such adjacent structures as the trachea sometimes develop. Tenderness and lack of adherence to neighboring structures as well as evidences of hypothyroidism may help to distinguish thyroiditis from thyroid gland malignancy.[30] However, certification of the diagnosis by biopsy should be undertaken in questionable cases.

Subtotal thyroidectomy (isthmectomy) should be performed if pressure symptoms develop. Thyroid hormone therapy may be given as for adolescent goiter.

REFERENCES

General Reference
MEANS, J. H. *The Thyroid and Its Diseases*. 2d ed. Philadelphia, J. P. Lippincott, 1948.

Specific References

1 (a) DU BOIS, E. F. *Basal Metabolism in Health and Disease*. 3d ed. Philadelphia, Lea & Febiger, 1936.
  (b) HOUSSAY, B. A. The action of the thyroid on diabetes. In *Recent Progress in Hormone Research*. Vol. II. Edited by G. Pincus. New York, Academic Press, 1948.
  (c) WHITE, A. Integration of the effects of adrenal cortical, thyroid and growth hormone in fasting metabolism. In *Recent Progress in Hormone Research*. Vol. IV. Edited by G. Pincus. New York, Academic Press, 1949.

2 TALBOT, N. B. and SOBEL, E. H. Endocrine and other factors determining the growth of children. In *Advances in Pediatrics*. Vol. II. Edited by S. Z. Levine, *et al*. New York, Interscience Publishers, 1947.

3 (a) WINKLER, A. W., LAVIETES, P. H., ROBBINS, C. L. and MAN, E. B. Tolerance to oral thyroid and reaction to intravenous thyroxine in subjects without myxedema. *J. Clin. Invest.* 22:535, 1943.
  (b) RIGGS, D. S., MAN, E. B. and WINKLER, A. W. Serum iodine of euthyroid subjects treated with desiccated thyroid. *J. Clin. Invest.* 24:722, 1945.

4 (a) SEIDELL, A. and FENGER, F. Seasonal variation in the iodine content of the thyroid gland. *J. Biol. Chem.* 13:517, 1912-13.
  (b) CRAMER, W. On the biochemical mechanism of growth. *J. Physiol.* 50:322, 1916.
  (c) WOLF, O. and GREEP, R. O. Histological study of thyroid gland of hypophysectomized rats exposed to cold. *Proc. Soc. Exper. Biol. & Med.* 36:856, 1937.
  (d) DEMPSEY, E. W. and SEARLES, H. F. Environmental modification of certain endocrine phenomena. *Endocrinology* 32:119, 1943.
  (e) LE BLOND, C. P., GROSS, J., PEACOCK, W. and EVANS, R. D. Metabolism of radio-iodine in the thyroids of rats exposed to high or low temperatures. *Am. J. Physiol.* 140:671, 1944.

(f) DEMPSEY, E. W. and ASTWOOD, E. B. Determination of the rate of thyroid hormone excretion at various environmental temperatures. *Endocrinology* 32:509, 1943.

(g) RAND, C. G., RIGGS, D. S. and TALBOT, N. B. The thyroid gland in body homeostasis. (Unpublished observations.)

(h) D'ANGELO, S. A. The effect of acute starvation on the thyrotrophic hormone level in the blood of the rat and mouse. *Endocrinology* 48:341, 1951.

5 (a) TALBOT, F. B., WILSON, E. B. and WORCESTER, J. Standards of basal metabolism of girls (new data) and their use in clinical practice. *J. Pediat.* 7:655, 1935.

(b) TALBOT, N. B., WORCESTER, J. and STEWART, A. New creatinine standard for basal metabolism and its clinical application. *Am. J. Dis. Child.* 58:506, 1939.

(c) TALBOT, N. B. and WORCESTER, J. The basal metabolism of obese children. *J. Pediat.* 16:146, 1940.

6 (a) WILKINS, L., FLEISCHMANN, W. and BLOCK, W. Hypothyroidism in childhood; the basal metabolic rate, serum cholesterol and urinary creatine before treatment. *J. Clin. Endocrinol.* 1:3, 1941.

(b) WILKINS, L., FLEISCHMANN, W. and BLOCK, W. Hypothyroidism in childhood; sensitivity to thyroid medication as measured by the serum cholesterol and the creatine excretion. *J. Clin. Endocrinol.* 1:14, 1941.

(c) WILKINS, L. and FLEISCHMANN, W. Hypothyroidism in childhood; the effect of withdrawal of thyroid therapy upon the serum cholesterol; relationship of cholesterol, basal metabolic rate, weight and clinical symptoms. *J. Clin. Endocrinol.* 1:91, 1941.

7 (a) ESCAMILLA, R. F. Carotinemia in myxedema: explanation of typical slightly icteric tint. *J. Clin. Endocrinol.* 2:33, 1942.

(b) RADWIN, L. S., MICHELSON, J. P., MELNICK, J. and GOTTFRIED, S. Blood lipid partition in hypothyroidism of childhood. *Am. J. Dis. Child.* 60:1120, 1940.

8 TALBOT, N. B., HOEFFEL, G., SHWACHMAN, H. and TUOHY, E. L. Serum phosphatase as an aid in the diagnosis of cretinism and juvenile hypothyroidism. *Am. J. Dis. Child.* 62:273, 1941.

9 (a) ALBRIGHT, F. Changes simulating Legg-Perthes' disease. (osteochondritis deformans juvenilis) due to juvenile myxoedema. *J. Bone & Joint Surg.* 20:764, 1938.

(b) WILKINS, L. Epiphyseal dysgenesis associated with hypothyroidism. *Am. J. Dis. Child.* 61:13, 1941.

10 TODD, T. W., ET AL. *Atlas of Skeletal Maturation.* St. Louis, C. V. Mosby, 1937.

11 PONCHER, H. G., BRONSTEIN, I. P., WADE, H. W. and RICEWASSER, J. C. Creatine metabolism in hypothyroid infants and children. *Am. J. Dis. Child.* 63:270, 1942.

12 (a) KEATING, F. R., JR., POWER, M. H., BERKSON, J. and HAINES, S. F. The urinary excretion of radioiodine in various thyroid states. *J. Clin. Invest.* 26:1138, 1947.

(b) MEANS, J. H. The use of radioactive iodine in the diagnosis and treatment of thyroid diseases. *Bull. New York Acad. Med.* 24:273, 1948.

(c) SKANSE, B. N. Radioactive iodine: its use in studying urinary excretion of iodine by humans in various states of thyroid function. Preliminary report. *Acta med. Scandinav.* 131:251, 1948.

(d) RAWSON, R. W. The use of radioactive iodine in studying the pathologic physiology of thyroid disease. *J. Clin. Invest.* 28: 1330, 1949.

(e) RABEN, M. S. and ASTWOOD, E. B. The use of radioiodine in physiological and clinical studies on the thyroid gland. *J. Clin. Invest.* 28:1347, 1949.

13 (a) RIGGS, D. S., GILDEA, E. F., MAN, E. B. and PETERS, J. P. Blood iodine in patients with thyroid disease. *J. Clin. Invest.* 20:345, 1941.

(b) MAN, E. B., CULOTTA, C. S., SIEGFRIED, D. A. and STILSON, C. Serum precipitable iodines in recognition of cretinism and in control of thyroid medication. *J. Pediat.* 31:154, 1947.

(c) DANOWSKI, T. S., JOHNSTON, S. Y., PRICE, W. C., MC KELVY, M., STEVENSON, S. S. and MC CLUSKEY, E. R. Protein-bound iodine in infants from birth to one year of age. *Pediatrics* 7:240, 1951.

(d) RAPPORT, R. L. and CURTIS, G. M. The clinical significance of the blood iodine. *J. Clin. Endocrinol.* 10:735, 1950.

(e) STARR, P., PETIT, D. W., CHANEY, A. L., ROLLMAN, H., AIKEN, J. B., JAMIESON, B. and KLING, I. Clinical experience with PBI as a routine procedure. *J. Clin. Endocrinol.* 10:1237, 1950.

14 ENGELBACH, W. *Endocrine Medicine.* Vol. I: General Considerations. Springfield, Ill., C. C. Thomas, 1932.

15 (a) TREDGOLD, A. F. *Mental Deficiency (Amentia).* 5th ed. New York, W. Wood, 1929.

(b) GESELL, A., AMATRUDA, C. S. and CULOTTA, C. S. Effect of thyroid therapy on the mental and physical growth of cretinous infants. *Am. J. Dis. Child.* 52:1117, 1936.

(c) BRUCH, H. and MC CUNE, D. J. Mental development of congenitally hypothyroid children; its relationship to physical development and adequacy of treatment. *Am. J. Dis. Child.* 67:205, 1944.

16 PONCHER, H. G. and WOODWARD, H. Pathogenesis and treatment of myotonia congenita. *Am. J. Dis. Child.* 52:1065, 1936.

17 BRONSTEIN, I. P. and BARATZ, J. J. Hypothyroidism and cretinism in childhood; enlargement of the heart with hirsuties (myxedema heart). *Am. J. Dis. Child.* 52:128, 1936.

18 BENDA, C. *Mongolism and Cretinism: A Study of the Clinical Manifestations and the General Pathology of Pituitary and Thyroid Deficiency.* New York, Grune & Stratton, 1946.

19 (a) CASTLEMAN, B. and HERTZ, S. Pituitary fibrosis with myxedema. *Arch. Path.* 27:69, 1939.

(b) LERMAN, J. and STEBBINS, H. D. The pituitary type of myxedema. *J. A. M. A.* 119:391, 1942.

20 (a) BAIRD, F. and NEALE, A. V. A case of exophthalmic goiter. *Arch. Dis. Childhood* 5:229, 1930.

(b) ELLIOT, P. C. Exophthalmic goiter before one year of age. *J. Pediat.* 6:204, 1935.

(c) CRILE, G., JR. and BLANTON, J. L. Exophthalmic goiter in a boy two-and-one-half years of age. *Am. J. Dis. Child.* 53:1039, 1937.

(d) ATKINSON, F. R. B. Exophthalmic goiter in children. *British J. Child. Dis.* 35:165, 1938.

(e) REILLY, W. A. Thyrotoxicosis. *Am. J. Dis. Child.* 60:79, 1940.

(f) KERLEY, C. G. Hyperthyroidism in children. *Am. J. Dis. Child.* 60:452, 1940.

(g) KENNEDY, R. L. J. Results of surgical and medical treatment of exophthalmic goiter of children. *Am. J. Dis. Child.* 60:1002, 1940.

21 MEANS, J. H. Hyperophthalmopathic Graves' disease. *Ann. Int. Med.* 23:779, 1945.

22 (a) RAWSON, R. W. and MC ARTHUR, J. W. What has thiouracil contributed to the management of Graves' disease? *New York State J. Med.* 46:2733, 1946.

(b) BARKER, W. H. and WOOD, W. B., JR. Severe febrile iodism during the treatment of hyperthyroidism. *J. A. M. A.* 114:1029, 1940.

(c) HILLS, S. R., REISS, R. S., FORSHAM, P. H. and THORN, G. W. The effect of adrenocorticotrophin and cortisone on thyroid function: thyroid-adrenocortical interrelationships. *J. Clin. Endocrinol.* 10:1375, 1950.

23 (a) ASTWOOD, E. B. Chemotherapy of hyperthyroidism. In *The Harvey Lectures, 1944-45.* Series 40:195. Lancaster, Science Press, 1945.

(b) BARR, D. P. and SHORR, E. Observations on the treatment of Graves' disease with thiouracil. *Ann. Int. Med.* 23:754, 1945.

(c) MC CULLAGH, E. P., HIBBS, R. E. and SCHNEIDER, R. W. Propyl thiouracil in the treatment of hyperthyroidism. *Am. J. M. Sc.* 214:545, 1947.

(d) WHITELAW, M. J. Thiouracil in the treatment of hyperthyroidism complicating pregnancy and its effect on human fetal thyroid. *J. Clin. Endocrinol.* 7:767, 1947.

(e) JACKSON, A. S. and HALEY, H. B. Exophthalmic goiter in children: Treatment with propylthiouracil. *Am. J. M. Sc.* 218:493, 1949.

(f) WILLIAMS, L. P. and JANNEY, F. F. Thiouracil in childhood hyperthyroidism. *J. Pediat.* 30:370, 1947.

(g) KUNSTADTER, R. H. and STEIN, A. F. Treatment of thyrotoxicosis in children with thiouric derivatives. *Pediatrics* 6:244, 1950.

24 (a) CHAPMAN, E., SKANSE, B. N. and EVANS, R. D. Treatment of hyperthyroidism with radioactive iodine. *Radiology* 51:558, 1948.

(b) SOLEY, M. H. and FOREMAN, N. Radioiodine therapy in Graves' disease. *J. Clin. Invest.* 28:1367, 1949.

25 MOORE, F. D. Toxic manifestations of thiouracil therapy. *J. A. M. A.* 130:315, 1946.

26 (a) MOORE, F. D., SWEENEY, D. N., COPE, O., RAWSON, R. W. and MEANS, J. H. The use of thiouracil in the preparation of patients with hyperthyroidism for thyroidectomy. *Ann. Surg.* 120:152, 1944.

(b) RAWSON, R. W., MOORE, F. D., PEACOCK, W., MEANS, J. H., COPE, O. and RIDDELL, C.B. Effect of iodine on the thyroid gland in Graves' disease when given in conjunction with thiouracil—a two-action theory of iodine. *J. Clin. Invest.* 24:869, 1945.

27 DRILL, V. A. Interrelations between thyroid function and vitamin metabolism. *Physiol. Rev.* 23:355, 1943.

28 (a) CROTTI, A. *Thyroid and Thymus.* Philadelphia, Lea & Febiger, 1922.

(b) PARMALEE, A. H., ALLEN, E., STEIN, I. F. and BUXBAUM, H. Three cases of congenital goiter. *Am. J. Obst. & Gynec.* 40:145, 1940.

(c) WHEELER, R. S. and HOFFMAN, E. Influence of quantitative thyroprotein treatment of hens on length of incubation period and thyroid size of chicks. *Endocrinology* 43:430, 1948.

29 GREER, M. A. and ASTWOOD, E. B. The antithyroid effect of certain foods in man as determined with radioactive iodine. *Endocrinology* 43:105, 1948.

30 HARE, H. F. Cancer of the thyroid in children. *Radiology* 28:131, 1937.

THE PARATHYROIDS

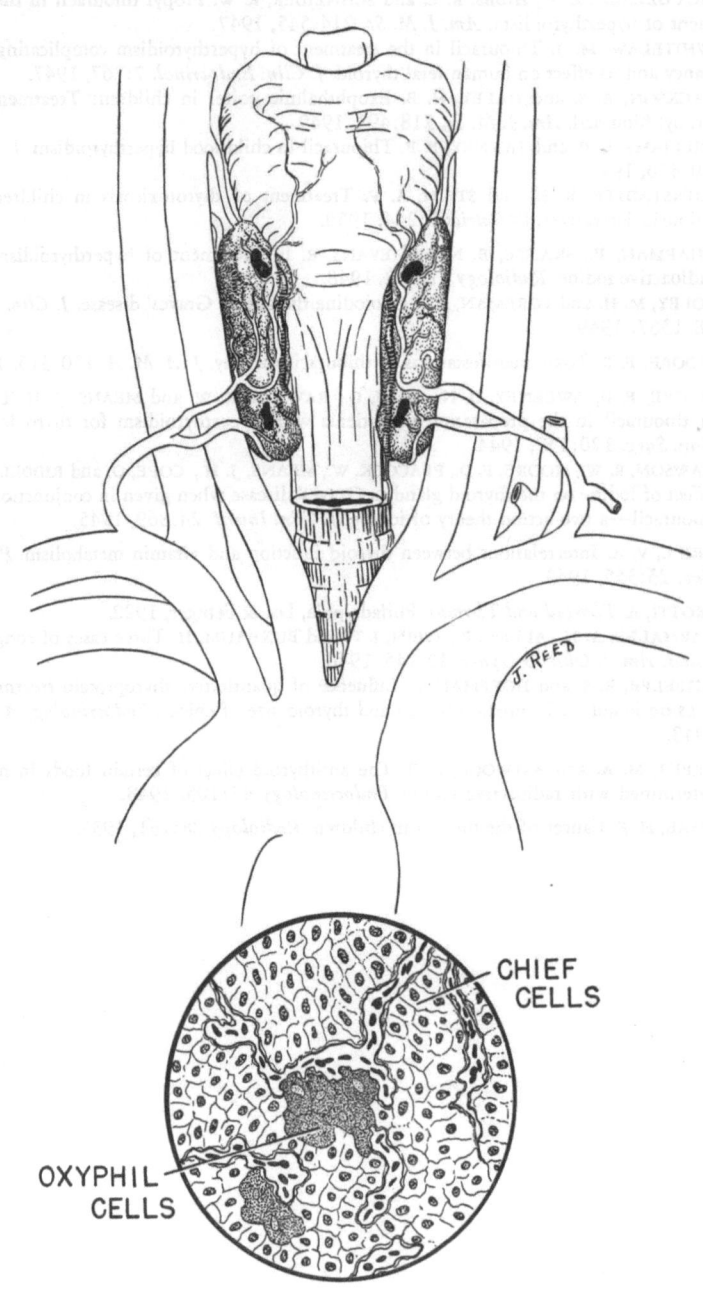

CHIEF CELLS

OXYPHIL CELLS

CHAPTER II

THE PARATHYROIDS

BASIC CONSIDERATIONS

THE HORMONE AND ITS SITES OF ACTION[1-4]

The parathyroid glands produce a protein or protein-linked hormone which exerts a major influence on calcium and phosphorus metabolism. Though their active principle has been extracted in crude form, it has not been isolated or identified in any detail. As a protein, the hormone is destroyed by pepsin digestion. Inactivation by ketene acetylation indicates that free amino groups are necessary for physiologic activity. Studies with the ultracentrifuge suggest the presence of two molecular species, one with a molecular weight of approximately 20,000; the other, a much larger particle, with a molecular weight in the neighborhood of 500,000.[5]

The possibility that there may be two distinct parathyroid hormones is suggested by chemical as well as histologic and physiologic evidence. Three morphologically distinct cell types are represented in the normal parathyroid gland: chief, clear and oxyphil cells,[6a] the numerical distribution of which normally undergoes considerable change with advancing age. Marked secondary alterations are found in patients with diseases involving derangements in calcium and phosphorus metabolism.[6b]

Histologic studies show that clear cells become predominant in the hyperplastic glands of patients suffering from base-losing nephritis and rickets due to vitamin D lack. Chief cells, on the other hand, become the predominant type in the hyperplastic glands of patients suffering phosphorus retention as a result of renal glomerular disease and in the glands of experimental animals subjected to high phosphorus feeding. The significance of these cytologic alterations is poorly understood and needs further investigation.

Physiologic information is supplied by studies of the effects of parathyroid extracts upon the kidneys and skeleton. Generally speaking, these extracts prompt an increase in urinary phosphorus excretion, a decrease in urinary calcium excretion and a release of calcium and phosphorus from bone. The action upon the kidney has been shown to be independent of changes in the calcium and phosphorus content of the blood perfusing it.[7a, b] The action upon bone has been shown to continue following removal of the kidneys.[7 c-f]

PHYSIOLOGY OF THE PARATHYROID ENDOCRINE SYSTEM

Introductory Comments on Renal Excretory Mechanisms.[8] Consideration of the renal effects of parathyroid hormone may be aided by a brief preliminary review of certain renal excretory phenomena.

Glomerular filtration of calcium and phosphorus. The renal glomeruli filter in an almost mechanical manner a portion of the blood plasma which runs through their vascular channels. This filtrate is nearly protein free, but does contain electrolytes having concentrations equal to the respective concentrations of the same electrolytes in the circulating blood plasma (or serum). Thus, inorganic phosphorus appears in glomerular fluid at a concentration approximately equal to that measured in serum. Since about 50 per cent of the calcium in the serum is non-ionized and bound to protein molecules too large to pass the glomerular filter, only the ionized fraction appears in glomerular fluid. The diffusible portion of serum calcium can be estimated roughly on the basis of total serum calcium and protein concentrations with the aid of the nomogram of McLean and Hastings (Figure 1). This derivative may be used under ordinary circumstances to estimate the calcium concentration of glomerular fluid. Biologic assay methods must be used to determine accurately the concentration of ionized calcium in blood under unusual experimental circumstances.

Having arrived at an estimate of the concentrations of phosphorus and calcium in the glomerular fluid, the amounts of these substances filtered over a given period of time may be found by multiplying the concentration in glomerular fluid by the glomerular filtration rate. Glomerular filtration rate can be determined by inulin or other suitable clearance measurements. In most normal individuals the values found are essentially constant at about 100,000 cc. per m^2 per 24 hours. Thus, for a normal adult of 70 kg. (1.7 m^2) with a serum phosphorus of 4.0 mg. per cent (0.04 mg/cc.), phosphorus filtered at the glomerulus will be 6,800 mg. per day (1.7 m^2 x 100,000 cc. x 0.04 mg.). Figure 1 shows that when calcium is present in serum at a concentration of 10 mg. per cent, with a total protein of 6.5 gm. per cent, 46 per cent of the serum calcium is ionized. This ionized portion is filterable and yields a glomerular fluid concentration of

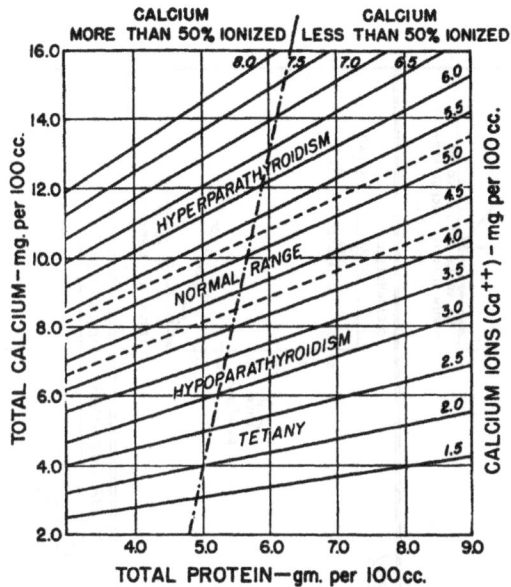

FIGURE II—1. Nomogram for the derivation of serum "ionized" calcium concentration from total calcium and total protein concentrations. The left-hand ordinate gives values for total calcium concentration; the abscissa, values for total protein concentration. Ionized calcium concentration is found by locating the intersection between a horizontal line drawn from the left-hand ordinate and a vertical line drawn from the abscissa. The position of the intercept is then extended by drawing a line to the right-hand ordinate parallel to the nearest of the slanted lines running from the lower left to the upper right-hand portion of the figure. Note that at any given total calcium concentration, ionized calcium varies inversely with total protein concentration. From F. C. McLean and A. B. Hastings, *Am. J. M. Sc.* 189:601, 1935.

4.6 mg. per cent. Hence, in the normal adult approximately 7,800 mg. of calcium ($1.7 \text{ m}^2 \times 100{,}000 \text{ cc.} \times 0.046 \text{ mg.}$) pass the glomerular filter in the course of 24 hours.

Such calculations of the amounts of calcium and phosphorus appearing in glomerular fluid yield figures which represent maximum quantities of these substances available for excretion in urine, for there is no convincing evidence that the glomerular filtrates of either calcium or phosphorus are normally augmented by contributions from the renal tubules. The usual quantities of calcium and phosphorus appearing in urine, while quite variable, are far below the maximal quantities indicated above. It follows that portions of the quantities filtered at the renal glomerulus are subsequently reabsorbed by the renal tubules.

Continued on page 60

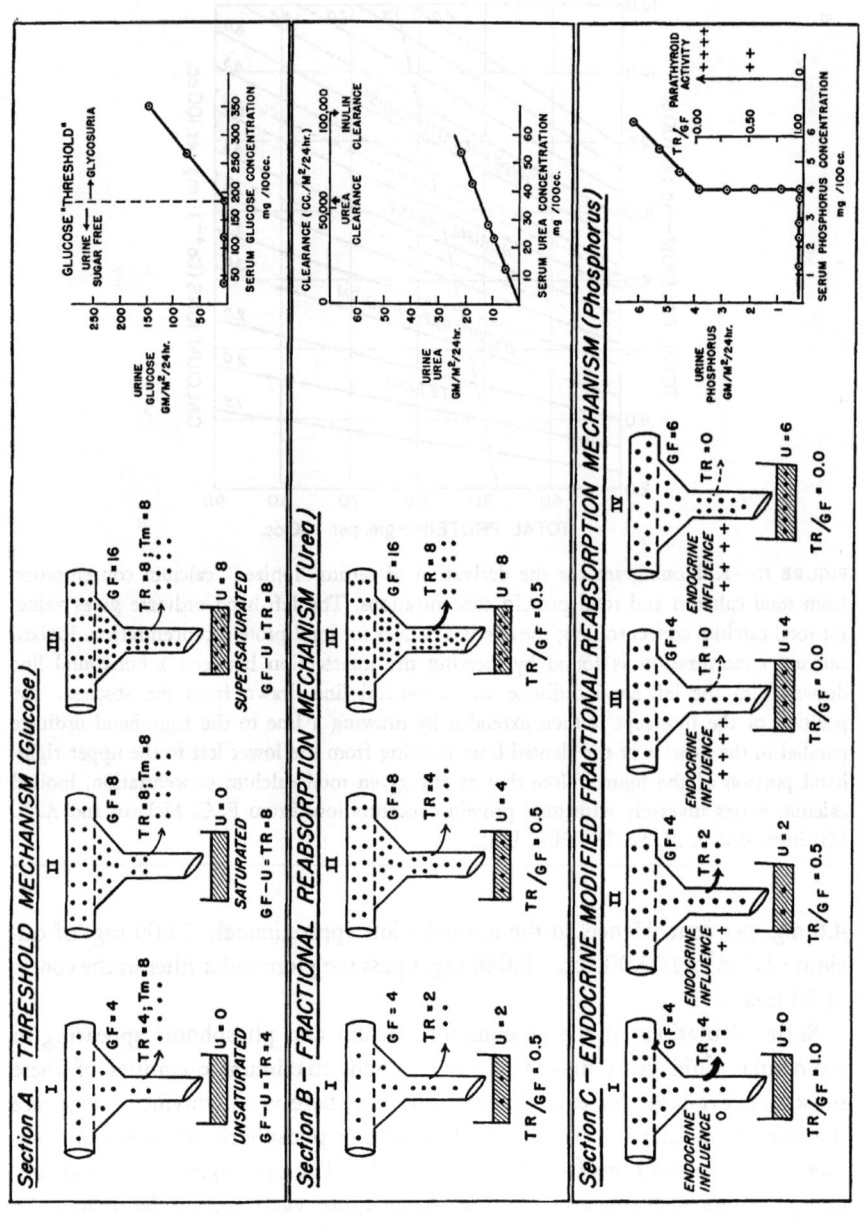

FIGURE II—2. Simplified diagrams of renal tubule reabsorption mechanisms and of the influence of endocrine factors upon them. The left-hand group of schematic diagrams are constructed to show a blood vessel from which material (black dots) escapes into a glomerular filter (funnel). The material then passes down the renal tubule (funnel stem) from which variable amounts are reabsorbed. The residue (urine) passes down into a vessel at the bottom of the system. The number of dots in the various parts of the system represents the concentration or quantity of the substance in question. The abbreviations used have the following meanings: GF=Glomerular filtrate; TR=Tubular reabsorbate; Tm=Tubular maximal reabsorptive capacity; U=Urine content; TS=Tubular secretion.

In the schematic diagrams units or quantities of material have been indicated by arbitrarily chosen small numbers. The graphs at the right of the schematic diagrams represent certain of the relations shown in the diagrams. However, the values assigned to the coordinates of these graphs are in keeping with quantitative clinical measurements.

SECTION A: *Threshold Mechanism*. The schematic diagrams illustrate the effect of changing serum glucose concentration on the glomerular filtration, tubular reabsorption and urinary excretion of glucose. Note that the urine is sugar free until the amount of filtered glucose exceeds glucose Tm ("threshold"). At higher serum glucose concentrations urine glucose content increases in proportion to the increase in serum glucose concentration. The graph at the right indicates that the serum glucose concentration equivalent of Tm is approximately 180 mg. per cent.

SECTION B: *Fractional Reabsorption Mechanism*. The schematic diagrams show the effect of changing serum urea concentration on the glomerular filtration, tubular reabsorption and urinary excretion of urea. Note that, in this instance, tubular reabsorption removes a constant fraction of filtered urea (TR/GF=approximately 0.5). There is no maximal tubular reabsorptive capacity. The urine contains urea at both high and low serum urea concentrations, the amount being a constant fraction of the quantity filtered. The graph at the right indicates the direct relationship between serum urea concentration and urinary urea excretion. At the top of the graph the horizontal scale shows the relation of urea clearance to inulin clearance or glomerular filtration rate. Note that approximately half the urea in 100,000 cc. of glomerular filtrate is "cleared" and appears in the urine (U/GF=approximately 0.5).

SECTION C: *Endocrine Modified Fractional Reabsorption Mechanism*. In this section the effect of an endocrine influence (parathyroid hormone) on the renal excretion of phosphorus is shown. Note that in instances I, II and III a constant serum phosphorus concentration is indicated. The effect of increasing endocrine influence is reduction of the fraction of filtered phosphorus reabsorbed by the tubules (TR/GF=1). When the endocrine influence is absent (instance I), essentially all the filtered phosphorus is reabsorbed (TR/GF=1). Moderate endocrine influence results in reabsorption of half the filtered phosphorus (TR/GF=0.5), and maximal endocrine influence reduces the amount of phosphorus reabsorbed relative to the amount of phosphorus filtered essentially to zero (TR/GF=0). Thus increasing endocrine activity provides for urinary excretion of increasing amounts of phosphorus without change in serum phosphorus concentration. On the other hand, it is evident by comparison of instances III and IV that at a constant level of endocrine influence urine phosphorus excretion varies in direct proportion to serum phosphorus concentration (compare mechanism of Section B). The graph

FIGURE II—2 (continued)

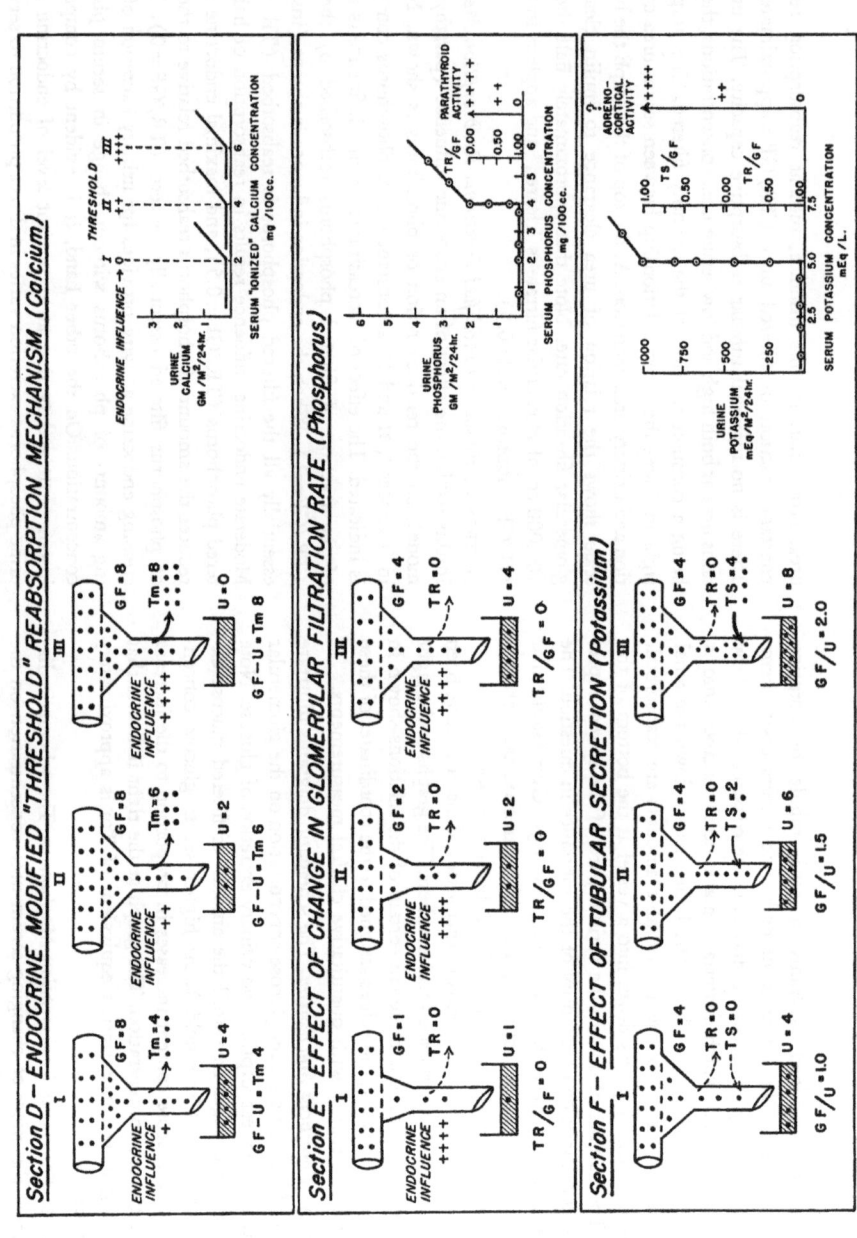

illustrates these relations again. The homeostatic responsibility of the parathyroid gland appears to be the maintenance of constancy of serum phosphorus concentration. Hence, endocrine influence is indicated as absent at serum phosphorus concentrations below average normal values. When serum phosphorus concentration rises to the average normal value of 4 mg. per cent, endocrine influence is shown to increase in proportion to needs for phosphorus elimination. This permits urine phosphorus excretion to rise from negligible quantities to 4 gm. per m² per 24 hours without a change in serum phosphorus concentration. The range through which urine phosphorus excretion varies as a result of changes in parathyroid influence is seen to be limited at the upper end of the scale by the rate of glomerular filtration (see also Section E). At this point endocrine influence can effect no further increase in urinary phosphorus excretion. Renal phosphorus excretion, however, may increase if filtration of phosphorus is augmented by an elevation of serum phosphorus concentration. Such increases in urinary phosphorus excretion will be proportional to increases in serum phosphorus concentration (see Section B).

SECTION D: *Endocrine Modified "Threshold" Reabsorption Mechanism.* In contrast to its inhibitory effect on tubular phosphorus reabsorption, increasing parathyroid influence acts to augment tubular calcium reabsorption. Furthermore, renal excretion of calcium at a constant level of endocrine influence depends upon filtration of sufficient calcium to surpass the maximal reabsorptive capacity of the tubules (see "Threshold" mechanism, Section A). When the amount of calcium is less than Tm, the urine is nearly calcium free. When the amount exceeds Tm, the excess calcium spills quantitatively into the urine. In the three instances shown by the schematic diagrams, serum-filterable or ionized calcium concentration is shown constant. In all instances sufficient glomerular filtrate calcium is indicated to saturate the tubular reabsorptive capacity. In instance I the tubular reabsorptive capacity is low as a result of minimal endocrine influence. Filtered calcium markedly exceeds the reabsorptive capacity of the tubules and large quantities spill into the urine. In instance II endocrine influence has increased the tubular reabsorptive capacity, and a smaller quantity of calcium appears in the urine. In instance III, where endocrine influence has caused an increase in tubular reabsorptive capacity sufficient to permit total reabsorption of the filtered calcium, there is no spill over into the urine. These relations are illustrated again in the graph at the right of the schematic diagrams. Here the effect of the endocrine influence on the serum calcium equivalent of Tm or threshold is to be contrasted with the graph of similar relations for glucose in Section A.

SECTION E: *Effect of Change in Glomerular Filtration Rate.* This section shows the effect of changes in glomerular filtration rate on the upper limit of urinary excretion of phosphorus at a constant, normal serum phosphorus concentration. Note that endocrine influence is represented as maximal in all the instances illustrated by the schematic diagrams. Under these circumstances urinary phosphorus excretion is directly dependent upon the rate of glomerular phosphorus filtration. In the graph at the right glomerular filtration rate is shown as half that indicated in Section C. Note that in comparison with the graph in Section C the range through which urine phosphorus excretion may vary without change in serum phosphorus concentration is reduced by 50 per cent. Except for this difference, the graphs of Sections C and E are nearly identical.

SECTION F: *Effect of Tubular Secretion.* The three schematic diagrams illustrate the way in which urinary excretion of a substance like potassium may be increased by tubular secretion. Such a mechanism augments the range of urinary excretion without change in serum concentration provided by the variable tubular reabsorption mechanism shown in Section C. The range is indicated in the graph at the right.

Values representing quantities absorbed by the tubules are found by subtracting amounts appearing in the urine from amounts filtered.

Tubular reabsorption mechanisms. Several different mechanisms of tubular reabsorption have been described. These are reviewed briefly in the following sections with the aid of Figure 2.

"Threshold" reabsorption (Figure 2, Section A). The most familiar mechanism is that which pertains to the reabsorption of glucose. In this instance the tubular cells appear to have a certain maximal capacity for reabsorption. When this maximal capacity, or threshold, is exceeded, excess filtered glucose appears quantitatively in the urine. The tubular maximum, frequently abbreviated Tm, is found by elevating serum glucose concentration until glucose begins to spill in the urine. The difference between glucose filtered at the glomerulus and glucose appearing in the urine then yields a nearly constant value, which represents the maximal capacity of the tubules for glucose reabsorption or glucose Tm.

"Fractional" reabsorption (Figure 2, Section B). A second familiar reabsorption mechanism, termed here "fractional" reabsorption to distinguish it from the threshold type, is that by which urea is reabsorbed. With respect to urea the tubular cells show no maximal capacity for reabsorption. Instead they reabsorb an essentially constant fraction of the urea presented them by glomerular filtration. In the normal adult this fraction relating urea reabsorbed by the tubules to urea filtered at the glomerulus (expressed in abbreviated form, TR urea/GF urea) has an average numerical value of approximately 0.56. Because urea is eliminated by this mechanism, appreciable quantities are always contained in the urine, the amount varying directly with serum urea concentration.

Fractional reabsorption of urea fails to provide for constancy of serum urea concentration in the face of a variable intake or load. In the case of this relatively inert substance, a variable blood concentration is apparently unimportant to the body. On the other hand, constancy in the concentrations of the various serum electrolytes appears to be of vital importance. If this is to be achieved by either threshold or fractional reabsorption, the threshold quantity or the fraction of the electrolyte which is reabsorbed from the glomerular filtrate must undergo certain homeostatic variations.

Endocrine-influenced fractional reabsorption (Figure 2, Section C). Here are shown diagrammatically the effects of endocrine-influenced alterations in fractional reabsorption of a substance appearing in glomerular filtrate. Serum concentration, glomerular filtration rate and hence glomerular filtrate content are represented as constant in the four hypothetical situations. In the first situation the endocrine influence is minimal and tubular reabsorption is equal to the filtration rate of the substance in question. The value for the fraction relating

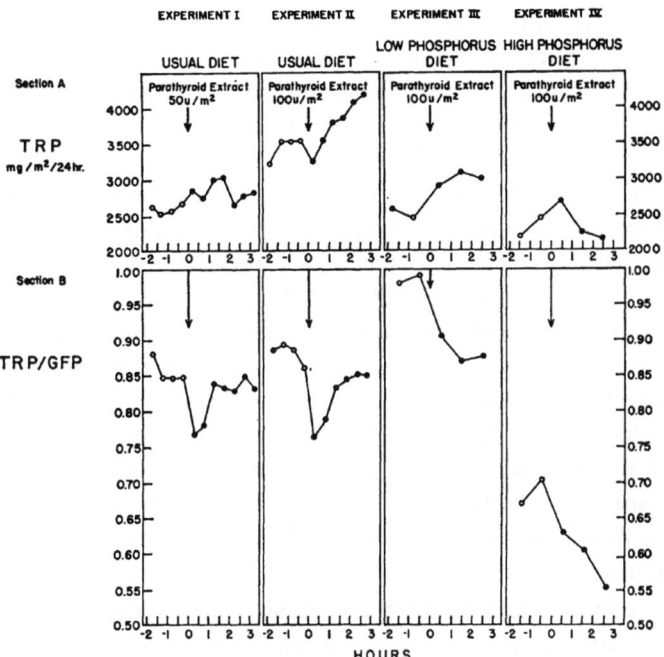

FIGURE II—3. Effect of parathyroid extract on the absolute value for tubular phosphorus reabsorption (TRP, Section A) and on the ratio between TRP and glomerular filtrate phosphorus (TRP/GFP, Section B). The abscissa gives time in hours in both sections. Note that while parathyroid extract causes irregular behavior of the value for TRP, it regularly causes a depression of the ratio TRP/GFP. This depression in the ratio value is seen both when control values are high (Experiment III) and when they are low (Experiment IV). From J. D. Crawford, M. M. Osborne, N. B. Talbot and M. L. Terry, *J. Clin. Investigation* 29:1448, 1950.

---

tubular reabsorption to glomerular filtration in this instance is 1.0 (TR/GF=1). Consequently, the filtered material is absent from the urine. In the second instance, where reabsorption has been partially inhibited by a moderate concentration of endocrine secretion, only half the filtered material is reabsorbed (TR/GF=0.5). Under this circumstance the urine contains appreciable quantities of the substance in question (half the amount filtered) with no change in serum concentration. In the third instance endocrine inhibition of tubular reabsorption is maximal and all the filtered material is rejected by the tubules (TR/GF=0). Now the urine contains the maximum quantity of the hypothetical substance possible under conditions of constant serum concentration and glomerular filtration rate (i.e., the entire amount in the glomerular filtrate). A further increase in urine excretion is possible only if either or both the serum concentration and the glomerular filtration rate are increased. The effect of elevating serum concentration is shown in the last instance of Section C. The effects of changes in glomerular filtration are shown in Section E.

Endocrine-influenced "threshold" reabsorption (Figure 2, Section D). The way in which constancy of serum concentration of a filterable substance might be achieved by endocrine-influenced reabsorption of the threshold type is shown by this portion of the diagram. In the first instance, where the endocrine influence is depicted as minimal, the quantity that the tubules can reabsorb is shown to be low. Under this circumstance there is a tendency for urine output to be large. Unless a correspondingly large amount of the substance is entering the blood stream from the alimentary tract or elsewhere, there will be a tendency for serum concentration to fall. Alternatively, a stable serum concentration might be effected if the endocrine influence were increased. This would result in an augmented capacity of the tubules to reabsorb the material (increased values for Tm) with diminution in the rate of renal loss. The effects of a rising threshold are illustrated by instances II and III in Section D.

The Parathyroids and Phosphorus Metabolism. Available evidence indicates that the parathyroid glands provide the major endocrine influence governing phosphorus reabsorption by the renal tubules. As will be shown below, parathyroid hormone exerts this influence by determining what portion of glomerular filtrate phosphorus shall be reabsorbed by the renal tubules (endocrine modification of fractional reabsorption, Figure 2, Section C).

Effect of parathyroid hormone on renal phosphorus excretion. When parathyroid activity is minimal (as after parathyroidectomy), essentially all of the phosphorus filtered at the glomerulus is reabsorbed by the tubules (TRP/GFP* $=1.0$).[9a] When parathyroid activity is increased, as by parathyroid extract administration,† the TRP/GFP ratio consistently falls (Figure 3). When parathyroid activity is maximal, tubular phosphorus reabsorption is completely inhibited and phosphorus appearing in urine is equal to that filtered at the glomeruli (TRP/GFP$=0.0$). These relations seem to hold regardless of relatively large changes in serum phosphorus concentration and in absolute values for filtered and reabsorbed phosphorus.

* TRP$=$absolute value for phosphorus reabsorbed by the renal tubules; GFP$=$absolute value for glomerular filtrate phosphorus.

† Administration of parathyroid extract fails to lower the TRP/GFP ratio when endogenous parathyroid hormone influence on the kidneys is already maximal. For example, in intact subjects fed very high phosphorus diets, the ratio may be found to have a value of zero (see Figure 6). Introduction of exogenous hormone under these circumstances can produce no further lowering of the TRP/GFP ratio. Increased urinary phosphorus excretion can occur, however, if serum phosphorus concentration is elevated (see Figure 2, Section C).

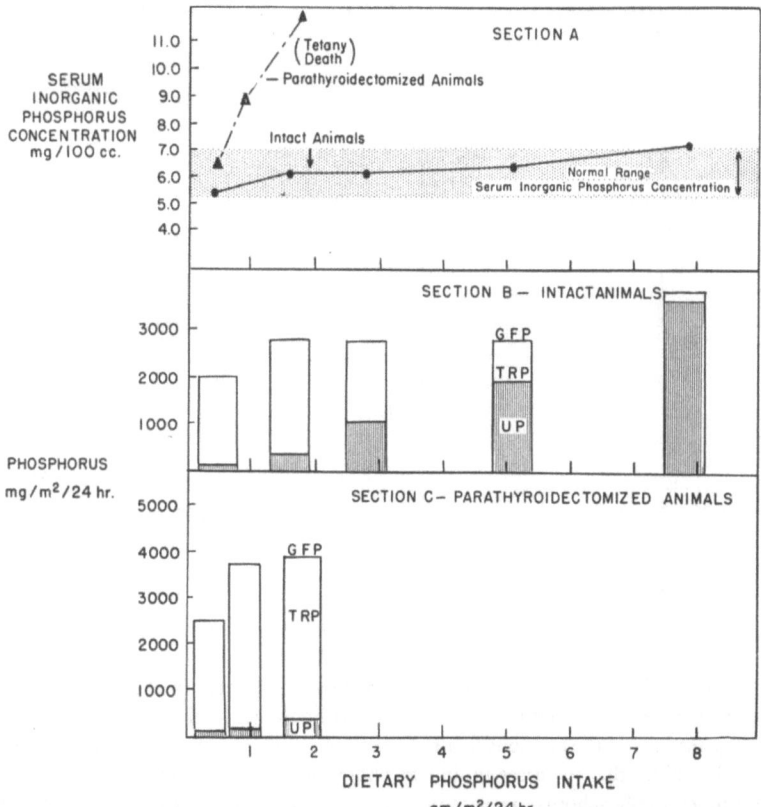

FIGURE II—4. The influence of changes in dietary phosphorus intake on intact and parathyroidectomized rats. Dietary phosphorus intake expressed as gm. per m² per day is shown on the abscissa. The ordinate of Section A gives plasma phosphorus concentration. The ordinates of Sections B and C give values in terms of mg. of phosphorus per m² per day corresponding to the heights of the vertical columns; the total height of each column indicates the value for glomerular filtrate phosphorus (GFP); the shaded portion, phosphorus excreted in the urine (UP), while the unshaded portion of the column represents phosphorus reabsorbed by the renal tubules (TRP). Note that, as dietary phosphorus intake is increased, the intact rats show minor changes in serum phosphorus concentration (Section A) and increases in urinary phosphorus excretion proportional to the increases in dietary phosphorus intake (Section B). By contrast, increases in dietary phosphorus intake cause marked hyperphosphatemia in the parathyroidectomized animals (Section A). However, their urinary phosphorus excretion (Section C) is similar to that of intact rats (Section B) on a given phosphorus intake. Increases in phosphorus excretion are dependent upon decreases in renal tubular phosphorus reabsorption in the intact animals (Section B) and to increases in phosphorus filtered at the glomerulus in the operated animals (Section C). From J. D. Crawford, M. M. Osborne, N. B. Talbot and M. L. Terry, *J. Clin. Investigation* 29:1448, 1950.

[64]   CHAPTER II:

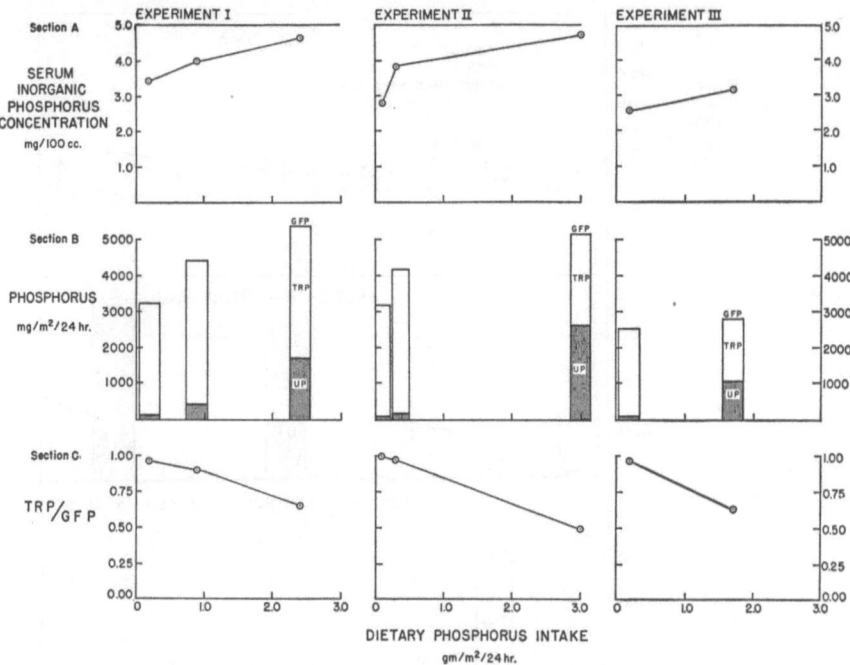

FIGURE II—5. The influence of changes in dietary phosphorus intake on normal human subjects. The designs of Sections A and B of this figure are similar to those of the corresponding sections of the previous figure. In Section C the ordinate gives values for the ratio TRP/GFP. Note that increases in dietary phosphorus intake prompt relatively small increases in serum phosphorus concentration (Section A), marked rises in urinary phosphorus excretion (Section B) and a decrease in value for the ratio TRP/GFP (Section C). From J. D. Crawford, M. M. Osborne, N. B. Talbot and M. L. Terry, *J. Clin. Investigation* 29: 1448, 1950.

It appears then that the value for the ratio may be used as an inverse index of parathyroid gland activity: high values for TRP/GFP indicate diminished parathyroid activity, low values indicate high degrees of gland activity.

The parathyroids and phosphorus homeostasis. The following phenomena are observed when *normal animals or humans* are given diets containing varying amounts of phosphorus (Figures 4 and 5):

1. Serum phosphorus concentration remains within the rather narrow limits of normal but varies within that range in the same direction as dietary phosphorus intake* (Figures 4 and 5, Section A).

* No reduction in either total or ionized calcium concentration results from high phosphorus diets when adequate calcium intake is maintained (see Table 1).

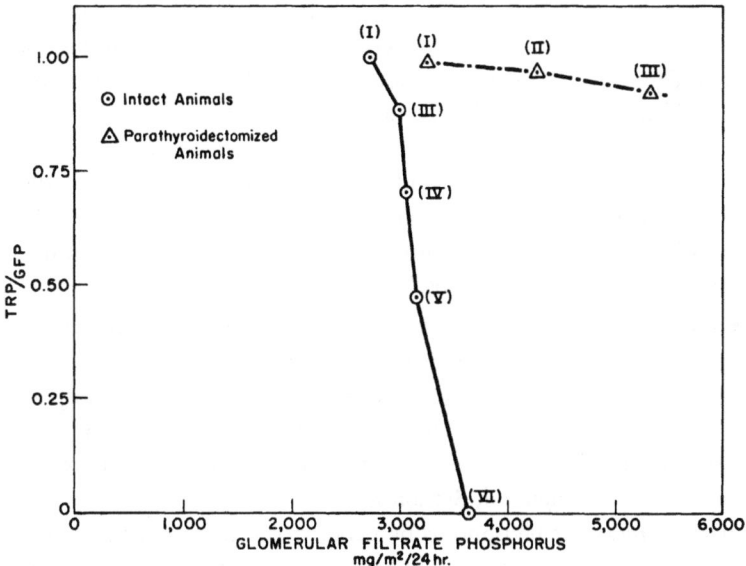

FIGURE II—6. Relations between GFP and the ratio TRP/GFP. The meaning of the abbreviations, TRP and GFP is given in the legend to Figure 3. The points enclosed in open circles represent observations on the intact rats while those enclosed in triangles represent observations on the parathyroidectomized animals of Figure 4. The roman numerals refer to the dietary regimen. Roman numeral I denotes a diet containing a minimal quantity of phosphorus (< 0.5 gm. per m^2 per day). The roman numerals of higher value refer to diets of progressively greater phosphorus content (II=1.0, III=2.0, IV=3.0, V=5.0 and VI=8 gm. per m^2 per day). Note in the data representing the intact animals that, while the value for GFP remains nearly constant, the ratio TRP/GFP falls rapidly from a value close to 1.0 to a value of zero. The data of the parathyroidectomized animals, by contrast, show little fall in the TRP/GFP value as marked increases in GFP occur. A high TRP/GFP value is characteristic of both pathologic and physiologic hypoparathyroidism; the value of this ratio falls as parathyroid hormone activity increases. From J. D. Crawford, M. M. Osborne, N. B. Talbot and M. L. Terry, *J. Clin. Investigation* 29:1448, 1950.

2. Urinary phosphorus excretion is roughly proportional to dietary phosphorus intake. On diets low in phosphorus there is marked reduction of urinary phosphorus. Phosphaturia proportional to the dietary phosphorus content is observed as intake is increased (Figures 4 and 5, Section B).
3. The increase in urinary phosphorus excretion prompted by increased dietary phosphorus intake is accomplished by adjusting the amount of phosphorus reabsorbed by the tubules in relation to that filtered at the glomeruli (TRP/

GFP) (Figure 2, Section C). The ratio TRP/GFP is found to have values approaching unity in subjects given diets providing minimal quantities of phosphorus. The ratio falls to very low values or zero when diets high in phosphorus are provided (Figures 4 and 5, Section C; Figure 6).

4. Parathyroid gland size bears a direct relation to the amount of phosphorus in the diet (Figure 7).[9] Assay of parathyroid hormone concentration in the blood of animals fed high phosphorus diets reveals considerable activity. Little or no parathyroid activity is demonstrable in blood samples taken from animals fed diets restricted in phosphorus.[9 b]

If similar phosphorus-loading experiments are performed on *animals after parathyroidectomy*, certain differences in response become evident.

1. Serum phosphorus concentration rises sharply when dietary phosphorus intake is but slightly increased. The moderate-to-high phosphorus intake which is well tolerated by normal animals results in marked hyperphosphatemia, tetany and death (Figure 4, Section A).
2. Urinary excretion of phosphorus by parathyroidectomized animals is quantitatively equal to that of normal animals on diets of comparable phosphorus content, although a period of several days is required for the parathyroidectomized animal to attain phosphorus equilibrium after an increase in dietary phosphorus intake. Increases in phosphorus excretion in response to increases in dietary phosphorus intake are accomplished by elevating serum and hence glomerular filtrate phosphorus concentration. The value for the TRP/GFP remains essentially constant (see Figure 2, Section B; Figure 6).
3. As in intact individuals, parathyroid extract administration regularly results in a prompt fall in the value of the ratio, TRP/GFP, and in an increase in urinary excretion of phosphorus (Figure 24).

These findings are interpreted to mean that the parathyroid glands normally respond to a rise in serum phosphorus concentration by increased hormone elaboration. Conversely, they respond by diminishing hormone production when serum phosphorus concentration falls. Thus, a state of physiologic hyperparathyroidism develops when phosphorus intake is increased; physiologic hypoparathyroidism develops when phosphorus intake is reduced. Variations in hormone production act at the kidney tubule to cause variations in phosphorus excretion proportional to the changes in intake. These adaptive changes in parathyroid activity have the apparent purpose of maintaining serum phosphorus concentration within narrow physiologic limits. The constancy of serum phosphorus concentration, despite considerable day-to-day variation in phosphorus intake, is evidence of the dynamic, homeostatic role played by the parathyroid glands in the healthy individual.

Continued on page 70

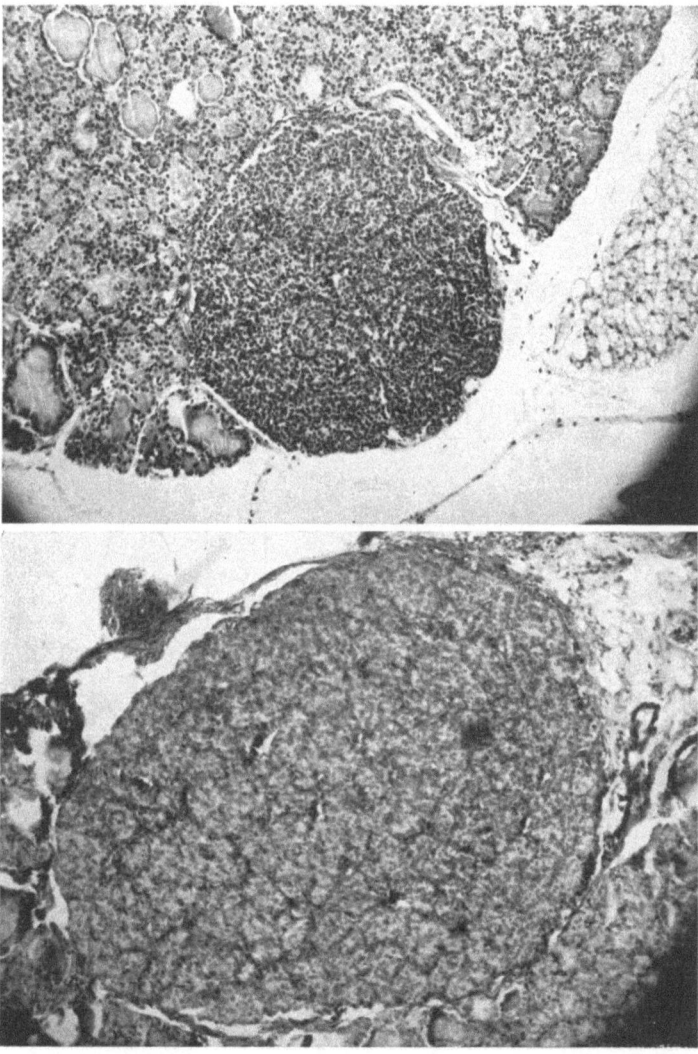

FIGURE II—7. Effect of dietary phosphorus intake on the size of the parathyroid glands. The photograph at the top shows an equatorial section from the gland of a rat receiving 0.5 gm. per m^2 per day of phosphorus in the diet. The serum phosphorus concentration was 5.5 mg. per cent at the time of removal. The photograph at the bottom shows a similar section from the gland of a rat receiving 6 gm. per m^2 per day of phosphorus in the diet. Serum phosphorus concentration was 6.9 mg. per cent. Note the larger total size of the gland of the animal receiving the higher phosphorus intake. Measurements indicate an increase both in size of individual cells and in the total number of cells in the gland. Magnification x 150. From J. D. Crawford, M. M. Osborne and N. B. Talbot. Unpublished observations.

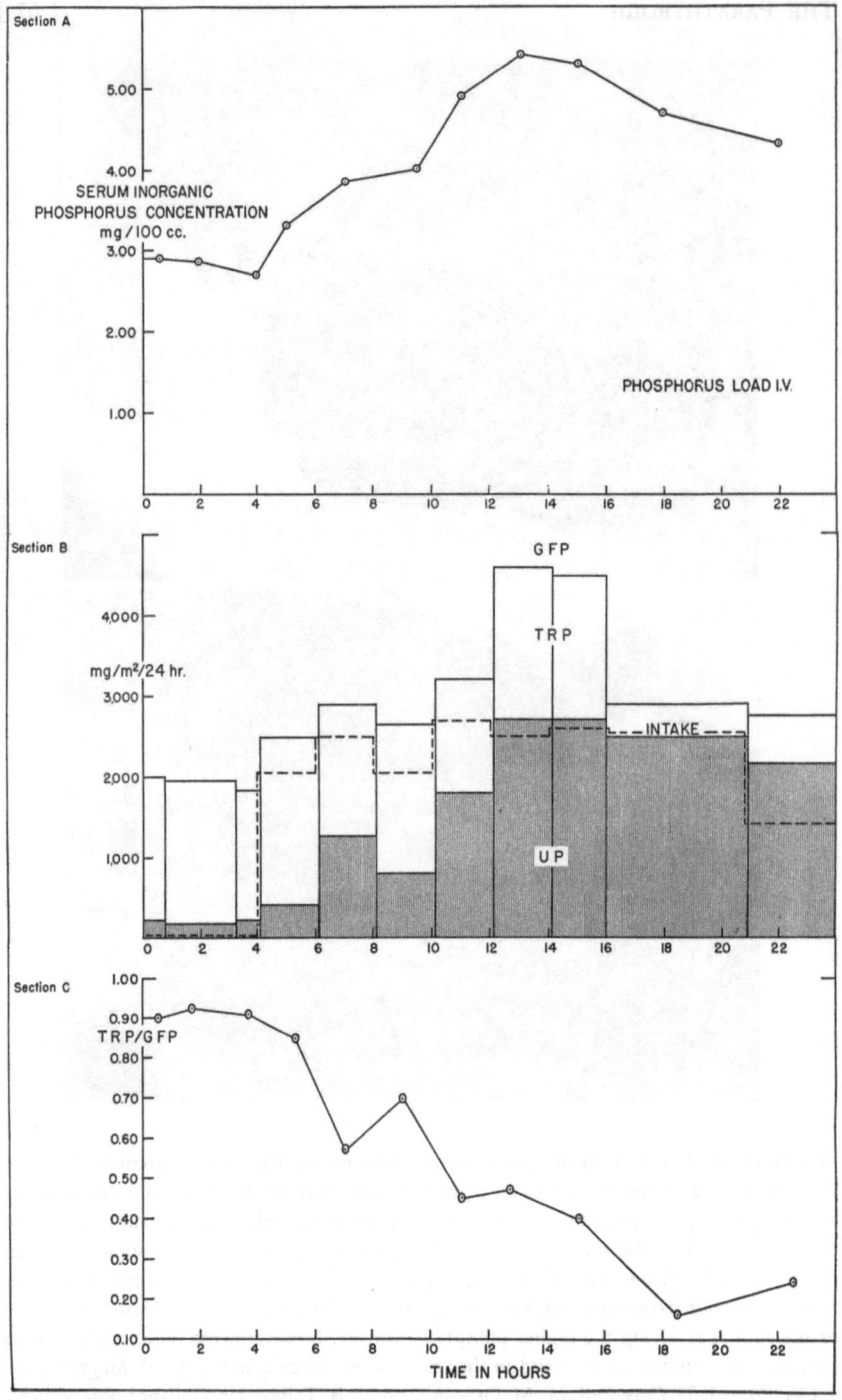

FIGURE II—8. The rapidity of parathyroid adaptative response to phosphorus loading. The design of this figure is similar to that of Figure 5. The subject of the experiment was a normal individual whose phosphorus intake was abruptly increased from a low to a high level.

SECTION A: Note that serum phosphorus concentration rises quite sharply when the phosphorus load is first imposed. A peak is reached within 8 to 12 hours, and thereafter serum phosphorus concentration begins to fall toward the control levels.

SECTION B: It is seen that urine phosphorus initially rises in rough proportion to the rise in serum phosphorus concentration. Thereafter a dissociation between serum concentration and renal excretion of phosphorus becomes evident—the rate of urinary excretion eventually reaches and exceeds the rate of phosphorus intake. As a result there is a fall in serum phosphorus concentration despite a continued rapid rate of phosphorus intake.

SECTION C shows the prompt fall in the ratio TRP/GFP, which follows the beginning of high phosphorus intake. This fall is interpreted to mean that there has been an increase in parathyroid activity in response to the homeostatic need for an increased rate of phosphorus elimination. The beginning of this homeostatic response is evident within 2 to 4 hours of the start of phosphorus loading. Adaptation to the elevated rate of phosphorus intake is essentially complete at the end of the periods of observation.

From J. D. Crawford, M. M. Osborne, N. B. Talbot and M. L. Terry, *J. Clin. Investigation* 29:1448, 1950.

Temporal and quantitative aspects of the parathyroid adaptative response. Adaptative changes in parathyroid activity are not instantaneous but take time to develop. The rapidity with which changes can occur is indicated by the experiments of Figure 8. In such experiments beginning adaptation may be evidenced by a fall in the TRP/GFP ratio value shortly after a sudden increase in phosphorus intake (from one to three hours). Full adaptation to the new level of phosphorus intake, evidenced by stabilization of the TRP/GFP ratio at a new value, usually occurs within 12 to 24 hours. Before and, to a diminishing extent, during adaptation, phosphorus balance is disturbed by an inequality between the rate of intake and the rate of elimination. This inevitably results in a temporary deviation of serum phosphorus concentration from the range which the homeostatic mechanism is designed to protect.

Deviations in serum phosphorus concentration may occur when phosphorus intake is either decreased below or increased above certain easily defined limits.

The *lower limit* of serum phosphorus homeostasis is defined by the maximal physiologic hypoparathyroidism occurring when phosphorus intake is restricted. This provides for complete tubular reabsorption and return to the body of all the phosphorus in the glomerular filtrate. While this renal phosphorus economy is sufficient to prevent a fall of serum concentration under most circumstances, there are conditions* in which the phosphorus of serum or extracellular fluid can undergo depletion even when urinary phosphorus excretion has ceased entirely. This is explained by the fact that appreciable amounts of phosphorus may be drained from extracellular fluid for protoplasmic anabolism and be lost in intestinal secretions. When no phosphorus is entering the body, such losses defeat the best efforts of the parathyroid-renal mechanism to prevent hypophosphatemia.

The *upper limit* of serum phosphorus homeostasis is defined as the point beyond which the parathyroid glands can no longer make adjustments to prevent an abnormal rise in serum phosphorus concentration when the phosphorus intake or load is increased. This point is determined largely by glomerular filtration rate (see Figure 2, Sections C and E). As shown in Figure 2, maximal parathyroid hormone effect on the kidney results in complete inhibition of tubular phosphate reabsorption and hence in the excretion of all the phosphorus contained in the glomerular filtrate. When more phosphorus must be excreted than

---

* These include extreme restriction of phosphorus intake in the normal and rapid skeletal remineralization after parathyroidectomy in osteitis fibrosa patients. Marked hypophosphatemia of the former type was encountered in the animal experiments of Figure 4. Intact animals maintained on the lowest phosphorus intake for one, two and three weeks showed serum phosphorus concentrations averaging 5.38, 2.90 and 1.97 mg. per cent, respectively. During this period there was essentially no loss of phosphorus in the urine.

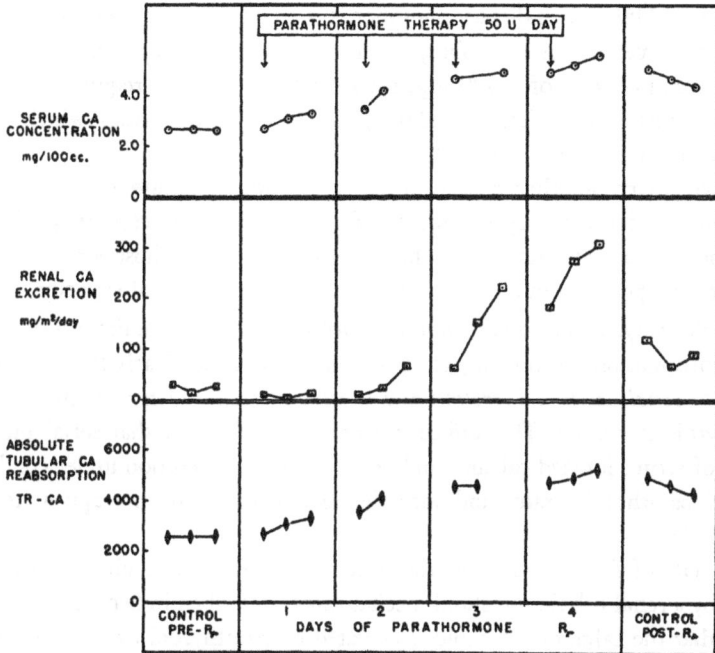

FIGURE II—9. The renal "threshold" for calcium excretion. The subject of this experiment was a patient with pathologic hypoparathyroidism. Serum ionized calcium concentration is shown by the upper ordinate, renal calcium excretion by the middle ordinate and values for renal tubular calcium reabsorption by the lower ordinate. Note that administration of parathyroid extract caused a progressive increase in serum calcium concentration (upper portion of figure). Essentially no calcium appeared in the urine until serum calcium reached certain critical values. When serum calcium concentration exceeded these values, urinary calcium excretion increased rapidly (middle portion of figure). The lower portion of the figure shows the increase in tubular calcium reabsorption (calcium "threshold") which occurred under the influence of parathyroid hormone. Recalculated from data of F. Albright and R. Ellsworth, *J. Clin. Investigation* 7:183, 1929, assuming a glomerular filtration rate of 100,000 cc. per m² per day.

is provided for by glomerular filtration of serum containing normal quantities of phosphorus, it can be eliminated only by increasing serum phosphorus concentration (Figure 2, Section C; Figure 4).

These limits beyond which the parathyroids can no longer maintain constancy of serum phosphorus concentration present no problem to the normal individual taking an ordinary diet. Our usual diets provide from 500 to 800 mg. per m² per day of phosphorus, of which approximately 70 per cent is excreted by the renal route. Only when dietary phosphorus is reduced below approximately 300 mg. per m² per day is hypophosphatemia likely to develop. Diets containing phosphorus in excess of 6,000 mg. per m² per day may be required to prompt hyperphosphatemia. Diets providing phosphorus in quantities which exceed either of these extremes are most unusual.

Viewed from another aspect, these calculations indicate that the normal individual under ordinary conditions of living maintains constancy of serum phosphorus concentration with his parathyroid-renal phosphorus excretory mechanism operating in a range not exceeding 10 per cent of capacity.

The Parathyroids and Calcium Metabolism. Though the literature contains much information on this subject, it is difficult to define clearly the exact mechanism of *renal calcium excretion* and the manner in which it is influenced by parathyroid hormone. This difficulty stems from the fact that serial measurements of serum ionized calcium and urinary calcium excretion under conditions of fixed parathyroid status and variable calcium intake do not appear to have been made.

The data of Figure 9 suggest that calcium, in contrast to phosphorus, is excreted by a renal tubule threshold mechanism as described in Section A of Figure 2 and that the calcium threshold is elevated by parathyroid extract administration as described in Section D.

Calcium Tm* is higher in patients with primary hyperparathyroidism (8.0 gm. per m² per day)[10 a-c] than in normal subjects (5.0 gm. per m² per day)[10 d] or patients with primary hypoparathyroidism (2.0 gm. per m² per day).[10 e,f] Incidentally, the relatively high tubular calcium reabsorption values observed in hyperparathyroid patients may explain their tendency to show calcification of the renal tubules.

Relations between parathyroid activity and renal tubule reabsorption of calcium (TRCa) and phosphorus (TRP). Figure 10 shows the effect of parathyroid extract administration upon the values for renal tubule reabsorption of calcium and phosphorus in a patient with primary hypoparathyroidism. Here is seen a tendency for TRCa to fall as TRP rises. An approximately similar relation is evident in isolated observations on other individuals with primary hyper- and hypoparathyroidism. As shown by the data of Figure 11 (see also Table 1), this is not an obligatory relationship. When parathyroid activity is altered in response to a change in phosphorus intake, there is a large change in values for tubular phosphate but little change in values for tubular calcium reabsorption.

It is difficult to explain these observations on the basis of a single parathyroid

---

* These Tm values have been calculated from the data of the literature assuming normal glomerular filtration values.

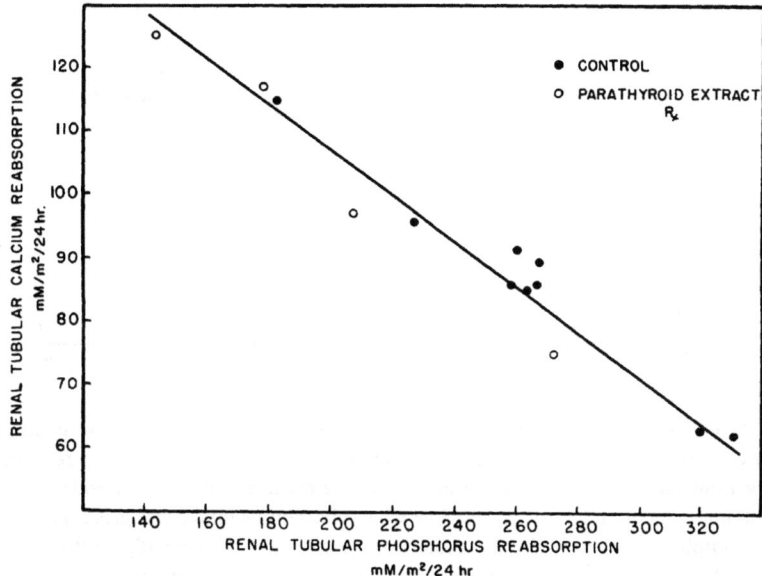

FIGURE II—10. Reciprocal relations between renal tubule calcium and phosphorus reabsorption under conditions of parathyroid extract treatment. The subject of this diagram was a patient with primary hypoparathyroidism. The black circles represent observations on the patient before and after treatment, the white circles observations during administration of 50 units of parathyroid extract daily for four days. During treatment there was a progressive increase in tubular calcium reabsorption and a reciprocal fall in phosphorus reabsorption. When treatment was discontinued, the reciprocal relationship continued in evidence as calcium reabsorption fell and phosphorus reabsorption rose to control levels. Recalculated from data of F. Albright and R. Ellsworth, *J. Clin. Investigation* 7:183, 1929. Results expressed in millimoles per m² per day.

---

hormone. On the other hand, they can be explained by postulating the existence of two parathyroid principles, one regulating tubular calcium, the other tubular phosphorus reabsorption. If this thesis is correct, it must further be assumed that, although parathyroid extract contains both principles, they are normally secreted by the gland at independent rates in accordance with need.

If calcium intake is varied from high to low levels while phosphorus intake is essentially constant, serum calcium concentration undergoes only a relatively slight fall.[11 a, b] Urinary calcium excretion, however, drops to very low levels.*[11 c]

* Despite an adequate intake, serum phosphorus concentration is apt to fall concomitantly to low or subnormal levels while moderate amounts of phosphorus continue to appear in the urine. This appreciable excretion of phosphorus in the urine at a time when serum phosphorus concentrations are reduced describes a low value for the ratio, TRP/GFP.

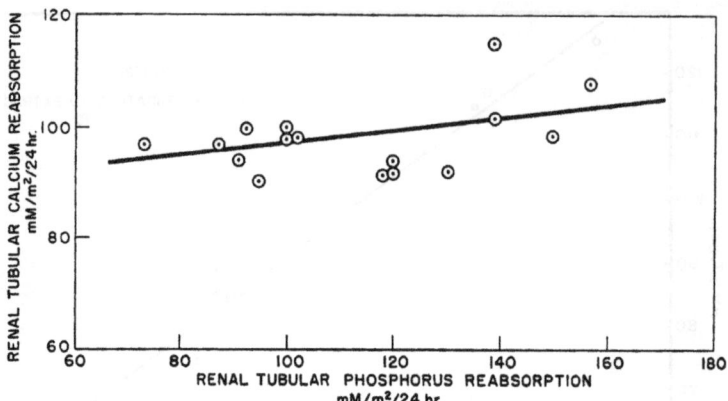

FIGURE II—11. Relations between renal tubule reabsorption of calcium and phosphorus under conditions of changing dietary phosphorus intake. The points in the figure represent observations on a normal individual given diets of constant calcium and widely variable phosphorus content. TRP values were low when phosphorus intake was great and elevated when phosphorus intake was small. Note that, in contrast to Figure 10, TRP values vary widely while TRCa remains essentially constant. In this experiment the observed values for GFP were nearly constant. Hence TRP values taken by themselves may be used instead of the ratio TRP/GFP as an inverse index of parathyroid activity. Thus the data suggest that, under physiologic conditions, phosphorus loading may stimulate the parathyroids to produce a hormone which decreases tubular phosphorus reabsorption without inducing a significant increase in tubular calcium reabsorption. From J. D. Crawford, M. M. Osborne, N. B. Talbot and M. L. Terry. Unpublished data.

Examination of the parathyroids of animals whose dietary intake has thus been manipulated shows variations in gland size inversely correlated with calcium intake.[11 d, e]

Parathyroidectomy results in an inability to support serum calcium concentration in the face of calcium restriction.[4] Doses of parathyroid extract act to boost the lowered serum calcium concentration toward normal, in part by increasing the efficiency of calcium reabsorption by the renal tubules (Figure 9).[10 e]

These data indicate that hypocalcemia, like hyperphosphatemia, prompts a physiological increase in parathyroid activity. Presumably, it is a fall in serum ionized calcium rather than total serum calcium which provides the stimulus. Hypocalcemia activates the parathyroids whether serum phosphorus concentration is normal or not.

Summary Comments on the Probable Nature of Physiologic Factors Influencing Parathyroid Activity. The parathyroids normally tend to be quiescent unless stimulated to activity either by hyperphosphatemia or by hypocalcemia. In this connection it is of interest that completely parathyroidectomized rats can

TABLE II—1. The effect on serum calcium concentration of increases in dietary phosphorus intake without change in dietary calcium intake.

	Dietary P intake gm/m²/24 hr.	Total serum Ca mg/100 cc.	Serum protein gm/100 cc.	Serum ionized Ca mg/100 cc.
Experiment I (normal adult)	0.1	8.2	7.2	3.5
	0.3	8.7	7.6	3.6
	3.3	8.3	6.8	3.7
Experiment II (infant—7 mo. amaurotic idiot)	0.2	7.1	5.8	3.3
	0.5	7.3	5.8	3.5
	0.7	7.9	5.8	3.8
	1.0	8.8	5.4	4.4
Experiment III (normal adult)	0.2	9.8	7.2	4.2
	1.7	10.3	7.1	4.5

survive over long periods if they are fed a diet which is of sufficiently low phosphorus and sufficiently high calcium content to prevent the development of hyperphosphatemia and hypocalcemia.[11 f, g]

Hypercalcemia does not deter the parathyroids from attempting to overcome hyperphosphatemia; as shown in Table 1, a slight rise in serum ionized calcium concentration may be observed when the phosphorus intake of a normal individual is raised from low to moderately high levels. Likewise, hypophosphatemia does not deter them from attempts at overcoming hypocalcemia; a tendency to marked hypophosphatemia is observed frequently in patients who suffer diseases tending to deplete body calcium stores (see page 82).

Consideration of the foregoing makes it appear likely that hyperphosphatemia need not induce hypocalcemia in order to prompt increased parathyroid activity. Parathyroid hormone secreted as a result of hyperphosphatemia alone tends to cause a decrease in the TRP/GFP ratio and hence an increase in urinary phosphorus output without prompting any major alteration in calcium metabolism. By contrast, when the parathyroids are stimulated to activity by hypocalcemia, the parathyroid hormone or hormones secreted have multiple actions. They cause increased phosphaturia as described above and in addition a tendency to increased renal tubule calcium reabsorption and to skeletal calcium phosphate catabolism.

While hyperphosphatemia and hypocalcemia may constitute the chief physiologic factors which normally act to determine parathyroid activity, it is probable that other factors may be of some importance (for examples, see page 78).

Parathyroid Hormone and Bone Catabolism. Demineralization of bone is a frequent occurrence in patients with primary hyperparathyroidism. There are two explanations for this finding: (a) unsaturation of body fluids with respect to calcium and phosphorus and (b) direct action of parathyroid hormone on bones.

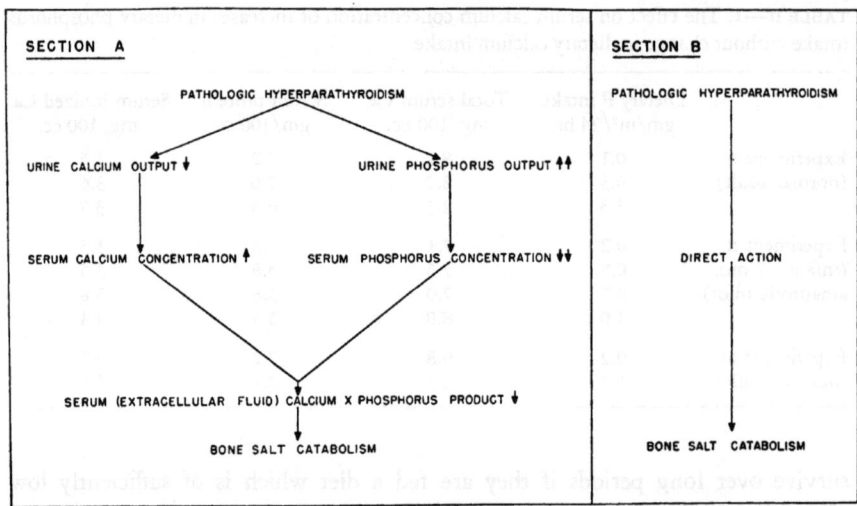

FIGURE II—12. Mechanisms for demineralization of bone by parathyroid hormone. In Section A it is indicated that parathyroid hormone acting at the kidney may cause a relatively greater increase in phosphorus excretion than calcium retention. As a result the decrease in serum phosphorus is more important than the increase in serum calcium concentration and hence the "calcium x phosphorus product" is lower. This situation favors the release of calcium and phosphorus from bone. In Section B the direct action of parathyroid hormone on bone is shown.

The first of these is expressed diagrammatically in Section A of Figure 12. Here it is seen that parathyroid hormone by its renal action may cause a proportionately greater lowering of serum phosphorus than elevation of serum calcium concentration. As a result, the calcium x phosphorus product is depressed below normal (Ca x P=35-40 in normal adults) and extracellular fluids become unsaturated with respect to calcium and phosphorus. To restore equilibrium, skeletal salt catabolism occurs.[12 a]

This theory is strongly supported by the observation that bone salt catabolism (osteomalacia) develops in experimental animals fed a diet low in phosphorus and high in calcium.[9 c, 12 b] The serum values of these animals are similar to those found in certain cases of hyperparathyroidism.[12 b] The parathyroid glands, however, are small and apparently functionally inactive.[11 d, 12 b]

The direct action of parathyroid hormone on the skeleton is indicated diagrammatically in Section B of Figure 12. Evidence in support of this thesis is provided by the observation that administration of parathyroid hormone causes skeletal salt catabolism in nephrectomized animals.[7]

TABLE II—2. The relative effect of vitamin D, dihydrotachysterol (A.T.-10) and parathyroid extract on gastrointestinal calcium absorption and urinary phosphorus excretion. Modified from F. Albright and E. C. Reifenstein, *The Parathyroid Glands and Metabolic Bone Disease*, Baltimore, Williams & Wilkins, 1948.

	Calcium absorption	Phosphorus excretion
Vitamin D (small doses)	++	−
A.T.-10	++	++
Vitamin D (large doses)	++++	++
Parathyroid extract	+	++++

Both the foregoing explanations for bone catabolism in primary hyperparathyroid disease are probably correct—one mechanism being predominant under some circumstances, the other under different circumstances.

Comparison of the Effects of Vitamin D, Dihydrotachysterol and Parathyroid Extract.[7a, 10f, 13a] The relative actions of these three substances are indicated in Table 2. Vitamin D has been listed twice because its action in large doses differs qualitatively and quantitatively from its action in small doses.[7a]

All three agents increase the absorption of calcium from the gastrointestinal tract. In this respect, parathyroid extract is the least effective agent. Vitamin D in large doses, dihydrotachysterol, (A.T.-10) and parathyroid extract all act to increase renal phosphorus excretion. Here, however, parathyroid extract is the most potent agent. Vitamin D in small doses actually diminishes rather than increases renal phosphorus excretion.

These slight differences in action help to explain three otherwise puzzling clinical observations. First, patients with primary pathologic hypoparathyroidism treated with A.T.-10 or large doses of vitamin D are observed to show persistent elevation of serum phosphorus concentration even after return of serum calcium to normal (Figure 25). This is explained by the fact that neither agent is as effective as parathyroid hormone in promoting renal phosphorus excretion. Secondly, patients with vitamin D deficiency rickets tend to develop tetany most frequently in the spring of the year, when increasing exposure to sunlight induces endogenous production of small amounts of the vitamin.[13b] Small quantities of vitamin D apparently produce this phenomenon by inhibiting renal phosphorus excretion.* Finally, neither parathyroid extract nor A.T.-10 is effective

---

* In experimental animals treatment of rickets due to vitamin D lack produces evidence of reduced renal phosphate excretion and of diminished parathyroid gland activity.[13c] Tetany incidental to such treatment responds to administration of parathyroid extract.[13d] These observations suggest that the paradoxical action of vitamin D in large and small doses is explained by postulating that in small doses the vitamin causes parathyroid inhibition with renal phosphate retention secondary thereto; in large doses the vitamin acts directly at the kidney in a manner similar to parathyroid hormone.[13a]

in healing osteomalacia,* though the condition is rapidly improved by a large dose of Vitamin D.[13 c] The explanation for this lies in the fact that neither A.T.-10 nor parathyroid extract can facilitate adequate calcium absorption from the gut without simultaneously prompting marked hyperphosphaturia. Consequently they do not create conditions favorable for mineralization of osteoid.

Relation of the Parathyroids to Other Endocrine Systems. Certain observations provide a hint that the activity of the parathyroids is influenced directly or indirectly by changes in function of other endocrine systems. Changes in the cytology of the gland are seen coincident with the various phases of normal growth and maturation.[6 a] Enlargement of the parathyroids is regularly observed during pregnancy[14 a-c] and is also frequently found in patients with acromegaly due to eosinophilic adenomas of the pituitary.[14 d-f] Parathyroid enlargement has been induced experimentally by administration of certain anterior pituitary extracts,[14 g, h] while partial involution has been noted in both clinical anterior pituitary deficiency and experimental hypophysectomy.[14 g, i]

Granted that such observations suggest interesting correlations, our present information on this subject is so limited that the topic is mentioned only to point out an area in which further research is needed.

CLINICAL CONSIDERATIONS

The preceding section serves as a basis for clinical consideration of patients with diseases which involve the parathyroids secondarily as well as of those with primary disturbances of parathyroid function. The conditions to be discussed in the present section are outlined in Tables 3 and 4. These tables are intended to give approximate information for purposes of orientation rather than detailed, unequivocal data.

PHYSIOLOGIC PARATHYROIDISM

This includes conditions in which normal parathyroid glands are called into action to maintain homeostasis. The average normal person receiving an ordinary amount of vitamin D in his diet is used as a point of reference in Table 3, Condition 1. The various other conditions listed in the table may be considered as follows:

Effect of Variations in Phosphorus Intake (Table 3, Condition 2). This topic has been discussed at some length in the preceding section. Since variations in

---

* In large doses, however, A.T.-10 is effective in preventing the development of rickets in experimental animals fed high phosphorus–low calcium diets.[12 b]

phosphorus intake are encountered daily by the normal individual and do not *per se* result in clinical pathology, the subject will not be dealt with further here.

Effect of Variations in Calcium Intake (Table 3, Condition 3). Under ordinary conditions of living, persons take a moderate excess of calcium in the diet. Only a fraction of this calcium intake is assimilated by the gastrointestinal tract, the major portion being excreted in the stool. Even so, the portion of dietary calcium which does gain entrance to the body is usually slightly in excess of anabolic needs, so that small amounts are excreted by the kidneys. A further small fraction of the calcium assimilated is re-excreted into the bowel as a constituent of bile salts.[15a]

Excess calcium intake. Marked excesses in calcium intake produce a tendency to hypercalcemia and physiologic hypoparathyroidism.* Significant hypercalcemia occurs only when the rate of calcium intake exceeds the ability of the kidneys to eliminate the surplus.

Hypercalcemia sometimes results from ingestion of large quantities of milk plus sodium bicarbonate or other alkali as part of the treatment of peptic ulcer.[15b] Possibly the simultaneous ingestion of other fixed bases (sodium or potassium) also requiring renal elimination reduces the ability of the kidneys to eliminate calcium and thus explains the development of this syndrome. Ordinarily, calcium intake from a milk diet is insufficient to tax the renal excretory capacity. We have seen only one such case in a child. More may be encountered as the syndrome becomes generally recognized.

Hypercalcemia secondary to massive doses of vitamin D may occur at any age.[15 c-e] Here, a normal dietary intake of calcium is almost totally assimilated from the gut. This creates a marked surplus of calcium in body fluids over and above anabolic needs. When the unneeded calcium exceeds the capacity of the kidneys for its elimination, hypercalcemia and metastatic calcification occur. The diagnosis of this condition rests upon eliciting a history of excessive vitamin D intake. Reduction of vitamin therapy, omission of calcium-containing foods and provision of a generous fluid intake constitute the appropriate treatment.

Finally, excessive quantities of calcium may be presented to the body fluids from endogenous sources—that is, skeletal catabolism. Usually this is a concomitant of primary parathyroid hyperfunction. In certain instances it may result from another cause, such as acute atrophy of bone due to disuse. This

---

* Excess calcium in the diet tends not only to elevate serum calcium concentration directly but also to diminish phosphorus assimilation from the gut by the formation of insoluble calcium phosphate combinations. Consequently both the stimuli to increased parathyroid activity, hypocalcemia and hyperphosphatemia, are absent.

TABLE II—3. Conditions prompting physiologic (or homeostatic) variations in the parathyroid activity of persons with normal parathyroid glands.

Condition	Serum concentration			Urinary excretion		Parathyroid activity	Bone pathology	Comments
	Ca	P	P-ase	Ca	P			
1. Average normal	N*	N*	N*	N	N	N	None	This is the point of reference for other conditions
2. (a) High P intake	N	N+	N	N	++	++	None	Note that serum values are essentially undisturbed by variations in P intake
(b) Low P intake (in presence of adequate calcium and vitamin D intake)	N	N−	N	N	=	−	None	
3. (a) High Ca intake	N	N	N	++	N	−	None	Note that serum Ca is maintained approximately normal at expense of low serum P when Ca intake is low
(b) Low Ca intake (vitamin D deficiency, steatorrhea)	N−	−	+	=	+	++	Osteomalacia; rickets	
4. Glomerular nephritis with ± normal tubules	Total− Ionized N	N+	N	N	N	++	None	Total serum Ca may be low because of diminished total protein concentration. Ionized Ca concentration is normal
5. Tubular nephritis with ± normal glomeruli	N−	−	+	+	+	++	Osteomalacia; rickets	See text for description of subtypes
6. Pannephritis	−	+	+	+	+	++	Osteomalacia; rickets plus tendency to fibrosis	Serum P may be + despite physiologic hyperparathyroidism, because glomeruli fail to filter P. Serum Ca is − because urine Ca is + and serum P is + (Figure 2, Section D)

In this table N denotes average normal; +, increased above average normal; −, decreased below average normal. * See Appendix.

TABLE II—4. Pathologic parathyroidism: characteristics of primary hypoparathyroidisim, primary hyperparathyroidism and related conditions.

Condition	Serum concentration			Urinary excretion		Parathyroid activity	Bone pathology	Comments
	Ca*	P*	P-ase*	Ca	P			
1. Average normal	N	N	N	N	N	N	None	As in Table 3, this is the point of reference for other conditions
2. Primary hypo-parathyroidism	=	++	N−	N−	N− (Clearance − −)	=	Possibly increased density	Parathyroid activity relative to physiologic need is grossly deficient
3. Pseudo-hypo-parathyroidism	=	++	N−	N−	N− (Clearance − −)	N	Tendency to congenital malformations	Owing to congenital malformation, the kidneys fail to respond normally to parathyroid hormone
4. Primary hyper-parathyroidism with normal renal function	++	=	+	++	++ (Clearance ++)	++	Osteitis fibrosa	Parathyroid activity relative to physiologic need is grossly excessive
5. Primary hyper-parathyroidism with impaired renal function	++	N or +	+	++	+	++	Osteitis fibrosa	Parathyroid activity relative to physiologic need is grossly excessive. Note, however, that serum P is up because renal ability to excrete P is abnormally decreased

* Normal values are given in Appendix.

condition will be considered in a later section dealing with the differential diagnosis of pathologic hyperparathyroidism.

Calcium deficiency. Calcium deficiency results in a tendency to hypocalcemia. This in turn prompts a physiologic increase in parathyroid activity. Physiologic hyperparathyroidism in turn prompts osteoclastic activity, skeletal catabolism, increased urinary phosphorus excretion and decreased urinary calcium excretion. The calcium made available to the body fluids by skeletal catabolism is largely retained. As a result, serum calcium is sustained at only slightly subnormal levels. The phosphorus derived from the skeleton is rapidly eliminated by the kidneys. This results in hypophosphatemia. Serum alkaline phosphatase concentrations are elevated because of a compensatory increase in osteoblastic activity.[16 a]

ETIOLOGY. It has been stated that calcium deficiency due *solely* to inadequate calcium intake has yet to be demonstrated in clinical medicine.[1] In the strictest sense this is unquestionably true. However, inadequate calcium intake may constitute a major factor in the pathogenesis of clinical calcium deficiency.

Primary deficiency of dietary calcium. This condition is most unusual in persons receiving an adequate caloric intake in the form of both vegetable and animal food. In this country calcium deficiency is occasionally seen in children suffering gross neglect. In China primary calcium deficiency resulting from the dietary habits peculiar to that area has been observed in large numbers of persons.[16 b-d]

Vitamin D resistance.[16 f] There are certain persons who, for unknown reasons, fail to respond to the usual doses of vitamin D. Fortunately, however, patients with vitamin D resistant rickets respond to massive doses of the vitamin (Figure 13).

Steatorrhea.[16 g] Calcium deficiency may result from diseases in which there is faulty gastrointestinal absorption of fat. These conditions are grouped under the term steatorrhea because of the soft, bulky stools of high fat content which are characteristically seen. They may be the result of pancreatic enzyme deficiency (cystic fibrosis of the pancreas), acholia or chronic intestinal insufficiency as it occurs in association with chronic infection, congenital malformations and other poorly understood disturbances (celiac syndrome). The steatorrheas interfere with calcium assimilation in two ways: First, insoluble fatty acid soaps are formed with calcium, binding it in such a way that it becomes unavailable for intestinal absorption. Secondly, vitamin D, being an oil soluble substance, is poorly absorbed and is therefore apt to be lost in the stools. Vitamin D deficiency results.

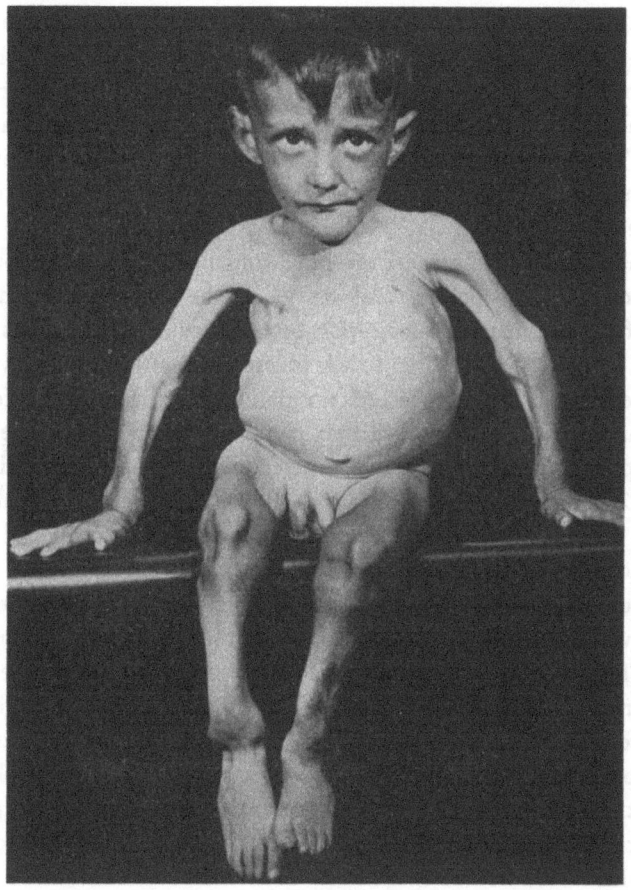

FIGURE II—13. Vitamin D resistant rickets. This boy was apparently normal until the age of 20 months, when it was noted that he was developing marked bowing of the legs. This became so extreme at the age of three that bilateral tibial osteotomies were performed. The photograph shows the patient at the age of seven, when the nature of his disease was first clarified. Note the short extremities, flaring in the region of the epiphyses of the wrists and ankles and the deformed chest. Costochondral beading appears in exaggerated form. Serum analysis at this time showed calcium concentration to be 9.2 mg. per cent, phosphorus 2.0 mg. per cent and alkaline phosphatase 20 B.U. per cent. Treatment with 200,000 units per day of vitamin D corrected the chemical abnormalities of the serum and led to improvement in general nutrition and growth. Two younger siblings have the same disease. Early institution of treatment in the latter patients has prevented the development of serious deformities. We are indebted to Dr. A. M. Butler for permission to record this case.

EFFECTS OF CALCIUM DEFICIENCY ON THE SKELETON. Calcium deficiency results in a deficiency of skeletal minerals. In growing children, where needs for calcium for tissue and skeletal anabolism are particularly great, the lack of skeletal calcium and phosphorus becomes clinically manifest more rapidly than in adults. The descriptive term commonly applied to this condition is *osteomalacia* in the adult. When osteomalacia occurs in the growing individual, it is called *rickets*.

Osteomalacia and rickets are to be distinguished from two other types of bone disease, osteoporosis and scurvy. In the former conditions there is no lack of protein matrix; calcification proceeds when the minerals are made available. In the latter conditions lack of protein matrix or framework is the primary defect; calcification proceeds normally as soon as osteoid is formed.

Osteomalacia and rickets have two metabolic components. The first is a catabolic phenomenon directly under the influence of a parathyroid hormone (Figure 12, Section B). The second is a disorder in skeletal salt anabolism occurring as a result of a decrease in the concentration of calcium and especially of phosphorus in extracellular fluids (Figure 12, Section A).

In calcium deficiency states support of serum calcium concentration at nearly normal levels eventually becomes impossible, even with maximal parathyroid activity. This is because the osteoblasts attempt to compensate for the failure of already formed matrix to calcify by laying down even more osteoid tissue. This excess osteoid eventually "insulates" much of the calcified skeleton against further rapid demineralization. When readily available calcium phosphate stores become exhausted, serum calcium concentration can no longer be supported at nearly normal levels by increased parathyroid gland activity. Marked hypocalcemia results.

Roentgenograms of patients suffering osteomalacia reveal cortical thinning and a decrease in the size and number of trabeculæ in the spongiosa of the long bones (Figure 14). In children rickets becomes evident in direct proportion to the velocity of growth. The failure of newly formed cartilage to calcify is most clearly evident at the distal ends of the tibia and fibula in the ankle. The characteristics of rickets by x-ray are irregularity of mineralization, fraying and a tendency to cupping and spreading of the epiphyseal plates (see Figure 15).

CLINICAL MANIFESTATIONS. The clinical picture in the foregoing types of disturbance varies with the specific cause. When there is calcium starvation due to dietary lack, there are apt to be other evidences of dietary deficiency. General nutrition usually is satisfactory when rickets is the only evidence of vitamin D deficiency. Not infrequently rickets and scurvy are observed together, but sometimes the simultaneous occurrence of the two conditions may

FIGURE II—14. Roentgenographic appearance of osteomalacia. X-ray of the arm bones of the patient shown in Figure 18, who developed osteomalacia as a result of excessive losses of calcium in the urine. Note the thinning of the cortical bone and coarse trabeculation. Increased radio-lucency of diseased bone as compared to normal bone gives an index of the degree of calcium loss.

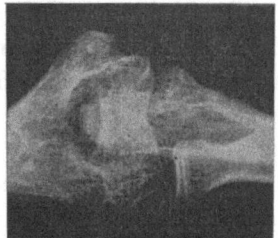

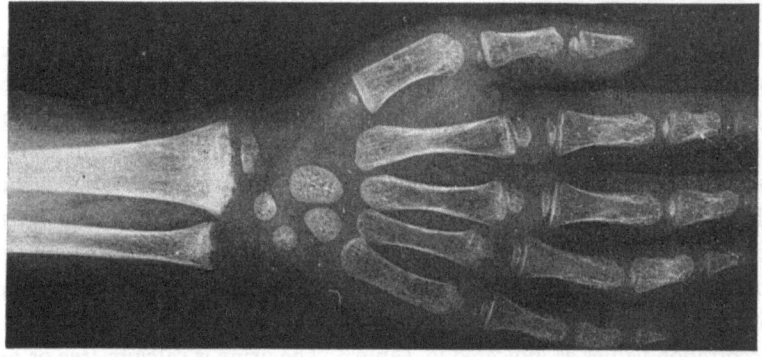

FIGURE II—15. Roentgenographic appearance of vitamin D lack rickets. Note the irregularity of mineralization, fraying and cupping of the epiphyseal plates. The carpals, metacarpals, and phalanges show coarse trabeculation and thin cortices, characteristics of both osteomalacia and rickets.

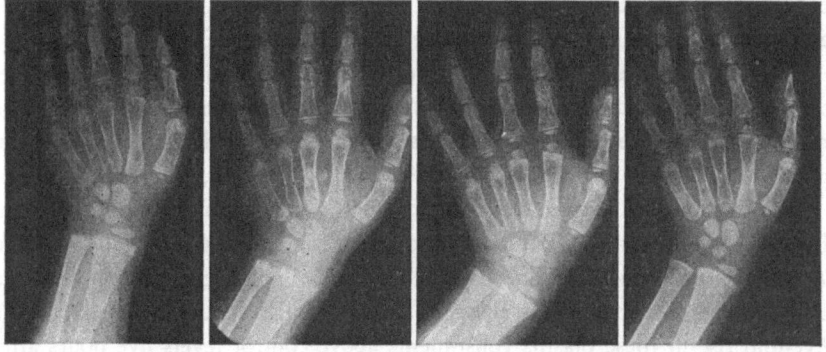

FIGURE II—16. Progress of healing in renal rickets. Series of x-rays representing the appearance of the rachitic bone lesions in a patient with base-losing nephritis (hyperaminoaciduria type—see Figure 20) taken at the start of therapy and at weekly intervals during treatment. Rapid healing was accomplished by the provision of sodium and potassium salts for replacement of fixed-base losses and vitamin D to promote gastrointestinal absorption of calcium.

result in a picture indistinguishable from that seen in scurvy alone. Presumably because vitamin C deficiency precludes the production of osteoid by the osteoblasts, patients suffering from both rickets and scurvy are apt to show little or no elevation of the serum alkaline phosphatase. By x-ray the features of scurvy may predominate.

Steatorrhea is suggested by a history of large, gray, foul-smelling, greasy stools, though occasional patients suffering from steatorrhea pass stools which are nearly normal in appearance.

Growth cannot proceed normally in the presence of chronic calcium deficiency, and children who suffer this condition over prolonged periods are stunted in stature. The skeleton becomes fragile when poorly mineralized, and fractures may occur repeatedly and on slight provocation. Bowing of the legs, craniotabes, flaring of the metaphyses of the long bones, smooth beading of the costochondral junctions and other skeletal deformities develop as a consequence of skeletal softening, or osteomalacia (see Figure 13). Tetany ordinarily is not seen while the disease is active.

DIAGNOSIS. The diagnosis of calcium lack is made from roentgenograms and chemical determinations of serum calcium, phosphorus and phosphatase concentration values as indicated in Table 3. The urine is calcium free or nearly so in these types of patients.

Vitamin D resistant rickets should be suspected when rickets appears between the age of one and two years despite adequate intake of dietary calcium and vitamin D and in the absence of steatorrhea. This diagnosis is confirmed by ruling out large losses of calcium by the renal route, as discussed in subsequent sections, and by a favorable response to massive doses of vitamin D.

The specific cause is often evident from the history alone. Steatorrhea sometimes can be diagnosed upon gross inspection of feces. On the other hand, a much more accurate appraisal of fat absorption can be made by use of the vitamin A tolerance test or by measuring the total fat absorption, or by both methods.

The vitamin A tolerance test is performed by oral administration of halibut liver oil containing 45,000 units of vitamin A per gm. The rise in serum vitamin A and carotene concentration observed after a dose of 3 gm. per m^2 yields an index of the efficiency of fat absorption. A normal response is indicated by a five-fold rise in these plasma constituents above control levels five hours after administration.

The diagnosis of steatorrhea is made by placing the patient on an approximately normal diet of known fat content. After two or three days on the diet all stools are collected for a period of three to five days. An aliquot of the total sample is then analyzed for fat. The stool fat content is referred to the dietary fat intake. Ordinarily not more than 10 per cent of the intake is lost in the stools, though slightly higher losses may be encountered in young infants. Under these standardized conditions losses of 20 or 30 per cent of the intake constitute evidence of steatorrhea.

DIFFERENTIAL DIAGNOSIS. The most important distinction is between calcium lack due to failure of assimilation as described above and calcium lack due to excess calcium loss as described below. Another condition to be differentiated is skeletal demineralization occurring in association with atrophy of disuse. This is noted in patients who are immobilized because of a fracture, severe burn or other illness. In this condition immobilization as viewed by x-ray occurs only in those parts of the skeleton which have been immobilized; the remainder of the skeleton appears normal. There is no evidence of rickets. Serum calcium concentration may be elevated but phosphorus and phosphatase values are normal.

TREATMENT. Correction of the calcium lack due to failure of assimilation is directed toward the underlying defect. The diet should contain sufficient amounts of calcium. According to National Research Council recommendations, children should receive about 1.4 gm. and infants about 1 gm. daily. These are very generous allotments for maintenance, but may need supplementation for repair purposes. Supplementary calcium can be given by adding calcium lactate to the diet in amounts ranging between 0.5 and 3.0 gm. thrice daily. Inorganic calcium comprises 13 per cent of the total weight of hydrated calcium lactate, hence these doses give 0.2 and 1.2 gm. of calcium per day, respectively. Expressed differently, the dose is approximately 5 gm. of calcium lactate per m^2 per day. Because of its chalky texture it may have to be camouflaged with chocolate syrup or other tasty food.

The normal requirements for vitamin D are approximately 400 to 800 USP units daily. Patients recovering from ordinary vitamin D deficient states do best when given larger amounts (about 8,000 units daily) during the period of healing. Patients suffering from so-called vitamin D resistant rickets may need much larger amounts (between 25,000 and 100,000 USP units daily). Concentrates containing 50,000 units of vitamin D per capsule are available and provide a convenient means of giving these large doses. In patients with steatorrhea, one of the water-miscible preparations of vitamin D may be absorbed more satisfactorily than the ordinary oily preparations.

Adequacy of calcium and vitamin D dosage. Serial determinations of serum calcium, phosphorus and phosphatase values, serial roentgenograms* and measurements of urinary calcium output are used to measure adequacy of dosage.

* In intractable steatorrheas and in vitamin D resistant rickets, where many roentgenograms may be desirable to check the results of therapy, attention should be directed to the fact that repeated exposure to radiation may damage the growing epiphyseal cartilage. Hence, one site should not be used continually; instead the various sites where activity may be checked should be used in rotation.

A qualitative appraisal of urinary calcium excretion may be made with the aid of Sulkowitch reagent. Equal parts of the reagent and the urine to be tested are mixed in a test tube. Calcium-free urine gives no cloud; increasing amounts of calcium in the urine give increasing degrees of cloudiness in the solution. Ordinarily, urine contains sufficient calcium to give a fine opalescence with Sulkowitch reagent. Marked hypercalcuria gives a milky appearance with this reagent.[17]

Excess dosage is indicated by a tendency to hypercalcemia and hypercalcuria. If hypercalcuria is evident the fluid intake should be increased and therapy should be reduced. Calcium and vitamin D therapy also should be reduced or omitted temporarily if a patient requires immobilization because of a fracture or other condition. This is particularly important in patients suffering from vitamin D resistant rickets. In patients with these diseases immobilization results in marked skeletal catabolism just as in normal individuals. The calcium thus released prompts hypercalcemia and hypercalcuria. If such endogenous sources of calcium are augmented by large amounts assimilated from the gut under the influence of vitamin D therapy, calcium presenting for renal elimination may exceed the excretory capacity of the kidney. Nephrocalcinosis and renal tract calculi may result.

Healing. A rise in serum phosphorus concentration and the occurrence of moderate amounts of calcium in the urine are the first indications of healing. Improvement in roentgenographic appearance follows (Figure 16). The last value to return to normal is the serum alkaline phosphatase.

PROGNOSIS. With adequate therapy, the prognosis for repair in any of these conditions is good. In patients with chronic steatorrhea or with so-called vitamin D resistant rickets, therapy must be continued indefinitely if normal or nearly normal bone structure is to be maintained.

Effect of Kidney Disease on Calcium and Phosphorus Metabolism and on Parathyroid Status. Kidney disturbances which involve the parathyroid glands can be conveniently grouped under three main headings: (a) glomerular disease without tubular insufficiency, (b) tubular disease without glomerular insufficiency and (c) combined glomerular and tubular disease. Though the lines of demarcation between these conditions are not always sharp, they will be considered separately below.

The phrases "without tubular insufficiency" and "without glomerular insufficiency" are used in an approximate sense. Patients receiving normal diets have been considered to show no glomerular insufficiency when the blood nonprotein nitrogen was not increased even though measurement of glomerular filtration rate might show 50 per cent reduction from normal. Again, patients

TABLE II—5. Physiologic hyperparathyroidism in glomerular disease without tubular insufficiency. Data from an 8-year-old girl with rapidly progressing glomerulonephritis. Relatively good tubular function was indicated by urines ranging in specific gravity from 1.003 to 1.022 and in pH from 5.5 to 7.5. The small losses of calcium in urine suggest both that base conservation was good and that no appreciable skeletal catabolism was occurring. Roentgenograms showed no evidence of demineralization. Approximately the entire glomerular filtrate content of phosphorus was excreted in the urine, suggesting maximal parathyroid effect (TRP/GFP=0.0). In the absence of hypocalcemia, hyperphosphatemia presumably acted as the stimulus to increased parathyroid activity.

Date, 1948	GFR* cc./m²/ 24 hr.	Serum P mg/100 cc.	GFP† mg/m²/ 24 hr.	Urine P mg/m²/ 24 hr.	Serum-ionized Ca mg/100 cc.	Urine Ca mg/m²/ 24 hr.	NPN mg/100 cc.
8/20	20,000	8.98	1,800	1,770	4.90	1.0	45
8/23	17,000	9.27	1,580	1,517	—	<1.0	112
8/25	15,000	8.70	1,310	1,445	4.10	1.0	82
8/31	9,500	7.34	700	895	—	3.0	50
9/11	7,000	5.43	380	297	4.75	<1.0	70

* GFR = glomerular filtration rate.
† GFP = glomerular filtrate phosphorus. TRP = Tubular phosphorus reabsorption.

have been considered to show no tubular insufficiency when they were able to excrete urines showing an essentially normal range of variation in concentration, pH and ammonia content.

Glomerular disease without tubular insufficiency (Table 3, Condition 4). This group includes a relatively small number of patients who retain good renal tubular function despite marked reduction of glomerular filtration. The effects of reduced glomerular function on phosphorus metabolism are summarized in the following paragraphs.

In order to maintain serum phosphorus homeostasis and phosphorus balance on a moderate phosphorus intake the diseased and the normal kidney are called upon to excrete equal quantities of phosphorus in the urine. However, as indicated by Sections C and E of Figure 2 and its accompanying text, reduction in glomerular filtration rate limits renal capacity for phosphorus excretion and therefore tends to produce a rise in serum phosphorus concentration. By stimulating increased parathyroid activity, this rise causes a compensatory decrease in tubular phosphorus reabsorption. If the phosphorus load is kept sufficiently small, this adaptative reaction can prevent marked hyperphosphatemia. Loads which exceed the capacity of the parathyroid-renal mechanism regularly cause an abnormal elevation in serum phosphorus concentration. This elevation permits the kidneys to excrete more phosphorus. Thus it constitutes an extra-hormonal reserve mechanism for preventing lethal hyperphosphatemia.

The normal individual can excrete as much as 4 gm. of phosphorus per m² per day without showing a pathologic rise in serum phosphorus concentration. In patients with advanced nephritis 85 per cent reduction in glomerular filtration rate is not uncommon. In such patients the ingestion of as little as 0.5 gm. of phosphorus per m^2 per day may tax the homeostatic capacity of the parathyroid-renal system to the full.

The physiologic hyperparathyroidism of patients with glomerular disease is similar to the hyperparathyroidism observed when very large amounts of phosphorus are given the normal individual (see Figure 7). The increased parathyroid activity in both instances has the purpose of facilitating renal phosphorus excretion. Were this hyperparathyroidism simultaneously to prompt skeletal catabolism (see Figure 12), the release of phosphorus from bone salts would only add to the phosphorus load that the kidneys are required to excrete. In point of fact, however, there is no evidence of skeletal catabolism in the hyperparathyroidism of certain patients with glomerular disease without tubular insufficiency (see Table 5) just as there is none in the hyperparathyroidism of normal individuals receiving an increased phosphorus intake (see Figure 5 and Table 1).

The commonest *cause* of this condition is acute glomerular nephritis. Occasionally it is seen as the result of vascular disturbances, such as nephrosclerosis.

DIAGNOSIS AND DIFFERENTIAL DIAGNOSIS. Glomerular disease is suggested by the occurrence of hyperphosphatemia and elevated non-protein nitrogen without acidosis, depression of serum ionized calcium or hyperphosphatasemia. The urea clearance value will be lowered to approximately the same extent as the glomerular filtration rate. Coexistence of serious tubular disease is ruled out by the presence of normal ability to vary urine specific gravity and pH as well as by the absence of systemic acidosis. The diagnosis can be confirmed by observing the patient's response to variations in phosphorus intake. Hyperphosphatemia is aggravated by moderate increases in phosphorus intake; it is alleviated by restriction of phosphorus intake.

Simple dietary phosphorus excess in an otherwise normal individual is easily ruled out by an accurate dietary history; the various forms of hypoparathyroidism are characterized by lowering of both total and ionized serum calcium concentrations as well as by hyperphosphatemia.

TREATMENT. The dietary phosphorus intake should be sufficiently restricted to return the serum phosphorus concentration to normal. Milk usually constitutes the chief dietary source of phosphorus in younger children. Other animal proteins can provide large quantities of phosphorus in the diets of older children. Elimination of milk, meat, fish, cheese and eggs from a normal diet reduces the phosphorus content considerably. Alternatively, phosphorus absorption from an ordinary diet can be greatly reduced by the addition of aluminum hydroxide gel* in doses of 30 cc. per m² per day or by calcium lactate in doses of 8 gm. per m² per day. The intensity of the therapeutic program in an individual case will depend on the degree of glomerular insufficiency.

PROGNOSIS. The immediate prognosis for control of hyperphosphatemia is good. However, the general, long-term prognosis must be guarded if the underlying renal disease is progressive.

Tubular disease without glomerular insufficiency (Table 3, Condition 5). This group of kidney disturbances includes a larger number of patients than the category just described. It may be divided into three subgroups according to the functional nature of the tubular lesion: (a) patients whose lesion is characterized by loss of base economy, (b) patients whose lesion involves failure to reabsorb amino acids and (c) patients whose lesion is characterized by selective failure of calcium reabsorption.

Loss of tubular base economy.[16] An important function of the renal tubules is to permit excretion of an excess of acid radicals derived from various body metabolic processes while conserving the so-called fixed bases—sodium, potassium, magnesium and calcium. The normal tubule has two means of accomplishing fixed-base conservation.† By elaboration of urine which is acid in relation to plasma, the base equivalence of bicarbonate, phosphate and organic acids is reduced. The saving of base thus accomplished can amount to as much as 70 mEq. per day in a child of 12 years. This base-saving mechanism can be brought into operation within a few hours' time. It thus constitutes the kidney's first line of defense against acidosis.

The kidney's second means of achieving base economy is the ammonium mechanism. When there is a large and continuing excess of anions over cations to be excreted in urine, the renal tubule cells have the ability to manufacture ammonium from urea or amino acids. The ammonium ion thus produced can be substituted for fixed base in the tubular fluid. This permits the reabsorption of fixed base to maintain body stores. Excess acidic radicals are eliminated in company with the substituted ammonium. Approximately 100 mEq. of ammonium ion per m² can be elaborated in 24 hours, providing for an equivalent saving of fixed base. Hence the ammonium mechanism is quantitatively more important to the base economy of the body than the excretion of an acid urine. On the other hand, this mechanism may require as much as six days' time to

* Each cubic centimeter of 3 per cent aluminum hydroxide gel may be expected to adsorb approximately 15 mg. of dietary phosphorus to form a complex which resists gastrointestinal absorption and hence passes out in the stool.
† While other mechanisms may be involved in tubular base economy, the two described here appear to be quantitatively the most important and are easily appraised clinically.

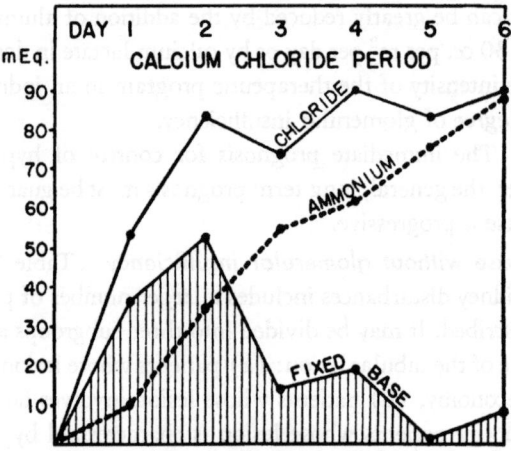

FIGURE II—17. Response of an individual with normal kidney function to chloride loading. The subject of this experiment was given 100 mEq. of chloride ion daily in the form of calcium chloride. A relatively insignificant quantity of the calcium was absorbed from the gastrointestinal tract, but most of the chloride gained entrance to the body and constituted a large increment in the acid radicles requiring renal elimination. The ordinate gives values for increments in urinary excretion of chloride and base over the fore-period levels. The abscissa gives time in days. In the first two days of chloride loading, ammonium production was small and large quantities of fixed base were expended by the kidney to neutralize the excess chloride ion. By the fifth or sixth day chloride excretion was almost entirely covered by ammonium ion; as ammonium production increased there was a diminishing need for fixed-base excretion. From J. L. Gamble, *Chem. Anat., Physiol. and Pathol. of Extracellular Fluid*. Cambridge, Harvard Univ. Press, 1950.

reach maximum efficiency (see Figure 17). Thus it constitutes in point of time a second line of defense against excessive fixed-base loss.

When these tubular mechanisms are rendered inoperative by disease, large quantities of the fixed bases appearing in glomerular filtrate must necessarily accompany the acid radicles in urine. Body stores are called upon to replace the resultant base depletion of plasma. Of the fixed bases mentioned above, only calcium is stored in quantities sufficient to fill more than temporary needs (see Table 6). Renal lesions which permit chronic loss of endogenous fixed base therefore tend to involve calcium eventually. When calcium is continuously lost from the body there develop the same tendencies to hypocalcemia, increased parathyroid activity, osteomalacia, hypophosphatemia and hyperphosphatasemia which have been described in connection with diseases of inadequate calcium intake (see page 82).

TABLE II—6. Distribution of body stores of fixed base. Results are for individuals over one year of age and are expressed as mEq. per kg. Data for exchangeable sodium from G. B. Forbes and A. M. Perley, *J. Lab. & Clin. Med.* 34:1599, 1949. Data for exchangeable potassium from L. Corsa, J. M. Olney, R. W. Steenberg, M. R. Bell and F. D. Moore, *J. Clin. Invest.* 29:1280, 1950. Data for total body content of sodium, potassium, magnesium and calcium and for body solid content of magnesium and calcium from A. T. Shohl, *Mineral Metabolism*, New York, Reinhold, 1939.

	Na+	K+	Mg++	Ca++
Total exchangeable contents	42	46	—	—
in $[H_2O]_E$	24	1	0.5	1
in $[H_2O]_I$	18	45	10.5	0
In solids	14	0	14	819
In total body	56	46	25	820
Per cent of total body base	6	5	3	86

The figures for the sodium and potassium contents of body solids were calculated as the difference between the total body and exchangeable contents of these elements. The figures for magnesium and calcium in body water were calculated as the difference between the amounts found in the total body and the amounts found in body solids.

The volume of $[H_2O]_E$ was estimated by using the average figure of 17 per cent of body weight for $[H_2O]_E$ as determined by inulin space. The sodium and potassium contents of $[H_2O]_E$ were calculated as the product of $[H_2O]_E$ volume and average sodium and potassium concentrations in $[H_2O]_E$ of 140 and 5 mEq. per liter respectively. The sodium and potassium contents of $[H_2O]_I$ were estimated as the difference between the respective total exchangeable values and the values calculated for $[H_2O]_E$ contents. The values for magnesium and calcium in body water were partitioned by calculating the $[H_2O]_E$ volume and average $[H_2O]_E$ concentration values of 2 and 5 mEq. per liter, respectively. Finally, the $[H_2O]_I$ content values for magnesium and calcium were estimated as the difference between the total body water and $[H_2O]_E$ contents, respectively.

Loss of the ammonia production mechanism may be the only discernible defect in occasional patients. In such cases, the ability to vary concentration, pH and titratable acidity of the urine is intact. These patients show no systemic acidosis under ordinary circumstances (see Figure 18). In other, unusual patients the base economy provided by acid urine formation is lost even though ammonia production may be nearly normal.

The large majority of patients who fall into this category of tubular (base-losing) nephritis have lost part of the function of both renal base-economy systems and show gross signs of tubular disease.

The *cause* of base-losing nephritis usually is not clear. Occasionally, cultures of the urine will reveal staphylococcus albus or other organisms of possible significance.

DIAGNOSIS. A variety of chief complaints suggest the diagnosis. These include anorexia, failure to grow and gain normally, skeletal fractures or deformi-

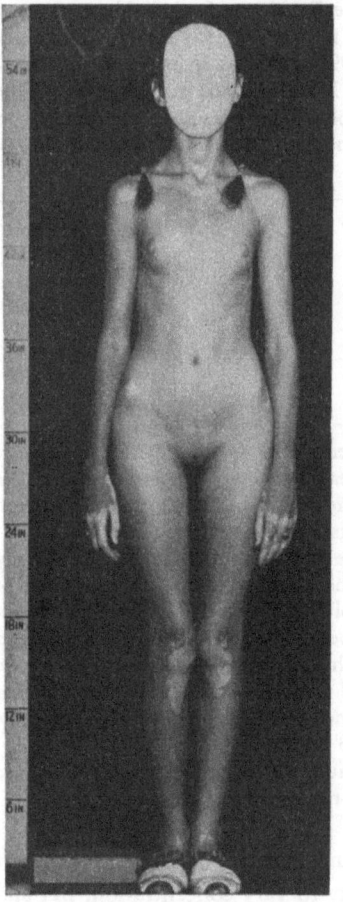

(Left)
FIGURE II—18. Physical appearance of a 14-year-old girl with loss of renal tubule base economy.

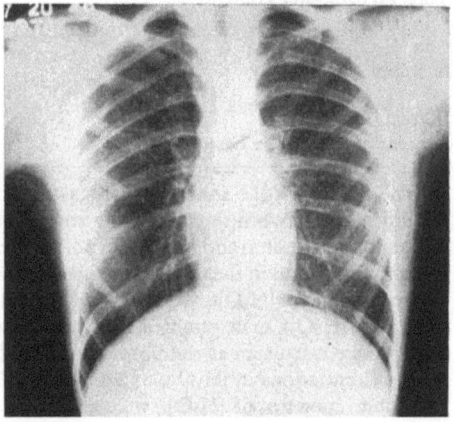

(Right)
FIGURE II—19. Roentgenogram of the chest of the patient of Figure 18, taken for heart size. The film was obtained before treatment and shows a significant degree of microcardia.

CASE HISTORY

The patient gave a history of multiple fractures after minor trauma. Laboratory studies showed slight hypocalcemia (9.0 mg. per cent) and hypophosphatemia (3.5 mg. per cent). There was moderate elevation of serum alkaline phosphatase concentration (15 B.U. per cent). Studies of the urine showed a normal range of variation in specific gravity and pH and no albumin or formed elements. Urea clearance was normal. The patient's ability to respond to chloride loading by urinary ammonium production was pathologically limited (see Figure 20). It appeared that this defect occasioned a slow drainage of calcium from the skeleton with resultant osteomalacia (see Figure 14). Treatment with sodium citrate resulted in a diminution in urinary calcium losses and healing of the osteomalacia. Note the generalized pigmentation and localized area of depigmentation of the skin over bony prominences. Vitiligo of this type is seen quite frequently in patients with base-losing nephritis. Partial to nearly complete clearing of the skin may be seen after institution of appropriate therapy.

ties (these may be grossly evident or evident only in roentgenograms), polyuria, polydipsia, renal calculi, vitiligo, weakness or lassitude.

Serum chemical studies show a tendency to slight lowering of both total and ionized calcium concentration values, moderate-to-marked hypophosphatemia and marked elevation of serum alkaline phosphatase concentration (see Table 3). Ordinarily there is no elevation of non-protein nitrogen concentration. Systemic acidosis may be absent. When present, it is usually of mild degree.

Roentgenograms show evidence of osteomalacia or rickets. Pseudofractures may be evident in the scapula just below the glenoid cavity as well as in long bones. Nephrocalcinosis and renal tract calculi may be evident in films of the abdomen.

The diagnosis is confirmed by studies of the urine. Gross tubular damage is indicated by the excretion of urine of fixed specific gravity (at about 1.010) and fixed nearly neutral pH (6.5 to 7.5).

The presence of bacterial organisms which hydrolize urinary urea to ammonia will invalidate measurements of pH, ammonia and titratable acidity; measurements of pH and titratable acidity are also invalidated by escape of volatile components from urine allowed to stand uncovered at room temperature. Hence pyelonephritis should be eradicated by appropriate chemotherapy, and all urine samples should be protected from bacterial contamination and loss of volatile components by collection under mineral oil in chilled containers to which 1 cc. of chloroform or toluol has been added.

In the presence of chronic acidosis a 24-hour urine sample which shows less than 70 mEq. of ammonium and 40 mEq. of titratable acidity per m^2 is indicative of at least partial loss of tubular base economy.

As indicated above, many of these patients may show no systemic acidosis under ordinary conditions. Evidence of gross tubular damage may be absent. In such cases detection of the functional disability is possible only by subjecting the renal base-economy system to stress. This can be done by the administration of "free" chloride* requiring renal excretion.

The patient is placed on a constant, normal diet. While this regimen is in force, a control 24-hour urine specimen is obtained, with proper precautions against bacterial contamination and escape of volatile components (see above). Thereafter the patient is given 6 gm. of ammonium chloride per m^2 per day (which provide 113 mEq. of free chloride), administered in divided oral

* The term "free" chloride is used to refer to chloride in combination with a cation that is metabolized to an electrically neutral substance (i.e., ammonium chloride → urea) for renal excretion. Chloride ion is thus rendered free to tax the renal base-economy defenses.

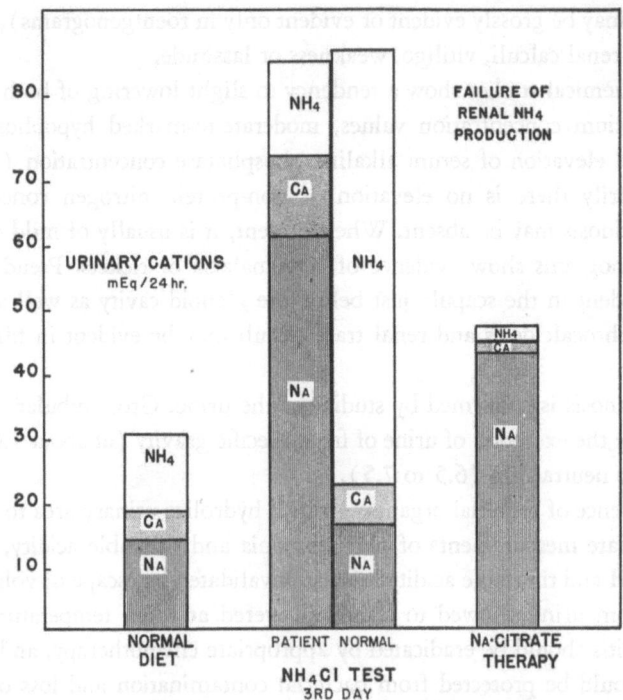

FIGURE II—20. Urinary losses of calcium and sodium in base-losing nephritis. This figure represents data obtained on the subject of the previous figures. The urinary excretion of ammonium, calcium and sodium during a control period on a normal diet are shown by the columns on the left. The paired columns in the center of the figure show the excretion of the same ions by the patient (left-hand column) and by a normal control (right-hand column) after three days on ammonium chloride (6 gm. per m² per day). Note the patient's failure to increase ammonium production and the compensatory increase in calcium and sodium in the urine. This behavior is to be contrasted with normal behavior, where increases in urinary ammonium prevent losses of fixed base during chloride-loading. At the right of the figure the single column indicates the saving of calcium which resulted when the patient was given 50 mEq. per m² per day of sodium in the form of sodium citrate.

---

doses at six-hour intervals. After three days on this test regimen,* during which the patient is observed carefully for signs of serious acidosis, such as dehydration and hyperpnea, a second 24-hour urine sample is collected.

The two urine collections are analyzed for pH, titratable acidity, ammonium and chloride. The chloride contents of the control and test specimens are com-

---

* It will be remembered (see Figure 17) that five or six days may be required for maximum increases in tubular ammonium production. However, for clinical purposes the increment is so small after the third day as to be relatively unimportant.

TABLE II—7. Free base equivalence of commonly used alkaline salts. The anions of these salts are metabolized and excreted by the lungs. This frees the cations for use by the kidneys in the excretion of other anions.

Salts	mEq. of free base per gm.
Sodium citrate	8.4
Sodium bicarbonate	12.0
Potassium citrate	9.3
Calcium lactate	6.5

pared as a check on chloride intake. Absorption of ammonium chloride is rapid and the amount administered should appear almost quantitatively in the urine. If the chloride increment of the second urine specimen is not approximately equivalent to the quantity of chloride administered, one suspects that the patient failed to take the full dosage recommended.

If the increase in chloride excretion correlates well with the recommended dosage of chloride, a calculation is made of the ammonium increment of the second specimen as compared with the first. When tubular function is normal, the ammonium increment will be found equal to 75 per cent or more of the chloride increment (see Figure 17). A fall in pH of the second specimen as compared with the first signifies increase in titratable acidity. The measured increase in titratable acidity will normally be found to cover excess chloride remaining after subtracting the quantity covered by increased ammonium production. A final check on the adequacy of tubular base economy under test circumstances is made by re-determination of the patient's serum pH and bicarbonate before discontinuation of ammonium chloride. Patients show stability of these serum constituents at nearly normal levels if tubular function is adequate.

When tubular base economy is deficient, analyses of the control and test urine collections for sodium, potassium and calcium may be of value. Demands for fixed base are met by increases in the urine of sodium, potassium, calcium and magnesium. The relative proportion of these substances gives information as to the appropriate distribution of the same substances in replacement therapy.

TREATMENT of this condition is designed to prevent further losses of body stores of fixed base and to replace losses which have already occurred. The first purpose is accomplished by administration of certain salts that provide free basic ions, which the kidney can use instead of body stores of fixed base. Table 7 lists a number of commonly used salts with their free-base equivalence.

Sodium citrate or bicarbonate is usually effective in eliminating the drain on body stores of all four major fixed bases. Use of sodium salts over extended periods, however, may result in intracellular potassium depletion. Hence we have been accustomed to provide a mixture of both sodium and potassium salts.

Use of potassium salts is not dangerous when glomerular function is good. It may cause potassium intoxication in patients with seriously diminished glomerular filtration rate (see below under treatment of pannephritis). Potassium should not be included in the therapeutic regimen until it has been established by measurement of serum potassium concentration or absence of the electrocardiographic signs of potassium intoxication that a patient can tolerate a prescribed dose of potassium salt.

Potassium depletion may be detected at an early stage by the flattening of the T-wave in the electrocardiogram (Chapter III, Figure 35). Other early symptoms are weakness and lassitude; later diarrhea and polyuria may be seen.

Administration of approximately 50 mEq. of free base per m^2 per day will serve to prevent losses of body stores of fixed base in most patients. Twenty-five mEq. each of sodium and potassium are contained in 15 cc. of the following quite palatable prescription:

Sodium citrate	68 gm.
Potassium citrate	62 gm.
Water to	350 cc.

The daily dose is divided into three parts and is taken with meals. The taste of this mixture may be almost completely hidden by dilution with citrus fruit juice.

The therapy outlined above not only prevents further losses of sodium and potassium but also serves to correct any deficiencies of these elements. When skeletal stores of calcium have been depleted by chronic base-losing nephritis, recalcification will proceed very slowly unless expedited by an adequate dietary intake of calcium plus therapeutic doses of vitamin D. Once skeletal calcium losses have been made up, however, there is no further need for therapeutic quantities of vitamin D, because the primary defect here is an abnormal, unselective loss of base rather than a defect in calcium assimilation. When skeletal repair is complete, vitamin D dosage should be reduced to maintenance levels.

Response to therapy can be judged in several ways. There may be a considerable improvement in the patient's general health and sense of well-being. Gains in height and weight may occur. A remarkable degree of healing of the skeletal lesions may be noted by x-ray within a few weeks. Serum analyses show rapid return of calcium, phosphorus, carbon dioxide and chloride concentrations to normal. Serum alkaline phosphatase values, however, return to normal only after osteomalacia or rickets has completely healed.

Therapy is inadequate unless acidosis is relieved. On the other hand, the development of alkalosis may indicate administration of base in excess of needs or provision of sodium in amounts sufficient to displace intracellular potassium.

This latter complication is suggested by characteristic changes in the electrocardiogram as previously indicated.

PROGNOSIS. There is an excellent prognosis for the healing of bones and the return of serum chemical values to normal. However, since the underlying renal effect is apt to be permanent, it is usually necessary to continue treatment indefinitely. As long as the tubular disability persists, withdrawal of therapy results in prompt redevelopment of skeletal lesions.

Hyperaminoaciduria (Fanconi's syndrome).[18a] The outstanding abnormality of this rare condition is the presence in the urine of abnormally large amounts of organic acids, including several of the α-amino acids. Cystine appears in large quantities in certain patients, and aceto-acetic acid may also appear. The presence of these acids is reflected by an abnormally high value for urinary titratable acidity and by a tendency for the average value of urine pH to be low (± 5.5). The value for titratable acidity averages approximately 25 mEq. per m^2 per day. The concentration of serum amino acids is not increased. As a rule, ammonia production is not grossly limited, but acidosis with hyperchloremia and decreased serum carbon dioxide content may occur. Other characteristics of the present condition are acetonuria and glycosuria. Since blood sugar values are not abnormally elevated, the glycosuria is considered to be a result of impaired tubular capacity for reabsorbing glomerular filtered glucose. The cause of acetonuria is not clear.

Finally, certain patients with the foregoing metabolic disturbances show a variety of congenital malformations including mental deficiency, buphthalmos and cataracts (see Figure 21).[18b] Autopsy findings in one such patient were consistent with cystinosis.

DIAGNOSIS. The distinguishing features of Fanconi's syndrome have been given above. Other symptoms and signs suggestive of the diagnosis are the same as those outlined in the preceding section.

TREATMENT and PROGNOSIS. Figure 16 shows that fixed base plus vitamin D treatment effectively corrects the skeletal disturbances (see also above, under loss of tubular base economy).

Idiopathic hypercalcuria.[1] This condition is said to be characterized by an isolated defect in tubular capacity for calcium reabsorption. Base conservation by increasing urinary titratable acidity and ammonium production is supposedly normal. Because of the selective nature of the lesion, treatment by provision of free sodium or potassium would not be expected to reduce hypercalcuria. On the other hand, calcium and vitamin D therapy might be anticipated to increase hypercalcuria, and hence the risk of stone formation.

[100] CHAPTER II:

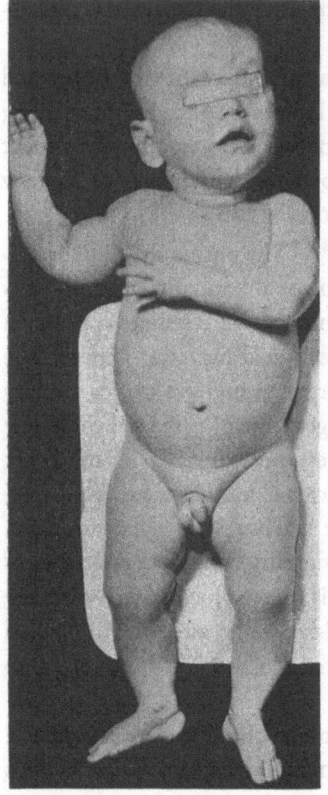

FIGURE II—21. Hyperaminoaciduria with buphthalmos and congenital cataracts in a child of 11 months.

CASE HISTORY

The patient was brought to the hospital because of searching nystagmus and failure to sit. Examination showed marked muscular hypotonia and bilateral buphthalmos and nuclear cataracts. Urine examination showed acetone, reducing substances, a pH of 4.5 and a strongly positive Sulkowitch test for calcium. X-rays of the epiphyses showed advanced rickets. General nutrition was good and calcium and vitamin D intake had always been adequate. Rapid healing of rickets was observed after beginning treatment with sodium and potassium citrate (see Figure 16).

Reports of the occurrence of this selective lesion in adults have aroused such interest that we have long sought to discover a case in the pediatric age group. To date we have not seen an actual case or the report of one in a child. Studies of our cases of base-losing nephritis have shown them all to belong in one of the previously described groups.

Combined glomerular and tubular insufficiency (pannephritis) (Table 3, Condition 6). In this condition reduction in glomerular filtration and loss of tubular base economy result in tendencies to hyperphosphatemia and hypocalcemia, respectively. Hence two stimuli to increased homeostatic parathyroid activity are present (see page 74). The response is evident functionally in low TRP/GFP ratios (see Figure 2, Section C) and rapid skeletal catabolism (see Figure 12). Pathologic enlargement of the parathyroid glands is grossly visible at anatomic dissection.

In the foregoing sections it was shown that a tendency to acidosis due to a lesion in the renal glomeruli may be compensated by normal tubular function. With combined insufficiency, systemic acidosis is regularly present.

The acidosis of pannephritis is of importance to the patient because of its effects on skeletal catabolism and serum calcium ionization. Acidosis promotes skeletal catabolism by increasing the solubility of bone salts.[1] Hence it predisposes to the development of osteomalacia and rickets. Simultaneously, acidosis increases the ionization of calcium in serum.[19] This action tends to protect patients from tetany despite profound lowering of total serum calcium concentration.

DIAGNOSIS. As a rule the diagnosis is obvious. Glomerular insufficiency is indicated by elevation of serum non-protein nitrogen and phosphorus and by diminished values for urea clearance. Tubular insufficiency is suggested by the excretion of urine of fixed specific gravity (± 1.010), neutral pH (6.5-7.5) and low ammonium content (less than 15 mEq. per m^2 per day).

TREATMENT. Correction of pannephritis is aimed at reducing the load of phosphates and other acid metabolites requiring glomerular filtration and at providing free base to replace losses secondary to tubular insufficiency. These measures have been discussed separately under glomerular and tubular insufficiency occurring independently. When used in combination to treat patients with pannephritis certain modifications may be necessary.

Phosphorus assimilation may be reduced by the use of aluminum hydroxide gel or calcium lactate. In pannephritis it is advisable to give calcium salts in doses of 3 to 6 gm. per m^2 per day because they not only render a portion of dietary phosphorus unavailable for gastrointestinal absorption, but also supply a cation which can be used by the body to replace fixed-base losses. The intake of phosphorus and, incidentally, of precursors of sulfates, organic acids and non-protein nitrogen may be further reduced to advantage by restricting the intake of milk, cheese, meat, fish and other animal proteins. Provided the patient's caloric requirement is met, a total protein intake of 30 gm. per m^2 per day is sufficient. An inadequate intake of calories results in endogenous catabolism of protein. If this is permitted to occur, it defeats the physician's best efforts to limit the nitrogenous waste load by reducing protein intake from exogenous sources.

Provision of base to replace tubular losses is complicated by the fact that the reduced glomerular filtration rate may contraindicate sodium salts, which aggravate tendencies to hypertension and edema. Finally, by correcting acidosis or causing alkalosis, treatment with either potassium or sodium salts may produce a depression of serum ionized calcium concentration which is sufficient to cause clinical tetany. Hence these salts should be used with caution and the patient carefully observed for untoward results. As requirements differ, doses should be slowly increased from very low to effective levels. Provision of 50 mEq. of base per m² per day in the form of sodium and potassium salts (see Table 7) is usually sufficient to correct acidosis.

As for phosphorus, marked reduction in glomerular filtration rate may seriously impair the kidney's ability to prevent toxic hyperkalemia. We have seen one patient with marked renal disease develop fatal hyperkalemia as a result of drinking large quantities of orange juice which contained 45 mEq. of potassium per liter.

The use of calcium lactate not only has advantages from the point of view of reducing phosphorus assimilation, but, as indicated above, is also a good source of base. Absorption of orally administered calcium is facilitated by the inclusion of relatively large doses (10,000 units or more per day) of vitamin D.

If tetany is encountered in a patient with pannephritis, from 1 to 1.5 gm. of calcium gluconate per m² may be given intravenously. This substance is about one-tenth calcium by weight and is dispensed in 10 per cent aqueous solution in 10 cc. vials. It should be given very slowly (± 1.0 cc. per minute) in order to avoid bradycardia. Failure to respond suggests that some condition other than hypocalcemia is responsible for the symptoms and signs.

Treatment of pannephritis includes many measures not mentioned here. Since they do not bear directly upon the parathyroid status of the patients under consideration, they are beyond the scope of this chapter.

Adequacy of therapy is judged by the return of serum calcium and phosphorus concentrations to normal, correction of acidosis and nitrogen retention and repair of skeletal lesions.

PROGNOSIS. The long-range prognosis in pannephritis must be guarded. However, the regimen outlined above, when combined with therapeutic measures such as sodium chloride restriction, iron therapy, abdominal paracentesis and transfusions, may greatly increase the patient's comfort and prolong his life.

PATHOLOGIC PARATHYROIDISM

This heading includes conditions in which phosphorus and calcium homeostasis by the parathyroid glands is deranged, so that production of parathyroid hormone is out of keeping with physiologic needs. The diseases to be considered are listed along with certain of their chief characteristics in Table 4.

Primary Hypoparathyroidism (Table 4, Condition 2). This disease occurs in several forms: (a) as a transient or permanent phenomenon in patients with damaged parathyroid glands (simple hypoparathyroidism), (b) as a transient semi-physiologic phenomenon in the newborn (tetany of the newborn) and (c) as a somewhat similar phenomenon in patients recovering from vitamin D resistant rickets (tetany of healing rickets). Because these conditions have somewhat different clinical characteristics, they will be considered separately.

Simple hypoparathyroidism. This heading includes all types of hypoparathyroidism not covered specifically in other sections of the chapter. It is seen occasionally in children and adolescents. Its various and many manifestations are due almost exclusively to hypocalcemia.

The *cause* of primary hypoparathyroidism is often obscure. It may be the obvious consequence of intentional surgical parathyroidectomy, as in patients with primary hyperparathyroidism, or it may be accidental as in patients subjected to thyroidectomy. A transient state of hypoparathyroidism may occur in patients recently subjected to surgical thyroidectomy as a consequence of hemorrhage into the parathyroid glands. Aplasia of the glands has been described.[20a] Hypoplasia and fibrosis of unknown cause have also been noted.[20b]

There is an interesting, though poorly understood, relation between primary hypoparathyroidism and generalized Monilia albicans infection. In two patients studied in this clinic, chronic moniliasis of the mouth, respiratory tract and fingernails preceded the onset of clinical hypoparathyroidism (and incidentally of hypoadrenocorticism) by a matter of months to years.[20c] It is not known whether the fungus caused these glandular defects or developed as a result of them.

CLINICAL MANIFESTATIONS. The symptoms and signs of hypocalcemia secondary to hypoparathyroidism are listed in Table 8. Here it is seen that the clinical manifestations are diverse and that they include such common complaints as epileptiform seizures and upper respiratory obstruction. Individual patients do not always show all the abnormalities listed. Indeed, cases of primary hypoparathyroidism may be encountered in which symptoms are mild or absent. In general, patients are apt to fall into one or the other of two broad groups. In one, central nervous system disorders predominate; in the other, respiratory difficulties are most prominent.

Neurologic signs. The central nervous system signs may be difficult to distinguish from those seen in patients with primary intracranial disease. Even such a classic sign as carpopedal spasm may be misleading. Occasionally it is not evident in persons suffering from hypocalcemia even when the tourniquet test for carpopedal spasm (Trousseau test)* is employed. Furthermore, certain pa-

* This test is performed by placing a sphygmomanometer cuff on the upper arm and inflating the cuff to a point just above systolic blood pressure. A positive result is indicated by the development of tetanic flexion of the wrist and hand within a period of three minutes of sustained pressure by the cuff.

TABLE II—8. Clinical manifestations of primary hypoparathyroidism in children and adolescents.

System or organ	Symptoms	Signs	Related findings
Personality	Irritable, unmanageable; emotionally unstable, tantrums	*Sensorium clear;* alert	
Nervous system	Dizziness; unsteadiness; loss of coordination; *tingling, numbness* of hands and feet; *painful twitchings; epileptiform seizures*, petit mal	*Spastic stiffness* of muscles with trismus of jaw, boardlike abdomen; carpopedal spasm, spontaneous or elicited by tourniquet test; facial twitching on tapping region over facial nerve; reflexes hyperirritable	Cracked-pot resonance of skull. Separation of cranial sutures seen by x-ray. Sometimes pathologic calcifications of the basal ganglia and cerebral hemispheres. Tests of cerebellar function usually give normal results. Electroencephalographic findings compatible with idiopathic epilepsy (diffuse slow-wave activity). Spinal fluid under increased pressure, but otherwise normal
Eyes	Blurred vision	Punctate opacities of lenses, bilateral	Papilledema
Respiratory tract	Inspiratory crow, tendency to *upper respiratory obstruction*, especially with pharyngeal infections	Evidences of upper respiratory obstruction (dyspnea, retraction of intercostal spaces, cyanosis, etc.)	On laryngoscopy, spasm of vocal chords
Gastro-intestinal system	Nausea, vomiting, *intermittent* diarrhea and abdominal pain		
Other findings, including chemical measurements	Urinary retention	Moniliasis of the mouth and fingernails occasionally seen	*Hypocalcemia* (serum ionized calcium); tendency to *hyperphosphatemia;* tendency to hypocalciuria. In *electrocardiograms*, abnormally long S-T (or Q-T) interval with normal P-R interval

tients with basal ganglia derangements due to anoxemia or other disturbance may suffer athetoid spasms of the hands and feet which are nearly identical to the carpopedal spasm of hypocalcemia. A valuable test is that performed by tapping lightly over the facial nerve just anterior to the ear (Chvostek test). A strongly positive result is indicated by a twitching of the muscles innervated by all three motor divisions of the nerve (i.e., muscles of the mouth, nose and eyelids). Twitching of the muscles of the upper lip only is a weak positive response and is often obtainable in normal individuals, particularly in infants.

Convulsive seizures without loss of consciousness are quite suggestive of hypocalcemic tetany, but typical epileptic seizures, particularly of the petit mal type, may be seen. Convulsions with maintenance of a clear sensorium are also occasionally observed in patients suffering from tetanus infection, from strychnine poisoning and from certain types of brain damage.

The reflexes of hypocalcemic patients vary with relation to the degree of hypocalcemia. With moderate hypocalcemia, tendon reflexes become hyperactive. When hypocalcemia is profound, tendon reflexes disappear; under these circumstances the bellies of the various muscles are hyperirritable and contract vigorously when tapped.

Respiratory system signs. Patients with chronic hypocalcemia may present no signs of laryngeal spasm and obstruction until they develop an upper respiratory infection. Then the picture may so closely resemble that seen in patients with ordinary respiratory tract infections or with congenital malformations of the larynx that the true nature of the underlying disease is missed, sometimes for periods of years. A number of patients have been unnecessarily subjected to tracheotomy on this account.

Miscellaneous signs. As stated above, moniliasis may involve the fingernails, the mouth or the throat. The infection may be self-evident, as in Figures 22 and 23, and in cases of infantile thrush, when plaques of white exudate appear in the tongue and buccal membranes. Otherwise, diagnosis may escape detection unless smears and cultures are made.

DIAGNOSIS. The diagnosis of pathologic hypoparathyroidism depends upon chemical measurements. Serum analysis shows a lowered total and ionized calcium concentration. Hyperphosphatemia may be moderate or marked, depending upon phosphorus intake. The serum alkaline phosphatase is found normal or slightly low. Other serum values, including total protein, non-protein nitrogen, carbon dioxide and pH are normal. Although the urinary output of phosphorus is small in proportion to the rise in serum concentration (phosphorus clearance is very low), renal excretion of phosphorus by hypoparathyroid patients is roughly equivalent to that of normal persons on a similar diet. The urine is apt to be calcium free as judged by the qualitative Sulkowitch test (see Appendix, page 590). The occasional cases in which considerable calcium is present in the urine are explained by the tendency of the kidney to waste this substance in the absence of parathyroid hormone (see page 72). Hypoparathyroidism is

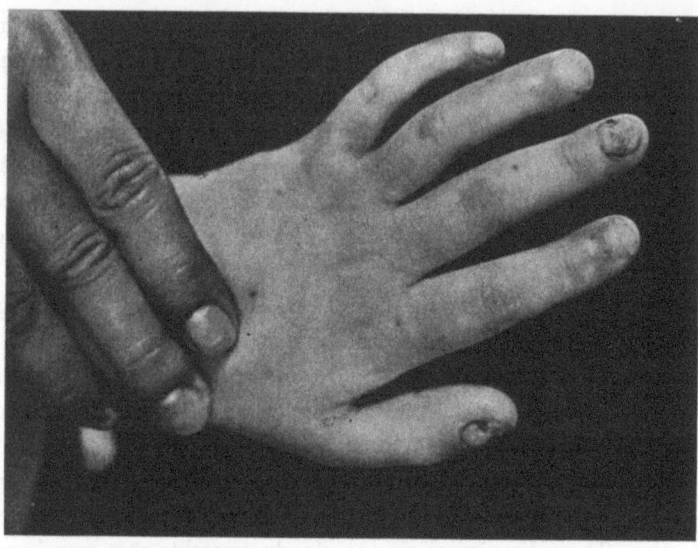

FIGURE II—22. Monilia albicans of the fingernails in hypoparathyroidism. The consistency of the nails is soft and spongy, and the nail beds frequently become discolored. Note the irregularity of the deformity.

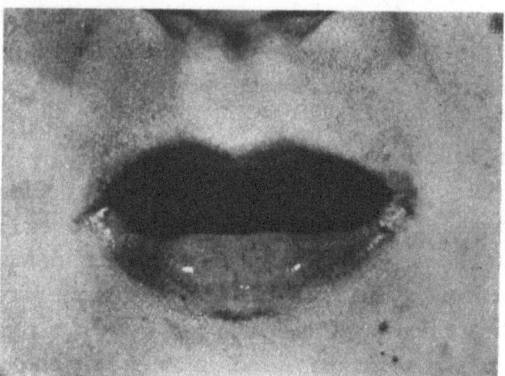

FIGURE II—23. Monilia albicans of the mouth in hypoparathyroidism. Typical plaques of white exudate are sometimes found on the hard palate. The tongue may be swollen, abnormally smooth and of a magenta color. Note the chielosis reminiscent of riboflavin deficiency.

characterized roentgenographically by hyperossification. This is evident as a thickening of cortical bone and metastatic calcification of soft tissues.

DIFFERENTIAL DIAGNOSIS. Table 9 indicates the differential diagnosis of hypocalcemia. In older children the conditions most likely to cause confusion at the onset are idiopathic epilepsy, expanding intracranial lesion and tetanus. In infants and younger children laryngeal obstruction due to croup, laryngotracheitis, or congenital laryngeal and tracheal defects are to be distinguished.

These conditions need give little difficulty if the possibility of hypocalcemia is investigated. When venous blood is withdrawn from a patient with possible hypocalcemia, much can be learned by introducing calcium intravenously through the same needle. If the patient is suffering from hypocalcemia, the slow intravenous administration of 50 to 100 mg. of calcium (as 10 per cent calcium gluconate in water) will bring striking benefit almost immediately. Such signs of tetany as carpopedal spasm, painful muscle twitchings and inspiratory crow are clearly alleviated for a period of one to several hours. Little if any benefit accrues from calcium therapy to patients who are not suffering from hypocalcemia.

Hypoparathyroidism is distinguished from alkalosis by the total serum calcium value and the serum pH measurement.* Clinically, alkalosis often can be alleviated long enough to make a tentative diagnosis by asking the patient to hold his breath or to re-breathe air in a bag. This inhibits pulmonary carbon dioxide excretion. The retained carbon dioxide corrects the alkalosis and thereby relieves tetany. This manœuvre is of practical importance particularly in patients who develop signs of tetany following surgical removal of a toxic goiter. They may, of course, be suffering from true hypoparathyroidism secondary to parathyroid hemorrhage or accidental parathyroidectomy. On the other hand, they may have developed tetany solely as a result of hyperventilation and alkalosis.

If a patient falls into the hypoparathyroid group (Table 9, Condition 1), it may still be necessary to demonstrate whether the difficulty is due to lack of parathyroid hormone (Condition 1 a) or to inability to respond to this hormone (Condition 1 b). Responsiveness versus resistance to parathyroid hormone can be determined with the aid of the parathyroid hormone test.[21] As used in this clinic, the test is performed as follows:

The patient is prepared by an overnight fast (this is not necessary in the case of small infants). In the morning a moderate diuresis is established by giving 500 cc. of water per m^2. A large urine volume is maintained for the duration of the test by subsequently administering 200 cc. of water per m^2 every hour. One

---

* The pH measurement indicates alkalosis regardless of its cause. The serum bicarbonate value alone is not a trustworthy index of alkalosis (see Chapter IX, page 557).

TABLE II—9. Characteristics of conditions resulting in decreased serum ionized calcium.

Condition	Total calcium	Total protein	Ionized calcium	Serum concentrations					
				Inorganic phosphorus	Alkaline phosphatase	Non-protein nitrogen	pH	HCO$_3$	Cl
1. (a) Hypoparathyroidism	−	N		+	N to −	N	N	+	N
(b) Pseudo-hypoparathyroidism	"	"		"	"	"	"	"	"
2. Pannephritis	−	−		+	+	+	−	−	+
3. Severe osteomalacia (healing rickets, after removal of parathyroid tumor)	−	N		N+	+	N	N	N	N
4. Alkalosis			Apparently normal, but actually low						
(a) Vomiting	N	N		N	N	N	+	+	−
(b) Alkali intoxication	N	N		N	N	N+	+	+	N
(c) Hyperventilation	N	N		N	N	N	+	−	N

N denotes normal; + = increased above average normal; − = decreased below normal.

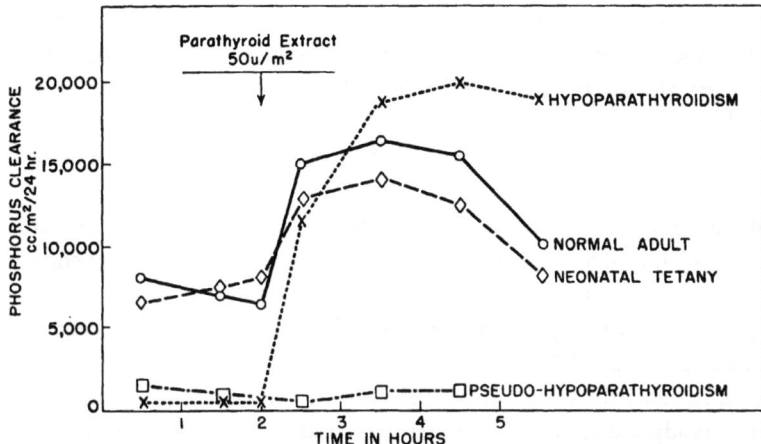

FIGURE II—24. Response to parathyroid extract in neonatal tetany, pathologic hypoparathyroidism and pseudo-hypoparathyroidism. Phosphorus clearance values are given on the ordinate; time in hours is shown on the abscissa. Parathyroid extract, approximately 50 units per m², was administered (arrow) after a two-hour control period. The responses of a healthy individual (solid line), an infant with neonatal tetany (broken line) and a patient with pathologic hypoparathyroidism (dotted line) are in sharp contrast to the response of the patient with pseudo-hypoparathyroidism. From J. D. Crawford, M. M. Osborne and N. B. Talbot. Unpublished observations.

---

hour after beginning the administration of fluid the bladder is emptied and thereafter six consecutive hourly urine specimens are obtained. Serum samples for inorganic phosphorus determination are obtained at the beginning of the test and at the end of the second, fourth and sixth hours. At the beginning of the third hour parathyroid extract in a dose of 50 units per m² is given intravenously. Because of the variability which is encountered in different lots of parathyroid extract, it is desirable to perform the test simultaneously on a normal control patient.

The serum and urine specimens are analyzed for inorganic phosphorus. Clearances are calculated by dividing the phosphorus content of each hourly urine specimen by the serum phosphorus concentration pertaining over that period of collection. For purposes of comparison it has been found convenient to re-express results in terms of one square meter of body surface area per 24 hours.

Responsiveness to parathyroid hormone is indicated by an increase of 100 per cent or more in the value for renal phosphorus clearance (Figure 24). Such a response indicates that the kidneys are capable of reacting to parathyroid hormone by decreasing tubular phosphate reabsorption, which one would expect in patients with primary hypoparathyroidism. Unresponsiveness is characteristic of patients with pseudo-hypoparathyroidism (see below) and of patients whose kidneys are already maximally stimulated by parathyroid hormone as a result of renal disease.

TREATMENT. The management of primary hypoparathyroidism is as follows:

Initially, for the prompt relief of tetany, the patient should be given intravenous calcium, calcium by mouth and large doses of vitamin D. Dietary phosphorus should be restricted.

Depending on the response of the patient, 10 to 20 cc. of a 10 per cent solution of calcium gluconate (the equivalent of 100 to 200 mg. of calcium) are administered intravenously at the rate of 0.5 to 1 cc. per minute. Too rapid infusion results in bradycardia. This therapy may be repeated after a few hours if necessary.

For oral administration the calcium salt of choice is calcium chloride, which not only satisfies the calcium requirement, but also prompts a mild acidosis (since chloride is absorbed in excess of calcium). This alleviates the hypocalcemia by increasing serum calcium ionization. Incidentally, calcium chloride is appropriate for the treatment of tetany due to alkalosis, although ammonium chloride serves equally well in the latter condition.

The daily dosage of calcium chloride is approximately 3.5 gm. per m^2 divided into three or four parts. Because the salt is irritating to the gastric mucosa, it should be administered in dilute solution (1 to 2 per cent) in water or fruit juice. If given for more than 24 hours, calcium chloride is apt to cause vomiting, severe acidosis and dehydration. Acidosis of undesirable severity is evidenced by hyperpnea, hyperchloremia, low serum bicarbonate and pH. If this condition develops, it is treated by discontinuing the calcium chloride and by providing a large fluid intake (about 2,000 cc. per m^2 per day). If parenteral fluids must be given, Solution 2 (see Chapter IX, Table 8) is satisfactory.

Initial treatment also includes oral administration of vitamin D or dihydrotachysterol (A.T.-10). Approximately the same results are to be obtained from 20,000 I.U. of crystalline vitamin D and 0.1 mg. of A.T.-10, but vitamin D is to be preferred because it is less expensive and because patients sometimes show increasing resistance to A.T.-10. The dose used at the start of treatment is approximately 200,000 I.U. of vitamin D. During the initial period of therapy it is also advisable to restrict the intake of milk and cheese, because of their high phosphorus content, or to administer aluminum hydroxide (see page 91). Milk formulas made up with aluminum hydroxide are well taken by infants. Elimination of high phosphorus foods from the diet does not pose a serious problem in older persons.

After the first day or two of treatment, a maintenance program is begun (see Figure 25). Calcium lactate in doses of 6 gm. per m^2 per day may be substituted for calcium chloride as an oral source of extra calcium. If calcium lactate proves objectionable because of its chalky texture and taste, calcium chloride may be continued at about half the initial dose schedule. However, it must be discontinued if it upsets the digestion or causes clinical evidence of acidosis or dehydration.

After the first few days, the dose of vitamin D (or A.T.-10) may also need adjustment. Doses are judged according to serum and urine calcium content. The least dose which will maintain serum calcium concentration values at normal or slightly subnormal levels is optimum. Usually a total serum calcium concentration of about 9.0 to 9.5 mg. per cent is satisfactory. With respect to the urine, it is important if possible to avoid gross hypercalcuria because of the danger of renal tract calcification. Urine calcium can be estimated with the aid of the Sulkowitch reagent (see Appendix, page 590). As the relation between serum and urine calcium varies from person to person, this interrelation must be studied in each individual before urine calcium is used even as an approximate index of serum calcium concentration.

Failure to adjust the dose of vitamin D carefully can result in marked hypercalcemia. Diffuse, metastatic calcification will follow if gross hypercalcemia is allowed to continue. When the concentration of total serum calcium reaches or exceeds 16 mg. per cent, death may occur suddenly.

Parathyroid extract is used relatively little in the therapy of chronic primary hypoparathyroidism. Even in the treatment of transient hypoparathyroidism, such as that seen occasionally following thyroid gland operations, it cannot be recommended without reservation because of the risk of inducing parathyroid intoxication through overdosage. When an excess of parathyroid hormone is given, marked hypercalcemia and hypercalcuria and sometimes hyperphosphatemia ensue, with effects similar to those described above in connection with vitamin D intoxication.

PROGNOSIS. With respect to therapeutic relief of hypocalcemic symptoms the prognosis is excellent. However, except for patients with transient hypoparathyroidism such as may be seen following surgery in the region of the parathyroid glands, the outlook with regard to spontaneous remission of the parathyroid deficient state is very poor.

Pseudo-hypoparathyroidism.[22] This is a rare clinical entity characterized by hypocalcemia and hyperphosphatemia. It has many clinical features in common with true hypoparathyroidism, since hypocalcemia, regardless of its cause, gives

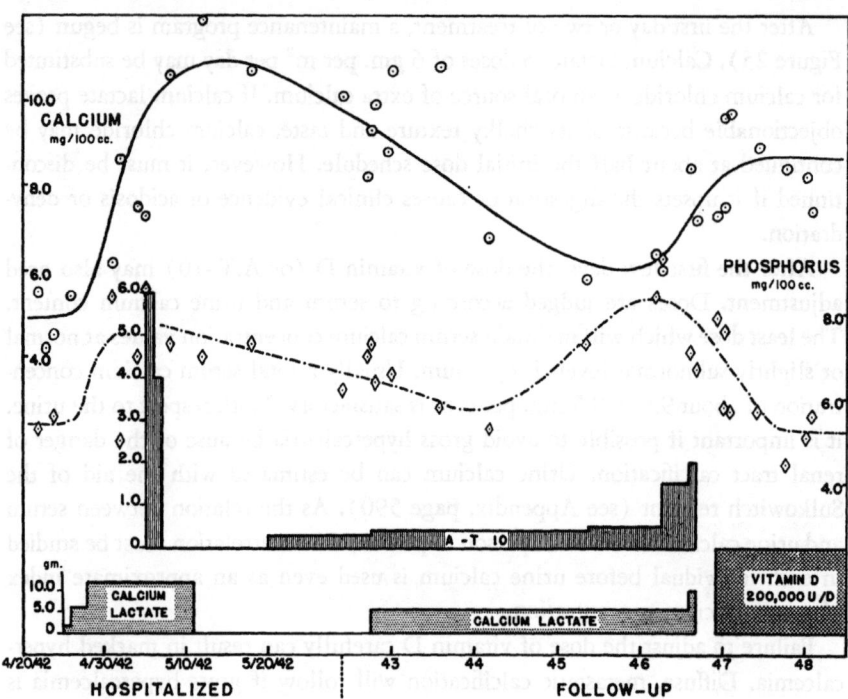

FIGURE II—25. Response to therapy in hypoparathyroidism. The data presented here are from a patient with pathologic hypoparathyroidism, with onset at 11 years of age. The left-hand ordinate gives values for serum calcium; the right-hand ordinate, values for serum inorganic phosphorus concentration. Note that the abscissa has two scales; the portion at the left gives intervals of 10 days, while the portion at the right gives yearly intervals.

CASE HISTORY

During the period of hospitalization values for serum calcium rose rapidly from tetany levels to supranormal values on large doses of A.T.-10 and calcium lactate. Therapy was discontinued for one week until serum calcium concentration had returned to normal. After the patient left the hospital, the doses of A.T.-10 and calcium lactate were increased gradually over the next four years. Despite this, values for serum calcium and phosphorus eventually returned toward pretreatment levels. In 1947 vitamin D in doses of 200,000 units per day was substituted for A.T.-10. Thereafter, calcium and phosphorus concentration values reverted toward normal, where they have been successfully maintained since. Note that, on both A.T.-10 and vitamin D therapy, serum inorganic phosphorus concentrations fail to fall to normal levels, presumably because neither agent is as effective as parathyroid hormone in promoting urinary phosphorus excretion.

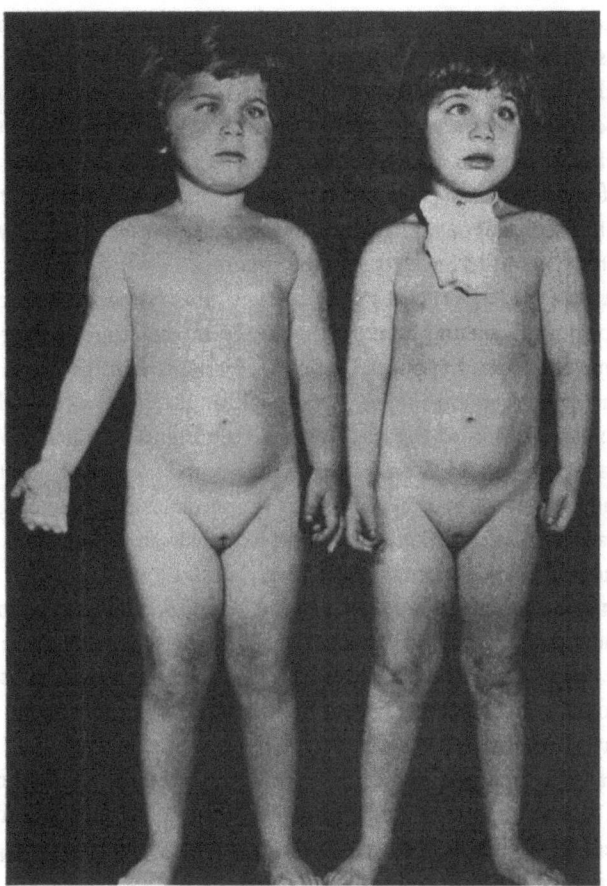

FIGURE II—26. Pseudo-hypoparathyroidism in twin sisters of five years. Note the moon-shaped faces, internal strabismus and moderate generalized obesity.

CASE HISTORY

Subcutaneous calcium plaques were observed in the abdominal walls of these children at birth. In the neonatal period they suffered tetanic convulsions, which were relieved by the administration of calcium. Later, with respiratory infection, they developed serious croup as a result of laryngeal spasm. Tracheotomy was performed on the girl at the right, after choking and cyanosis had been relieved by treatment. When the patients were admitted to the clinic one year later, serum analyses showed inorganic phosphorus concentrations of about 8 mg. per cent and calcium concentrations of about 6 mg. per cent. No increase in urinary phosphorus excretion occurred on administration of parathyroid extract (see Figure 24). Treatment with 1 cc. of A.T.-10 daily resulted in marked clinical improvement and return of serum chemical values to the normal range.

rise to certain symptoms (see Table 8). The pathogenesis of the two conditions, however, is quite distinct.

In pseudo-hypoparathyroidism there is no failure of the parathyroid glands. This has been demonstrated by biopsy of the glands of two patients.* Rather, there is refractoriness of the end organs, both renal and skeletal, to normal amounts of endogenously produced hormone. This is indicated by the fact that patients with pseudo-hypoparathyroidism fail to respond even to very large doses of administered parathyroid extract (see Figure 24).†

CLINICAL MANIFESTATIONS. Pseudo-hypoparathyroidism is characterized by a number of developmental defects which help in the clinical differentiation of the syndrome from true hypoparathyroidism. Patients with pseudo-hypoparathyroidism tend to have moon-shaped faces, strabismus, short necks and brachydactylia due to early fusion of the metacarpals (see Figures 26 and 27). They are obese and short in stature. Respiratory system signs are apt to be prominent in infancy, and central nervous system signs to appear as the patient grows older. Mental retardation is common, and, when coupled with strabismus and moon-face, produces in these patients a particularly stupid look.

Symptoms of hypocalcemia** usually date from the neonatal period. Palpable subcutaneous plaques and calcification of peripheral tendons are frequently found (see Figure 28). Roentgenograms reveal the bones to be coarsely trabeculated and sometimes considerably demineralized. On the other hand, the cortical shadow may be unusually dense, as in true hypoparathyroidism.

Incidentally, congenital defects are apt to be present in other members of the family. In one reported case deformities of the metacarpals similar to those of the patient were present in the mother. The family history of twin girls treated in this clinic included deaf-mutism in a maternal uncle.

DIAGNOSIS. The diagnosis of pseudo-hypoparathyroidism is confirmed by demonstrating refractoriness to administered parathyroid extract. The details of the test are outlined in the section dealing with the diagnosis of true hypoparathyroidism (see page 107). In pseudo-hypoparathyroidism parathyroid extract

---

* In one case the biopsy showed histologic evidence of normal activity; in the other, evidence of hyperfunction. In the first case the biopsy was obtained six months after the abnormal serum calcium and phosphorus concentrations had been corrected by appropriate therapy. Thus the stimuli to increased parathyroid function had long been absent. In the second case, where the biopsy was obtained very soon after treatment had been started, hyperplasia was in evidence.

† Comparable instances of end organ refractoriness are encountered in patients with "nephrogenic diabetes insipidus" (Chapter VIII) and in the failure of beard development in the American Indian (Chapter VI).

**The cerebral edema accompanying hypocalcemia may be responsible, at least in part, for the mental retardation. Marked convergent strabismus may result from pressure on the sixth oculomotor nerve in its exposed course over the base of the skull.

The Parathyroids

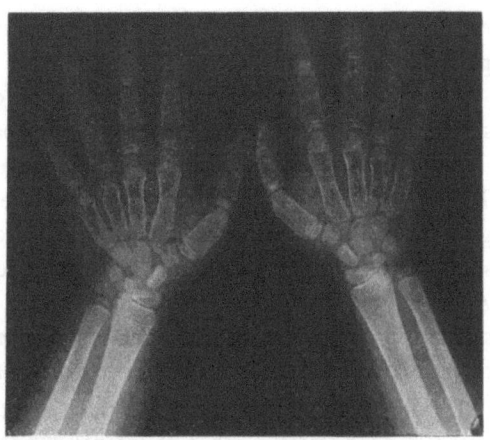

FIGURE II—27. Roentgenograms of the hands in pseudo-hypoparathyroidism. The trabeculation of all the bones is coarse. Note the beginning fusion of the metaphyses and epiphyses of the fourth metacarpals.

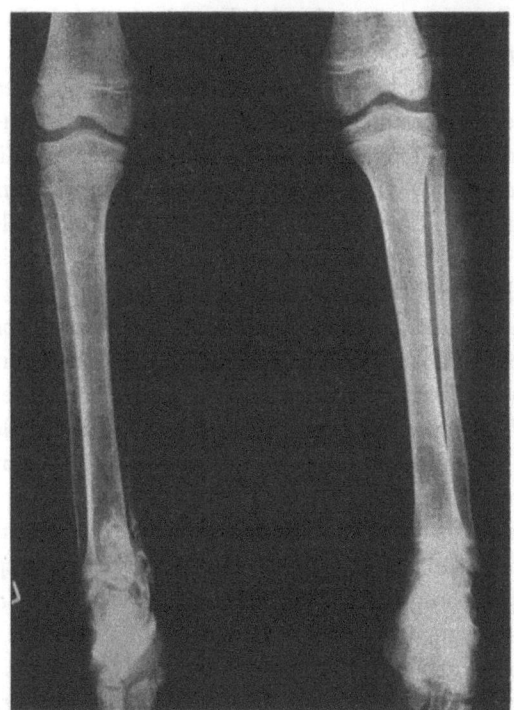

FIGURE II—28. Metastatic calcification in pseudo-hypoparathyroidism. Note the irregular calcium deposits in the tendons of the calf muscles of the leg at the left. The tendons of the other leg are not involved.

causes essentially no change in phosphorus clearance or urinary calcium and phosphorus content.

TREATMENT. In all respects treatment of pseudo-hypoparathyroidism is similar to that discussed earlier for true hypoparathyroidism.

PROGNOSIS. If adequate therapy is given, the prognosis for life is good. Tetanic seizures and croup may confidently be expected to disappear. The twin girls treated in this clinic have been relieved of petit mal epileptic attacks and show marked improvement in mentality as judged by the IQ determinations. Another child, in whom treatment was begun earlier in life, has failed to show satisfactory improvement in mental ability even though the cerebral edema incident to decreased serum calcium concentration has been relieved.

Tetany of the newborn.[23 a-c] This is a transient, semipathologic condition noted in a moderate number of infants during the neonatal period. Though it usually occurs within the first week of life, it has been reliably reported as early as the day of birth and as late as the eighth week after birth. In our experience it has occurred most commonly at about the seventh day of life.

The clinical manifestations of the disease are due to hypocalcemia. In association with this there is often a marked tendency to hyperphosphatemia. Incidentally, while hyperphosphatemia of some degree is a common finding in newborn infants, tetany occurs only when there is simultaneous hypocalcemia. The serum alkaline phosphatase and non-protein nitrogen concentration values are normal or nearly so and roentgenograms reveal no abnormalities in the skeleton.

ETIOLOGY. In size fetal parathyroid glands vary inversely with maternal serum calcium and directly with maternal serum phosphorus concentration.[23 d] In maternal hypoparathyroidism (parathyroidectomy) the serum calcium concentrations of the fetus are maintained at more nearly normal levels than those of the mother.[23 e] Parathyroid extract prompts marked hypercalcemia[23 f] when injected into the fetus, but has little effect on fetal serum calcium concentration when injected into the mother.[23 g]

These observations suggest the following conclusions: (1) the parathyroid gland of the fetus, like that of fully developed individuals, responds to hypocalcemia and hyperphosphatemia by increased secretory activity. (2) Under certain circumstances such secretory activity may be called upon to regulate the concentrations of calcium and phosphorus in the fetal circulation. (3) Although maternal parathyroid hormone fails to pass the placental barrier, maternal and fetal serum calcium and phosphorus are in equilibrium. (4) Hence little parathyroid activity ordinarily is required of the fetus, because maternal factors act to maintain fetal serum calcium and phosphorus concentrations within physiologic limits. More activity is demanded of the fetal parathyroids in maternal hypoparathyroidism; essentially none is required in maternal hyperparathyroidism.

As a result of the fact that there is essentially no load on the fetal parathyroids during normal pregnancy, the glands are relatively atrophic at birth.[23 h] This anatomic observation is supported by metabolic studies which indicate that the parathyroid glands of the newborn infant have only a very limited ability to correct tendencies toward hyperphosphatemia or hypocalcemia by increased parathyroid hormone production. Administration of a high phosphate meal to a newborn infant fails to increase renal phosphorus clearance sufficiently to prevent marked hyperphosphatemia.[23 c, i] However, clearance can be increased by administration of parathyroid extract (see Figure 24). This finding is interpreted to mean that the failure of the newborn to show a rise in phosphorus clearance upon developing hyperphosphatemia is due to failure to increase parathyroid hormone production rather than to renal refractoriness to parathyroid hormone action. Incidentally, even though the glomerular filtration rate of the newborn (50,000 cc. per m^2 per day)[23 j] is only half that of older children and adults, it potentially allows for the urinary excretion of 3,000 mg. of phosphorus per m^2 per day at a serum phosphorus concentration of 6 mg. per cent under conditions of maximal parathyroid hormone effect (TRP/GFP=0, see page 61).

Immediately after birth the infant's parathyroid glands must assume the major responsibility for maintaining serum calcium and phosphorus concentrations within their normal ranges. However, before they reach full efficiency in this regard the glands must develop anatomically and functionally under the stimuli provided by postnatal living. When the infant is breast-fed, this postnatal adaptation usually proceeds without noteworthy incident. When cow's milk is used instead of human milk, serious disturbances in calcium and phosphorus homeostasis can occur.

These differences in infantile response to feeding are explained by differences in the chemical composition of human and cow's milk. Human milk contains about 340 mg. of calcium and 150 mg. of phosphorus per liter. In cow's milk there are about 1,220 mg. of calcium and 900 mg. of phosphorus per liter. The calcium to phosphorus ratio of human milk (2.25 to 1) is considerably higher than that of cow's milk (1.35 to 1).

Infants fed adequate calories in the form of human milk take in about 350 mg. of phosphorus per m^2 per day. If cow's milk is substituted for human milk the phosphorus intake is increased to about 1,600 mg. per m^2 per day. Of the phosphorus ingested, a smaller portion is assimilated when the Ca/P ratio is high than when it is low. An estimate of phosphorus assimilation can be had by assuming that values for urine phosphorus output are roughly proportional to values for phosphorus absorption. The urinary excretion of breast-fed babies is about 120 mg. of phosphorus per m² per day, while that of formula-fed babies is about 1,200 mg.[23 k, 1] Thus breast-fed infants actually assimilate only about one-tenth as much phosphorus as infants fed cow's milk.

Clinical studies indicate that the normal breast-fed infant is not apt to develop hyperphosphatemia or hypocalcemia. By contrast, babies given cow's milk formulas during the neonatal period frequently show a marked elevation in serum inorganic phosphorus concentration. When this is accompanied by marked hypocalcemia, tetany becomes clinically evident.

The selective occurrence of neonatal tetany is of interest in these connections. It is met with much more frequently in formula-fed than in breast-fed infants. We have seen two infants born of hyperparathyroid mothers develop the syndrome early (on the second day of life) and in unusually severe form. Other instances are reported in the literature.[23 m, n] We have been unable to find reports of any cases occurring in infants born of hypoparathyroid mothers.

It is concluded that full-term infants are meant to ingest human, not cow's milk. If they are given human milk they rarely develop signs of hypocalcemic tetany. Thus, in the strictest sense, they rarely suffer from lack of parathyroid hormone. Moreover, it appears that during the neonatal period, the parathyroid glands, like the central nervous system, kidneys and other organs, may be functionally immature and incapable of adult-type activity. As a result, when infants are placed under the unnatural strain of a high phosphorus cow's milk regimen, their parathyroid glands may for a time be unable to accomplish their normal homeostatic purpose of preventing hyperphosphatemia and hypocalcemia.

CLINICAL MANIFESTATIONS. The symptoms and signs of tetany in newborn infants are fundamentally those outlined above for older children with primary hypoparathyroidism (page 103). Central nervous system signs, including hyperirritability, jitteriness, localized twitchings or generalized convulsions predominate. Laryngeal signs are uncommon.

DIAGNOSIS. The diagnosis is established by the chemical measurements as outlined above (see Table 9).

Whenever an infant is suspected of hypocalcemic tetany in the neonatal period, very rapid confirmation of the diagnosis usually may be had by (a) obtaining blood for serum phosphorus, total protein and NPN analysis, (b) obtaining an electrocardiogram and (c) administering by slow intravenous injection from 5 to 10 cc. of calcium gluconate (10 per cent solution). The former chemical determinations can be completed in the course of 30 minutes. Incidentally, blood should be obtained at the same time for calcium analysis, but this determination cannot be made accurately in so short a period as half an hour.

In tetany of the newborn the serum phosphorus is often 10 mg. per cent or higher, the NPN is 70 mg. per cent or lower and the electrocardiogram shows prolongation of the Q-T interval (see Figure 29). In addition, the serum ionized calcium as determined from total serum calcium and protein measurements is in the tetany range (see Figure 1). Intravenous administration of calcium (page 110) to patients with this condition causes the signs of tetany to disappear within a few minutes. It fails to exert a definite beneficial influence in the absence of hypocalcemia.

DIFFERENTIAL DIAGNOSIS. In young infants the differential diagnoses to be considered relate largely to other causes of convulsions and other causes of hypocalcemia.

In the neonatal period intracranial hemorrhages including subdural hematoma may give a similar picture. The symptoms of meningitis also may be confused with hypocalcemic seizures. These intracranial diseases are ruled out by lumbar puncture and subdural taps. Occasional infants are found to be suffering from both tetany of the newborn and a condition such as subdural hematoma. In one instance the latter condition was suspected by an alert house officer because the infant failed to become normally responsive following correction of his hypocalcemia. A sizable hematoma was discovered by subdural taps. In these connections it is interesting to note that quite typical carpopedal spasm has been noted in infants suffering from meningitis without hypocalcemia.

The chief alternate cause of hyperphosphatemia and hypocalcemia during the neonatal period is renal failure. These changes may be due simply to dehydration with circulatory collapse and functional impairment of renal activity (so-called pre-renal azotemia). It may also be a manifestation of congenital renal deformities such as polycystic or atretic kidneys. Under these circumstances the serum non-protein nitrogen is apt to be elevated to values of 80 mg. per cent or more. When renal failure is a result of dehydration, restoration of fluid balance will bring about a subsidence of the azotemia and hyperphosphatemia within one or two days.

The possibility of hypocalcemia should be thought of in infants with laryngeal stridor. Congenital defects and deformities such as redundant aryepiglottic folds, micro-larynx, vascular ring about the trachea, micrognathia, faulty regulation of the swallowing reflexes due to severe central nervous system defects and laryngeal infections are more likely diagnoses. However, they may be simulated in many respects by hypocalcemic laryngospasm. They occasionally occur in combination.

TREATMENT. Since the condition is self-limited in duration, treatment is relatively easy. At first 10 cc. of 10 per cent calcium gluconate may be given intravenously over a period of several minutes (see also page 110).

The purpose of subsequent therapy is to reduce the quantity of phosphorus and increase the quantity of calcium absorbed from the gastrointestinal tract. The intake of phosphorus in formula-fed infants can be reduced by substituting human for cow's milk. Alternatively, it can be managed by diluting cow's milk and adding to it calcium lactate or aluminum hydroxide (see also page 91), which tend to increase fecal phosphate excretion. Satisfactory diets for infants with neonatal tetany are as follows:

1. Human milk
2. Modified formula:

Whole cow's milk	250 cc.
Water	250 cc.
Sugar	40 gm.
to which is added either	
(a) calcium lactate	4 gm.
(b) aluminum hydroxide gel	15 cc.

The addition of calcium chloride to the foregoing regimen ordinarily is not necessary. In cases of unusual severity it may be added to the daily formula in doses of 1 to 1.5 grams. In young infants, as in older patients, it is likely to cause marked acidosis and hence to produce diuresis and dehydration. It should not be used for more than 24 hours without checking for these disturbances. Heavy vitamin D or A.T.-10 treatment appears unnecessary, but prophylactic doses of vitamin D (600 to 800 I.U. daily) should be given.

PROGNOSIS. In most cases the prognosis is probably excellent, since the normal infant's capacity to handle large phosphorus loads increases rapidly during the first months of life. However, it is possible that severe, prolonged episodes of hypocalcemic convulsions occurring during the transient period of neonatal hypoparathyroidism may, by inducing anoxemia of several minutes' duration, lead to permanent brain damage.

Tetany of healing rickets. This is now an uncommon disease. Its physiology has already been discussed in an earlier section (page 77). It is enough to say here that when small doses of vitamin D are given in active vitamin D deficiency rickets they suppress parathyroid function without prompting sufficient extra gastrointestinal calcium assimilation and renal phosphorus excretion to maintain normal serum concentrations of these elements. Hypocalcemia, hyperphosphatemia and tetany develop in consequence. The clinical manifestations of this form of tetany bear a close resemblance to those of primary hypoparathyroidism

The Parathyroids

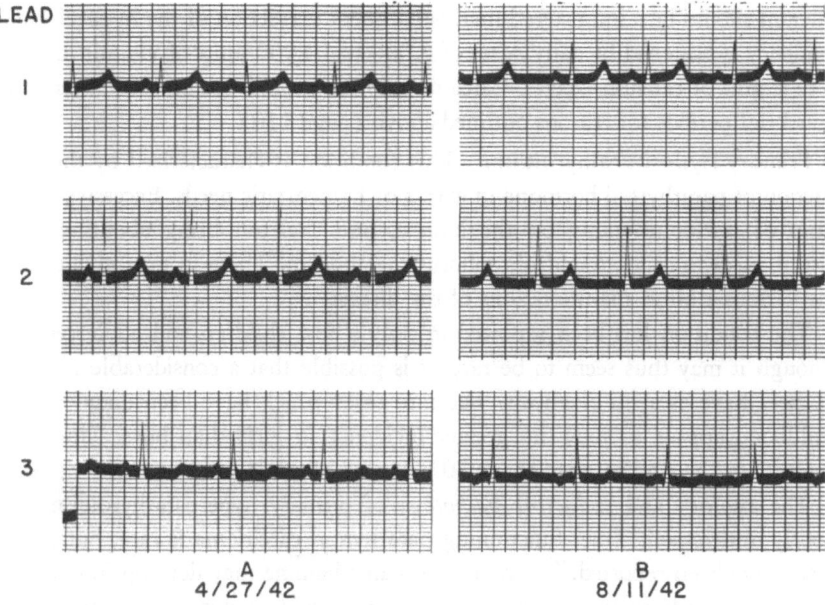

FIGURE II—29. Electrocardiographic changes in hypocalcemia (serum calcium 6.5 mg. per 100 cc.): The Q-T interval is prolonged in hypocalcemia and returns to normal when hypocalcemia is corrected. The time of the Q-T interval must be related to the cardiac rate for interpretation in any given case. A convenient nomogram is available for this purpose; see Kissin et al., Am. Heart J. 35:990, 1948. Serial electrocardiograms taken during return of serum calcium from low to normal levels are illustrated in a publication of Barker et al., Am. Heart J. 14:82, 1937.

(Table 8). Convulsive seizures and laryngeal disturbances predominate. Roentgenograms indicate osteomalacia and rickets.

The chemical picture differs from that found in active rickets. The serum total calcium and serum ionized calcium values fall from the normal to the slightly subnormal levels which usually prevail during active, untreated rickets to definitely low levels. On the other hand, the serum inorganic phosphorus concentration simultaneously rises from the abnormally low levels characteristic of active rickets to normal or supranormal levels. The serum alkaline phosphatase activity remains elevated. The resultant picture is one of hypocalcemia, normal or elevated serum phosphorus concentration and hyperphosphatasemia. The serum non-protein nitrogen concentration is normal.

The management of this condition is much the same as that outlined above for childhood hypoparathyroidism. When clinical tetany is found, intravenous calcium should be administered first. Subsequent correction of the hypocalcemic tendency is hastened by daily doses of 8,000 to 10,000 units of vitamin D plus 3 to 6 gm. of calcium lactate. Calcium chloride should not be used except for very brief periods for reasons outlined above (page 110).

Primary Hyperparathyroidism. This condition is characterized by the production of parathyroid hormone in excess of homeostatic needs. Excessive quantities of hormone acting on the kidneys and skeleton bring about marked disturbances in calcium and phosphorus metabolism. These in turn give rise to the various clinical manifestations of the disease.

The condition has been reported in only a few children and adolescents.[24] Though it may thus seem to be rare, it is possible that a considerable number of cases have escaped diagnosis. The rare cases which have been diagnosed in childhood appear to show no greater incidence in girls than boys. This is in contrast to the finding that about 70 per cent of adult cases occur in women.

The *etiology* and *endocrine pathology* of primary hyperparathyroidism are poorly understood. True, functioning parathyroid carcinoma is rare, but a few cases have been reported.[24 b, c] Sometimes an adenoma may develop in one and very occasionally in two or more of the parathyroid glands and, alternatively, diffuse hyperplasia of all parathyroid tissue may develop without adenoma formation. Marked differences in cytology appear in individual cases of adenoma or diffuse hyperplasia. The occurrence of the latter suggests that the term "primary" hyperparathyroidism may be a misnomer and that hyperfunction in these cases is secondary to extrinsic factors. Some still obscure relations between parathyroid function and other endocrine systems have been discussed previously (page 78). The possibility that abnormal diets taken over prolonged periods play a role in the pathogenesis of hyperparathyroidism is indicated by the experiments discussed in the introductory sections (page 66 and Figure 7).

CLINICAL MANIFESTATIONS. The symptoms and signs of hyperparathyroidism can be divided into groups as they relate to (a) manifestations of hypercalcemia, (b) urinary tract disturbances, (c) skeletal defects and (d) miscellaneous findings.

Hypercalcemia leads to hypotonia, lassitude, a sense of mental depression, constipation and a vague sense of ill health. In addition, if hypercalcemia becomes marked, there may be slowing of the heart, irregularity of the pulse beat, vomiting, dizziness and coma. The latter manifestations may terminate fatally. Minimal symptoms are produced when total serum calcium concentration values exceed about 11.5 mg. per cent; they increase in severity as the serum calcium concentration climbs to levels of about 16 mg. per cent.

Urinary tract disturbances may be divided into two groups, those due to effects of the hormone on the renal tubule epithelium and those due to stone formation in the urinary collecting passages. The most prominent symptoms of the former group are polyuria and polydipsia.

There is a poorly understood tendency for parathyroid hormone to increase the urinary excretion of water, inorganic base (in addition to calcium) and chloride. This action is seen in normal individuals after administration of parathyroid extract, as well as in some patients with pathologic hyperparathyroidism. The increased output of water is manifested by a very low urine specific gravity. This hyposthenuria appears to be relatively unresponsive to posterior pituitary extract. In this connection it is of interest to speculate whether these phenomena in hyperparathyroidism are in any way related to similar phenomena observed in hyperadrenocorticism (see Chapter III, page 153).

Formation of stones in the urinary collecting passages is variable and dependent not only upon the amount of calcium and phosphorus being excreted, but upon the alkalinity and volume of the urine as well. Stones form most readily when the concentrations of calcium and phosphorus are high and the urine is of alkaline pH.

Renal colic due to calcium phosphate stone formation may be a prominent complaint in hyperparathyroidism. Calcium phosphate and calcium oxalate stones are common in hyperparathyroid patients. In x-ray films calcium phosphate stones may be of staghorn appearance, filling the major and minor renal pelvices. Occasionally, staghorn stones are composed chiefly of cystine. By x-ray cystine stones have a homogenous, waxlike appearance. They occur in patients with cystinuria, which can be detected by appropriate analysis of the urine (see Appendix). Phosphate stones are apt to grow by surface apposition. Hence in x-rays they often show a lamellar structure. Calcium oxalate stones have a snowflake appearance, with spicules radiating from a central focus. Uric acid stones do not show up in x-ray films.

Infection of the urinary tract secondary to stone formation is common. Stone formation, infection and calcification of the renal parenchyma together may produce gross limitation in renal function. The resultant clinical manifestations are like those of any patient with shrunken, scarred kidneys (pannephritis).

Skeletal disturbances may or may not be evident. When present they may be characterized by tenderness and pain over bones and joints like those observed in patients with arthritis or neuritis. The legs and hips are especially apt to be involved. Moreover, marked bony deformities of the legs, pelvis and arms may occur as a result of skeletal decalcification. Knock-knee has been a chief present-

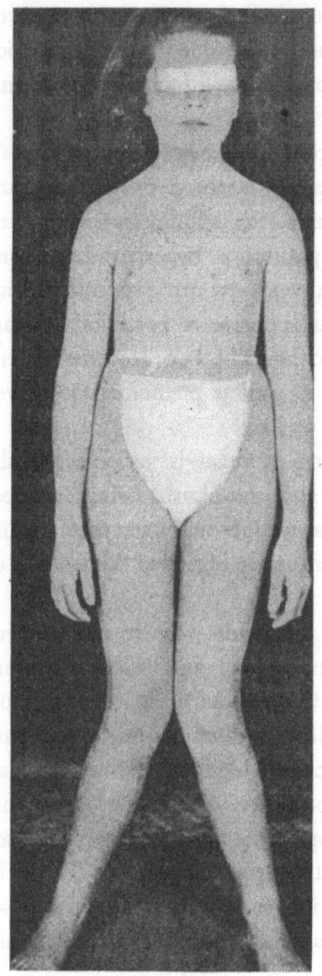
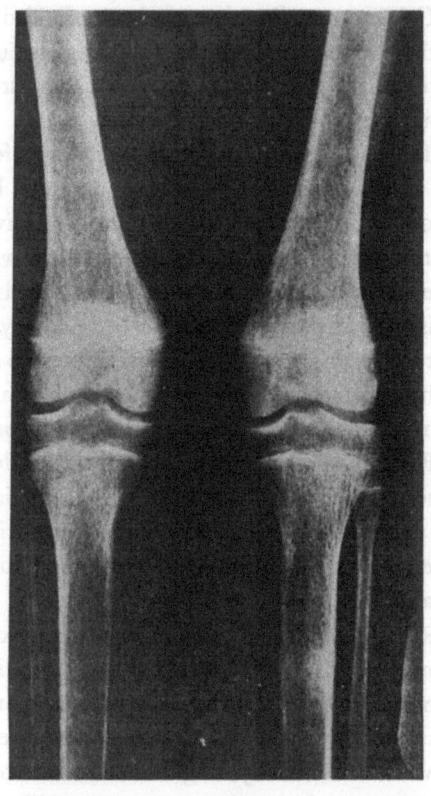

(Right)
FIGURE II—31. Roentgenogram of the knees of the patient in Figure 30, showing diffuse skeletal demineralization. The loss of bone salt from the fibulæ has been so marked that the x-ray shadow is barely visible.

(Left)
FIGURE II—30. Skeletal deformities in primary hyperparathyroidism in a girl of 12 years.

CASE HISTORY

The patient developed the severe genu valgum deformity illustrated within approximately one year. Serum analysis on hospital admission showed values of 15.3 mg. per cent for serum calcium, 2.61 mg. per cent for serum inorganic phosphorus, and 6.37 B.U. per cent for alkaline phosphatase concentration. Roentgenograms showed diffuse skeletal demineralization (see Figure 31). At operation a parathyroid adenoma was found and removed. Follow-up studies showed return to normal of serum calcium and phosphorus concentration values. Correction of the deformity at the knees occurred spontaneously over a five-year period.

Figures 30 and 31 are from R. D. McClure and C. R. Lam, *Ann. Surg.* 121:454, 1945.

ing complaint (see Figure 30). Kyphosis and scoliosis may be noted and with them shrinkage of stature. Bony tumors are seen. Spontaneous fracture may result from an underlying bone cyst.

Miscellaneous clinical findings include loss of hair, palpable tumor in the region of one of the parathyroid glands, purpura, cessation of menstrual periods, laxness of tendons and a wobbly gait.

ROENTGENOGRAPHY. Valuable additional information may be obtained from roentgenograms. In some patients the skeleton is found to be free from obvious defects. In others there is gross decalcification, the degree of which varies with the severity and duration of the disease.

Skeletal demineralization is always diffuse. This is evident in films of long bones, pelvis, spine and skull (Figure 31). The epiphyses and also the shafts of the long bones can be almost completely decalcified. Coarseness of trabeculation is characteristic. Displacement of the epiphyses may be evident. The skull and pelvis are apt to have a finely granular appearance with miliary areas of decalcification on the one hand and of nearly normal calcium deposition on the other. The spinal vertebræ may show relatively dense lines adjacent to the intervertebral discs while their midportions are unusually radiant. Loss of the lamina dura about the teeth is another familiar sign. This is not pathognomonic of primary hyperparathyroidism, however, since it may be observed in patients who have suffered demineralization for other reasons. Finally there may be multiple bone cysts, tumors, fractures and gross deformities of the skeleton.

Roentgenograms of the abdomen may reveal renal tract calculi. Punctate deposits of calcium salts are often visible in the renal parenchyma. Barium studies of the esophagus may aid in localizing mediastinally located parathyroid tumors.

LABORATORY STUDIES. Certain laboratory tests are necessary to the diagnosis. These include determinations of serum phosphorus and calcium concentration values. Except when renal function is impaired by diminution in glomerular filtration rate (Figure 2, Section E), or the phosphorus from dietary intake or from skeletal catabolism is extraordinarily large (Figure 2, Section C), patients with primary hyperparathyroidism are hypophosphatemic.

In adults with uncomplicated primary hyperparathyroidism serum phosphorus values range between about 1.5 and 3.5 mg. per cent. In children, whose serum phosphorus values (3.5 to 4.5 mg. per cent) are normally a little higher than those of adults (3.0 to 4.0 mg. per cent), values up to 3.8 or 3.9 mg. per cent may be considered unusually low. It is important to use blood samples collected under conditions of fasting for these determinations, because changes in glycogenesis and glucose metabolism occurring after meals can cause an appreciable lowering of serum phosphorus values.

The renal impairment can be recognized by measurement of the urea clearance and may be reflected by the presence of acidosis and nitrogen retention. When one wishes to determine whether, as a consequence of a renal excretory limitation, the serum phosphorus is elevated above the level intended by the parathyroids, the patient should be placed on a low but adequate phosphorus diet (300 mg. of phosphorus per m^2 per day) for several days.

Where no limitation in renal phosphorus excretion is present, there will be initially a rapid fall in serum phosphorus concentration, sometimes to very low levels. This is a consequence of the period of time (24 hours or more) necessary for the glands to complete adaptation to a marked change in phosphorus intake (see Figure 8). The first fall in serum phosphorus concentration normally will be superseded by a gradual rise to a stable level. This equilibration should be complete within three days. A latent tendency to hypophosphatemia in a patient with pathologic hyperparathyroidism and severe renal disease becomes manifest in the course of such a test.

The occurrence of hypophosphatemia indicates hyper-parathyroid-hormonism. Whether this is of the physiologic rather than the pathologic type is indicated by the serum calcium concentration. In patients with pathologic primary hyperparathyroidism, total serum calcium values are abnormally elevated to levels which range from 11.5 to about 17 mg. per cent. The calculated values for serum ionized calcium also are pathologically high and in the hyperparathyroid range (see Figure 1). By contrast, total serum calcium is either normal or abnormally low in patients with physiologic hyper-parathyroid-hormonism (see page 84).

Urine phosphorus clearance values are apt to be unusually high in patients with hyperparathyroidism. This results in a large phosphorus output despite a low serum phosphorus concentration. Urine calcium excretion values also are apt to be large (> 200 mg. per m^2 per day) even after the calcium intake has been restricted for three or more days by omission of fish, milk and all milk products (see Table 10).

The serum alkaline phosphatase activity is abnormally elevated when skeletal disease is present (osteoblastic activity $++$). Except when there is renal impairment, serum total protein and non-protein nitrogen values are normal. Anemia and leukopenia secondary to fibrosis of the bone marrow may be present.

Examination of the urine will give variable results, depending upon the degree of renal tract damage. There are apt to be calcium phosphate casts in the urine. In addition, if calculi or infections are present, red cells, white cells, bacteria and albumin may be found.

DIAGNOSIS. The diagnosis is suggested by any one or more of various sets of symptoms: (a) skeletal deformities, cysts, tumors, fractures, (b) renal colic,

TABLE II—10. Low calcium diet. From F. Albright and E. C. Reifenstein, *The Parathyroid Glands and Metabolic Bone Disease,* Baltimore, Williams & Wilkins, 1948.

    Morning: Orange juice—1 small glass
                Cooked farina or rice—⅓ cup after cooking
                Oleomargarine
                3 strips of crisp bacon
                Gingerale, coffee, or tea
                Salt and sugar

    Noon: Lean meat—medium-sized serving
            Potato—1 medium-sized
            White corn—½ cup
            4 Uneeda biscuits
            Oleomargarine
            Applesauce—½ cup; or 1 medium-sized apple
            Gingerale or tea
            Salt, pepper, sugar

    Night: Chicken—1 medium-sized serving
             Macaroni—⅓ cup (cooked)
            Canned tomato—½ cup
            4 Uneeda biscuits
            Oleomargarine
            Banana—1 medium-sized
            Gingerale, tea, or coffee
            Salt, pepper, sugar

Note: Use oleomargarine and sugar generously to keep up weight. Eliminate butter, milk, cheese and cream. This diet contains approximately 0.137 gm. of calcium. Caution must be exercised to avoid cereals and oleomargarine that have been fortified with additional calcium.

renal insufficiency, dysuria, polyuria, polydipsia or (c) unexplained lassitude, weakness and fatigue. The important point is that the disease varies widely in its manifestations. Patients may have only subtle and seemingly minor symptoms even when gross lesions are demonstrable in the skeleton or renal system. Thus primary hyperparathyroidism is a disease that easily can be missed unless specific steps are taken to establish the diagnosis, by means of the clinical, roentgenographic and chemical studies described in foregoing paragraphs.

DIFFERENTIAL DIAGNOSIS. Several of the diseases to be differentiated are indicated in Table 3. In addition, the following conditions should be considered. They may be grouped approximately according to serum calcium values.

Group A: Serum Calcium Normal

"Solitary," *idiopathic or congenital bone cysts* are distinguished from those due to hyperparathyroidism by the fact that the skeleton is otherwise normal. Paradoxically, these "solitary" bone cysts may be multiple.

Polyostotic fibrous dysplasia is a rare, non-metabolic bone disease seen in childhood. It is characterized by bone cysts and localized areas which show either demineralization or excess mineralization. The lesions tend to have a segmental distribution. The presence of some normal bone sharply distinguishes the condition from hyperparathyroidism, in which bone involvement is always generalized. Areas of cutaneous and buccal pigmentation also may be present. Female children with this disease usually show precocious sexual development (see Chapter V, page 327).

Solitary, benign giant-cell tumor is similarly distinguished by the absence of generalized demineralization and fibrosis.

Erythroblastic anemia. The roentgenographic appearance of the bones of patients with this condition may be confused with that of hyperparathyroidism. The diagnosis of the blood dyscrasia, however, should be obvious on inspection of stained smears of peripheral blood or bone marrow.

Osteogenesis imperfecta is a hereditary generalized bone disease in which multiple fractures often occur. Congenital defects including blue sclerae and deafness are present. It is characterized by a pathologic decrease in the rate of bone formation with a normal rate of bone absorption. Accordingly, bone biopsy specimens show no fibrosis of the type seen in the osteitis fibrosa of hyperparathyroidism.

Group B: Serum Calcium Elevated

Acute osteoporosis. Immobilization can result in such rapid release of calcium from affected areas that the excretory capacity of the kidneys is exceeded. Hypercalcemia results, but there is no deviation from normal of serum phosphorus or alkaline phosphatase values.

Vitamin D intoxication and the syndrome of hypercalcemia secondary to excessive milk and alkali intake are considered elsewhere (page 79). In these conditions serum calcium is elevated and serum phosphorus concentration is either normal or elevated.

Metastatic bone lesions are most commonly due to neuroblastoma. Renal cell carcinoma and multiple myeloma are other malignancies giving a similar picture. Sarcoidosis, though not strictly a metastatic bone lesion, is also included here. These conditions may be accompanied by marked hypercalcemia. In the last two conditions this is accompanied by an abnormal rise in serum protein and frequently, also, by slight elevation in serum phosphorus concentration. Unusual cases are encountered in which the serum phosphorus concentration is abnormally low. This type of disease is likewise differentiated from primary hyperparathyroidism by the localized character of the bone lesions as seen in roentgenograms and by biopsy examination.

TREATMENT. Attempts at medical therapy have been unrewarding. While administration of calcium may inhibit the development of bone disease, it automatically increases the likelihood of renal disease. The administration of phosphorus fails to produce an increase in serum phosphorus concentration or in body phosphate stores unless the amount given is so large as to exceed renal capacity for phosphorus excretion by normal means (see Figure 2, Section C). At high levels of intake phosphorus may cause renal stone formation. Attempts to bring about sustained improvement by x-ray treatment have been disappointing. Accordingly, the treatment of choice is surgical. It must be remembered, however, that parathyroid surgery requires expert and experienced personnel. The important thing from the medical point of view is not to remove too much parathyroid tissue.

Postoperatively, a marked drop in urine calcium and phosphorus excretion values is to be expected. This takes place within a few hours and persists for weeks or months until the bones become normally mineralized. The concentration of calcium in the serum also falls rapidly, and temporarily there may be a slight fall in serum phosphorus concentration. Patients with marked bone disease may pass through a transient phase of severe hypocalcemic tetany. Therapy for this complication is the same as that outlined above under neonatal tetany and tetany of healing rickets (page 120).

PROGNOSIS. Though the condition may recur, the prognosis following subtotal parathyroidectomy is usually quite good. There is marked improvement in general health and in sense of well-being. Improved appetite, weight gain and increase in energy, and loss of constipation, bone pain and bone tenderness are to be expected within a short time. Over a period of months there is likely to be a marked spontaneous improvement in skeletal deformities. For this reason, corrective orthopedic surgery should be postponed. Osteomas disappear slowly; bone cysts remain indefinitely. The prognosis for return of normal renal function must be guarded. Calcium deposits in the kidneys are reabsorbed very slowly if at all.

REFERENCES

General References
See below numbers 1-4.

Specific References

1   ALBRIGHT, F. and REIFENSTEIN, E. C., JR. *Parathyroid Glands and Metabolic Bone Disease.* Baltimore, Williams & Wilkins, 1948.

2   PINCUS, G. and THIMANN, K. V. *The Hormones: Physiology, Chemistry and Applications.* Vol. I. New York, Academic Press, 1948.

3   POPE, A. and AUB, J. C. Medical progress: the parathyroid glands and parathormone. *New Eng. J. Med.* 230:698, 1944.

4   SHELLING, D. H. *The Parathyroids in Health and Disease.* St. Louis, C. V. Mosby, 1935.

5 (a) ROSS, W. F. and WOOD, T. R. Partial purification and some observations on nature of parathyroid hormone. *J. Biol. Chem.* 146:49, 1942.
  (b) WOOD, T. R. and ROSS, W. F. Ketene acetylation of parathyroid hormone. *J. Biol. Chem.* 146:59, 1942.

6 (a) CASTLEMAN, B. and MALLORY, T. B. The pathology of the parathyroid gland in hyperparathyroidism; study of twenty-five cases. *Am. J. Path.* 11:1, 1935.
  (b) CASTLEMAN, B. and MALLORY, T. B. Parathyroid hyperplasia in chronic renal insufficiency. *Am. J. Path.* 13:553, 1937.

7 (a) HARRISON, H. E. and HARRISON, H. C. Renal excretion of inorganic phosphate in relation to action of vitamin D and parathyroid hormone. *J. Clin. Invest.* 20:47, 1941.
  (b) BRULL, L. and CARBUNESCU, G. L'Action de la parathyroide sur le rein. *Compt. rend. Soc. de biol.* 131:800, 1939.
  (c) ELLSWORTH, R. and FUTCHER, P. H. Effect of parathyroid extract upon serum calcium of nephrectomized dogs. *Bull. Johns Hopkins Hosp.* 57:91, 1935.
  (d) COLLIP, J. B., PUGSLEY, L. I., SELYE, H. and THOMSON, D. L. Observations concerning the mechanism of parathyroid hormone action. *Brit. J. Exper. Path.* 15:335, 1934.
  (e) MC JUNKIN, F. A., TWEEDY, W. R. and MC NAMARA, E. W. Effect of parathyroid extract and calciferol on tissues of nephrectomized rats. *Am. J. Path.* 13:325, 1937.
  (f) INGALLS, T. H., DONALDSON, G. A. and ALBRIGHT, F. Locus of action of parathyroid hormone: experimental studies with parathyroid extract on normal and nephrectomized rats. *J. Clin. Invest.* 22:603, 1943.

8   SMITH, H. W. *The Physiology of the Kidney.* New York, Oxford Univ. Press, 1937.

9 (a) CRAWFORD, J. D., OSBORNE, M. M., TALBOT, N. B. and TERRY, M. L. The parathyroid glands and phosphorus homeostasis. *J. Clin. Invest.* 29:1448, 1950.
  (b) BAUMAN, E. J. and SPRINSON, D. B. Hyperparathyroidism produced by diet. *Am. J. Physiol.* 125:741, 1939.
  (c) HAM, A. W., LITTNER, N., DRAKE, T. G., ROBERTSON, E. C. and TISDALL, F. F. Physiological hypertrophy of parathyroids; its cause and its relation to rickets. *Am. J. Path.* 16:277, 1940.
  (d) DRAKE, T. G., ALBRIGHT, F. and CASTLEMAN, B. Parathyroid hyperplasia in rabbits produced by parenteral phosphate administration. *J. Clin. Invest.* 16:203, 1937.

10 (a) BAUER, W., ALBRIGHT, F. and AUB, J. C. A case of osteitis fibrosa cystica (osteomalacia?) with evidence of hyperactivity of the parathyroid bodies; metabolic study. *J. Clin. Invest.* 8:229, 1930.
   (b) ALBRIGHT, F., BAUER, W., CLAFFLIN, D. and COCKRILL, J. R. Studies in parathyroid physiology; the effect of phosphate ingestion in clinical hyperparathyroidism. *J. Clin. Invest.* 11:411, 1932.
   (c) PEMBERTON, J. J. and GEDDIE, K. D. Hyperparathyroidism. *Ann. Surg.* 92:202, 1930.
   (d) ALBRIGHT, F., BAUER, W., ROPES, M. and AUB, J. C. Studies of calcium and phosphorus metabolism; the effects of the parathyroid hormone. *J. Clin. Invest.* 7:139, 1929.
   (e) ALBRIGHT, F. and ELLSWORTH, R. Studies on the physiology of the parathyroid glands; calcium and phosphorus studies on a case of idiopathic hypoparathyroidism. *J. Clin. Invest.* 7:183, 1929.
   (f) ALBRIGHT, F., BLOOMBERG, E., DRAKE, T. G. and SULKOWITCH, H. W. A comparison of the effects of A.T. 10 (dihydrotachysterol) and vitamin D on calcium and phosphorus metabolism in hypoparathyroidism. *J. Clin. Invest.* 17:317, 1938.

11 (a) TEMPLIN, V. M. and STEENBOCK, H. Vitamin D and the conservation of calcium in the adult; effect of vitamin D on calcium conservation in adult rats maintained on low calcium diets. *J. Biol. Chem.* 100:209, 1933.
   (b) BAUER, W. and MARBLE, A. Studies on the mode of action of irradiated ergosterol; its

effect on the calcium and phosphorus metabolism of individuals with calcium deficiency diseases. *J. Clin. Invest.* 11:21, 1932.
- (c) BAUER, W., ALBRIGHT, F. and AUB, J. C. Studies of calcium and phosphorus metabolism; the calcium excretion of normal individuals on a low calcium diet; also data on a case of pregnancy. *J. Clin. Invest.* 7:75, 1929.
- (d) STOERK, H. C. and CARNES, W. H. The relation of the dietary Ca:P ratio to serum Ca and to parathyroid volume. *J. Nutrition* 29:43, 1945.
- (e) CARNES, W. H., PAPPENHEIMER, A. M. and STOERK, H. C. Volume of parathyroid glands in relation to dietary calcium and phosphorus. *Proc. Soc. Exper. Biol. & Med.* 51:314, 1942.
- (f) LUCKHARDT, A. B. and GOLDBERG, B. Preservation of the life of completely parathyroidectomized dogs. *J. A. M. A.* 80:79, 1923.
- (g) BODANSKY, M. and DUFF, V. B. Effects of parathyroid deficiency and calcium and phosphorus of diet on pregnant rats. *J. Nutrition* 21:179, 1941.

12 (a) HOWLAND, J. and KRAMER, B. Factors concerned in the calcification of bone. *Tr. Am. Pediat. Soc.* 34:204, 1922.
- (b) SHOHL, A. T., FAN, C. H. and FARBER, S. Effect of A.T. 10 (dihydrotachysterol) on various types of experimental rickets in rats. *Proc. Soc. Exper. Biol. & Med.* 42:529, 1939.

13 (a) ALBRIGHT, F., SULKOWITCH, H. W. and BLOOMBERG, E. Comparison of effects of vitamin D, dihydrotachysterol (A.T. 10), and parathyroid extract on disordered metabolism of rickets. *J. Clin. Invest.* 18:165, 1939.
- (b) GUILD, H. G. Infantile tetany. In *Brennemann's Practice of Pediatrics*. Edited by I. McQuarrie. Hagerstown, Md., W. F. Prior, 1948.
- (c) ROBERTIS, E., DE Cytology of parathyroid and thyroid glands of rats with experimental rickets. *Anat. Rec.* 79:417, 1941.
- (d) LIU, S. H. A comparative study of the effects of various treatments on the calcium and phosphorus metabolism in tetany. *J. Clin. Invest.* 5:259, 1927.

14 (a) BODANSKY, M. Changes in serum calcium, inorganic phosphate and phosphatase activity in the pregnant woman. *Am. J. Clin. Path.* 9:36, 1939.
- (b) SINCLAIR, J. G. Size of parathyroid glands of albino rats as affected by pregnancy and controlled diets. *Anat. Rec.* 80:479, 1941.
- (c) OPPER, L. and THALE, T. Influence of pregnancy, hypervitaminosis-D and partial nephrectomy on volume of parathyroid glands in rats. *Am. J. Physiol.* 139:406, 1943.
- (d) ERDHEIM, J. Zur normalen und pathologischen Histologie der Glandula thyreoidea, parathyreoidea, und Hypophysis. *Beitr. z. path. Anat. u. z. allg. Path.* (Jena) 33:158, 1903.
- (e) CLAUDE, H. and BAUDOUIN, A. Étude histologique des glandes à sécrétion interne dans un cas d'acromégalie. *Compt. rend. Soc. de biol.* 71:75, 1911.
- (f) CUSHING, H. and DAVIDOFF, L. M. The pathological findings in four autopsied cases of acromegaly with a discussion of their significance. *Monographs of Rockefeller Inst. Med. Res.* No. 22, 1927.
- (g) HOUSSAY, B. A. Relations between the parathyroids, the hypophysis, and the pancreas. In *The Harvey Lectures, 1935-36*. Series 31:116. Lancaster, Science Press, 1936.
- (h) HERTZ, S. and KRANES, A. Parathyreotropic action of anterior pituitary: histologic evidence in rabbit. *Endocrinology* 18:350, 1934.
- (i) CASTLEMAN, B. and HERTZ, S. Pituitary fibrosis with myxedema. *Arch. Path.* 27:69, 1939.

15 (a) SHOHL, A. T. *Mineral Metabolism*. New York, Reinhold, 1939.
- (b) BURNETT, C. H., COMMONS, R. R., ALBRIGHT, F. and HOWARD, J. E. Hypercalcemia without hypercalcuria or hypophosphatemia, calcinosis and renal insufficiency. *New Eng. J. Med.* 240:787, 1949.

(c) TUMULTY, P. A. and HOWARD, J. E. Irradiated ergosterol poisoning; report of two cases. *J. A. M. A.* 119:233, 1942.
(d) FREEMAN, S., RHOADS, P. S. and YEAGER, L. B. Toxic manifestations associated with prolonged ertron ingestion. *J. A. M. A.* 130:197, 1946.
(e) KAUFMAN, P., BECK, R. D. and WISEMAN, R. D. Vitamin D (ertron) therapy in arthritis; treatment followed by massive, metastatic calcification, renal damage and death. *J. A. M. A.* 134:688, 1947.

16 (a) ROBISON, R. The possible significance of hexosephosphoric esters in ossification. *Biochem, J.* 17:286, 1947.
(b) HANNON, R. R., LIU, S. H., CHU, H. I., WANG, S. H., CHEN, K. C. and CHOU, S. K. Calcium and phosphorus metabolism in osteomalacia; the effect of vitamin D and its apparent duration. *Chinese M. J.* 48:623, 1934.
(c) LIU, S. H., HANNON, R. R., CHU, H. I., CHEN, K. C., CHOU, S. K. and WANG, S. H. Calcium and phosphorus metabolism in osteomalacia; further studies on the response to vitamin D of patients with osteomalacia. *Chinese M. J.* 49:1, 1935.
(d) MAXWELL, J. P. The modern conception of osteomalacia and its importance to China. *Chinese M. J.* 49:47, 1935.
(e) ELIOT, M. M. and PARK, E. A. Rickets. In *Brennemann's Practice of Pediatrics*. Edited by I. McQuarrie. Hagerstown, Md., W. F. Prior, 1948.
(f) ALBRIGHT, F., BUTLER, A. M. and BLOOMBERG, E. Rickets resistant to vitamin D therapy. *Am. J. Dis. Child.* 54:529, 1937.
(g) PARSONS, L. G. The bone changes occurring in renal and coeliac infantilism and their relationship to rickets; coeliac rickets. *Arch. Dis. Childhood* 2:198, 1927.

17 BARNEY, J. D. and SULKOWITCH, H. W. Progress in the management of urinary calculi. *J. Urol.* 37:746, 1937.

18 (a) MC CUNE, D. J., MASON, H. H. and CLARKE, H. T. Intractable hypophosphatemic rickets with renal glycosuria and acidosis (the Fanconi syndrome); report of case in which increased urinary organic acids were detected and identified, with review of literature. *Am. J. Dis. Child.* 65:81, 1943.
(b) LOWE, C. U., TERRY, M. L. and MAC LACHLAN, E. A. Organic aciduria, systemic acidosis, hydrophthalmia and mental retardation complicated by rickets: a clinical entity. (To be published.)

19 MC LEAN, F. C. and HASTINGS, A. B. The state of calcium in the fluids in the body. *J. Biol. Chem.* 108:285, 1935.

20 (a) ROSSLE, R. Das Verhalten von Syphilis und Tuberkulose in Familien. *Schweiz. med. Wchnschr.* 68:3, 1938.
(b) DRAKE, T. G., ALBRIGHT, F., BAUER, W. and CASTLEMAN, B. Chronic idiopathic hypoparathyroidism; report of six cases with autopsy findings in one. *Ann. Int. Med.* 12:1751, 1939.
(c) TALBOT, N. B., BUTLER, A. M. and MAC LACHLAN, E. A. The effect of testosterone and allied compounds on the mineral, nitrogen, and carbohydrate metabolism of a girl with Addison's disease. *J. Clin. Invest.* 22:583, 1943.

21 ELLSWORTH, R. and HOWARD, J. E. Studies on the physiology of the parathyroid glands; some responses of normal human kidneys and blood to intravenous parathyroid extract. *Bull. Johns Hopkins Hosp.* 55:296, 1934.

22 ALBRIGHT, F., BURNETT, C. H., SMITH, P. H. and PARSON, W. Pseudo-hypoparathyroidism—an example of Seabright-Bantam syndrome; report of three cases. *Endocrinology* 30:922, 1942.

23 (a) GARDNER, L. I., MAC LACHLAN, E. A., PICK, W., TERRY, M. L. and BUTLER, A. M. Etiologic factors in tetany of newly born infants. *Pediatrics* 5:228, 1950.

(b) DODD, K. and RAPOPORT, S. Hypocalcemia in the neonatal period. *Am. J. Dis. Child.* 78:537, 1949.
(c) BAKWIN, H. Pathogenesis of tetany of the newborn. *Am. J. Dis. Child.* 54:1211, 1937.
(d) SINCLAIR, J. G. Fetal rat parathyroids as affected by changes in maternal serum calcium and phosphorus through parathyroidectomy and dietary control. *J. Nutrition* 23:141, 1942.
(e) SATO, Y. Calcium metabolism of the fetus. *J. Chosen M. A.* 28:44, 1938.
(f) HOSKINS, F. M. and SNYDER, F. F. Calcium content of maternal and foetal blood serum following injection of parathyroid extract in foetuses in utero. *Proc. Soc. Exper. Biol. & Med.* 25:264, 1928.
(g) HOSKINS, F. M. and SNYDER, F. F. Placental transmission of parathyroid extract. *Am. J. Physiol.* 104:530, 1933.
(h) KAPLAN, E. Parathyroid gland in infancy. *Arch. Path.* 34:1042, 1942.
(i) DEANE, R. F. and MC CANCE, R. A. Phosphate clearances in infants and adults. *J. Physiol.* 107:182, 1948.
(j) BARNETT, H. L. Kidney function in young infants. *Pediatrics* 5:171, 1950.
(k) CZERNY, A. and KELLER, A. *Des Kindes Ernährung, Ernährungsstörungen und Ernährungstherapie.* 2d ed. Leipzig and Vienna, F. Deuticke, 1928.
(l) NELSON, M. V. K. Calcium and phosphorus metabolism of infant receiving undiluted cow's milk. *Am. J. Dis. Child.* 42:1090, 1931.
(m) FRIDERICHSEN, C. Hypocalcämie bie einem Brustkind und Hypercalcämie bie der Mutter. *Monatschr. f. Kinderh.* 75:146, 1938.
(n) SCHWARTZER, K. Uber die Blutkalkregulation beim Neugeborenen. *Klin. Wchnschr.* 19:107, 1940.

24 (a) PHILLIPS, R. N. Primary diffuse parathyroid hyperplasia in an infant of 4 months. *Pediatrics* 2:428, 1948.
(b) MEYER, K. A., ROSI, P. A. and RAGINS, A. B. Carcinoma of parathyroid gland. *Surgery* 6:190, 1939.
(c) GENTILE, R. J., SKINNER, H. L. and ASHBURN, L. L. Parathyroid glands; malignant tumor with osteitis fibrosa cystica. *Surgery* 10:793, 1941.

THE ADRENAL CORTICES

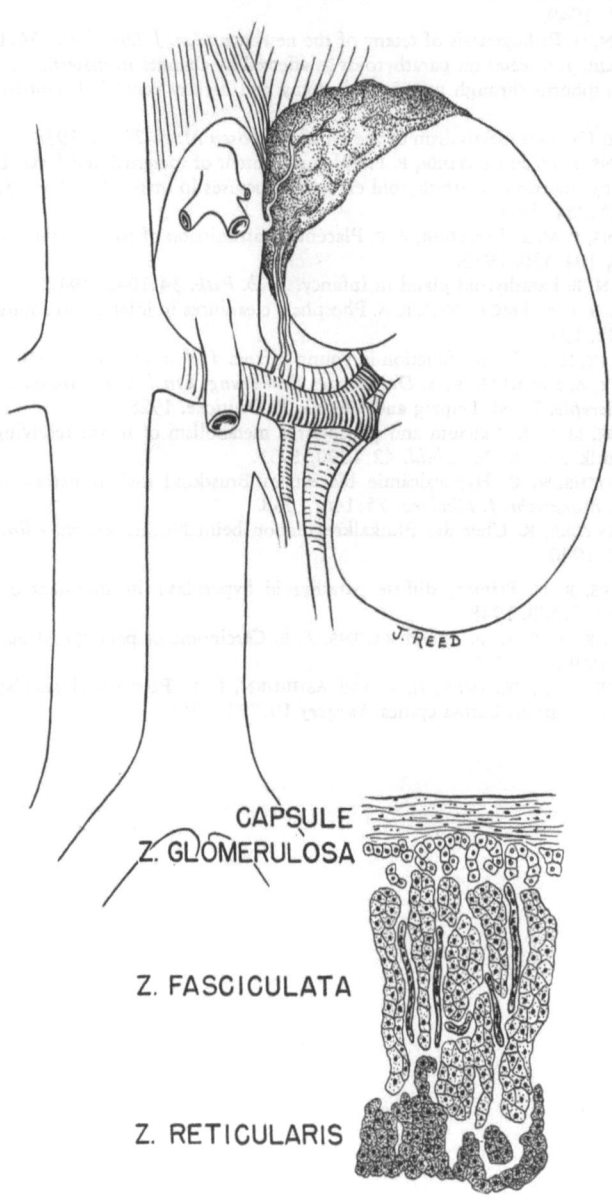

CHAPTER III

THE ADRENAL CORTICES

BASIC CONSIDERATIONS

The adrenal cortex is comprised of three approximately defined zones: the glomerulosa (outer), fasciculata (middle) and reticularis (inner layer). In broad terms, adrenocortical hormones also can be separated into three chief types, namely, those which (a) influence the metabolism of certain electrolytes and water, (b) alter sugar, fat and protein metabolism and (c) induce sex hair growth and acne. Under abnormal circumstances the adrenal cortices also may secrete appreciable amounts of androgens, estrogens and other types of hormone. There is some evidence that type (a) originates in the zona glomerulosa, type (b) in the fasciculata, and type (c) in the reticularis. Thus, this gland almost can be considered as three organs in one, each with a special function.

The adrenal cortex bears an important relation to the anterior pituitary, which secretes one and possibly two adrenocorticotropic hormones (ACTH). In the absence of ACTH the adrenal cortex involutes and becomes inactive; when stimulated by ACTH, it enlarges and secretes its hormones into the circulation.

CHEMISTRY OF THE HORMONES

Adrenocortical hormones have a steroidal configuration like that of cholesterol, from which they are probably derived. Over 30 different but closely related steroids have been isolated from animal adrenal glands.[1] Only a few of the compounds are of current clinical interest. Representative formulas are given below.

Compound I is 11-desoxycorticosterone. As shown in the figure the 11-desoxy designation indicates that this compound has no oxygen atom attached to carbon 11. Its acetate is desoxycorticosterone acetate, or DOCA, which can be synthesized and is available commercially. Substances of this type are also contained in aqueous adrenocortical extracts. DOCA acts almost exclusively on sodium, potassium, chloride and water metabolism. For purposes of abbreviation, the hormones of this group will, therefore, be labeled Na-K hormone.

I. 11-DESOXYCORTICOSTERONE

II. CORTICOSTERONE

III. 17-OH-11-DEHYDROCORTICOSTERONE

IV. TESTOSTERONE

V. ADRENOSTERONE

VI. 17-KETOSTEROID

Compounds II and III differ from Compound I in that they have an oxygen attached to carbon 11. Compound II is called corticosterone, and Compound III is called 17-hydroxy-11-dehydrocorticosterone (cortisone). Inspection of Compound III will show that it differs from Compound II in having a hydroxyl, or OH, group attached to carbon 17. Small amounts of these substances are contained in adrenocortical extract preparations. Physiologically speaking, they have relatively little action on electrolyte metabolism.* Instead they exert an important influence on sugar, fat and nitrogen metabolism. Hence, for purposes of abbreviation, hormones of this type will be labeled S-F-N hormones. Because the most potent members of this hormone type have as described above oxygen atoms attached to carbons 11 and 17 (Compound III), they may also be labeled 11-17-oxycorticosteroids, or 11-17-OCS for short.

The foregoing adrenocortical hormones may be contrasted with the testicular androgen, testosterone (Compound IV), which has not been found in adrenal extracts. Note that it lacks an oxygen on carbon 11 and that it has a hydroxyl (OH) group instead of a 2-carbon ketolic ($COCH_2OH$) side chain attached to carbon 17. Compound V is adrenosterone, a substance with weak androgenic activity which has been isolated from adrenocortical tissue. Note its general re-

* Compound II has weak activity of the Na-K hormone type; the actions of Compounds III (cortisone) tend to negate the action of Na-K hormone on the kidneys; in large amounts cortisone *per se* exerts some Na-K type of hormone action. Thus cortisone can paradoxically have anti-Na-K as well as Na-K action.

semblance to Compound IV. It is not certain whether adrenosterone is produced normally or is just a degradation product of substances like Compounds II and III.

Compound V has a ketone (C=0) instead of a hydroxyl (C-OH) group at carbon 17. It is, therefore, a 17-ketosteroid (17-KS). Compound VI is representative of 17-KS found in extracts of human urine. It is known that such urinary 17-KS are formed when substances similar to Compounds III, IV and V are injected into human beings.* In other words, urinary 17-KS are excretory transformation products of certain types of adrenocortical and testicular steroids. The 17-KS shown here are neutral in the sense that they are of neither acid nor alkaline reaction.

In addition to crystallizable hormones of the types indicated above extracts of adrenocortical material contain amorphous material of high biologic potency with respect to maintenance of life.

PHYSIOLOGIC ACTIONS OF THE HORMONES

The physiologic actions of the hormones will be considered under several somewhat arbitrary headings: (a) electrolyte and water metabolism, (b) sugar-fat-nitrogen metabolism and (c) dermatotropic and androgenic actions. Animal experiments indicate that distinctions could also be made on the basis of capacity to maintain life and to increase work capacity.

Electrolyte and Water Hormone (Na-K Hormone). At present it appears that the Na-K hormone acts chiefly at three sites, the renal tubules and the sweat and salivary glands. Figure 1 sets forth in diagrammatic form the effect of Na-K hormone on the renal tubules. It is seen that, as Na-K hormone concentration increases, the tubular reabsorption of glomerular filtrate sodium tends to increase while tubular reabsorption of glomerular filtrate potassium tends to decrease.[3]

Under normal circumstances glomerular filtration rate is approximately 100,000 cc. per m^2 per 24 hours. The concentrations of sodium, potassium, chloride and other freely diffusable electrolytes are about the same in the glomerular filtrate as in the serum. The daily glomerular filtrate content of any of these electrolytes can be found by multiplying its serum concentration value by the number of liters of glomerular filtrate. Because the glomerular filtrate contents of sodium and potassium are directly proportional to the respective serum concentration values of these electrolytes, an increase in Na-K hormone will give (a) a decrease in urine sodium excretion relative to serum sodium concentration

* Compounds IV and V yield much more urinary 17-KS than does Compound III, of which relatively large amounts must be administered to cause a significant increase in urinary 17-KS output.[2]

[138] CHAPTER III:

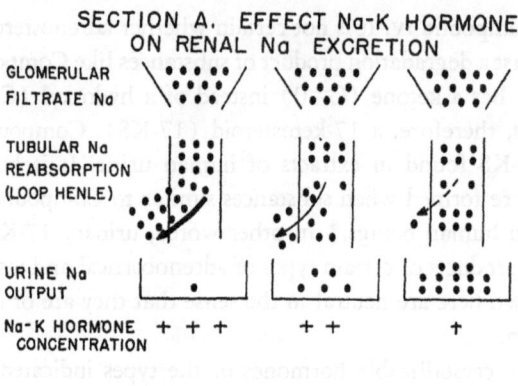

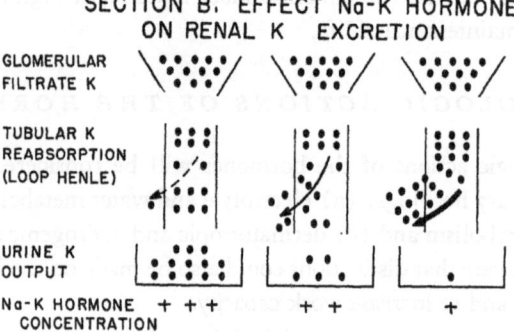

FIGURE III—1. Diagrammatic representation of probable relations between Na-K hormone and renal excretion of sodium and potassium. See text for other comments.

---

and (b) an increase in urine potassium excretion relative to serum potassium concentration. As would be expected, opposite changes take place when Na-K hormone concentration falls, as in patients with Addison's disease.

Figure 2 gives information concerning the effect of Na-K hormone on sweat composition. The sweat of patients with hypoadrenocorticism contains sodium and chloride in high and potassium in low concentrations relative to those found for normal persons and persons with hyperadrenocorticism of the Cushing's syndrome type.[4] Administration of Na-K hormone (DOCA) results in a fall in sweat sodium and chloride and a rise in sweat potassium concentration. In terms of total body balances of sodium, potassium and chloride, under most circumstances the effects which Na-K hormone has on sweat composition are quantitatively insignificant compared to those it has on urine composition. Nonetheless, they are of potential qualitative interest, since they may serve as an index of the Na-K hormone status of an individual.

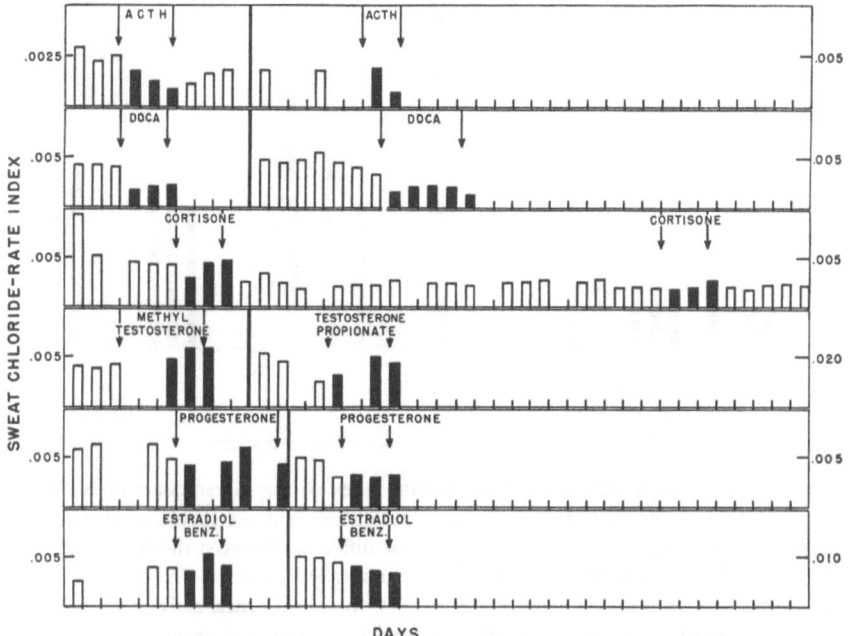

FIGURE III—2. Effect on the sweat chloride–rate index of various hormones. Note that ACTH and desoxycorticosterone acetate (DOCA) prompted a fall in index values. The other agents shown exert little or no effect. In hypoadrenocorticism index values tend to be abnormally high. Thus it appears that sweat chloride–rate index values bear an inverse relation to adrenocortical activity. From W. Locke, N. B. Talbot, H. Jones and J. Worcester, *J. Clin. Investigation* 30:325, 1951.

Presently available information suggests that the effects of Na-K hormone on salivary gland behavior is qualitatively similar to that observed for sweat glands. To what extent this hormone also directly influences the functional behavior of other types of body cells has long been debated and still remains an unsettled question of considerable interest.

Excess of Na-K hormone. When an excess of Na-K hormone results in a positive sodium and a negative potassium balance, the course of events outlined in Figure 4 takes place.[3, 5] The negative potassium balance produces a tendency to low serum potassium (hypokalemia) and to intracellular potassium depletion; the positive sodium balance produces a tendency to elevated serum sodium (hypernatremia) and especially to an overexpansion of extracellular water volume with edema, hypertension, and so forth. Further, sodium tends to migrate into cells and to replace or displace potassium.[6]

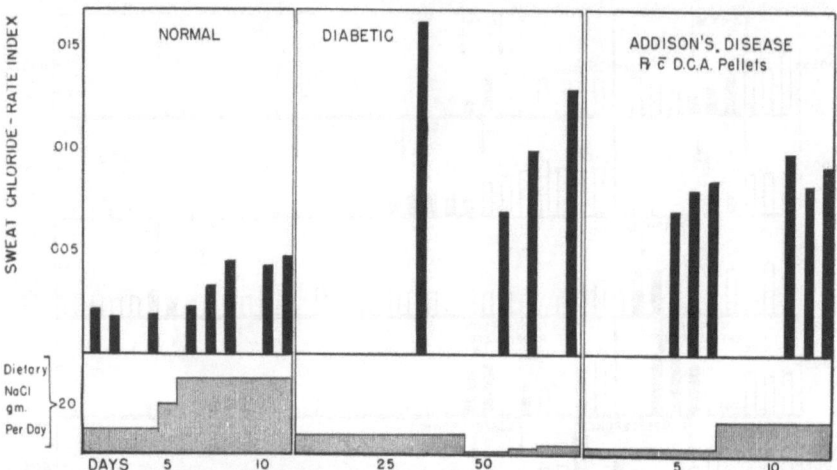

FIGURE III—3. Effect on the sweat chloride–rate index of varying amounts of NaCl in the diet. Differences noted in the normal and the diabetic subject following changes in dietary NaCl intake are statistically significant; the difference between the two groups of values obtained in the Addisonian patient is not statistically significant. These observations suggest that there tends to be a homeostatic decrease in adrenocortical activity when NaCl intake is augmented, and conversely an increase in adrenocortical activity when NaCl intake is diminished. Data from W. Locke, N. B. Talbot, H. Jones and J. Worcester, *J. Clin. Investigation* 30:325, 1951.

The exchange of sodium for potassium within the cells can be of considerable magnitude. Normally, intracellular water of muscle contains about 8 mEq. of sodium and about 150 mEq. of potassium per liter. Under conditions of abnormal sodium retention and potassium depletion, intracellular sodium of muscle may rise to levels as high as 50 mEq. per liter and potassium may fall to levels of 100 mEq. per liter or thereabouts (see Figure 4).*

* Isotopic studies of the body as a whole, first performed by Dr. F. D. Moore and now being carried out by our group, yield a picture which differs quantitatively though not qualitatively from the foregoing. In these studies intracellular water is determined as the difference between total body water, measured with deuterium oxide, and extracellular water, measured with inulin. Intracellular potassium is determined as the difference between total exchangeable potassium and extracellular potassium. Available data indicate that from 90 to 95 per cent of total body potassium exchanges with administered K^{42} in 20 to 40 hours.[6 i] Intracellular sodium is found as the difference between total exchangeable sodium and extracellular sodium. Current data indicate that all the sodium in the body except that bound with calcium salts in bone will exchange with administered Na^{24} in about 20 hours.[6 j] Data obtained with aid of these techniques indicate that the concentration of potassium approximates 105 while that of sodium approximates a value of 35 mEq. per liter of intracellular water.[6 k, l] In these connections it is known that the sodium per kilogram of total body weight is much larger in infants (about 100 mEq.) than in children and adults (about 50 mEq.).[6 m] It remains to be determined whether these differences are due entirely to differences in extracellular sodium content.

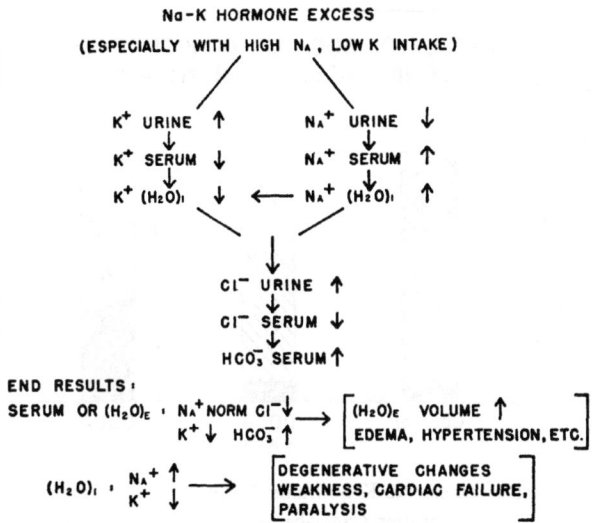

FIGURE III—4. Effect of excess Na-K hormone (DOCA) on body water and electrolyte composition. See text for further comments.

These changes in intracellular electrolyte pattern create disturbances in intracellular-extracellular ionic equilibrium with a resultant tendency to hypochloremic alkalosis (serum bicarbonate concentration and pH elevated; serum chloride depressed). With extension of sodium retention and potassium depletion, slight hypernatremia and hypokalemia are also likely to develop. The combination of low serum chloride and potassium, normal or elevated serum sodium and elevated serum bicarbonate is considered diagnostic of intracellular potassium lack. At the same time it must be emphasized that intracellular potassium deficiency is not necessarily accompanied by these particular changes in extracellular electrolyte composition. For example, serum sodium values may be grossly depressed and serum potassium values may be elevated at times when cellular stores of potassium appear to be significantly reduced as evidenced by electrocardiographic and balance studies.[6 g, h]

When intracellular potassium deficiency develops, muscular weakness or paralysis develops. Moreover, striking morphological abnormalities in skeletal and cardiac musculature and in the renal parenchyma become evident (see Figure 6). The cardiac changes somewhat resemble those seen in rheumatic carditis.

The middle section of Figure 5 calls attention to the fact that excessive amounts of Na-K hormone do not produce the metabolic and anatomic defects just described if the individual's intake of potassium chloride is generous and his sodium

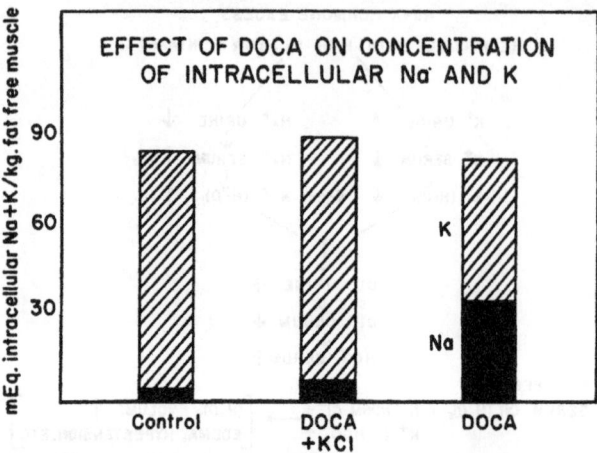

FIGURE III—5. Effect of excess Na-K hormone (DOCA) on the muscle composition of normal dogs receiving ordinary diet (right-hand column) or ordinary diet fortified with KCl (middle diagram). Note that the intracellular replacement of K ion by Na ion in the muscles of normal dogs receiving DOCA is approximately 1:1. This replacement of K by Na is inhibited by the administration of KCl. From R. F. Loeb, *Bull. New York Acad. Med.* 18:263, 1942.

---

intake is restricted.* Such a dietary regimen protects the individual from these pathologic changes by preventing potassium depletion and sodium retention. As might be expected from the foregoing, changes very much like those described above can be produced experimentally without the aid of administered Na-K hormone by feeding animals diets of very low potassium, but of normal or high sodium content.[6 c] They also may be observed in patients suffering from the effects of chronic diarrhea or from base-losing nephritis.[6 d]

As an incidental additional action of interest, it may be mentioned that toxic doses of Na-K hormone cause dogs to develop a condition reminiscent of diabetes insipidus. For further comments on this subject, see Chapter VIII.

Na-K hormone deficiency. This condition results in the abnormalities indicated in Figure 7,[3] which are by and large the reverse of those outlined for Na-K hormone excess. Potassium is retained with resultant tendency to hyperkalemia and to intracellular potassium storage and edema. Somatic and cardiac muscle weakness results. The latter can be fatal to the subject. There also is a tendency for sodium and chloride to be lost from the body in abnormal amounts.

* They also fail to produce these effects under conditions of anuria.[6 e] Recent studies suggest that the depletion of the body's potassium stores which ordinarily results from excessive Na-K hormone activity can be prevented by sodium restriction alone.[6 f]

The Adrenal Cortices

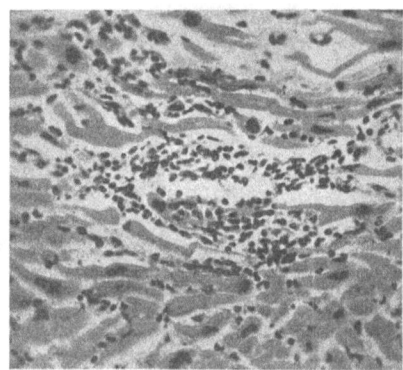

FIGURE III—6. A focus of necrosis in cardiac muscle caused by intracellular potassium depletion which followed Na-K hormone poisoning. From G. MacBryde, *J. Clin. Endocrinol.* 4:30, 1944.

In addition there is a possibility that sodium may leave the extracellular compartment and enter the bones.[6 1] As a result of this loss of extracellular osmoles, there is a shrinkage of extracellular fluid volume, with consequent extracellular dehydration, decrease in plasma and blood volume, anhydremia, hypotension and microcardia. Hyponatremia and hypochloremia also are prone to develop. Moreover, because of circulatory failure, renal function becomes impaired. This can result in the pathologic retention of such other blood constituents as non-protein nitrogen, inorganic phosphorus and sulfate (so-called prerenal azotemia).

Na-K hormone deficiency, like Na-K hormone excess, must be viewed with relation to total body balances of sodium and potassium. A low sodium–high potassium intake aggravates the effects of Na-K hormone lack. The opposite type of regimen ameliorates and even can largely eliminate most of the signs of Na-K hormone deficiency.[7]

Dehydration secondary to Na-K hormone lack. The disturbances in sodium and potassium metabolism resulting from this condition are apt to interfere seriously with body water and electrolyte homeostasis and to make the hypoadrenocortical individual unusually vulnerable to water and salt deprivation. This phenomenon can perhaps be illustrated best by comparing the events which occur when a normal dog is thirsted and fasted to death with those seen when an adrenalectomized dog is deprived of Na-K hormone therapy while receiving food and water.

Figure 8 presents electrolyte balance data pertinent to this subject. As seen in the left-hand section, the thirsting and fasting normal dog initially loses both sodium and potassium. However, after about three to five days, losses of sodium essentially stop while losses of potassium continue. By contrast, as illustrated by the right-hand section of the figure, Na-K hormone withdrawal results not only

[144]

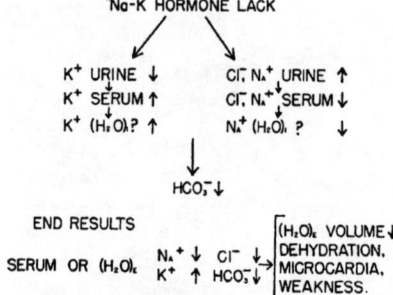

FIGURE III—7. Effect of Na-K hormone deficiency on body water and electrolyte composition under conditions of normal or low sodium and normal or high potassium intake. See text for further comments.

in a sizable loss of sodium but also in the retention of appreciable amounts of potassium.* That is, when Na-K hormone is withdrawn, the adrenalectomized dog no longer is able to retain the necessary amount of dietary sodium or to eliminate unneeded amounts of dietary potassium.

These balance phenomena have interesting significance with relation to changes in body water and electrolyte content. Figure 9 shows that in the thirsting, intact dog, the brunt of the dehydration is borne initially by extracellular compartment fluid. Subsequent lethal reduction in extracellular volume is delayed extensively (i.e., by about 10 days) by replacement of water from the intra- to the extracellular compartment. This replacement occurs because osmolar concentration (or osmotic pressure) outside the cell becomes slightly higher than that inside the cell (see Figure 10, middle section). It appears that this osmotic relationship develops in part as a consequence of the elevation in serum sodium concentration shown in the upper section of Figure 9 and in part as a result of excretion, by way of the kidneys, of an amount of intracellular potassium beyond the quantity released by protoplasmic catabolism secondary to fasting (see Figure 9, lower section).

In the hypoadrenocortical animal the situation was quite different. As a consequence of the primary renal sodium loss there was a considerable fall rather than a rise in serum sodium concentration. This resulted in a fall in extracellular osmotic concentration and a tendency for water to migrate from the extra- to the intracellular compartment, as shown in the right-hand diagram of Figure 10. This tendency was augmented by the factor of potassium retention, which acted to increase intracellular osmotic concentration and hence further to increase the osmotic gradient in favor of the intracellular compartment. As substantiated by

* While these observations are not strictly comparable to those shown on the normal thirsting dog, they show the approximate differences in dehydration between normal and hypo adrenocortical individuals. Strictly comparable experiments could not be found.

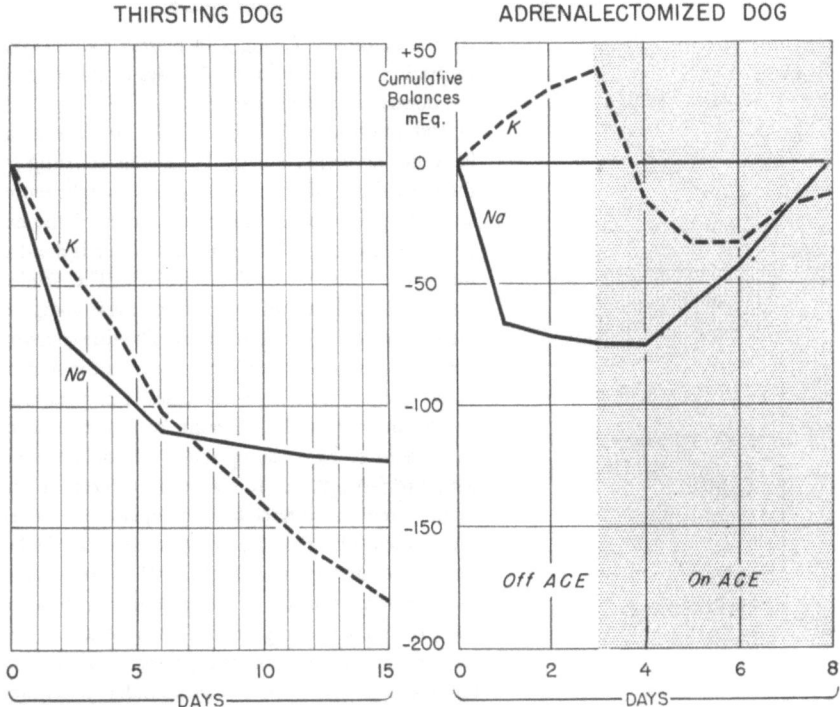

FIGURE III—8. Comparison of sodium and potassium losses by a thirsting and fasting normal dog and an adrenalectomized dog whose ACE therapy was discontinued while he was receiving a constant mixed dietary intake. Data on the thirsting dog from J. R. Elkinton and M. Taffel, *J. Clin. Investigation* 21:787, 1942; data on the adrenalectomized dog from G. A. Harrop, W. M. Nicholson and N. Strauss, *J. Exper. Med.* 64:233, 1936.

muscle tissue studies, the end result of adrenocortical hormone lack is marked extracellular dehydration in the presence of intracellular edema.[8]

Stated in other words, the foregoing indicates that the normal individual is able to survive conditions of water deprivation for an extended period by conserving extracellular sodium and eliminating intracellular potassium and thus creating osmotic relations which prompt a transfer of some water from the cells to the interstitial spaces. This support of extracellular water is vitally necessary to the maintenance of a minimally adequate blood volume. The individual with adrenal insufficiency can no longer retain extracellular sodium and excrete intracellular potassium in accordance with need. Consequently, extracellular water is lost with sodium by way of the kidneys and also migrates into the cells. Extra-

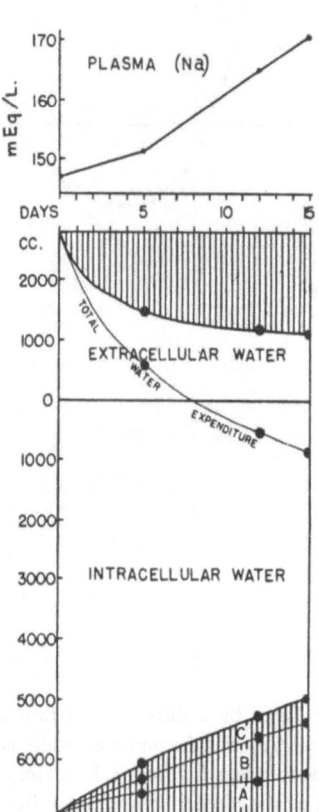

FIGURE III—9

UPPER DIAGRAM: Changes in plasma sodium concentration occurring during 15 days of thirsting by the normal dog of Figure 8.

LOWER DIAGRAM: Changes in extra- and intracellular water occurring during 15 days of thirsting by the normal dog of Figure 8. The total height represents the total body water at the onset of the experiment. Note that the total body water is divided into extra- and intracellular phases. The shaded areas indicate losses of water from these compartments during the period of thirst. The line coursing downward from left to right represents the sum of extra- plus intracellular water losses or expenditure. At the bottom of the diagram, area A represents water released by consumption of protoplasm incidental to fasting; area B is water transferred to the extra- from the intracellular compartment under the osmotic effect of the increase in extracellular ionic concentration (see Figure 10); area C shows the additional transfer of water from the intra- to the extracellular compartment as a result of decreased intracellular osmotic pressure incident to removal and excretion of intracellular potassium beyond the quantity released by catabolism of protoplasm. Data of J. R. Elkinton and M. Taffel, *J. Clin. Investigation* 21:787, 1942, as set forth by J. L. Gamble, *Chem. Anat., Physiol. and Pathol. of Extracellular Fluid*, Cambridge, Harvard Univ. Press, 1950.

cellular dehydration and circulatory collapse therefore develop with great rapidity even though total body losses of fluid are relatively small.

Sodium-potassium homeostasis by the adrenal cortices. In the foregoing sections it was shown that there is an inverse relation between sodium intake and a direct relation between potassium intake and Na-K hormone requirements. Since the healthy individual tolerates diets of widely variable sodium and potassium content, it must be assumed that adrenocortical Na-K hormone production is normally varied in accordance with physiologic needs. While the mechanisms involved in this adaptation are not clearly understood, it appears from sweat electrolyte measurements that sodium lack is a more important stimulus to Na-K hormone production than is potassium excess.[4] (See also Figure 3.)

The Adrenal Cortices

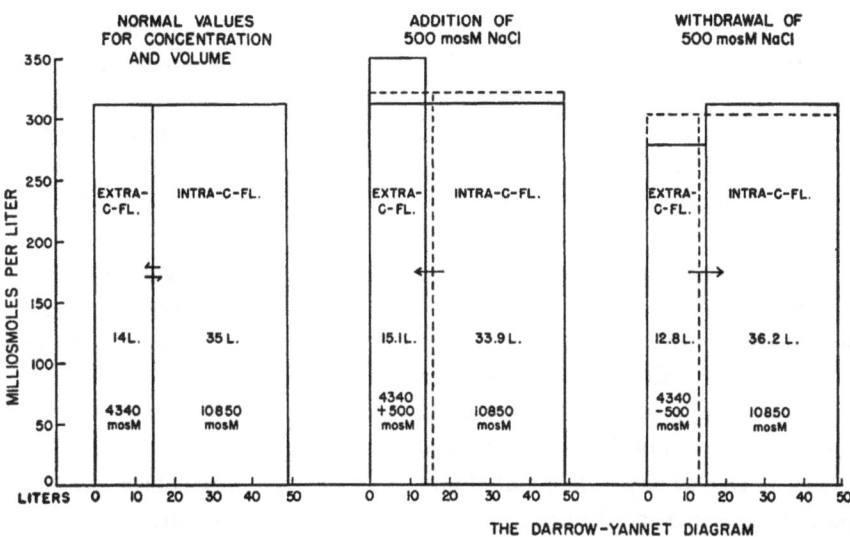

FIGURE III—10. Chart showing the effect of adding to or subtracting from the extracellular compartment a certain amount of NaCl without changing the volume of body water. The left-hand section of this diagram represents the normal for a 70 kg. adult. In the middle section the solid lines indicate that the addition of 500 mosM of NaCl to extracellular fluid would increase ionic concentration from 310 to 346 mosM per liter if no transfer of water from the intra- to the extracellular compartment took place under the influence of this osmotic gradient. By transfer of water from the intra- to the extracellular compartment, osmotic equilibrium (horizontal broken line) is established at an ionic concentration of 320 mosM per liter. The change in volume of extracellular fluid (vertical broken line) is from 14 to 15.1 liters. In the right-hand section of the diagram, the reverse is shown in that osmotic equilibrium is regained by a transfer of water from the extra- to the intracellular compartment. Data of D. C. Darrow and H. Yannet, *J. Clin. Investigation* 14:266, 1935, as set forth by J. L. Gamble, *Chem. Anat., Physiol. and Pathol. of Extracellular Fluid*. Cambridge, Harvard Univ. Press, 1947.

Sodium and potassium are not the only factors which determine Na-K hormone production. Stress acting via the hypothalamic–pituitary–adrenocorticotropic hormone mechanism (see Figure 17) also can cause increased production of adrenocortical hormones having Na-K activity. Presumably this reaction is intended to support the vitally important extracellular fluid volume under conditions where stress results in water deprivation.

Stress can override the sodium-potassium status of the body as a determinant of Na-K hormone production. This is of clinical importance, for it means that individuals under stress may lose their normal ability to eliminate administered sodium in accordance with physiologic needs. Instead of being eliminated by way of the urine, surplus administered sodium may enter the intracellular compartment and displace potassium, which can be excreted readily. There result essentially the same derangements in extra- and intracellular composition that are described above in the section dealing with the Na-K hormone excess. They commonly occur in patients who have been given saline-dextrose solutions for several days. [6 g, h]

Sugar-Fat-Nitrogen ("S-F-N") Hormones or 11-17-Oxycorticosteroids (11-17-OCS).[3 c, d, 9] Such hormones exert a number of effects which can be demonstrated experimentally and at times clinically by appropriate measurements. Though it is probable that all these effects are intimately related, it is convenient to consider them under three main headings: sugar, fat and nitrogen. In addition, there are certain miscellaneous actions which deserve mention.

Effects on carbohydrate metabolism. Carbohydrate metabolism is a complex phenomenon and the literature contains a vast amount of information concerning it. A considerable number of the ideas recorded are currently the subject of vigorous debate. Accordingly, it is at present difficult to present more than a simplified picture of what is thought to be approximately true.

Figure 11 may aid in these considerations. Here are indicated potential sources of blood glucose and potential routes or mechanisms by which glucose may be withdrawn from the circulation.[3] It is seen that dietary carbohydrate is not the only source of circulating glucose. Glucose may be formed (gluconeogenesis) within the body from both amino and fatty acids. In addition, limited amounts of glucose can be released into the blood stream by lysis of hepatic glycogen stores. As described in Chapter IV, hepatic glycogen stores can be replenished in part by conversion of lactic acid originating in muscle glycogen. The foregoing are on the credit side of the blood glucose balance sheet. On the debit side are tissue utilization or oxidation, tissue fat deposition, muscle glycogen formation and hepatic glycogen deposition.

Next it will be noted that the S-F-N hormones are thought to accelerate certain of these reactions and to slow others. Thus, both gluconeogenesis from protein and mobilization of body depot fat proceed with increasing rapidity as the concentration of 11-17-OCS increases. Concomitantly there is a decrease in the rate at which the peripheral tissues utilize circulating glucose. Current information suggests that quantitatively the 11-17-OCS have a much more pronounced effect upon the rates of tissue carbohydrate utilization and depot fat mobilization than upon the rate of gluconeogenesis from protein (amino acids).

The diagram of Figure 11 illustrates an additional point, namely, that there are other factors which modify the rates at which glucose enters and leaves the

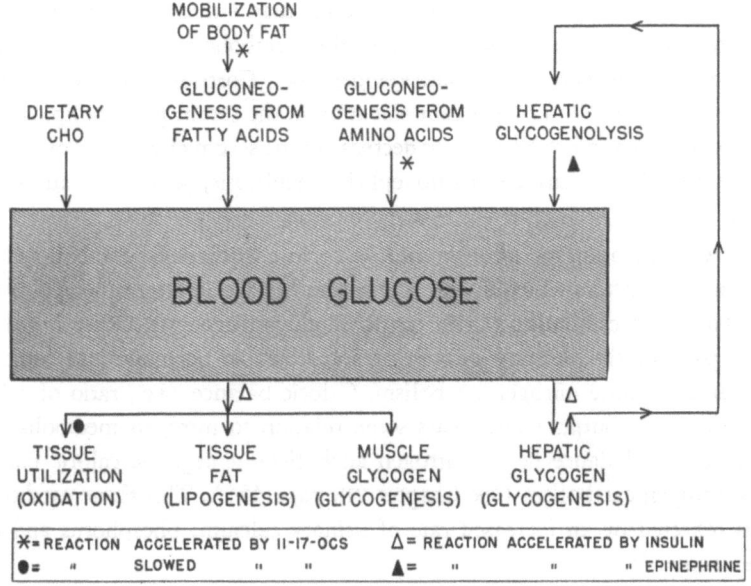

FIGURE III—11. Schematic representation of potential sources of blood glucose and potential routes or mechanisms by which glucose is withdrawn from the circulation. This diagram is largely self-explanatory. While gluconeogenesis from fatty acids is indicated, the proportion is probably very minor compared with that of gluconeogenesis from protein. From N. B. Talbot, *Pediatrics* 3:519, 1949.

blood stream. Only two factors are indicated, though others are known to exist. One of these, insulin, increases the rate at which circulating glucose is utilized for purposes of oxidation, lipogenesis and glycogenesis. The other, epinephrine, tends among other things to accelerate the rate at which hepatic glycogen is transformed into blood glucose (see Chapter IV).

S-F-N hormone excess results in a tendency to hyperglycemia, probably chiefly by inhibiting peripheral tissue glucose utilization. S-F-N hormone lack has the expected opposite effect of producing a tendency to hypoglycemia. It seems likely that this is due to an absolute increase in peripheral glucose utilization or to a combination of the latter and failure of gluconeogenesis from protein.

Effects on fat metabolism. In the absence of the S-F-N hormones, the organism loses its normal capacity to mobilize depot fat. Consequently, when a deficiency exists there is a lessened tendency to ketone-body formation and ketonuria under conditions of fasting. In the normal fasting ketotic subject ACTH produces a consistent and impressive fall in blood ketones. This has been interpreted to mean that adrenocortical hormones may either increase the rate at which ketone bodies are utilized or change the metabolic pathways of fatty acids in such a way as largely to eliminate ketogenesis.[9 i] Cortisone has been found to produce a gradual, 19 to 61 per cent elevation in the serum phospholipids and a slower, concomitant 4 to 53 per cent decrease in the serum cholesterol of patients with lupus erythematosus, glomerulonephritis, nephrosis, periarteritis and scleroderma.[9 j]

Effects on nitrogen metabolism and on certain body cells. S-F-N hormones are among the factors which in one way or another accelerate amino acid breakdown (nitrogen catabolism) with resultant gluconeogenesis. Other hormonal agents, particularly pituitary growth or somatotropic hormone and testicular androgens, promote nitrogen anabolism. Caloric balance (i.e., ratio of caloric intake to caloric output) also bears some relation to nitrogen metabolism. A positive caloric balance favors nitrogen anabolism, a negative caloric balance favors nitrogen catabolism (see Chapter VII, page 455). This tissue catabolism also is reflected by an increased rate of urinary calcium, phosphorus and uric acid excretion.[9 i, 2 b]

The over-all effect of S-F-N hormones on sugar, fat and nitrogen metabolism is illustrated by Figure 12. Here it can be seen that in S-F-N hormone-lack carbohydrate is the major source of calories. When the deficiency is corrected or an excess of the hormone is given, fat becomes a much larger and carbohydrate a much smaller source of calories. Protein metabolism is influenced to a much smaller degree than carbohydrate and fat metabolism. However, protein occupies a slightly greater portion of the total metabolic mixture when S-F-N hormones are present than when they are lacking.

Viewed with relation to the foregoing incomplete list of other factors which influence nitrogen metabolism, S-F-N hormones would not necessarily appear to be quantitatively very important, although it is noteworthy that over a long period a small change in balance can result in gross alterations in body composition. Qualitatively, however, S-F-N hormones are capable of producing interesting changes in certain tissues. In particular, the lymphoid structures (including the thymus) and circulating eosinophils undergo involution or lysis when S-F-N hormone concentration is increased.[9 g, h]

Fibroblastic proliferation in wounded experimental animals is inhibited by cortisone.[9 k] Experience with human subjects suggests, however, that this effect does not necessarily interfere with wound-healing in patients treated with therapeutic doses of cortisone or ACTH for short periods of time.[9 l]

Opposite effects are noted with respect to certain other cells. Cortisone can

The Adrenal Cortices

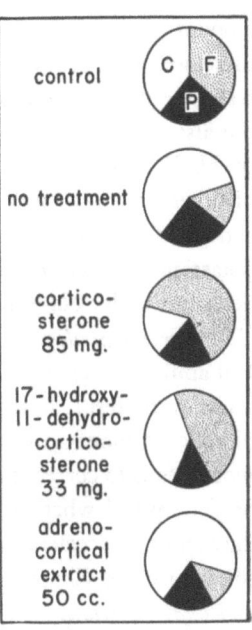

FIGURE III—12. Effect of S-F-N hormone on the relative amounts of carbohydrate, fat and protein which are oxidized to provide the organism with energy. The divisions of the various circles of the diagram indicate the approximate composition of the metabolic mixture from which calories were derived in a patient with hypoadrenocorticism. The white area stands for carbohydrate; the speckled for fat; the black for protein. Adapted from G. W. Thorn et al., *J. Clin. Investigation* 19:813, 1940.

produce transitory reticulocytosis[9 l] and relative erythrocytosis[2 b] and can result in increased growth of macrophages and increased phagocytosis.[9 m]

Miscellaneous effects. These are considered under several headings below.

Muscle fatigue. S-F-N hormones act via the metabolic pathways outlined above, or otherwise, to slow muscle fatigue and to aid in adaptation to a variety of stresses and strains.[10 a-e] There is some evidence that mitigation of muscle fatigue is accomplished largely by maintaining a satisfactory concentration of glucose in the blood stream.

Electrolyte metabolism. The fact that certain 11-17-OCS negate, cancel or in some manner neutralize the effect of Na-K hormone upon the kidneys has been mentioned before. This means that the 11-17-OCS type of S-F-N hormone (Compound III, page 136) may induce a sodium diuresis.[9 h] Its effect upon potassium metabolism is less readily evident, probably because more variables are involved.

Na-K hormone produces an increase in potassium excretion relative to serum potassium concentration. If Na-K hormone action is canceled out by S-F-N hormones there should result a tendency to decreased potassium excretion. But S-F-N hormones may cause protoplasmic catabolism with a resultant increase in the amount of potassium presenting for excretion on the one hand and may induce increased glycogenesis with increased potassium anabolism on the other. Potassium output and potassium balances are products not only of all these variables but also of intake. Hence the difficulty in assessing the effect of S-F-N hormones on Na-K hormone action with regard to potassium metabolism. In the absence of other adrenocortical hormones S-F-N hormones have weak Na-K hormone activity. Given in large doses, over a long period, they produce intracellular potassium deficiency and hypokalemic, hypochloremic alkalosis similar to that described under Na-K hormone excess.

Water metabolism. Individuals with adrenocortical insufficiency lose normal ability to increase their urinary output when given a water load (see below, under water test). In association with this disturbance there is an excess of antidiuretic hormone in blood and urine. While desoxycorticosterone (Na-K hormone) fails to correct this disturbance, cortisone apparently can.[9 l] It remains to be determined whether cortisone acts by depressing antidiuretic hormone production or by accelerating its utilization or inactivation. For other comments on this subject see Chapter VIII.

Renal function. As mentioned above, S-F-N hormones cause an increase in urinary uric acid output. This is due not only to protoplasmic catabolism, but also to increased renal uric acid clearance.[10 f]

Brain metabolism. In patients with Addison's disease the electroencephalogram is apt to show slowing of the alpha rhythm and a decreased number of beta waves.[10 g] These abnormalities are correctable with adequate doses of 11-17-oxycorticosteroids, but not with 11-desoxycorticosterone.[9 l]

Immunologic phenomena. Neither adrenocorticotropic hormone nor cortisone treatment appears to interfere with the capacity of human beings to produce antibodies to pneumococcus polysaccharides.[10 h] These hormones do not prompt an increase in gamma globulin or antibody levels in the blood.[9 l, 10 h] They produce only slight and irregular fluctuations in the titers of antiblood group substance, typhoid agglutinin and C-reactive protein.[10 h]

S-F-N-type hormones, however, do cause interesting alterations in antigen-antibody reactions. For example, cortisone sometimes depresses skin sensitivity to pneumococcus polysaccharide (Francis test) in individuals known to be producing high titers of antibody.[10 h] This hormone also can inhibit the intradermal tuberculin-test reaction in hyperimmune guinea pigs.[10 i] Similar loss of cutaneous hypersensitivity to tuberculin has been observed following ACTH therapy to human patients suffering advanced tuberculosis.[10 j] Reports concerning the ability of ACTH and cortisone to alter positive skin tests to various other bacterial antigens in man have been somewhat contradictory.[9 l]

Histamine metabolism. Following adrenalectomy in the rat, there is a marked increase in the histamine content of the gastrointestinal tract and a lesser increase in the histamine content of the liver and lung.[10 k] There also is a decrease in the histaminase content of the tissues. This decrease is eliminated by adrenal extract treatment. These findings may explain why adrenalectomized animals are more vulnerable to anaphylactic reactions and more sensitive to histamine than normal controls.[10 m, n] In most asthmatic patients it has been found that ACTH treatment results in an increase in urine histidine excretion and to a moderate or marked transient increase in urine histamine excretion. In association with this, asthmatic symptoms subside. By contrast, in some asthmatic and in most rheumatoid arthritis patients ACTH induces little or no change in urine histamine excretion.[10 o] It remains to be determined whether these effects should be attributed specifically to S-F-N hormones. It does appear, however, that adrenocortical hormones can "dissociate the harmful effects of hypersensitivity from the beneficial reaction of immunity."[9 l]

Other actions.[9 l] Current studies suggest that S-F-N hormones cause an increase in gastric pepsin, mucoprotein and mucoproteose secretion, and in patients with ulcerative colitis a decrease in the elevated lysozyme activity of the feces. The 11-17-OCS also inhibit hyaluronidase, an enzyme which facilitates the spreading of various substances in body tissues.

Adrenocortical hormones apparently bear some relation to the metabolism of compounds containing sulfhydryl (SH groups). These are known to be involved in many cellular enzyme systems. One such compound is glutathione. ACTH apparently causes a reduction in blood glutathione concentration.[10 q] In association with this there is observed the tendency to hyperglycemia and to insulin resistance described above. It has been suggested that the latter phenomena may be explained at least in part by reduced availability of free sulfhydryl groups. This suggestion is supported by observations indicating that ACTH-induced hyperglycemia and glycosuria can be lessened considerably for a short period by the intravenous administration of pure reduced glutathione.

Renal effects produced by ACTH treatment, but not yet known to be due specifically to a single type of adrenocortical hormone. ACTH in large doses causes an increase in the glomerular filtration rate (inulin clearance) of normal men.[10 p] ACTH in small doses and cortisone at all dose levels fail to produce this effect. Phosphate clearance also rises following large doses of ACTH or cortisone. Tubular secretion of para-amino-hippurate may be increased up to 35 per cent with cortisone, though not with ACTH. Finally, ACTH treatment has been noted to cause a lowering in the renal tubular threshold for glucose.[10 q] This phenomenon has been noted to occur spontaneously in a patient with severe

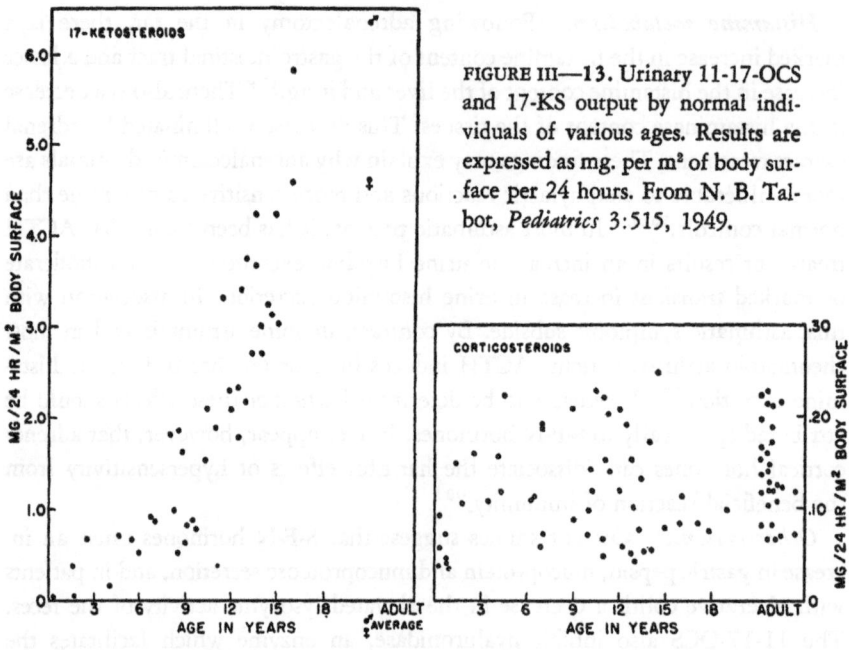

FIGURE III—13. Urinary 11-17-OCS and 17-KS output by normal individuals of various ages. Results are expressed as mg. per m² of body surface per 24 hours. From N. B. Talbot, *Pediatrics* 3:515, 1949.

diabetic acidosis and functional hyperadrenocorticism as evidenced by marked eosinopenia.[10 r]

Rate of S-F-N hormone production under normal conditions.[11] It is possible only to estimate production rates in a relative sense by indirect means. Measurements of the urinary output of 11-17-OCS make it appear that, with the possible exception of very young infants, the daily production of S-F-N hormones per square meter of body surface area is essentially the same in all healthy individuals regardless of sex or age (see Figure 13). The few urinary 11-17-OCS values obtained for healthy young infants suggest that they may be producing S-F-N hormones at a slower rate than normal older persons. However, some of these values in infants may be subject to errors of underestimation (see below under diagnostic methods). It remains to be determined whether the tendency of infants to have relative eosinophilia (see Figure 18), to develop hypoglycemia (see Chapter IX) and to show involution of the fetal zone of their adrenal cortices (see Figure 14) during the neonatal period is significantly related to the foregoing.[12] It is interesting to speculate on the possibility that the fetus has no need to elaborate adrenocortical S-F-N or Na-K hormones. Fetal life is presumably free from stress until the onset of labor, and it may be supposed that the mother's adrenocortical system maintains sugar and electrolyte homeostasis in the infant residing in utero. If this is correct, it follows that infants may be born

The Adrenal Cortices

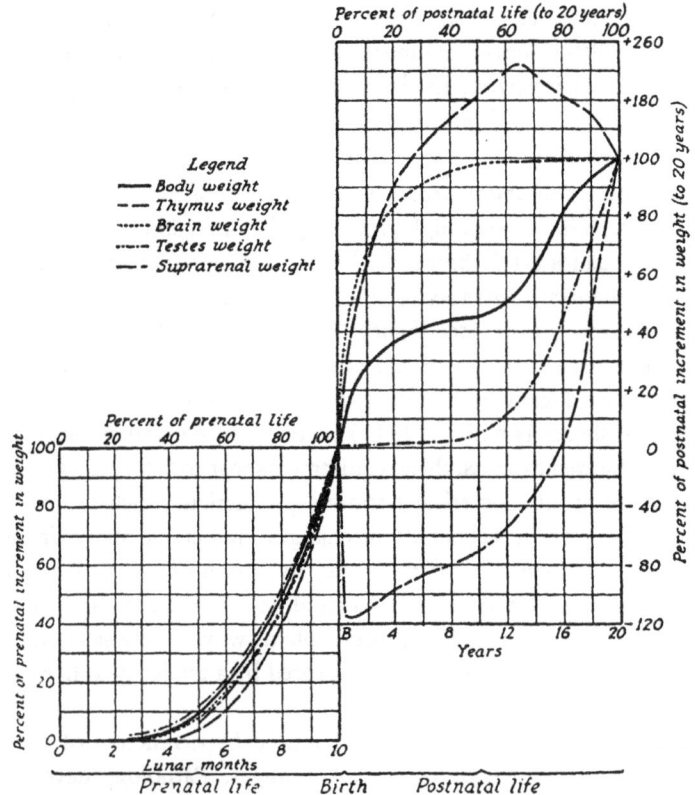

FIGURE III—14. Diagram illustrating the growth in prenatal and postnatal life of a series of structures. Note the marked postnatal involution in adrenal (suprarenal) weight which occurs during the first weeks of life. From J. A. Harris et al., *The Measurement of Man*. Minneapolis, Univ. of Minnesota Press, 1930.

---

with relatively inactive adrenocortical S-F-N and Na-K hormone mechanisms, just as, apparently, they are born with inactive parathyroid and posterior pituitary glands. In these connections, recent studies have revealed that the pituitary ACTH–adrenocortical system of the premature infant is incapable of responding to epinephrine and responds only poorly to ACTH.[12 b] It would seem that maturation must proceed to some critical point before this mechanism becomes fully operative.

While the urinary 11-17-OCS measurements probably provide relative information concerning S-F-N hormone production, they most certainly do not indicate absolute rates of production. In other words, the material which appears in the urine probably comprises but a small fraction of the material produced by the adrenal cortices. This is indicated by experiments wherein the effect upon urinary 11-17-OCS values of administering adrenocortical extract, corticosterone and 17-hydroxycorticosterone has been studied.[11] Such studies suggest that only 5 per cent or less of S-F-N hormone material presenting to the circulation ordinarily reaches the urine.

Rate of production under stress (alarm reaction of Selye). Stress of almost any sort (heat, cold, exercise, high protein intake, infection and trauma) creates an increased need for S-F-N hormones.[3 c, d, 10 c-e] As mentioned earlier, this need is met by spontaneous activation of the hypothalamic–pituitary–adrenocortical alarm reaction mechanism (see Figure 17). The order of magnitude of this reaction is indicated by studies of the adrenocortical hormone requirements of adrenalectomized dogs. Under ideal, stressless conditions of living, they can be maintained satisfactorily with 0.3 to 0.5 cc. of adrenocortical extract per kg. per day. When subjected to stress, their requirements soar to 5 cc. per kg. per day.[10 d]

The increase in adrenocortical hormone production which normally occurs in response to stress brings about all the changes enumerated above. Incidentally, it appears to be responsible for the acute involution of the thymus and other lymphoid structures seen in infants and children who die after an illness of two or three days' duration. It probably also explains why acutely sick patients have a diminished tolerance for glucose as evidenced by a tendency to hyperglycemia and glycosuria.

So far as is known at present, stress-induced hyperfunction of the adrenal cortices is not productive of pathologic changes. Pathology develops when adrenal hormone secretion is excessive or deficient in relation to physiologic needs.

Normal and Abnormal Adrenocortical Urinary 17-Ketosteroid Precursors (17-KS-Gens)—the So-called Adrenocortical Androgens. The adrenal cortices normally commence to produce urinary 17-KS-Gens in significant amounts between the eighth and tenth years of life (see Figure 13). Abnormally, in patients with adrenocortical virilism, 17-KS-Gens production may start at a much earlier age.

While the chemical nature of these 17-KS-Gens is known in general terms,*

---

* As stated earlier, it is known that 17-hydroxy and 17-ketosteroids may be metabolized and excreted as urinary 17-KS. Recent studies also have shown that the administration of large amounts of substances like Compound III may result in a small but definite rise in urinary 17-KS output.[2]

There is a possibility that the increase in urinary 17-KS seen during adolescence is due to a change in the intermediary metabolism of adrenocortical steroids during that period. Detailed information concerning this possibility is lacking. On the basis of unpublished observations it may be said, however, that the yield of urinary 17-KS following standard doses of testosterone propionate is the same in infants, children and adults.

it is not understood in precise detail. Lacking more specific information, one may infer the physiologic actions of these substances from clinically observed relations between urinary 17-KS excretion values and certain somatic changes. Table 1 sets forth in summary form such relations in various selected types of individuals. Similar information pertaining to the testicular male hormones is included for comparative purposes.

Table 1 suggests the following comments: (a) Normally produced adrenocortical 17-KS-Gens (i.e., Conditions 1 to 8) in contrast to the testicular androgens (right-hand section) and testosterone (Condition 9) do not cause development of the penis in the male or of the clitoris in the female.* Neither do they exert a measurable influence upon protoplasmic anabolism, as judged by rates of growth in stature or by degrees of muscular development.[14 a] However, they do appear to share with the natural testicular androgens and with testosterone the capacity to stimulate pubic and axillary hair growth and to produce acne. (b) Adrenocortical 17-KS-Gens produced by patients with adrenocortical virilism (Condition 10) in contrast to those elaborated normally appear to have an action very much like that of the testicular androgens and testosterone.[14 b, c, e] Such a difference in apparent biologic action might theoretically be due either to quantitative or qualitative phenomena. Pertinent quantitative information is set forth in Table 2, while qualitative observations are presented in Figure 15.

Table 2 shows that the urinary 17-KS output values of young patients with adrenocortical virilism (a) are higher than normal for their age (see Figure 13) but (b) are not necessarily appreciably higher than the values obtained for normal, non-masculinized women when considered either on the basis of absolute value or that of a per square meter of body surface area (see right-hand columns, Table 2).

On the other hand, chromatographic fractionation studies carried out here (see Figure 15) and elsewhere[2, 13 b] indicate that there are distinct qualitative differences between the 17-KS mixtures excreted by patients with adrenocortical virilism and by normal individuals. These differences are due both to alterations in the relative proportions of certain 17-KS which normally are present in extracts of adult urine and to the presence of 17-KS which are not normally present in appreciable amounts.

These findings suggest strongly that the 17-KS-Gens secreted by the adrenal cortices of patients with adrenocortical virilism differ qualitatively from those normally secreted. Incidentally, there also appear to be qualitative abnormalities in the appearance of adrenocortical zona reticularis cells of patients with adreno-

* Dr. F. Albright has seen a eunuchoid male who showed no evidence of masculinization despite the fact that his urinary 17-KS output was more than 30 mg. per day.

cortical virilism.[14 b] These findings provide a possible explanation for the clinical impression that normal adrenocortical 17-KS-Gens are not androgenic even when present in sizable amounts, whereas abnormal 17-KS Gens may be androgenic when present in relatively small amounts.

Factors Controlling Adrenocortical Activity.[15] The development and secretory activity of the adrenal cortices are determined largely by anterior pituitary adrenocorticotropic hormone (ACTH). ACTH is a protein substance the composition of which has been approximately, but not precisely, determined. Most preparations have a molecular weight of about 23,000. Polypeptide mixtures derived from ACTH protein are as potent as the parent substance.

When endogenous ACTH production is eliminated by hypophysectomy, the adrenal cortices undergo structural and functional atrophy.* Adrenocortical development and activity can be restored by pituitary tissue implants and by suitably prepared, parenterally administered anterior pituitary extracts. Orally administered ACTH is largely destroyed by digestive enzymes before it can reach the circulation.

It is possible that there is more than one type of ACTH. For instance, values of spontaneous urinary 17-KS and 11-17-OCS output can vary quite independently (see Figure 13) and even in opposite directions (see Figure 16). These phenomena suggest that production of the 17-KS-Gens is under the control of one, and that 11-17-OCS (or S-F-N hormone) production is determined by another ACTH. If this thesis is correct, it must be concluded that currently available ACTH preparations contain both types of tropic hormones, for they have been observed to increase both 17-KS and 11-17-OCS excretion values in patients of all ages.[15 h] These preparations appear, however, to be particularly rich in ACTH of the type which stimulates 11-17-OCS production, for they usually cause a much greater percentage increase in the output of urinary 11-17-OCS-like material than of 17-KS. In addition, it is known that adrenocortical responsiveness to ACTH as measured by changes in the urinary output of 11-17-OCS and 17-KS can vary markedly under certain circumstances. For example, ACTH administration causes a much greater increase in urinary 11-17-OCS and a much smaller increase in urinary 17-KS excretion in infants than it does in adults.[15 h]

As discussed elsewhere, trauma and stress of all sorts are apt to prompt increased ACTH production and hence increased adrenocortical activity. The

* In rodents the zona glomerulosa (together with Na-K hormone production) appears to be at least partially independent of ACTH control.[16] Hence this zone undergoes relatively little atrophy following hypophysectomy.

TABLE III—1. Apparent effects of normal or abnormal adrenocortical and testicular urinary 17-KS precursors on certain somatic phenomena.

Condition	17-KS output *	Apparent effect of adrenocortical 17-KS-Gens				Apparent effect of testicular 17-KS-Gens			
		Penile or clitoral enlargement	Acne	Pubic and axillary hair	Protoplasmic anabolism	Penile or clitoral enlargement	Acne	Pubic and axillary hair	Protoplasmic anabolism
1. Normal preadolescent	0	0	0	0	0	0	0	0	0
2. Normal adolescent girl	rising (Figure 13)	0	+	+	0?				
3. Castrate women and adolescent girls	± normal	0	+	+	0?				
4. Hypoadrenocortical adolescent girls	0	0	0	0	0				
5. Normal adolescent boy	About as no. 2	0	+	+	0	+	+	+	+
6. Castrate and eunuchoid boys of adolescent age	± normal	0	±+	+	0?	0	0	0	0
7. Hypoadrenocortical boys of adolescent age	low	0	0	0	0	+	+	+	+
8. Panhypopituitary boys of adolescent age	0	0	0	0	0	0	0	0	0
9. Testosterone therapy to patients of types 1, 2, 3, 4, 6, 8						+	+	+	+
10. Adrenocortical virilism in preadolescent children and in women	Higher than normal for age and of abnormal composition †	+	+	+	+	0	0	0	0

* See under diagnostic methods, Table 3.   † See Table 2 for example values.

TABLE III—2. Quantitative relations between total urinary 17-ketosteroid output of children with congenital adrenocortical virilism (due to adrenocortical hyperplasia) and maximum output of normal adult women.

Case no.	Sex	Age, yr.	Surface area, m²	Urinary 17-KS mg/24 hr.	Urinary 17-KS mg/m²/24 hr.	Ratio observed 17-KS output to adult normal* absolute value basis	Ratio observed 17-KS output to adult normal* per m² basis
1	M	2.5	.6	8	13	0.6	1.4
2	F	6	1.0	14	14	1.0	1.6
3	F	2.5	0.75	9	12	0.6	1.3
4	F	5	1.0	8	8	0.6	0.9
5	M	9	1.45	8	6	0.6	0.7
Average	—	—	—	—	—	0.7	1.2

* The maximum 17-KS output for normal adult women is taken to be 14 mg. per 24 hours. Assuming the average surface area of adult women to be 1.6 m², the maximum normal value on a surface area basis is 14 ÷ 1.6 = 9 mg. per m² per 24 hours.

manner in which stress occasions these changes is gradually becoming clarified. It now seems reasonably certain that the reaction to stress can be divided approximately into two response phases—acute and chronic. These phases may be independent or sequential.

Immediate response to acute stress is accomplished with the aid of the sympathetic-adrenomedullary system.[17] Thus released, epinephrine acts directly upon the anterior pituitary and so effects rapid production of ACTH. Animals which have been rendered incapable of secreting epinephrine are still capable of responding to stress, but they increase ACTH production only after a latent period of several hours. Hence it appears that the formation of epinephrine normally constitutes the mechanism initially responsible for augmenting ACTH secretion under sudden stress. On the other hand, it seems unlikely that epinephrine plays a major role in inducing the sustained overproduction of ACTH observed in individuals under chronic stress.

The explanation for sustained overproduction of ACTH in response to stress is less clearly evident. One or more factors other than epinephrine may play a role. For example, it is known that a rise in the concentration of adrenocortical hormones in the blood stream acts to inhibit ACTH production.[18] Hence it may be presumed that lowered adrenocortical hormone concentration in the blood should lead to increased ACTH secretion by the anterior pituitary. Stress leads to accelerated tissue utilization of adrenocortical hormones, a phenomenon which should result in a fall in adrenocortical hormone concentration and a compensa-

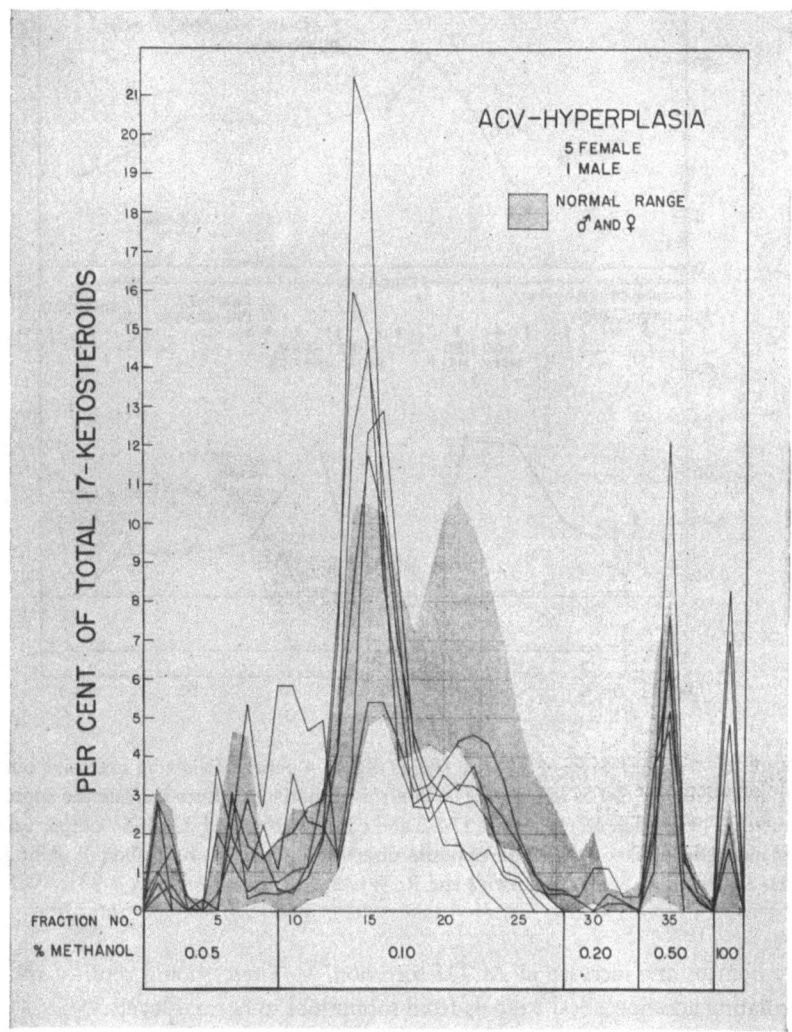

FIGURE III—15. Microchromatographic fractionation studies of the urinary 17-KS excreted by normal persons (shaded area) and by patients with adrenocortical virilism due to bilateral adrenocortical hyperplasia (individual curves). The eluate fraction number is indicated along the abscissa. The composition of the eluant is indicated in the adjacent lower area. The scale along the ordinate indicates the per cent of the total 17-KS material recovered in each of the 40 fractions eluted. Thus the sum of the individual points described by each curve equals 100 per cent. This fractionation was carried out with the aid of a procedure devised by A. S. Zygmuntowicz, M. Wood, E. Christo and N. B. Talbot, *J. Clin. Endocrinol.* 11:578, 1951.

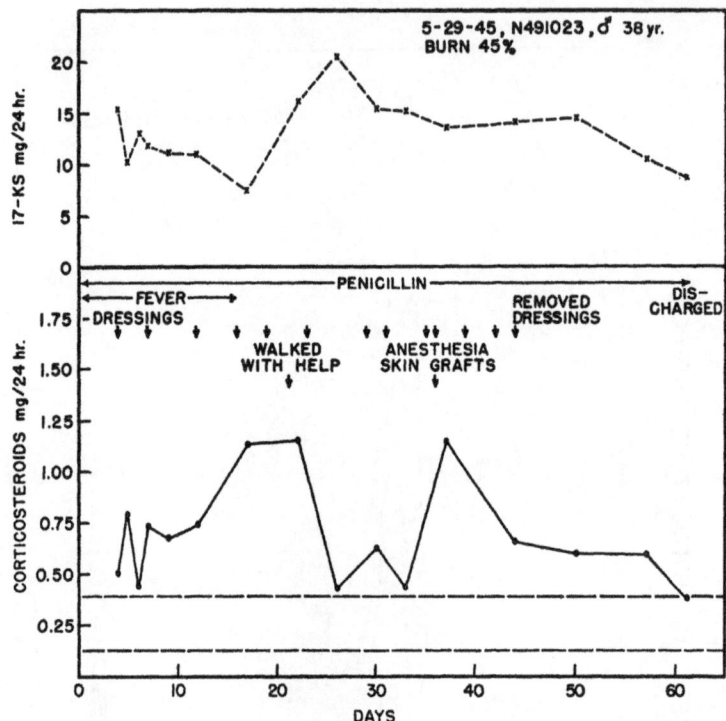

FIGURE III—16. Excretion of 11-OCS and 17-KS by a patient following extensive burns. Zero represents the day of the burn. The interrupted horizontal lines indicate the approximate limits of normal. Note that the 17-KS and corticosteroid (11-17-OCS) output values vary independently, sometimes in opposite directions. From N. B. Talbot, F. Albright, A. H. Saltzman, A. S. Zygmuntowicz and R. Wixon, *J. Clin. Endocrinol.* 7:331, 1947.

tory homeostatic increase in ACTH secretion.[14 e] There should result a rise of circulating adrenocortical steroids from subnormal to normal levels.

While this type of mechanism may be active in endocrinologically normal individuals, it fails to explain observations which indicate that stressed individuals normally have *hyper* -11-17-oxycorticosteroidemia as evidenced by eosinopenia, reduced glucose tolerance and hyper-11-17-oxycorticosteroiduria. These changes strongly suggest that stress activates some factor other than epinephrine or lowered corticosteroid concentration which is capable of stimulating increased ACTH secretion to such an extent that hyper-11-17-oxycorticosteroidemia develops despite an increased rate of tissue hormone utilization. The nature of this factor remains to be ascertained.

METHODS OF DIAGNOSIS

A list of procedures which gives information concerning the respective rates of production of the various types of adrenocortical hormone is given in Table 3. As the comments in the right-hand portion of the table briefly indicate, some of the tests are simple and particularly useful for screening purposes (for example, nos. 1, 2, 4), while others are more complex and in certain instances more specifically diagnostic. Each of these procedures is commented upon in turn in the following paragraphs.

Test 1—the Water Test for Adrenocortical Insufficiency.[19 a] This test has the advantage of being safe and simple to carry out and of being fairly reliable. It is performed as follows: Food and fluids are withheld after 6 p.m. on the evening preceding the test. The urine which the patient voids at 10 p.m. is discarded. All urine voided thereafter is saved, and the total volume passed between 10 p.m. and 7 a.m. inclusive is measured. After the 7 a.m. voiding, the patient is asked to drink 850 cc. of water per m^2 within approximately half an hour. Urine specimens are then collected at 8 a.m., 9 a.m., 10 a.m. and 11 a.m. In normal individuals the volume of urine passed during one of these periods exceeds the 10 p.m. to 7 a.m. volume. In patients with hypoadrenocorticism none of the hourly specimens exceeds the total overnight volume.

Generally speaking, about 90 per cent of patients with proven hypoadrenocorticism have abnormal responses to the water tests. This figure applies both to patients with primary hypoadrenocorticism and to patients with hypoadrenocorticism secondary to anterior pituitary insufficiency. While most normal persons have normal reactions, patients with various diseases (sprue, rheumatoid arthritis, ulcerative colitis, pulmonary tuberculosis and so forth) may give an abnormal response, even though they do not appear to be suffering from hypoadrenocorticism when more specific tests are applied. In other words, a normal test rules against though it does not rule out hypoadrenocorticism; an abnormal test indicates that the patient may be suffering from adrenocortical insufficiency and that he deserves more careful study (i.e., application of Tests 3, 5, 11 or 13).

Introductory Comments on Tests 2, 3 and 4.[9 h, 19 b-e] Figure 17 presents the basis for these tests in diagrammatic form. Section A shows the relations found in normal persons who are not under stress of any sort. It is seen that the anterior pituitary, perhaps under the influence of the hypothalamus, is producing some ACTH. This in turn causes the adrenals to secrete a "normal" amount of 11-17-OCS. The eosinophil count, and incidentally urinary steroid values are "normal" under these circumstances. Section B shows that stress of any sort, or

Continued on page 167

TABLE III—3. Summary of diagnostic methods.

Type of procedure or measurement	Condition designed to reveal						Comments
	Na-K		S-F-N		17-KS-Gens		
	Excess	Lack	Excess	Lack	Excess	Lack	
1. Water test	0	0	0	+	0	0	A nonspecific, approximate screening test for adrenocortical insufficiency
2. Epinephrine-eosinophil	0	0	0	+	0	0	An approximate screening test for adrenocortical and anterior pituitary insufficiency
3. ACTH-eosinophil (or 17-KS response)	0	0	0	0	0	0	A specific test for primary hypoadrenocorticism
4. Eosinophil count	0	0	+	0	0	0	A simple, though approximate means of judging adrenocortical status (Figure 17)
5. 24-hr. fast	0	0	0	0	0	+	A fairly specific test for S-F-N hormone lack
6. I. V. Glucose tolerance (a) Hypoglycemia unresponsiveness	0	0	0	0	0	0	(a) This test is most apt to be positive when adrenal medulla and cortex are both destroyed; also when hepatic glycogen stores are depleted.
(b) Hyperglycemia unresponsiveness	0	0	+	0	0	0	(b) This test also positive in diabetes mellitus.
7. Insulin tolerance	0	0	0	0	0	0	About the same as 6 (a)

TABLE III—3 (continued)

8. Urinary 11-17-OCS	0	0	+	0	0	Moderately reliable, direct (?) measure of S-F-N hormone production rate
9. Serum Na, Cl, K, HCO$_3$						
(a) Na↓, Cl↓, K↑, HCO$_3$↓	0	+	0	0	0	Suggestive of Na-K hormone lack
(b) Na±, Cl↓, K↓, HCO$_3$↑	+	0	0	0	0	Suggestive of Na-K hormone excess
10. Sodium deprivation	0	+	0	0	0	Moderately specific, moderately strenuous test
11. Sodium deprivation plus potassium feeding	0	+	0	0	0	Quite specific, potentially dangerous test—should be reserved for selected patients
12. Sweat Na, Cl, K	+	+	0	0	0	Potentially interesting, but as yet not thoroughly explored
13. Urinary 17-KS:						
(a) Hypo-17-ketosteroiduria	0	0	0	0	+	(a) Moderately specific test in males over 16 and quite specific in females over 16
(b) Hyper-17-ketosteroiduria	0	0	0	+	0	(b) Quite specific test in persons of both sexes regardless of age
(c) Qualitatively abnormal urinary 17-KS pattern	0	0	0	+	0	(c) Of some value for diagnosing presence of adrenocortical hyperplasia and carcinoma, but not yet fully developed

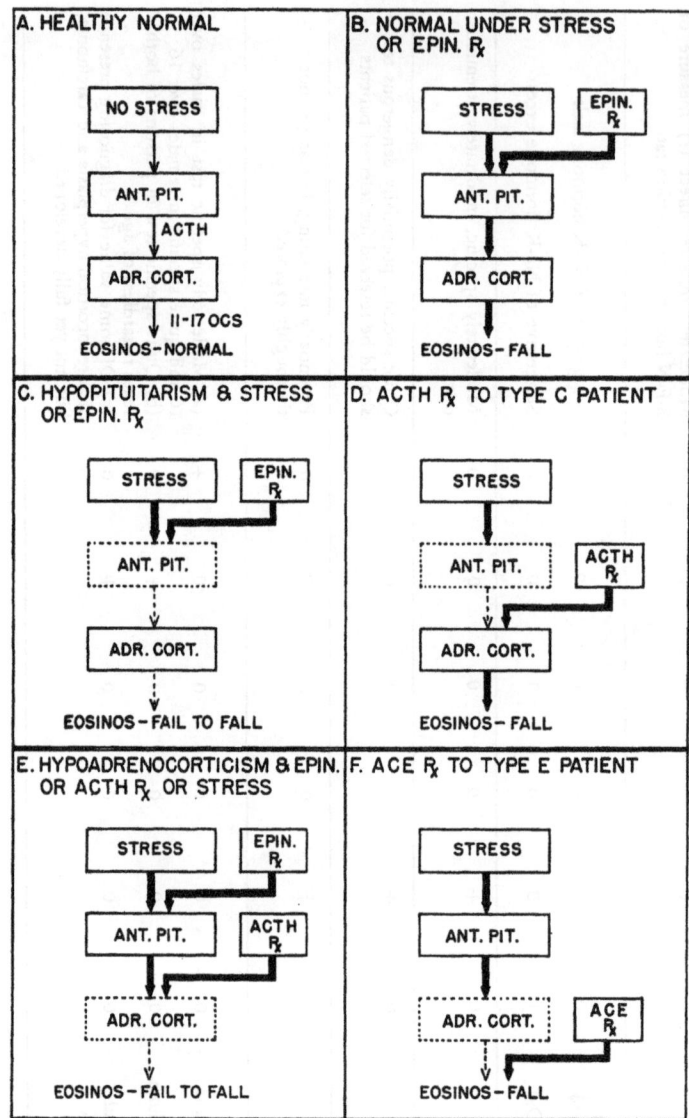

FIGURE III—17. Diagrammatic representation of factors involved in tests designed to give information concerning capacity for ACTH and 11-17-OCS (S-F-N hormone) production.

SECTIONS A AND B: Note that stress (or epinephrine treatment) stimulates ACTH secretion, ACTH activates 11-17-OCS production and 11-17-OCS induce eosinopenia.

SECTIONS C AND D: When the pituitary is destroyed or exhausted, neither stress nor epinephrine can elicit the changes shown in B, but the patient responds to exogenous ACTH.

SECTIONS E AND F: When the adrenals are destroyed, 11-17-OCS production is not stimulated by stress, epinephrine or ACTH. Hence, they fail to induce eosinopenia; the circulating eosinophils can be decreased by ACE or cortisone substitution therapy.

The Adrenal Cortices

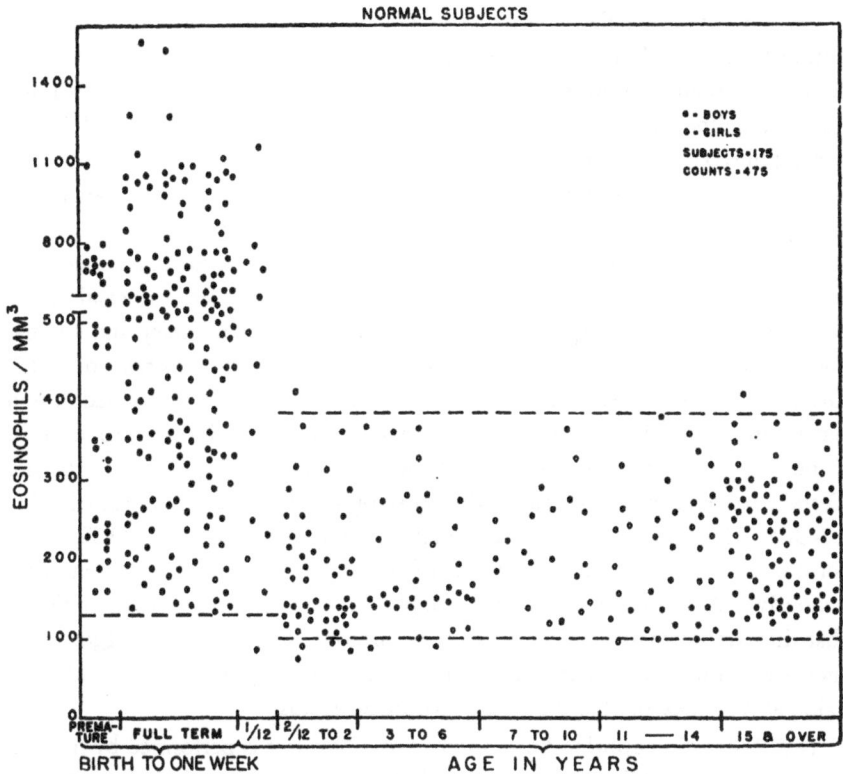

FIGURE III—18. Absolute eosinophil counts on normal subjects of various ages. The interrupted horizontal lines indicate approximate normal ranges. Data from C. Uribe R. and N. B. Talbot. Unpublished observations.

---

administered epinephrine, causes increased ACTH production in healthy individuals and hence an increase in 11-17-OCS production. As a consequence of the increase in 11-17-OCS, the eosinophil count falls. If stress is prolonged, the output of 11-17-OCS also rises.

Section C shows that in hypopituitary patients stress (or administered epinephrine) usually fails to prompt the fall in eosinophil count noted in Section B, because the anterior pituitary is incapable of secreting more ACTH. Occasionally in such patients epinephrine may induce eosinopenia. This suggests that epinephrine *per se* may be capable of causing lysis of circulating eosinophils. Section D shows that the adrenocortical activity of such patients can be increased by administered ACTH.

Section E indicates that neither stress (including epinephrine treatment) nor administered ACTH is capable of eliciting increased adrenocortical 11-17-OCS hormone production in patients with primary hypoadrenocorticism. Consequently, neither stress nor administered ACTH is followed by a fall in the eosinophil count (or a rise in urinary steroid output) in patients of this sort. Section F shows that eosinopenia can nonetheless be induced in such patients by giving appropriate amounts of the 11-17-OCS type of hormone.

In the paragraphs which follow, the manner in which these phenomena can be utilized as aids in clinical diagnosis are discussed. In brief, a normal epinephrine-eosinophil test response suggests that the anterior pituitary and adrenal cortices are functionally intact and that the eosinophils are sensitive to 11-17-OCS. If this test gives an abnormal result, the ACTH test can be applied to find out whether the adrenal cortices rather than the anterior pituitary are at fault. A normal response eliminates the possibility of primary hypoadrenocorticism. Certain patients may have circulating eosinophils which are not lysed by 11-17-OCS. This situation can be recognized by administering 11-17-OCS in the form of adrenocortical extract (30 cc. of aqueous extract per m^2 is given intravenously). A 50 per cent fall in eosinophil count within four hours indicates that they are normally susceptible to this hormone. Failure to fall suggests that they are resistant. Under the latter circumstance eosinophil counts are of little value as an index of changes in adrenocortical status.

Test 2—the Epinephrine-Eosinophil Test. This test is performed by making a series of eosinophil counts before and after the administration of a standard dose of epinephrine. The basis for this test is described by Figure 17 and its accompanying text. A method for counting blood eosinophils is given in the Appendix. Normal values are given in Figure 18. In this clinic 0.3 cc. of 1:1000 epinephrine solution* per m^2 is given subcutaneously. Eosinophil counts are made on capillary blood just before the injection and at intervals of half an hour, three hours and four hours afterwards. If the count at the third or fourth hour has remained above 60 to 70 cells per mm^3, a second similar dose of epinephrine is given and the count is repeated three to four hours later.†

Figure 19 sets forth results obtained for a series of normal individuals. It is seen that all the control values were within normal limits. Half an hour following

* Epinephrine solutions are apt to deteriorate when exposed to light and air. Confusion due to this can be minimized by using freshly opened vials containing 1 cc. of 1:1000 epinephrine for each injection.

† The Peter Bent Brigham Hospital group[19 d] prefers to administer the epinephrine diluted in salt solution intravenously over the course of 30 minutes. A 50 per cent or greater fall in the eosinophil count below the control level within four hours is considered a normal response. No attention is paid to absolute eosinophil values.

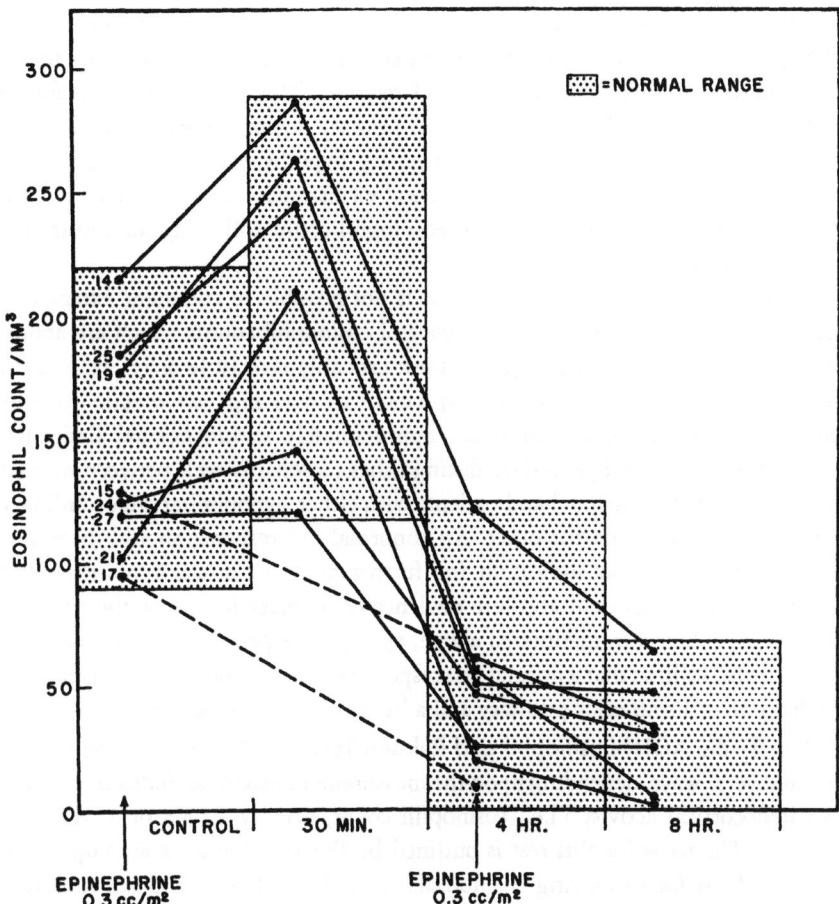

FIGURE III—19. Results obtained by application of the epinephrine-eosinophil test to normal individuals ranging in age between 3 months and 17 years. Expressed in terms of per cent fall in eosinophil count from control level, the least values obtained were 40 per cent at four hours and 70 per cent at eight hours. From observations by C. Uribe R. and N. B. Talbot. Unpublished observations.

the epinephrine dose the count rose somewhat. Thereafter, it tended to fall. In each case the eosinophils numbered less than 70 cells per mm^3 (usually less than 50 cells per mm^3) within four hours after the first or second dose. Expressed in relative terms, the fall in normal persons was at least 40 per cent at four hours and at least 70 per cent at eight hours.

Figure 20 shows that patients with hypopituitarism and hypoadrenocorticism failed to show a normal fall in the eosinophil count. Incidentally, it also indicates that patients with mild-to-moderate primary hypothyroidism responded to the epinephrine-eosinophil test in a normal manner. This is of interest because it suggests a way in which patients with primary hypopituitarism may be distinguished from most patients with primary hypothyroidism. The figure also shows that two patients with adrenocortical virilism due to bilateral adrenocortical hyperplasia had a normal fall in eosinophil count following administration of epinephrine.

Because this test is relatively new, it is not possible to comment extensively upon its reliability. In patients with control eosinophil counts which are abnormally elevated because of allergy, this test probably is of little or no value as an index of adrenocortical function. Experience to date suggests that in patients whose control eosinophil counts are approximately within normal limits the epinephrine-eosinophil procedure distinguishes reasonably well between normal individuals on the one hand and patients with either hypopituitarism or ordinary hypoadrenocorticism on the other. An abnormal test response should, however, be considered more as indication for further study of anterior pituitary and adrenocortical status than absolute evidence of a defect in one or the other of these organs. Since, as mentioned above, epinephrine *per se* may induce eosinopenia, it also follows that a normal test response should not be considered absolute evidence that the anterior pituitary and adrenal cortices are normal.

Test 3—the ACTH-Eosinophil and Related Tests. This test can be carried out in several ways, depending upon the measurement used as an index of changes in adrenocortical activity (i.e., eosinophil count, urinary 17-KS or 11-17-OCS output). The basis for this test is outlined by Figure 17 and its accompanying text. Methods for measuring eosinophils, 17-KS and 11-17-OCS are indicated in the Appendix.

When the eosinophil count is employed as the index, the procedure followed is the same as that described for Test 2 except that 15 mg. of ACTH (Armour Standard*) per m^2 is injected instead of epinephrine. A decrease of 50 per cent or more in eosinophil count by the fourth hour after injection is considered satisfactory evidence that the adrenal cortices are functionally normal. As was true for the epinephrine-eosinophil procedure, it appears probable that the test results

* The Armour Laboratories of Chicago have standardized the potency of their product by a bio-assay procedure. The doses recommended here are expressed, therefore, as so many milligrams of Armour Standard equivalent. The ACTH is dispensed as a sterile lyophilized powder which must be dissolved in sterile saline (about 10 mg. per cc.) and administered intramuscularly. To date no serious allergic sensitivity reactions have been observed in this clinic. However, a few patients have developed hives of moderate degree.

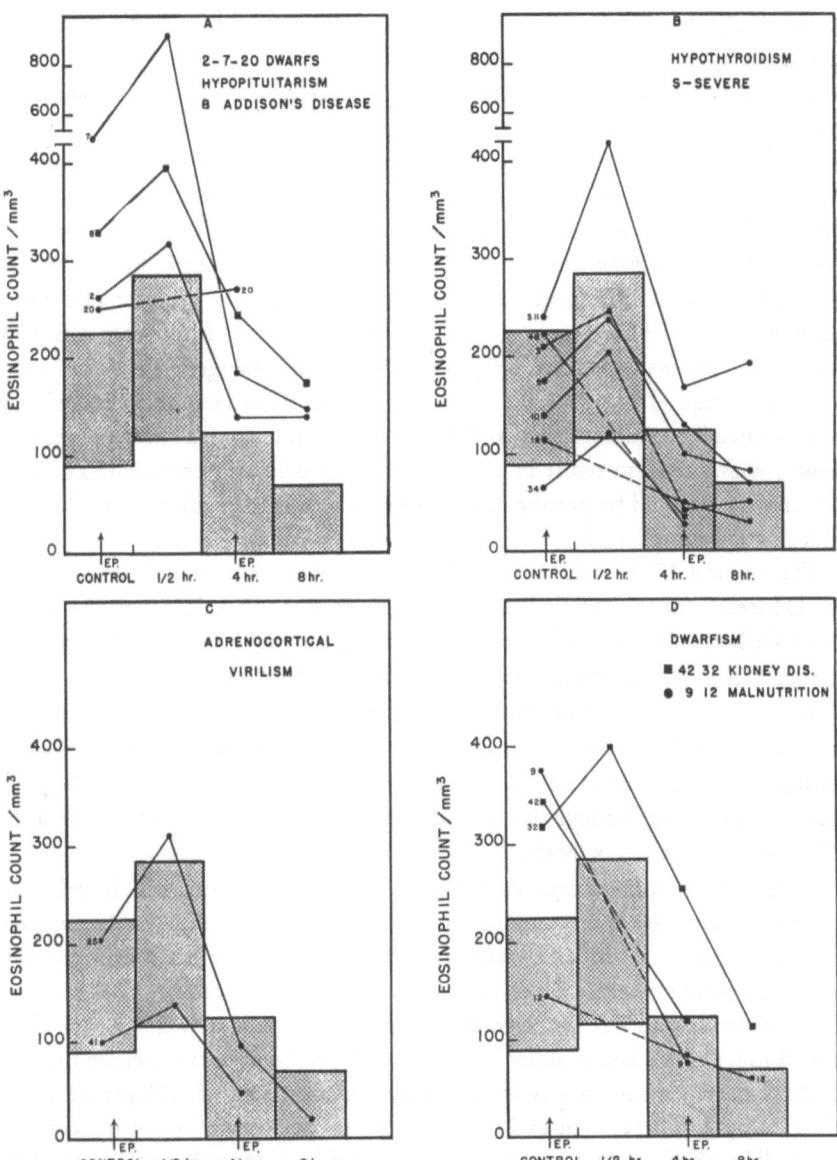

FIGURE III—20. Results obtained by application of epinephrine-eosinophil test to patients with various abnormal conditions. The shaded areas define the normal limits suggested by the data of Figure 19. From observations by C. Uribe R. and N. B. Talbot. Unpublished observations.

are most apt to be reliable in non-allergic patients whose control eosinophil counts are approximately within normal limits.

The urinary uric acid/creatinine ratio also can be used as an indication of increased 11-17-OCS hormone production, provided the purine intake is carefully controlled.[19 s] The test is performed under conditions of fasting by collecting a sample of urine between 6 and 8 a.m., before the administration of 15 mg. per m^2 of Armour's Standard ACTH, and a second sample between 9 a.m. and noon. The uric acid/creatinine ratio of both samples is determined. If the adrenals are normal, the ratio increases on the average 90 per cent following administration of ACTH (range +60 to +130 per cent). In patients with primary hypoadrenocorticism ACTH prompts little or no change in the ratio (average +16; range −14 to +59 per cent). The diagnostic value of the uric acid test is eliminated by conditions such as dehydration, gout, leukemia and renal insufficiency, which tend to result in abnormal urinary uric acid excretion. The test also may be negated by hepatic conditions which interfere with the metabolism or formation of uric acid.

The urinary 17-KS and 11-17-OCS output increases appreciably following ACTH treatment. However, from 7 to 15 mg. per m^2 of ACTH must be given every six hours for two to four days to elicit a clear-cut change in these urinary steroid values. Accordingly, the test is performed by (a) collecting the urine voided during the 24 hours before treatment, (b) administering ACTH for a period of 48 to 96 hours as outlined above, (c) collecting the urine voided during the second, third or fourth day after the inception of ACTH therapy and (d) analyzing the first and second collections of urine for their content of 17-KS or 11-17-OCS or both.

With the exception of patients with primary hypoadrenocorticism, individuals of all ages show rises in the output of both 17-KS and 11-17-OCS. On the average the 17-KS output of infants, children and adults alike increases over control levels by approximately 700 per cent within 2 to 12 days. Absolute 17-KS values attained during this interval average for infants approximately 2 mg., for children 3 mg. and for adults about 22 mg. per m^2 per day. On the average the 11-17-OCS output of infants is increased by approximately 4,000 per cent, of children by 2,000 per cent and of adults by 900 per cent over normal control levels. The absolute 11-17-OCS values attained by infants rise to remarkably high levels, averaging 4 mg. per day. In children average absolute values of about 1.5 mg., and in adults average absolute values of about 3.0 mg. per day are reached after a period of 2 to 12 days of ACTH treatment. These differences in response to ACTH by individuals of various ages suggest that either adrenocortical responsiveness to ACTH or the intermediary metabolism of adrenocortical steroids can be markedly affected by age and presumably by other factors as well.[15 h]

While a normal response to ACTH, as evidenced by an appropriate change in one or more of the foregoing indices, effectively rules out primary hypoadrenocorticism, an abnormal response does not necessarily rule in this condition. This qualification stems from the observation that it may take as long as a week of ACTH therapy to regenerate and reactivate adrenal cortices which have undergone marked functional and anatomic atrophy as a consequence of chronic, severe hypopituitarism. Thus, prompt response to ACTH by a hypopituitary patient suggests that the pituitary disease is mild or of very recent origin.

Test 4—the Eosinophil Count.* Tests 2 and 3 have indicated that artificially induced, increased adrenocortical activity usually results in eosinopenia. The eosinophil count also tends to fall when spontaneous physiologic or pathologic hyperadrenocorticism results in increased production of 11-17-OCS.

Figure 21 shows that when endocrinologically normal non-allergic persons are subjected to stress, such as acute infection, accident, operation, emotional upset or the like, they are very apt to have abnormally low eosinophil counts (i.e., less than 100 and usually less than 50 cells per mm^3; see Figure 18 for normal controls). By contrast, available evidence indicates that hypopituitary and hypoadrenocortical patients fail to develop eosinopenia under similar circumstances. In other words, when there is a question of adrenocortical failure in severely sick patients (i.e., the so-called Waterhouse-Friderichsen syndrome), the eosinophil count can be used as an approximate index of adrenocortical status.

If the patient has marked eosinopenia, there is little likelihood that adrenocortical failure has developed. But the possibility exists that infection or toxins, by suppressing leucocytogenesis, may occasionally cause granulocytopenia or pancytopenia and hence eosinopenia of non-endocrine origin. Moreover, it is to be remembered that the eosinophil count indicates the adrenocortical status of the patient three or four hours prior to the time of counting rather than his status at the time the count is made.

If, on the other hand, a severely sick patient fails to have an eosinophil count of less than about 50 cells per mm^3, serious consideration should be given to the possibility that his adrenocortical–anterior pituitary mechanism has failed and that he may therefore be in acute need of adrenocortical hormone therapy. In these connections it is noteworthy that the eosinophil count tends to rise to, and for a transient period above, normal levels as patients convalesce (see Figure 21). Therefore, a rising or normal count in a patient who is showing clinical

---

* See also preceding sections.

[174]   CHAPTER III:

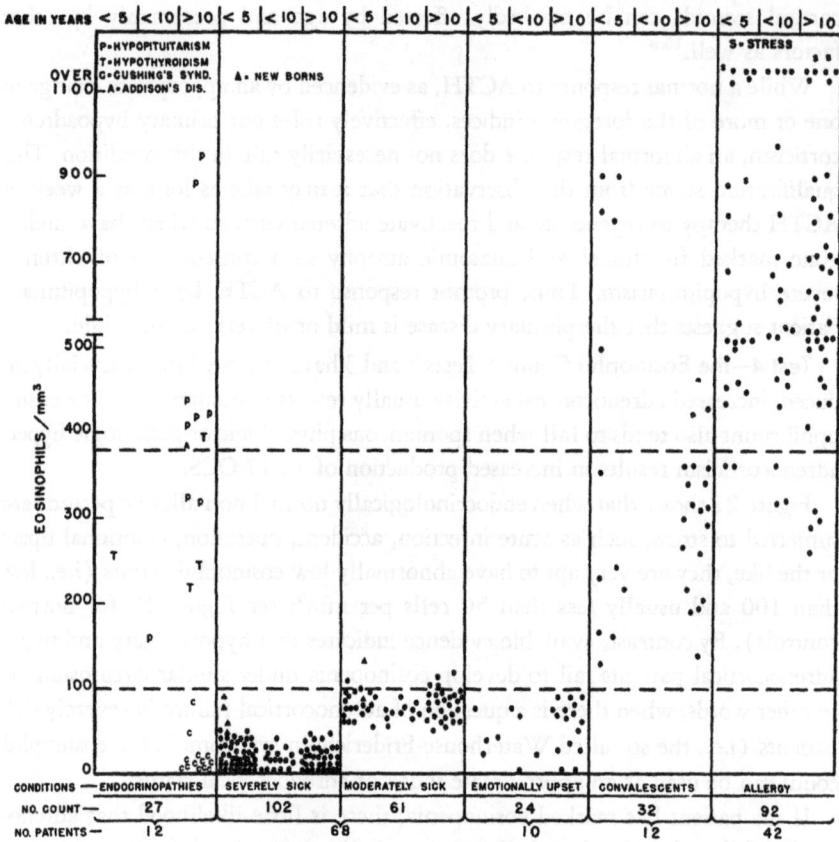

FIGURE III—21. Absolute eosinophil counts on patients with various primary endocrinopathies and on sick, convalescent and allergic individuals who were endocrinologically normal. The broken lines indicate the range of normal (see Figure 18). Points are distributed approximately according to age as indicated along the top margin of the chart. In the right-hand section allergic patients suffering marked stress are designated by the letter S. From observations by C. Uribe R. and N. B. Talbot. Unpublished observations.

signs of improvement has altogether different implications than it has in a patient whose clinical condition is deteriorating.

Incidentally, eosinopenia is a characteristic of patients with active Cushing's syndrome. A normal count in a non-allergic individual therefore rules against this diagnosis.

Test 5—the Twenty-four-Hour Fast.[9 b, 19 d] The purpose of this test is to determine whether a subject has lost his normal ability to fast for a prolonged period without becoming hypoglycemic. The physiologic concepts underlying this test are set forth by Figure 11 and its accompanying text.

The test is carried out by omitting all foods except water (and salt if desired) for a potential period of 24 hours, commencing after the evening meal. Starting at eight o'clock the next morning, blood sugar concentrations are determined at intervals of about two hours throughout the day. If the patient becomes faint or shows signs of developing hypoglycemic coma or convulsions before the 24-hour period of fasting is completed, the test may be terminated and the patient revived by the administration of sugar and, if necessary, adrenocortical extract or cortisone. Incidentally, additional information of interest may be had by testing specimens of urine voided during the latter part of the fast for acetone. Unlike normal persons, hypoadrenocortical patients are not apt to develop acetonuria during a 24-hour fast.[19 d]

Figure 22 diagrammatically illustrates the fact that under conditions of fasting (a) normal persons are able, with the aid of their 11-17-OCS, to maintain blood sugar concentrations within standard limits (80 to 120 mg. per cent) for long periods of time but (b) hypoadrenocortical persons tend to become hypoglycemic within 24 hours.

Though this test procedure is somewhat strenuous, it is of value for ruling adrenocortical insufficiency in or out in questionable cases. There are a few conditions which may confuse the meaning of the test. Coexistent diabetes mellitus due to insulin deficiency will lessen the tendency to develop hypoglycemia shown by patients with simple hypoadrenocorticism.[19 f] Contrariwise, patients suffering from hyperinsulinism secondary to pancreatic islet hyperplasia or tumor may show a striking tendency to fasting hypoglycemia even though their adrenal cortices are functionally intact. Such patients tend to have abnormally low rather than normal eosinophil counts when hypoglycemic. Hepatic diseases, including glycogen storage disease, may also be characterized by episodes of hypoglycemia which are not due to adrenocortical hormone lack. For other discussion of these problems see under hyperinsulinism, Chapter IX.

Tests 6 and 7—the Insulin and Glucose Tolerance Tests.[19 g, 9 b] The basis for these tests is given by Figure 11 and its accompanying text. They are applied to the various homeostatic mechanisms which normally act to keep blood sugar concentrations within certain limits (usually 80 to 120 mg. per cent). More specifically, both the insulin and the glucose tolerance tests may be used to find out whether an individual has an abnormal tendency to "hypoglycemia unresponsiveness." This can be due to a number of conditions, including primary liver disease (with fixation of or lack of glycogen), hyperinsulinism, possibly adrenal medullary failure (with epinephrine deficiency), possibly central nerv-

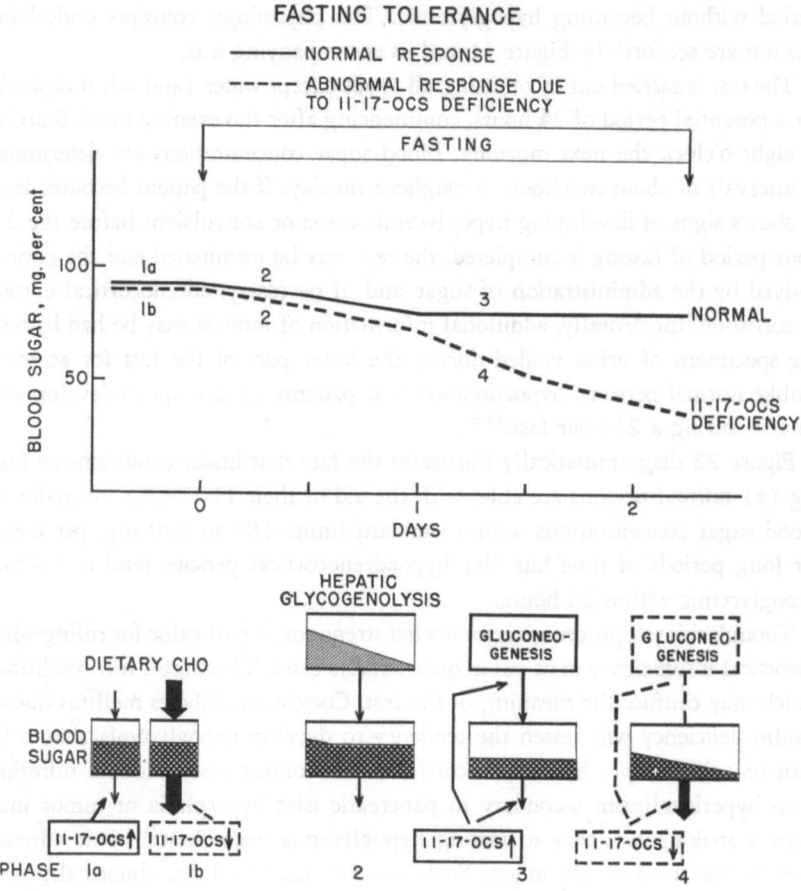

FIGURE III—22. Effect of fasting on blood sugar of a normal individual and a patient with 11-17-OCS hormone deficiency. The numbers shown adjacent to the blood sugar curves are phase numbers. In Phase 1 blood sugar is sustained by dietary carbohydrate. In the early hours of a fast (Phase 2) blood sugar is upheld both in normal and in hypoadrenocortical individuals by lysis of hepatic glycogen stores. When hepatic glycogen stores become depleted, the normal person maintains his blood sugar by forming new sugar from protein (gluconeogenesis) (Phase 3). By contrast, the patient with S-F-N hormone lack is unable to form sugar from protein at a normal rate (see Figure 11). In addition he tends to utilize available glucose at an abnormally rapid rate. Because of these disturbances glucose is withdrawn from the circulation more rapidly than it is being added. Consequently, the patient with S-F-N hormone deficiency becomes hypoglycemic within 18 to 48 hours of fasting (Phase 4). From N. B. Talbot, *Pediatrics* 3:519, 1949.

ous system disease (failure of production of hypothalamic ACTH stimulator?) and adrenocortical insufficiency (with S-F-N hormone lack). Alternatively, the glucose tolerance test may reveal "hyperglycemia unresponsiveness." This condition may be due either to pancreatic islet malfunction (with insulin deficiency), excess pituitary glycotropic factor or hyperadrenocorticism (with S-F-N hormone excess).

As the foregoing indicates, neither the insulin nor the glucose tolerance test alone can be expected to yield very specific information concerning adrenocortical status. On the other hand, they are relatively easy to perform and may be of considerable value in the negative if not in the positive diagnostic sense. It should be remembered that both tests can give rise to untoward reactions in patients with Addison's disease. The insulin tolerance test can cause severe hypoglycemia; the intravenous glucose tolerance test can give rise to high fever which develops about 12 hours after the infusion.[19 d] Accordingly, it is advised that these tests be omitted in patients known to have adrenocortical insufficiency.

To simplify the present discussion, it will be assumed that the pancreatic islets, liver and central nervous system are not diseased. However, because the adrenal medullæ may become damaged when the adrenal cortices are destroyed, attention will be given here to the adrenal glands as a whole. As an aid in presentation, "hypoglycemia unresponsiveness" and "hyperglycemia unresponsiveness" will be dealt with under separate subheadings. Both the insulin and the glucose tolerance tests will be mentioned under the former; only the glucose tolerance test will be considered under the latter heading.

Hypoglycemia unresponsiveness. The insulin tolerance test is performed in the morning following an overnight fast. Ideally, the patient should be prepared for this and the glucose tolerance test by being fed a diet containing about 175 gm. of carbohydrate per m^2 per day for three days prior to the test. This regimen assures that the liver will be well stocked with glycogen at the time the test is performed.[19 h]

After obtaining a sample of blood for sugar determination, from 1 to 4 units of regular crystalline insulin per m^2 are administered intravenously. Normal persons can tolerate 4 units per m^2 without excessive difficulty. Patients with marked anterior pituitary and adrenal insufficiency may, however, be very sensitive to insulin. Therefore, when there appears to be a real likelihood that a patient has one of these conditions, it is best to give 1 or 2 units per m^2 rather than the 4 units per m^2 dose. Samples of blood for glucose analysis are obtained 20, 30, 45, 60 and 90 minutes later. In 20 or 30 minutes the patient is apt to show clinical signs of hypoglycemia (pallor, nervousness, sweating). Normally these disappear rapidly within the ensuing 15 or 30 minutes. If they persist or appear

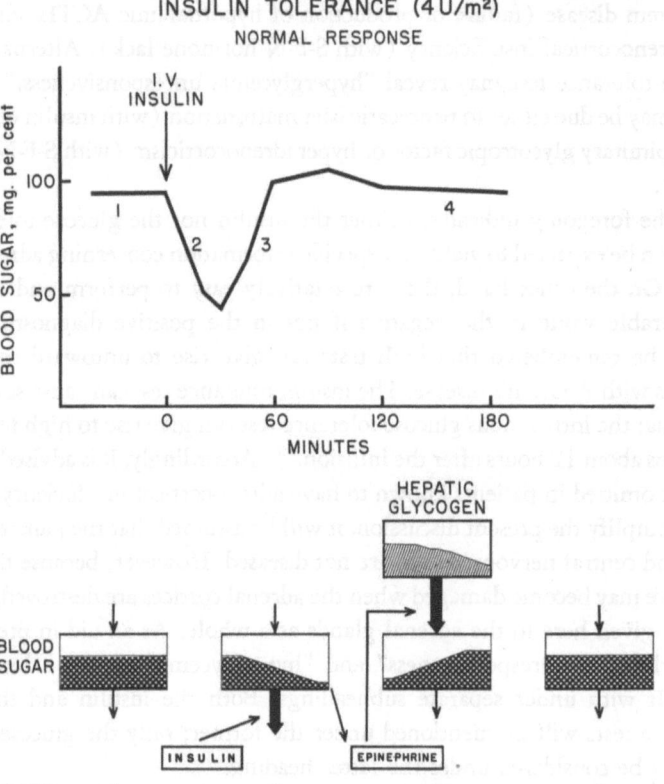

FIGURE III—23. Normal insulin tolerance test. Insulin accelerates tissue utilization of glucose. Under conditions of fasting, this results in hypoglycemia (Phase 2). Hypoglycemia stimulates release of epinephrine, which raises blood sugar concentration by causing hepatic glycogenolysis (Phase 3). Activation of the adrenocortical alarm reaction mechanism by epinephrine (see Figure 17) may facilitate this homeostatic response because S-F-N hormones tend both to block insulin action (see Figure 26) and to promote gluconeogenesis from protein (see Figure 11). From N. B. Talbot, *Pediatrics* 3:519, 1949.

---

to be progressing toward coma or convulsions, glucose should be given promptly by mouth or, if necessary, by vein. Incidentally, hypoadrenocortical patients often develop signs of hypoglycemia before blood sugar levels have fallen to levels productive of symptoms in normal persons.

As shown by Figure 23, insulin increases the relative rate at which glucose leaves the blood stream. Thus a single intravenous dose of insulin characteristically produces an acute fall in blood sugar concentration. Normally, the resultant

The Adrenal Cortices

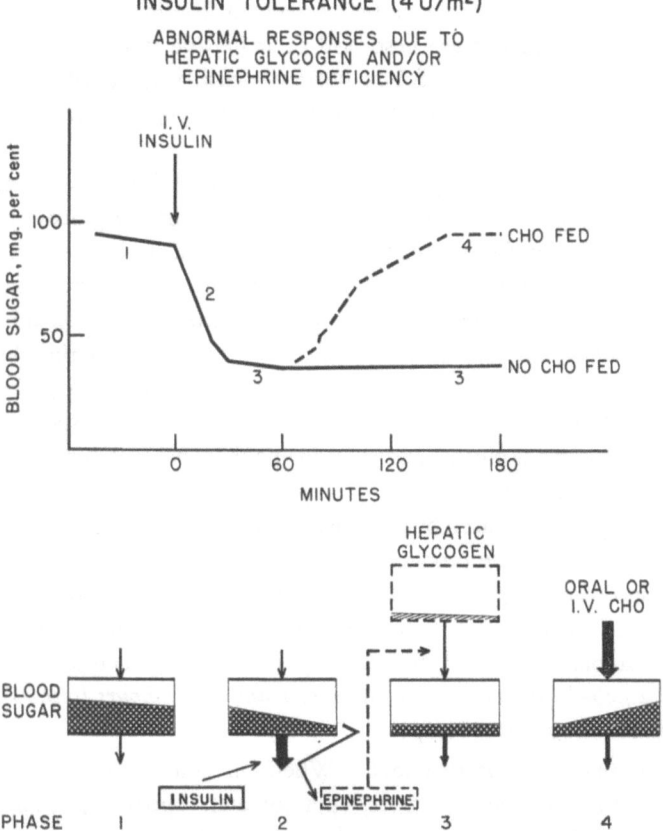

FIGURE III—24. Insulin tolerance test in adrenocortical insufficiency. S-F-N hormone lack results in increased insulin sensitivity. As a result, a standard dose of insulin causes an exceptionally large increase in glucose utilization by peripheral tissues and hence a sharp drop in blood sugar (Phase 2). If the adrenal medullæ are destroyed, the hypoglycemia cannot induce epinephrine release. More important, if liver glycogen stores are depleted as a result of S-F-N hormone deficiency, there is no possibility of elevating blood sugar by hepatic glycogenolysis. Under these circumstances hypoglycemia persists (Phase 3) until carbohydrate is administered (Phase 4). From N. B. Talbot, *Pediatrics* 3:519, 1949.

period of relative hypoglycemia is transient—probably because hypoglycemia stimulates the release of epinephrine by the adrenal medullæ. The epinephrine in turn induces hepatic glycogenolysis which serves to elevate blood sugar concentrations. If the adrenal medullæ are intact and glycogen stores in the liver are adequate, patients with hypoadrenocorticism may also respond in an essentially normal manner when subjected to the intravenous insulin tolerance test. However, if the adrenal glands are destroyed or if hepatic stores of glycogen are depleted, as a consequence of S-F-N hormone lack, insulin will cause hypoglycemia which cannot be corrected spontaneously (hypoglycemia unresponsiveness) (see Figure 24).

A closely similar picture may be evoked in patients with hypoadrenocorticism by administering glucose intravenously. Preparation for the glucose tolerance test is the same as for the insulin tolerance test. Blood is obtained for glucose determination just before and ½, 1, 2, 3, 4 and 5 hours after dextrose is administered. To avoid the unpredictable variability in glucose absorption inherent in the oral type of glucose tolerance test, it is recommended that the glucose be given intravenously. The dose (20 gm. per m^2) is given over a period of 30 minutes as a 10 to 20 per cent solution; it is calculated to correspond approximately to the amount of glucose absorbed during the same length of time following a normal carbohydrate meal.

The hyperglycemia induced by administration of glucose in the amount stated is thought to stimulate the production of endogenous insulin (see Figure 25). When the intravenous glucose infusion is stopped, this endogenous insulin sets off the train of events just outlined for parenterally administered insulin, but the time relations are spread out. *Consequently, hypoadrenocortical patients should be watched for evidences of hypoglycemia for six hours following cessation of intravenous glucose therapy.*

Hyperglycemia unresponsiveness. When, in contrast to the foregoing, S-F-N hormone is present in excess, approximately opposite phenomena are observed. As a rule, fasting does not induce abnormal consequence, presumably because increased gluconeogenesis from protein is not quantitatively sufficient to result in fasting hyperglycemia. However, when glucose is administered, a diabetic type of glucose tolerance curve may be produced, because excess 11-17-OCS tend to block insulin action (see Figure 26).

Test 8—Urinary 11-17-Oxycorticosteroid Measurements. Suitably prepared extracts of normal urine contain substances with biologic and chemical properties similar to those of known 11-17-OCS* (or S-F-N hormones).[11] The daily output of these substances can be measured by both bio-assay and chemical procedures. The former have the merit of measuring only substances which have S-F-N hormone activity; counterbalancing this attribute is the fact that they are difficult and expensive to carry out. The available chemical assay procedures have

* Alternative terms used in the literature are cortins, corticoids, neutral reducing lipids, formaldehydogenic substances and 11-oxysteroid-like substances.

the advantage of being comparatively easy to perform. On the other hand, they suffer from the disadvantage of being also less specific.*

As was illustrated by Figure 14, it appears that the urinary 11-17-OCS output normally ranges between 0.05 and 0.22 (average about 0.1) mg. per m^2 per day regardless of sex or age. While preliminary data suggest that the values obtained for infants under one or two months of age may average somewhat lower, there is a possibility that this finding is an artefact.† While there are moderate day-to-day fluctuations, it is unusual for the average value for two consecutive daily determinations to lie outside the normal range under normal circumstances.

Figure 27 gives information concerning the urinary output of 11-17-OCS in various conditions. Reading this chart from left to right, mean values for conditions up to and including osteoporosis may be considered low. The conditions bounded by essential hypertension on the left and allergy on the right give mean values falling within the normal range. Conditions falling to the right of allergy have mean values which are considered high. This classification is statistically significant in conditions where 10 or more observations are recorded, and probably significant in most of the others.

Several facts appear to be of interest. First, values tend to be low in patients with primary hypoadrenocorticism,** hypopituitarism and hypothyroidism. This lowering, though definite, is of limited diagnostic value because the space available for abnormally low values (i.e., the difference between nought and the lower limit of normal) is small.

* In these connections a word on chemical methodology may be in order. Generally speaking, two types of procedure are available. In one method the urine extract is rather extensively processed and purified.[19 i] The results obtained with this method compare reasonably favorably with the results obtained by bio-assay. In the other, the purification procedure is considerably abbreviated.[19 j] In consequence, the values thus obtained tend to be several-fold higher than those obtained by the more extensive method. When the urinary output of 11-17-OCS is high, both procedures give relatively similar information; when it is low, there is apt to be a considerable discrepancy in the results obtained by the two procedures. It is believed that the discrepancy reflects errors of overestimation due to the presence of interfering substances in the extracts, which have been only partially purified. Because experience in this clinic has been largely with urinary 11-17-OCS assays carried out with the aid of the more extensive chemical procedure mentioned above, results obtained thereby will form the basis for most of the comments which follow.

† The lower limit of sensitivity of the chemical procedure employed is about 0.05 mg. per urine sample analyzed. Inasmuch as the surface area of a newborn infant is only about 0.2 m^2, it is apparent that at least 48 and preferably 96 hours' worth of urine should be collected if valid information concerning urinary 11-17-OCS output is to be obtained. Only one of the values obtained on small infants and recorded in Figure 13 meets this qualification in full. This value is on the high rather than the low side of adult normal values.

** It is possible that the low normal values obtained on certain hypoadrenocortical patients are not in error but are real and indicative of some residual adrenocortical function.

Continued on page 185

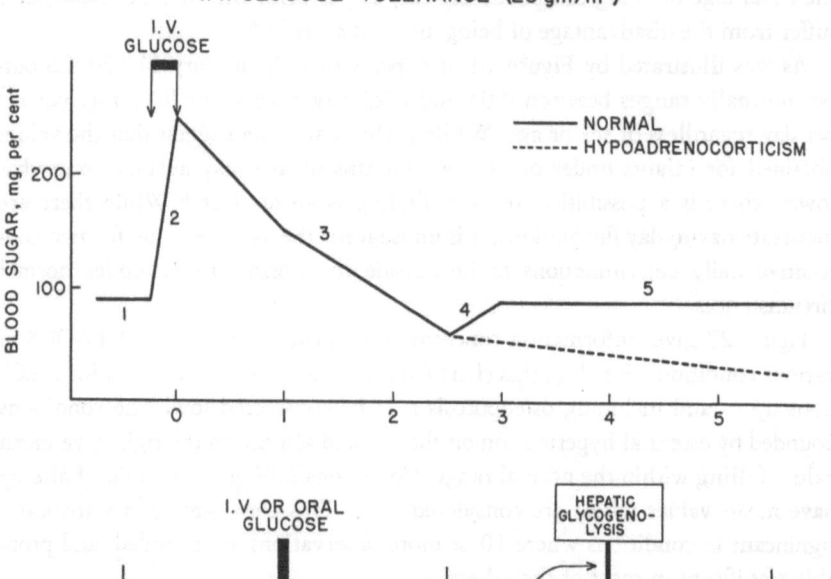

FIGURE III—25. Glucose tolerance test in a normal person and in a patient with hypoadrenocorticism (i.e., S-F-N hormone lack). Elevation of blood sugar by glucose administration (Phase 2) causes the pancreatic islets to secrete insulin. The insulin increases glucose utilization by the peripheral tissues and hence causes blood glucose to fall (Phase 3). In the healthy person, as blood sugar concentration reaches normal levels the stimulus to insulin secretion wanes. Nonetheless, insulin already released may cause blood sugar to fall to hypoglycemic levels. Hypoglycemia stimulates release of epinephrine, which raises blood sugar to normal by stimulating hepatic glycogenolysis (Phase 4). A state of euglycemia is finally regained (Phase 5). In the case of the hypoadrenocortical individual, hypoglycemia may follow hyperglycemia within three to six hours for several reasons. Lack of S-F-N hormone renders the individual unusually sensitive to insulin and can result in depletion of hepatic glycogen stores. As a result of these disturbances hypoglycemia persists until carbohydrate is fed (see Figure 24). From N. B. Talbot, *Pediatrics* 3:519, 1949.

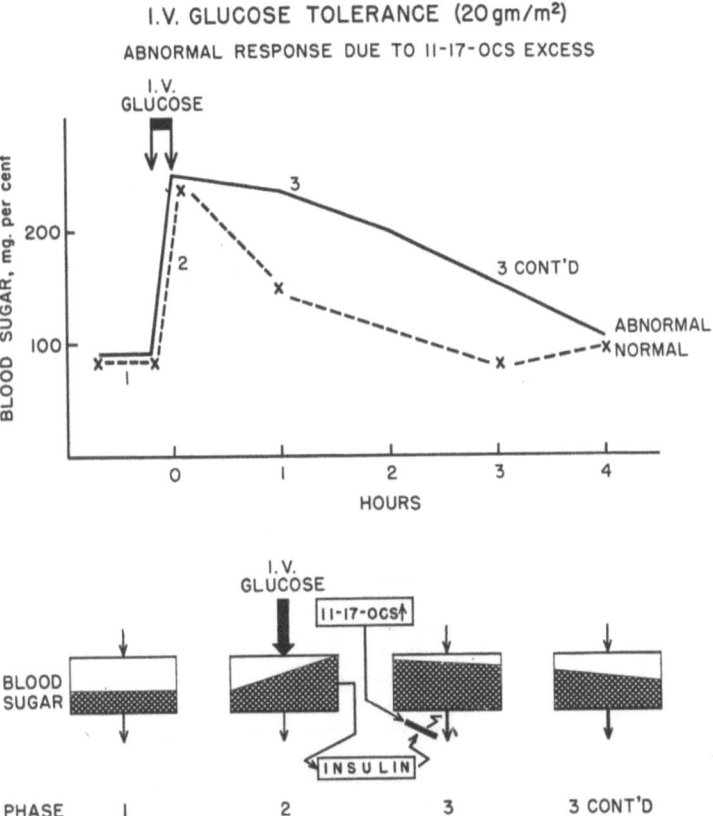

FIGURE III—26. Glucose tolerance test in a patient with hyperadrenocorticism (i.e., increased S-F-N hormone activity). In this diagram the broken line represents the normal as shown in Figure 25. The solid curve shows the tendency of hyperglycemia to persist which develops when S-F-N hormone (11-17-OCS) production is increased. During Phase 2 hyperglycemia stimulates insulin secretion in a normal manner. Increased S-F-N hormone activity partially prevents insulin from accelerating tissue utilization of glucose, and in consequence a diabetic type of glucose tolerance curve results (Phase 3). In diabetes mellitus this type of curve is thought to be due to insulin deficiency. However, when the stress of diabetic coma stimulates the adrenocortical alarm reaction (functional hyperadrenocorticism), increased S-F-N hormone activity aggravates the degree of insulin deficiency by producing the insulin resistance just described. From N. B. Talbot, *Pediatrics* 3:519, 1949.

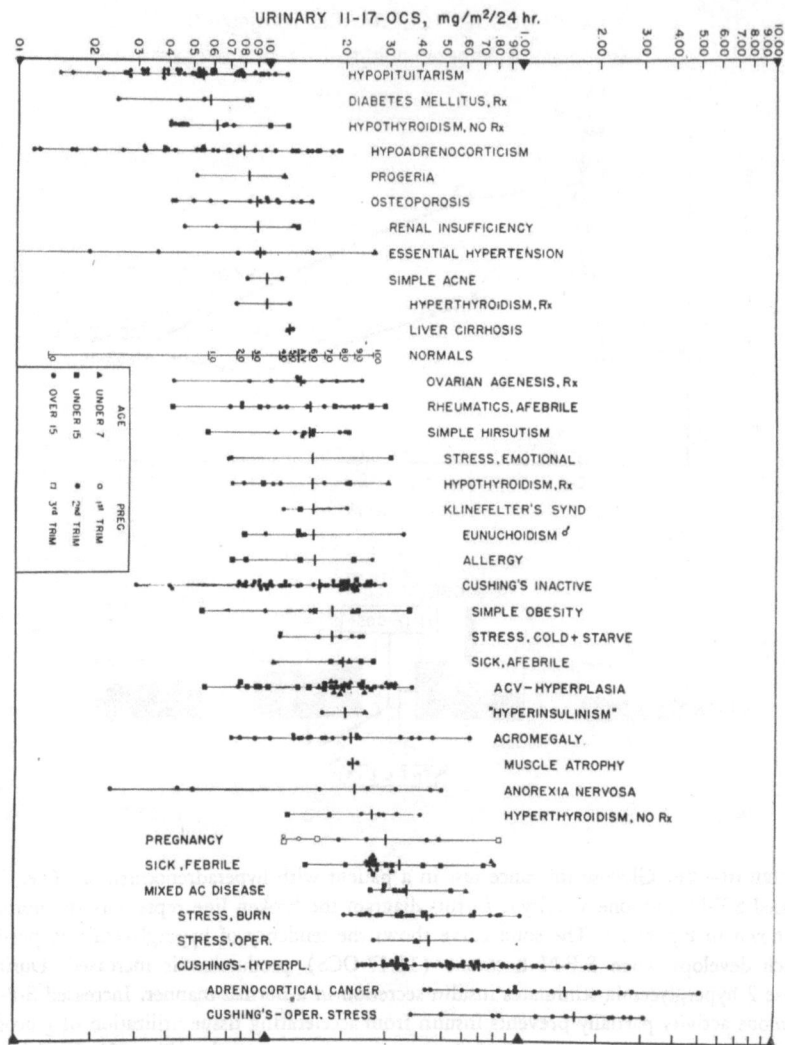

FIGURE III—27. Urinary 11-17-OCS values in patients with various conditions. Note that the results are expressed as mg. per m^2 of body surface per 24 hours. The numbers shown along the line representing normal individuals are percentile distribution values. One hundred per cent of normal persons have urinary 11-17-OCS values equal to or less than that indicated by the top of the normal line; 90 per cent have values equal to or less than the indicated level, etc. Average values for each condition are indicated by the short horizontal bars intersecting the vertical line representing each condition. Rx=treated; ACV= adrenocortical virilism; AC=adrenocortical; hyperpl=adrenocortical hyperplasia; CA= carcinoma; OP=operation. From N. B. Talbot, M. Wood, E. Christo and A. S. Zygmuntowicz, in *Proc. 1st Clin. ACTH Conf.*, J. R. Mote, ed. Philadelphia, Blakiston, 1950.

Second, the values obtained on patients with Cushing's syndrome are abnormally elevated. This is true whether the patient has adrenocortical hyperplasia or an adrenocortical cancer. Following removal of an adrenocortical cancer, the values return to normal or subnormal levels. On the other hand, in the case of patients with virilism due to hyperadrenocorticism, the values are apt to be normal or slightly elevated if the patient has bilateral adrenocortical hyperplasia and to be more markedly elevated if the patient has an adrenocortical cancer.

Third, it is especially noteworthy that there is likely to be a marked increase in the urinary 11-17-OCS output of endocrinologically normal persons when they become severely stressed as by accidents, operations or other acute illnesses. This increase is of the same order of magnitude as that seen in patients with Cushing's syndrome. In other words, an "abnormally" elevated urinary 11-17-OCS value does not necessarily mean that a patient has pathologic hyperadrenocorticism, for it is believed that the elevated values seen in severely sick patients should be considered as physiologic, or normal, for the abnormal circumstances. Such physiologic hyperadrenocorticism subsides when the stress ends.

Tests 9 to 11—Electrolyte Measurements.[19 k-n] Tests 9 to 11 have the purpose of attempting to define adrenocortical status with respect to the Na-K hormone. More specifically, they are intended to find out whether there is a tendency toward abnormal retention or loss of sodium and potassium. The basic considerations underlying these measurements have been set forth in Figures 1 to 5 and the text which accompanies them.

Serum electrolyte measurements. Section 9 of Table 3 indicates the most characteristic types of abnormality in serum electrolyte composition seen in patients with adrenocortical deficiency (i.e., serum sodium < 130 mEq. per liter, chloride < 90 mEq. per liter, bicarbonate < 23 mEq. per liter and potassium > 6 mEq. per liter). However, such abnormalities are not always evident. Moreover, quite similar deviations may be found in patients who do not have adrenocortical disease. On these accounts, serum concentration measurements by themselves cannot be considered very reliable indices of adrenocortical status.

The reasons for this can be outlined briefly. First, it will be remembered that development of changes in serum electrolyte concentrations depends in part upon the existing relations between electrolyte intake and output. Only the output is influenced by Na-K hormone. Second, serum concentrations are also dependent in part upon the existing relations between electrolyte balance on the one hand and water balance on the other. For example, if a patient with hypoadrenocorticism and initially normal extracellular electrolyte concentration values happens to lose sodium, chloride and water in normal extracellular fluid proportions (i.e., 140 mEq. Na and 100 mEq. Cl per 1,000 cc. H₂O), dehydration can develop while the serum sodium and chloride concentrations remain unchanged. Therefore, to obtain information concerning Na-K hormone status, it is necessary to find out whether sodium and potassium are being retained or rejected by the kidneys in accordance with the physiologic needs of the body. When there is a question of hypoadrenocorticism, this can be accomplished by applying a provocative test of the type outlined below. At the moment we lack a well-documented test having the opposite purpose of indicating hyperadrenocorticism with respect to Na-K hormone.

Provocative test for revealing hypoadrenocorticism. This test is based upon the fact that patients suffering from adrenocortical insufficiency lose their natural ability to conserve sodium and to eliminate potassium under conditions of relatively low sodium and relatively high potassium intake. The test consists in feeding the patient a special diet and observing him for signs of excess sodium loss and of potassium retention.* Inasmuch as these phenomena may result in hypoadrenocortical collapse or crisis, the test is not without risk. It should therefore be performed only if conditions permit keeping the patient under constant observation and if appropriate therapeutic measures can be instituted promptly should the need arise (see below under treatment of acute hypoadrenocorticism). Obviously, this type of test should not be employed in the case of patients who have already given clear-cut signs of hypoadrenocorticism. Rather, it should be reserved for patients with questionable evidences of adrenocortical insufficiency, being used more to rule out the disease than to rule it in.

The test† is carried out as follows: On the day before the first day of the standardized examination the subject is served an ordinary diet containing about 85 mEq. each of sodium and chloride and about 60 mEq. of potassium per m². He is allowed no extra sodium chloride. During the test the subject is given a diet such as that indicated in Table 4, which provides about 15 mEq. each of sodium and chloride and about 60 mEq. of potassium per m² per day. The fluid intake is maintained at about 1,500 cc. per m² per day. It is recommended that, except in patients strongly suspected of hypoadrenocorticism, the dietary potassium intake be fortified by daily administration of 30 additional mEq. of potassium per m². This is given in the form of potassium citrate (3.8 gm. per m² per day). The test ordinarily is continued for two and a half days. It may, however, become necessary to discontinue the examination sooner if signs of crisis (nausea, vomiting, weakness, weight loss, dehydration, hypotension,

---

* Because potassium is apt to be retained intracellularly, it is not always easy to demonstrate potassium retention by serum analysis.

† The original description[19][k] has been modified slightly for application to children.

TABLE III—4. Low sodium diet used in provocative Tests 10 and 11 (Table 3) for demonstrating adrenocortical Na-K hormone deficiency. This diet is designed for a child of 30 kg. (1 m^2). We are indebted to Miss Merme Bonnell, dietitian at the Massachusetts General Hospital, for the material used in the chart.

Food	Gm.	K/mEq.	Na/mEq.	Cl/mEq.	Calories
Breakfast:					
Farina (dry)	20	0.61	0.57	0.42	73
Sugar	15	—	—	—	60
Egg	50	1.76	3.05	1.72	75
Orange juice	100	4.63	0.52	0.14	40
Sugar	10	—	—	—	40
Salt-free bread	25	0.46	0.39	0.31	66
Salt-free butter	20	0.08	0.04	0.09	155
Honey	20	0.05	0.04	0.17	65
Lanalac + 120 H$_2$O	15	4.60	0.09	2.20	77
+ Vanilla + 10 sugar	—	—	—	—	40
Dinner:					
Beef	100	9.23	3.92	2.28	152
Rice (dry)	20	0.36	0.22	0.23	69
Salt-free peas	80	5.83	0.44	0.54	45
Salt-free bread	25	0.46	0.39	0.31	66
Salt-free butter	20	0.08	0.04	0.09	155
Lanalac + 120 H$_2$O	15	4.60	0.09	2.20	77
+ Vanilla + 10 sugar	—	—	—	—	40
Pears	100	3.38	0.44	0.14	75
Supper:					
Chicken	60	7.05	2.44	0.90	75
Green beans	60	3.43	0.57	0.82	25
Macaroni	20	0.67	0.09	0.42	72
Salt-free bread	50	0.90	0.78	0.62	132
Salt-free butter	20	0.80	0.04	0.09	155
Pure grape jelly	20	0.38	0.04	—	60
Lanalac + 120 H$_2$O	15	4.60	0.09	2.20	77
+ Vanilla + 10 sugar	—	—	—	—	40
Peaches	100	5.47	0.96	0.11	75

Totals:
CHO—261 gm.   K—1.5 gm. (59 mEq.)
P—82 gm.   Na—.66 gm. (15 mEq.)
F—82 gm.   Cl—.45 gm. (16 mEq.)
Calories—2,080

abdominal pain) set in. Occasionally, the examination must be prolonged for a week or more before clear-cut abnormalities due to mild adrenocortical insufficiency can be demonstrated.

On the morning of the last (usually the third) day of the test, the patient is asked to take half his daily fluid allowance before 11 a.m. Blood is drawn at 10 a.m. for serum sodium and chloride determinations. While serum potassium can also be measured, it usually proves to be normal. Urine is also collected for a four-hour period, starting at eight a.m. and ending at noon. The urine likewise is analyzed for its sodium and chloride content.

Table 5 sets forth representative results obtained for normal adults and for patients with authentic hypoadrenocorticism.[19 k] It is seen that hypoadrenocortical and normal persons cannot be distinguished clearly by measurements of serum sodium and chloride concentration values, for although average values differ, ranges overlap. However, both types show a marked difference in urine output values relative to serum concentration values. By the third day normal persons almost stop excreting sodium and chloride in the urine, but patients with adrenocortical insufficiency continue to excrete these electrolytes in the urine in sizable amounts. This phenomenon is evident in the clearance data shown in Table 5 (for comments on the meaning of clearance values see Chapter II, page 54). They show that sodium and chloride are being "cleared" by hypoadrenocortical patients at three or four times the normal rate.

In the foregoing comments no particular distinction has been made between sodium and chloride. Actually, there is extensive evidence (see above, page 137) that Na-K hormone exerts a direct controlling influence over sodium metabolism, but only an indirect and very variable influence upon chloride metabolism. Basically, therefore, sodium metabolism measurements are preferable to chloride as an index of adrenocortical status.

In closing, a few comments appear to be in order on the applicability of these considerations to random patients who are found to be suffering from hyponatremia. If the urine of such a patient is sodium free or nearly so, it is unlikely that he is suffering from Na-K deficiency. This idea can be expressed semiquantitatively on the basis of the sodium concentrations reported for the third day of the provocative test. At this time the urine sodium concentration of normal persons was found to average 10 mEq. per liter (range 3 to 37 mEq. per liter) and of hypoadrenocortical patients to average 90 mEq. per liter (range 72 to 123 mEq. per liter). Differences in urine chloride concentration values also were found (average normal 15, range 5 to 40 mEq. per liter; average for hypoadrenocortical patients 84, range 65 to 102 mEq. per liter). These urine concentration values were obtained under conditions of ample fluid intake and urine volume. They will, of course, tend to be higher when oliguria is present.

Though a low urine sodium value in association with hyponatremia rules against hypoadrenocorticism, it does not follow that the presence of larger quantities of sodium in the urine is necessarily suggestive of this condition. Even the strictly normal person takes about two full days to adjust his urine sodium output to a low sodium intake, even though his serum sodium concentration is markedly depressed during that interval.[19 o] Furthermore, abnormal sodium loss can

TABLE III—5. Representative average results obtained for normal and hypoadrenocortical patients on the second and third days of the low sodium provocative test. Adapted from data of H. H. Cutler, M. H. Power, and R. M. Wilder, *Proc. Staff Meet., Mayo Clin.* 13:244, 1938; *J. A. M. A.* 111:117, 1938.

		Sodium			Chloride		
Condition	Test day no.	Serum mEq/L.	Urine mEq/m²/ 24 hr. †	Clearance cc/m²/ 24 hr. **	Serum mEq/L.	Urine mEq/m²/ 24 hr.	Clearance cc/m²/ 24 hr.
Normal	2	135 (130 to 140) *	33	240	100 (95 to 106)	36	360
	3	133 (126 to 141)	21	160	98 (93 to 105)	32	330
Hypoadreno- corticism	2	130 (106 to 134)	117	900	96 (85 to 101)	87	910
	3	121 (107 to 127)	110	910	89 (77 to 96)	89	1,000

* The values in parentheses represent the ranges.

† It has been assumed that the adult subjects reported were of average size (70 kg., 1.7m²). The hourly urine excretion values given in the original report have been extrapolated to 24 hours.

** Clearance values were calculated by dividing urine output values (mEq. per m² per day) by serum concentration values (mEq. per cc.).

also develop as a consequence of primary renal disturbances (see under renal acidosis, Chapter II). Abnormal sodium diuresis due to adrenocortical hormone lack can be corrected by the administration of adrenocortical extract or DOCA. This therapy is ineffective when the sodium diuresis is caused primarily by renal disease.[19 p]

Test 12—the Sweat Test.[4] As commented upon in Table 3, Section 12, the possibility of assessing adrenocortical Na-K hormone status is being currently explored by many workers.

In persons of apparently steady endocrine status, the concentration of chloride, and also of sodium, may be altered to an important extent by factors related to the rate of sweating.[4 c] Consequently it appears that rate of sweating should be taken into account when the chloride or sodium concentration values of sweat are employed as an index of adrenocortical status. This can be done by application of a formula which yields sweat chloride–rate index values.[4 c] These index values bear an inverse relation to adrenocortical Na-K hormone activity, being high in patients with hypoadrenocorticism and low in individuals treated with DOCA. Index values fall within a day following administration of DOCA (see Figure 2), indicating that the index is promptly responsive to changes in Na-K hormone status. Cortisone, a predominantly S-F-N type of hormone, fails to induce a fall in index values within a period of three days. Possibly it would after more prolonged administration. ACTH induces as rapid a fall in index values as DOCA. Gonadal steroids produce, if anything, a rise in index values. These findings lend support to the thesis that the human adrenal cortex secretes a DOCA-like hormone and suggests that sweat chloride–rate index measurements may yield interesting information concerning bodily Na-K hormone status.

Like the urinary 11-17-OCS values, sweat chloride–rate index values undergo wide changes in subjects exposed to certain types of physiologic stress. For example, the values observed for normal persons receiving a high sodium chloride intake rise to levels comparable to those observed in patients with primary hypoadrenocorticism or hypopituitarism. This finding may be interpreted as suggesting that a high sodium chloride intake induces a physiologic, homeostatic decrease in adrenocortical Na-K hormone production. Conversely, values obtained on patients receiving a NaCl-poor or NaCl-free diet fall to levels equivalent to those found for subjects treated with DOCA or ACTH. It follows that sweat chloride–rate index values and, indirectly, adrenocortical status must be viewed with relation to the over-all status of the individual. Unusually elevated sweat chloride–rate index values do not necessarily mean that the subject has hypoadrenocorticism, for it appears that elevated values in patients receiving a high sodium chloride intake should be considered physiologic or normal for the particular circumstance. Unusually high values would, however, be abnormal for a person receiving an average or a low sodium salt intake.

Recent studies indicate that measurements of the concentration of sodium and potassium in saliva may yield information similar to that discussed above. It is not yet known whether rate of salivation is a factor of importance in appraising salivary electrolyte determinations.

Test 13—Urinary 17-Ketosteroid (17-KS) Measurements. Background information including normal standards for 17-KS output are given in Tables 1 and 2 and Figure 13 and its companion text. Numerous procedures for the colorimetric assay of urinary 17-KS have been reported in the literature. With a few exceptions, they are all fundamentally similar. The data discussed here were obtained almost exclusively by means of a method (see Appendix) designed to eliminate errors of overestimation due to interfering chromogens.

To recapitulate briefly, the evidence available today[13 a, 19 q] suggests that the urinary neutral steroids are excretory transformation products of certain adrenocortical steroid hormones and to a lesser extent of testicular hormones. Thus the 17-KS output may be considered a roughly proportional index of the secretory activity of these two glands. It appears that the adrenal cortices are a much more important source of 17-KS than the testes during childhood. Current information suggests that the testes are responsible for about a quarter or a third of the total 17-KS output in adults.

Variations in 17-KS excretion by children must be judged with relation to the individual's age. In this connection it is important to bear in mind that 17-KS excretion in adolescents is a function of physiologic rather than chronologic age. By definition the physiologic age or maturity status of the average healthy child is equal to his chronologic age. Viewed individually, however, many normal children will deviate in physiologic age from the average for actual age. Deviations of as much as two or three years are not unusual, and even greater deviations may not be indicative of disease.

Table 6 presents in summary form observations on 17-KS excretion by individuals with selected conditions. Further comments concerning most of the conditions listed there are given in the various clinical sections of this volume.

Earlier in the present chapter attention was called to the fact that qualitative analyses of urinary 17-KS may give valuable information concerning the possibility of abnormal adrenocortical steroid hormone production (see Figure 15). Moderately extensive experience has been had with a simpler method of qualitative analysis which is designed to separate 3-β-hydroxy-17-ketosteroids from 3-α-hydroxy and non-alcoholic 17-ketosteroids.[14 b]

In most normal subjects the 3-β-17-KS comprise not more than 15 or 20 per cent of the total urinary, neutral 17-KS output. Stated differently, the output of 3-β-17-KS does not often exceed about 3 or 4 mg. per day in normal persons; in patients with adrenocortical cancer, the 3-β-17-KS usually comprise a larger proportion of the total 17-KS output. Because the total 17-KS output is apt to be large, the absolute value for 3-β-17-KS also is apt to be increased, at times reaching values from 10 to 30 times normal. Occasional patients with adrenocortical hyperplasia also have abnormally high 3-β-17-KS values.

These observations have led to the following thoughts: If a patient with marked hyper-17-ketosteroiduria also has abnormally high 3-β-17-KS values, it is assumed that the patient has a cancer of the adrenal cortex until proved otherwise. A normal 3-β-17-KS value is more suggestive of adrenocortical hyperplasia than cancer, particularly in patients who give a history suggestive of adrenocortical virilism dating back to birth. However, it does not rule out adrenocortical cancer. In this connection, note in Table 6 that occasional patients with adrenocortical cancer can have only slightly elevated total 17-KS values.[13 c] In other words, one cannot count upon the urinary 17-KS measurement to rule out adrenocortical cancer.

TABLE III—6. Urinary 17-ketosteroid excretion in selected conditions. Adapted from N. B. Talbot and A. M. Butler, *J. Clin. Endocrinol.* 2:724, 1942.

Presenting symptom	Causes	Sex	Total 17-KS excretion
A. Precocious or abnormal masculinization (virilism)	1. Adrenocortical carcinoma	♂ and ♀	+ to +++
	2. Adrenocortical hyperplasia	♂ and ♀	++ to +++
	3. Testicular interstitial cell tumor	♂	+++
	4. Central nervous system lesion Physiologic accelerated adolescence	♂	+
	5. Ovarian arrhenoblastoma	♀	N
B. Precocious or abnormal feminization (gynecomastia)	1. Ovarian granulosa cell tumor	♀	N?
	2. Central nervous system lesion Physiologic accelerated adolescence	♀	+
	3. Associated skin pigmentation and bone cysts (one case)	♀	N
C. Retarded sexual development or hypogonadism	1. Hypopituitarism	♂ and ♀	≡
	2. Hypothyroidism	♂ and ♀	≡
	3. Castration Primary gonadal deficiency	♂ ♀	N to ≡ N to −
	4. Debility, malnutrition	♂ and ♀	N to =
D. Dwarfism	1. Hypopituitarism	♂ and ♀	≡
	2. Hypothyroidism	♂ and ♀	≡
	3. Familial or non-endocrine	♂ and ♀	N to −
	4. Associated with anovarianism	♀	− to =
E. Overweight	1. Cushing's syndrome:	♂ and ♀	
	(a) with adrenocortical carcinoma		N to +++
	(b) without adrenocortical carcinoma		N to +
	2. Dietary plus constitutional factors (children)	♂ and ♀	N to +
	3. Hypothyroidism	♂ and ♀	≡
F. Fatigability and weakness	1. Addison's disease	♂ ♀	− to = ≡
	2. Hypopituitarism	♂ and ♀	≡
	3. Hypothyroidism	♂ and ♀	≡
	4. Malnutrition Anorexia nervosa Chronic illness Non-endocrine carcinoma	♂ and ♀	N to =
	5. Cushing's syndrome (see E, 1 above)		

Key to symbols: N within normal limits; — low normal or slightly below normal limits; = definitely below normal limits, but more than 1 mg. per day (applies only to subjects over 12 years); ≡ very low, usually between 0.0 and 0.5 mg. and never over 1.0 mg. per day (application restricted to subjects over 12); + elevated to correspond to average normal for older children or adults (applies only to children); ++ moderately high (i. e. more than 6 mg. at 6 years, 10 mg. at 10 years, 15 mg. at 15 years, 18 mg. for adult women or 21 mg. for adult men); +++ very high (more than 35 mg. per day).

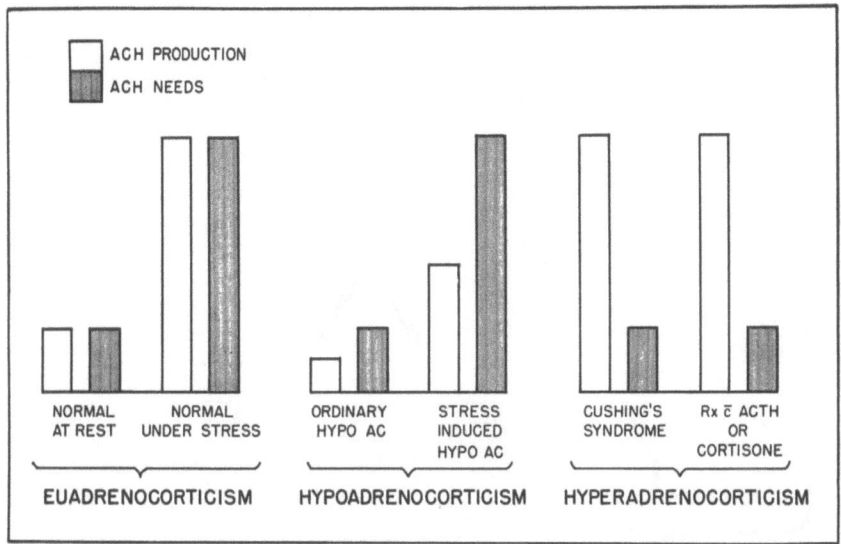

FIGURE III—28. Diagram indicating various possible relations between adrenocortical activity and body needs for adrenocortical hormones, particularly the Na-K and S-F-N types. In euadrenocorticism (left) production rate is geared to needs. Note that stress increases adrenocortical hormone requirements. In hypoadrenocorticism (center) production rate fails to keep up with needs. In hyperadrenocorticism (right) adrenocortical hormones are being produced in excess of needs. Note that absolute rates of adrenocortical hormone production by stressed endocrinologically normal persons may equal those of pathologically hyperadrenocortical persons (compare the 11-17-OCS values of burned and operated patients with Cushing's hyperplasia patients in Figure 27).

CLINICAL CONSIDERATIONS

Figure 28 indicates how physiologic (euadrenocorticism) differs from pathologic adrenocorticism. Adrenocortical activity is considered to be physiologic when adrenocortical hormone production is geared to needs, and pathologic when it is out of keeping with physiologic needs. Adrenocortical hormone requirements vary considerably according to circumstances and are apt to be markedly increased under conditions of stress. Hypoadrenocorticism may be absolute, as in patients with grossly defective adrenal cortices, or relative and clinically evident only when demands for adrenocortical hormone are increased as a consequence of stress. Hyperadrenocorticism is described as being relative and of two chief types. One occurs spontaneously in sporadic form as Cushing's syndrome or adrenocortical virilism or feminism. The other is seen in individuals treated with ACTH, cortisone or other adrenocortical hormone.

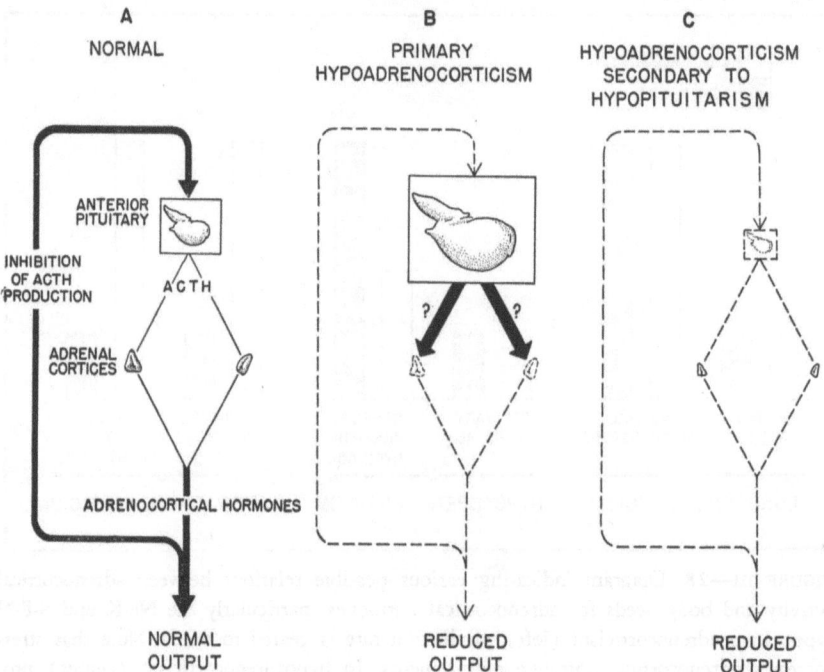

FIGURE III—29. Diagrammatic representation of the chief causes of hypoadrenocorticism.
SECTION A indicates normal relations. Note that the pituitary produces ACTH, which stimulates the adrenal cortices to produce their hormones. Note also that the adrenocortical hormones tend to inhibit ACTH production (see also Figure 38).
SECTION B indicates primary hypoadrenocorticism wherein the primary difficulty is characterized by loss or destruction of adrenocortical tissue. Here it is known that adrenocortical hormone output is reduced; it is presumed that there is a compensatory increase in ACTH production resulting from a lack of the inhibition shown in Section A.
SECTION C illustrates hypoadrenocorticism secondary to primary hypopituitarism. Here the difficulty originates in the pituitary which has been destroyed or otherwise damaged and fails to produce ACTH; lacking this stimulus the adrenal cortices secrete their hormones at a reduced rate.

For comments on physiologic adrenocortical hyperfunction, see above, page 156. Remarks on pathologic hypo- and hyperadrenocorticism are given below.

HYPOADRENOCORTICISM

This condition is caused by several types of disturbances, which may be divided into two chief groups (see Figure 29). In the first, there is a primary destructive lesion in the adrenal glands. In the second, the adrenal glands are intact and potentially capable of normal functional activity but are involuted and functionally hypoactive because of failure on the part of the pituitary to secrete adrenocorticotropin. ACTH deficiency (secondary hypoadrenocorticism) can be due either to primary pituitary lesions or to such extrapituitary conditions as athyrosis and malnutrition. These two types of hypoadrenocorticism will be considered separately below.

Primary Hypoadrenocorticism (Addison's Disease). This disease has not been recognized in children as frequently as in adult patients. However, though distinctly uncommon in pediatrics, it is not rare, for about 100 cases have been reported in the literature. Generally speaking, hypoadrenocorticism as it is seen in children is quite similar to the disease as it is seen in adults.[19 d]

ETIOLOGY. It is the exception rather than the rule to be able to find an adequate explanation for primary hypoadrenocorticism in children. Tuberculosis used to be the most frequently reported cause.[20 a] However, in our limited direct and indirect experience with nine cases over the past 15 years, tuberculosis was a factor in only one case. Two patients had generalized moniliasis, and one of these also had idiopathic hypoparathyroidism. A fourth patient had calcification of the adrenal glands, as shown by x-ray examination. In the remaining five no clue as to the cause could be found. Such patients are apt to show idiopathic adrenocortical atrophy.

CLINICAL MANIFESTATIONS. The following comments are based largely upon the findings obtained on eight of the previously mentioned cases of hypoadrenocorticism. It can be stated with reasonable assurance that the diagnosis in each instance was authentic. It also is believed that the symptoms and signs can be attributed solely to adrenocortical failure.

The relative frequencies with which the more striking symptoms and signs were encountered are set forth in Figure 30. The patients represented there were between 5 and 13 years of age when their disease first became evident. Of these children three were boys and five were girls. It is seen that the various symptoms and signs have been divided into several groups. This division is for purposes of convenience in presentation. It neglects quite arbitrarily the boundaries suggested by the physiologic characteristics of the three adrenocortical hormone types.

Neuromuscular signs. In these patients easy fatigability and muscular weakness developed rather insidiously. Neither the parents nor the children recognized that this complaint was truly significant when it first appeared. On the contrary, some parents thought that their previously vigorous and energetic

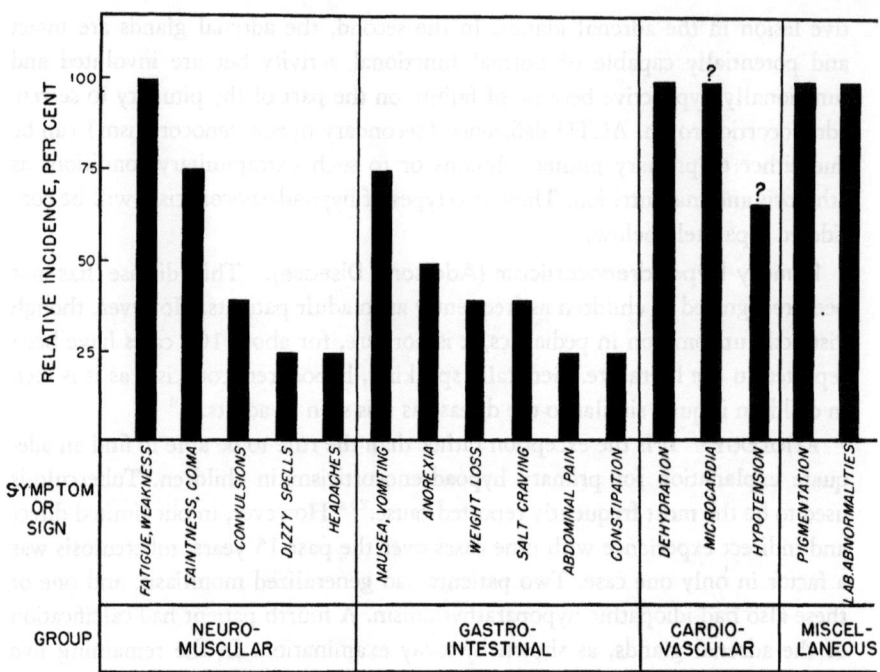

FIGURE III—30. Relative incidence of various symptoms and signs of primary hypoadrenocorticism in children.

children simply had discarded interest in sports and outdoor play in favor of sedentary indoor recreation. It was only later that they became aware of the fact that even a little physical exertion was very exhausting. Ultimately, most of these children rapidly became exceedingly weak, some to the point where they were unable to sit up or even elevate their heads or arms.

Faintness was most apt to develop for a few moments when a patient assumed upright posture, as after getting out of bed or rising from a chair. At times dizziness was an associated complaint, though usually it was not. The same may be said with respect to headaches. Coma was observed only with episodes of hypoadrenocortical crisis. In association with this manifestation convulsions occurred commonly. The convulsions usually were generalized and of the type seen in patients with idiopathic epilepsy. Lumbar punctures were performed in a few instances. Except for occasional lymphocytosis, no abnormalities were recorded. Unfortunately, the records do not indicate whether spinal fluid pressures and sugar values were normal. A few patients also become psychically disturbed as evidenced by disorientation, extreme restlessness and even mania.

Gastrointestinal manifestations. In these patients vomiting preceded by nausea tended to occur in spells of one to several days' duration. At the time there was nothing to distinguish these spells symptomatically from ordinary gastrointestinal upsets. In retrospect it seems likely that they represent one of the earliest manifestations of chronic hypoadrenocorticism.

In association with nausea and vomiting, anorexia was an early and common complaint. As a consequence of this, patients were apt to stop gaining or to lose in body weight.

Abdominal pain was sometimes severe, and particularly when accompanied by nausea and vomiting strongly suggested intestinal obstruction. In infants with mixed adrenocortical disease (see page 245) the clinical picture strongly resembled that seen in infants with hypertrophic pyloric stenosis. In these connections it is noteworthy that nausea, vomiting and abdominal pain usually subside rapidly after hypoadrenocortical patients are given isotonic saline intravenously.

Salt craving was an interesting symptom. It tended either to be definitely present or absent. When present, it was readily discernible because these patients were apt not only to salt their food rather heavily and to develop a taste for pickles, pretzels, potato chips and the like, but also to eat salt "straight" after pouring some on the hand or on cookies or apples. One mother became very much afraid that her son might harm himself by eating so much table salt. Acting on her concern, she forbade him to use the salt shaker. As a consequence, the boy rapidly developed an acute hypoadrenocortical crisis. Similar accidents have occurred to children with as yet unrecognized hypoadrenocorticism upon admission to a hospital ward. Being unable to obtain their usual quota of extra salt, they suffered the effects of abrupt sodium chloride deprivation.

Constipation, though not a common complaint, may be marked. Treatment with cathartics is apt to produce unexpectedly voluminous results.

Cardiovascular manifestations. Dehydration appeared in all the patients of this series. As might be expected, it varied in severity from time to time, but it was always at least moderately marked under conditions of hypoadrenocortical crisis. As in any dehydrated patient, there was a tendency to loss of skin elasticity, dryness of mucous membranes and softness of the eyeballs. Particularly when dehydration was of marked degree, the pulse was rapid and of thready character. At times the pulse became so weak that it could not be felt at the wrist when the patient's hand was raised a few centimeters off the bed. Under such circumstances the skin was cold, clammy, mottled and blue.

Microcardia[20 b] is thought to be a manifestation of extracellular dehydration and reduced blood volume (anhydremia). It has been noted in patients whose

Continued on page 202

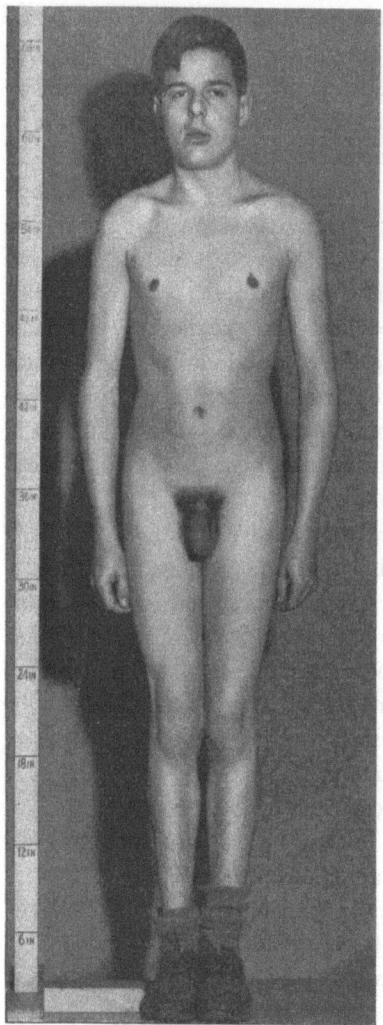

(Left)

FIGURE III—31. Idiopathic Addison's disease in a boy of 14½ years receiving DOCA therapy. Note that (a) his nutritional state, muscular development and genital development are good and (b) his nipples and genitalia are deeply pigmented.

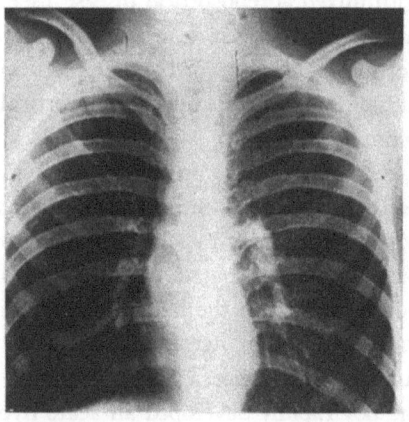

(Right)

FIGURE III—32. Roentgenographic demonstration of microcardia in the patient of Figure 31 at the time when he was first seen in hypoadrenocortical crisis. The cardiothoracic ratio was 0:31.

CASE HISTORY

The patient was admitted to the hospital with a story of having found it increasingly difficult during the past two or three years to keep up in physical activity with other children and of having noticed increasing pigmentation of his skin. About four months previously he had contracted "influenza," which lasted only three or four days but following which he failed to regain his usual strength and energy. The family history and the boy's own history were otherwise non-contributory. There was no record of salt-craving or of fainting, dizziness or convulsions.

CASE HISTORY (continued)

On physical examination he measured 68 inches in height (170 cm.) and weighed 97 pounds (44 kg.). He was a lean, well-developed boy who appeared to be moderately weak. His skin showed generalized pigmentation of a smoky brown color. It was most marked over the genitalia and nipples. In addition, there were numerous freckle-like spots, but none were observed on the mucous membranes. Dehydration was evidenced by loss of tissue elasticity and dryness of the mucous membranes. His heart was strikingly reduced in transverse diameter. Blood pressure was 80/40 mm. Hg. The remainder of the physical examination was not remarkable.

Laboratory studies showed his urine to be entirely negative. He had a mild leukocytosis. Fasting blood sugar was 60 mg. per cent, serum sodium 135 mEq. and serum chloride 108 mEq. per liter. The NPN was 46 mg. per cent and serum protein 7.4 gm. per cent. An x-ray taken at the time of admission confirmed the clinical impression that his heart was extremely small (see Figure 32). Subsequent studies showed that his urinary output of 17-KS (0.5 mg. for 24 hours) and of 11-17-OCS (.06 mg. for 24 hours) were abnormally low, but that his urinary gonadotropic hormone output (6.5 mouse units for 24 hours) was within normal limits. An insulin tolerance test yielded a normal result. A water diuresis test, however, yielded an abnormal result. An epinephrine-eosinophil count yielded an abnormal result (control count, 325; four hours after epinephrine, 260; four hours after a second dose of epinephrine, 190 cells per mm^3). A tuberculin test (1:1,000 dilution) was negative.

Initial therapy consisted in an intravenous infusion of 1 liter of 5 per cent glucose in normal salt solution, 20 cc. of aqueous adrenocortical extract and 10 mg. of DOCA. Because of restlessness he was also given 45 mg. of phenobarbital. When half the intravenous infusion had been administered (about one hour), he began to look better and asked for water. A definite improvement was noted in his pulse. Before receiving the infusion he had been too weak to sit up without help. Immediately afterwards he stated that he felt he could sit up and did so spontaneously. An hour after the infusion had been completed, he was found sitting up in bed full of pep and reading a book. He commented that he felt better than he had for weeks. Subsequent therapy consisted in the gradual institution first of a liquid and then of a house diet. In addition, he was given DOCA in approximately the manner described in the text of this chapter.

His course has since been largely uneventful. On two occasions all sodium chloride and DOCA therapy was discontinued for test purposes for periods of 48 and 72 hours. On each of these occasions he rapidly lost about 5 pounds (2.5 kg.) in weight and developed typical symptoms and signs of acute hypoadrenocorticism with respect to the Na-K hormone. For chronic maintenance he has been given daily 3 gm. of sodium chloride in the form of enteric-coated tablets and either 1.5 to 2 mg. of DOCA by daily intramuscular injection or 2 to 4 DOCA pellets of 125 mg. each by subcutaneous implantation, as described in the text of this chapter. Recently, cortisone therapy in daily oral doses of about 20 mg. has been added. This has appreciably increased his sense of well-being and capacity for work.

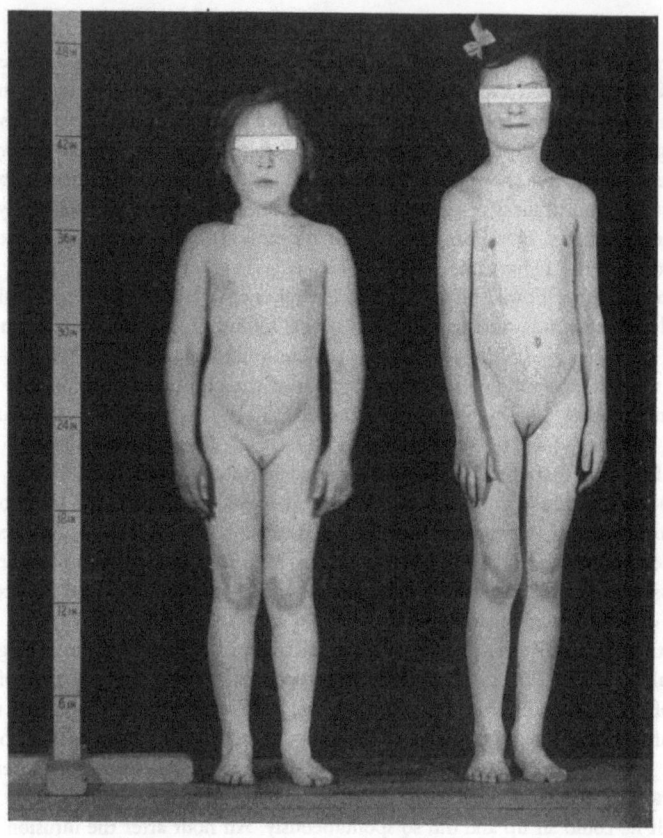

FIGURE III—33. Primary hypoadrenocorticism (Addison's disease), with hypoparathyroidism and moniliasis in a girl of eight years.

LEFT: Normal control.

RIGHT: The patient's appearance was essentially normal except for moderate pigmentation of the nipples and umbilicus and moniliasis of the mouth.

CASE HISTORY

On admission to the hospital the patient's chief complaint was occasional convulsions during the previous four years. Aside from these, she had been essentially well until the past year, when she began to have enuresis. Eight months before admission, she had come in from play one afternoon because of feeling tired and had gone to bed of her own volition

CASE HISTORY (continued)

Some time later, when she arose to go to another room, she experienced an episode of generalized clonic convulsions, with stiffened limbs, upward rolling of the eyes, frothing at the mouth and loss of consciousness. She recovered from this episode spontaneously, but subsequently experienced several more. At about this time she also developed anorexia and commenced to lose weight. Increasing pigmentation of the skin was then noted. She also developed a craving for salt and as a result made a practice of pouring salt on all her food, including cookies and other sweet things. During the few weeks prior to admission her thirst became more intense. On the day before admission she fell downstairs in school and, though apparently unhurt, came home at noon, complaining of exhaustion. She was put to bed and given an ordinary supper, which she ate well. That night she slept unusually soundly. On the morning of admission her mother heard her scream and found her kneeling in bed with her eyes turned upward. Although unaware of her surroundings, she was not convulsing. A short time later she was brought to the hospital because of a generalized convulsion.

Physical examination revealed her to be a fairly well-developed but thin and acutely ill child, who was lying in a bed in a semi-stuporous condition. She was markedly dehydrated, as evidenced by loss of tissue elasticity, dryness of the mucous membranes, softness of the eyeballs, a rapid, thready pulse and hypotension. At times no pulse was obtainable if her arm was raised above her body. There was definitely increased pigmentation of the skin and of the buccal mucous membranes. Her lips were dry and cracked and there were excoriations at the corners of her mouth which resembled cheilosis. The transverse diameter of the heart appeared to be smaller than normal. The rest of the physical examination was not remarkable.

Laboratory examinations revealed the blood sugar to be 35 mg. and NPN 40 mg. per cent, serum sodium 127, chloride 84 and bicarbonate 22 mEq. per liter, respectively. The urine was normal and free from acetone. The white cell count was 20,500 with a normal differential; the red cell count was 4,700,000. The spinal fluid was normal, and a blood culture was sterile. Hinton and 1:1,000 tuberculin tests were negative.

A diagnosis of hypoadrenocorticism was made, and the patient was treated with intravenously administered glucose and saline together with aqueous adrenocortical extract and DOCA approximately as outlined elsewhere in this chapter. On this therapy her condition improved gradually, so that within 36 hours she had partially recovered. Though she had been very irritable at first, on the afternoon of the second day she suddenly "woke up" and regained a rational sensorium. Thereafter her course was relatively uneventful until about a year later, when it was discovered that she also had idiopathic hypoparathyroidism. For a description of this aspect of her difficulties see Chapter II. It was also discovered that her mouth lesion was due to moniliasis. She died at the age of 10 with apparently disseminated moniliasis, hypoadrenocorticism and hypoparathyroidism. No post-mortem could be obtained.

pulse, blood pressure and other vital signs were not grossly abnormal. In other words, it is potentially an early manifestation of dehydration secondary to Na-K hormone deficiency. When present, percussion of the left border of the heart reveals it to lie appreciably within the midclavicular line and at times about at the border of the sternum. Palpation of the apical impulse yields similar information. By x-ray the transverse diameter of the heart is found to occupy a smaller than normal (0.4 to 0.5) fraction of the transverse diameter of the chest (see Figure 32).

As Figure 30 suggests, microcardia appears to be a very common finding in patients with hypoadrenocorticism. But in interpreting this sign it must not be overlooked that many factors besides the state of hydration can modify heart size and shape. For example, patients with long, narrow chests are apt to have unusually narrow heart shadows, as are patients whose intrathoracic pressure is increased because of emphysema or attempts to exhale with the glottis closed (Valsalva experiment). The heart is apt to appear narrower when the diaphragms are low than when they are elevated. Moreover, dehydration due to factors other than hypoadrenocorticism may result in apparent microcardia (see Chapter II, Figure 19). For such reasons as these, it is evident that this sign of hypoadrenocorticism must be interpreted with caution. Changes in heart size under the influence of therapy are noteworthy as evidence of changes in blood volume and extracellular hydration.

Pigmentary and other findings. Abnormal pigmentation was noted in every patient. It was most marked on the nipples, genitalia and over areas exposed to chronic friction such as the elbows, knuckles and palms, occasionally taking the form of freckle-like spots scattered over the body. The color varied from chestnut tan to bluish black. A few patients showed sizable vitiligo-like patches of depigmentation in the midst of areas of apparently increased coloration; about a third of them also had bluish black patches of pigment in the mucous membranes of the mouth. In every case the pigmentary changes tended to be subtle in early stages of the disease and to increase in intensity with passage of time.

The following *miscellaneous findings* may be mentioned. As a rule, the children tended to be underweight for height at the time of diagnosis. This probably was due in part to the previously mentioned tendency to anorexia and in part to the fact that most of the patients were dehydrated because of Addisonian crisis when the initial diagnosis was made. In the girls of adolescent age who showed definite mammary and vulval development, pubic and axillary hair growth was notably sparse or absent. No such digression from the normal pattern of adolescent sex development was noted in boys. Finally, it is important to remember that patients in hypoadrenocortical crisis may be extremely sensitive to apparently minor stresses. Thus passage of an urethral catheter or dosage with castor oil has been known to result in death.

LABORATORY STUDIES. In this series fewer laboratory examinations were performed than one might wish. Those obtained, however, support the theses presented above in the section on methods of diagnosis. Thus, in four patients the serum sodium concentrations ranged between 119 and 135 mEq. while the serum chloride ranged between 84 and 108 mEq. per liter. These data indicate, as explained previously, that patients in or on the verge of circulatory collapse because of adrenocortical insufficiency do not necessarily have low serum sodium and chloride values. For two patients with low sodium values, serum carbon dioxide content values of 12 and 14 mEq. per liter were obtained. Unfortunately, no serum potassium measurements were made prior to therapy. However, on subsequent occasions, following temporary withdrawal of specific treatment, values of 6 to 7 mEq. per liter were obtained. Blood nonprotein nitrogen values were elevated to levels of 40 to 50 mg. per cent. For the three patients tested, blood sugar values ranged between 35 and 60 mg. per cent. The expected results were obtained in the single case in which we applied other indices of adrenal function, such as the epinephrine-eosinophil test and urinary 17-KS and 11-17-OCS assays.

DIAGNOSIS. The symptoms and signs of adrenocortical insufficiency (see Figure 30) seldom suffice to certify a diagnosis. Certification is accomplished by application of one or more of the diagnostic tests listed in Table 3 or by careful observation of the effects of specific therapy. Objective information should be obtained about the patient's status with respect to each of the major types of adrenocortical hormone in Table 3: Na-K hormone (Tests 9-11), S-F-N hormone (Tests 2-5) and 17-KS-Gens (Test 13).

There are a variety of conditions which can simulate simple primary hypoadrenocorticism in whole or in part. For example, patients with primary kidney disease (base-losing nephritis or renal acidosis—see Chapter II, page 91) can have symptoms and signs which are somewhat suggestive of those caused by Na-K hormone lack. If simple clinical examinations are inconclusive, the two conditions can be distinguished with the aid of serum calcium, inorganic phosphorus, phosphatase, bicarbonate and pH (see page 95), by application of tests for S-F-N hormone status (see Table 3, Tests 2 to 7) and by observing the patient's response to DOCA. This hormone exerts a favorable influence upon the metabolic status of patients with adrenocortical insufficiency (expansion of extracellular fluid volume, weight gain, restoration of serum sodium concentration, etc.) but is without influence upon patients with renal acidosis.[19 p]

Patients with mixed adrenocortical disease have hyper- rather than hypoketosteroiduria (see below, page 245). Patients with hypoadrenocorticism secondary to hypopituitarism may be distinguished by application of the ACTH-eosinophil test (see Table 3, Test 3). Persons suffering circulatory collapse or shock secondary to overwhelming non-endocrine disease (see page 216) may be separated from hypoadrenocortical patients by means of the eosinophil count test (see Table 3, Test 4).

TREATMENT. In treating patients with hypoadrenocorticism it is to be remembered that they have lost their normal ability to retain sodium and reject potassium in accordance with need, to prevent the development of hypoglycemia under conditions of fasting and to overcome stress. It follows that their clinical and chemical status must be checked frequently, especially during the initial phase of treatment, in order that therapy may be modified according to changing needs.

From the over-all therapeutic point of view, the goal is to restore body fluid to normal volume and composition and to re-establish a reasonably stable carbohydrate metabolism. The former is accomplished by the administration of solutions containing sodium and chloride and by giving Na-K hormone (DOCA), and the latter by giving dextrose and S-F-N hormone in the form of aqueous adrenocortical extract or cortisone. There follow sections describing the salient characteristics of the agents used in therapy and the use and abuse of these agents.

Therapeutic Agents

Hormone preparations. The four types of presently available preparations have the following characteristics:

Aqueous adrenocortical extract, which is prepared by extraction of bovine adrenals, contains a balanced mixture of the various adrenocortical hormone types, including in each 100 cc. of extract, about 6 mg. of corticosterone and 2 mg. of 17-hydroxycorticosterone, as well as various unidentified substances.* Experience suggests that this mixture has a potency which is much greater than can be explained by the content of two of its constituents, 100 cc. being as effective as 170 mg. of corticosterone and 66 mg. of 17-hydroxy-11-dehydrocorticosterone (cortisone). In terms of Na-K hormone equivalents, 3 or 4 cc. of Wilson's, Armour's, Upjohn's, or Parke-Davis' aqueous adrenocortical extract given every six hours (12 to 16 cc. daily) have an effect equal to 1 mg. of DOCA given once a day.[19 d] The effect of aqueous adrenocortical extract given intramuscularly or subcutaneously is maximal in one or two hours and lasts about six hours.

* These values are based on studies of Wilson's extract by E. C. Kendall of the Mayo Clinic.[9 g]

Very large amounts of aqueous extract are needed to provide quantities of hormone equal to those produced by healthy adrenal glands. Thus, about 13 cc. of aqueous extract per m^2 per day are needed to maintain the health of an adrenalectomized dog under optimal conditions of living, while about 130 cc. per m^2 per day are needed under conditions of stress.[20 e] Expressed in terms of the 1.7 m^2 adult human, the former dose is the equivalent of 20 cc. and the latter dose of 200 cc. per day.

These values may be taken as rough guides to the therapeutic requirements of unstressed and severely stressed hypoadrenocortical humans. In the patient who is suffering from Addisonian crisis, 20 cc. of extract per m^2 are given intravenously at once and 3 to 5 cc. per m^2 are given via an intravenous drip or by the intramuscular or subcutaneous route each hour for the first few hours. As the patient improves, the injections can be spaced at longer intervals (i.e., two and later three hours). If the patient fails to respond satisfactorily, larger and more frequent doses usually are indicated. It is usually advantageous to give a minimum of three or four injections each day for at least two days after the patient has largely passed the crisis and recovered from any intercurrent infection or other traumatic condition.

Aqueous adrenocortical extract is safe to use, and when given in adequate amounts, it covers all the hormonal needs of a hypoadrenocortical organism. It is practically impossible to give a toxic overdose. For these reasons it provides a very good means of treating patients who are suffering from hypoadrenocortical crisis. The only important drawback with relation to use of adrenocortical extract is cost. At present the price of 100 cc. of this material is about $60.

Lipo-adrenocortical extract, which is obtained from pork adrenals, is dispensed in oily solution and must be given intramuscularly. Approximately speaking, 1 cc. of the lipo extract is equivalent to about 10 cc. of aqueous extract.[19 d] It is relatively weak with respect to Na-K hormone action on water and electrolyte metabolism. From 2 to 3 cc. per m^2 per day given in two or three divided doses will, after several days' administration, prevent fasting hypoglycemia in a hypoadrenocortical patient who is not suffering stress. Two or three times as much hormone is needed if the patient has an infection or other complication.

Compared with aqueous extract, this preparation has a slower but more prolonged action, reaching a peak within four to six hours and lasting eight to twelve hours. On these accounts it is less satisfactory than the aqueous extract in the treatment of Addisonian crisis and more valuable in preventing hypoglycemia.

Lipo extract also is expensive. Most of the effects produced by it can be accomplished at less cost with cortisone.

Desoxycorticosterone acetate (DCA or DOCA),[20 b-g] a synthetically prepared substance is dispensed commercially in sesame oil or peanut oil solution (5 mg. per cc.) for intramuscular administration* and in sterile pellets weighing either 75 mg. (Schering) or 125 mg. (Ciba). The 75 mg. pellets deliver about 0.25 of desoxycorticosterone to the organism per day, and the 125 mg. pellets about 0.5 mg., until they become nearly exhausted.[19 d] The pellets last approximately 300 days.

DOCA is pure Na-K hormone and therefore acts solely on electrolyte and water metabolism. It is a very potent hormone in this regard and when given in excess of needs is capable of producing serious, even fatal toxic changes (see page 139). The likelihood of producing these undesirable effects is greatest when the intake of sodium and chloride is high and that of potassium is low. The likelihood also increases in proportion to the size of the dose and the length of time it is given. With very large doses, toxic changes may be produced within a few days; with slightly excessive doses symptoms may not appear for two to six weeks.

The toxic manifestations caused by DOCA poisoning are as follows: headaches; peripheral edema (this may be noticeable first about the eyes); excessive weight gain (after initial rehydration the total weight may be increased by more than 1 per cent a day during the first week and more than 0.5 per cent a day during subsequent weeks of therapy); hypertension (this may not develop for four or even six weeks; in cases of severe poisoning hypotension may develop terminally); pulmonary edema and dilatation of the heart (see Figure 34); electrocardiographic changes (see Figure 35); cyanosis, coma and convulsions. Finally, there may be the serum electrolyte changes referred to in Figure 4 and Table 3, Section 9. In addition, weakness is apt to develop. Because this last sign can also be a manifestation of Na-K hormone lack, it may cause confusion concerning DOCA dosage unless considered in relation to the phenomena mentioned above. Another rare but interesting consequence of excess DOCA effect is painful and disabling contracture of thigh muscles and tendons. It is observed only after a prolonged period of therapy and in association with marked weakness and arthritic involvement of the knee joints.

DOCA intoxication is treated by unloading excess stores of sodium and extracellular water and replenishing intracellular stores of potassium. In instances of mild toxicity, it may suffice to decrease the dose of DOCA or sodium chloride. If the changes made are adequate, signs of toxicity should subside in a day or so. In more severe cases, DOCA and sodium salts must be discontinued altogether

---

* Occasionally patients develop local reactions to one or the other of these oils but rarely to both.

The Adrenal Cortices

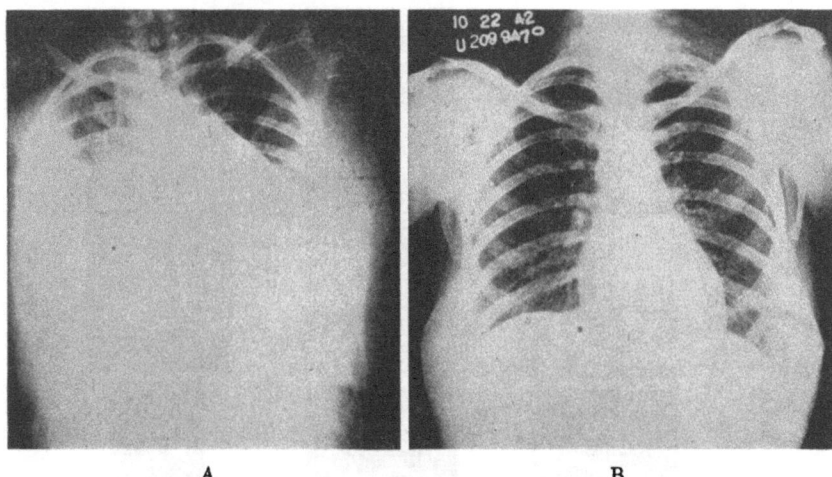

        A   B

FIGURE III—34. Cardiovascular effects of Na-K hormone (DOCA) intoxication. From J. H. Currens and P. D. White, *Am. Heart J.* 28:613, 1944.

SECTION A: Bedside roentgenogram showing cardiac enlargement and congestion of the lungs particularly on the right in an adult patient suffering from the effect of DOCA plus sodium salt intoxication.

SECTION B: Teleroentgenogram of the same patient following recovery from this intoxication. At this time the heart and lungs are normal.

---

pending recuperation. In very severe instances, where the patient is suffering acute cardiac failure and pulmonary edema, it may also be necessary to perform a phlebotomy and to administer digitalis, oxygen and mercurial diuretics. Under such circumstances it is likewise important to make sure that a reasonable amount of potassium is being received. This can be provided in the form of food of the types used in the provocative test (Table 4). If food is not tolerated, potassium may be given as potassium citrate ($K_3C_6H_5O_7H_2O$). Each cubic centimeter of a 10 per cent aqueous solution of this salt contains about 1 mEq. of potassium. From 20 to 30 mEq. of potassium per m^2 per day constitute a conservative dose. This amount is best given in three or four divided doses. Much larger doses have proved beneficial in cases of severe DOCA intoxication. As soon as it is feasible, the potassium citrate should be discontinued and a normal diet instituted. The electrocardiogram may be used as a guide to intracellular potassium status and needs (see Figure 35).

From the foregoing it can be seen that it is better to give too little than too much DOCA. For maintenance purposes, a dose of 1.0 to 1.5 mg. per m^2 per

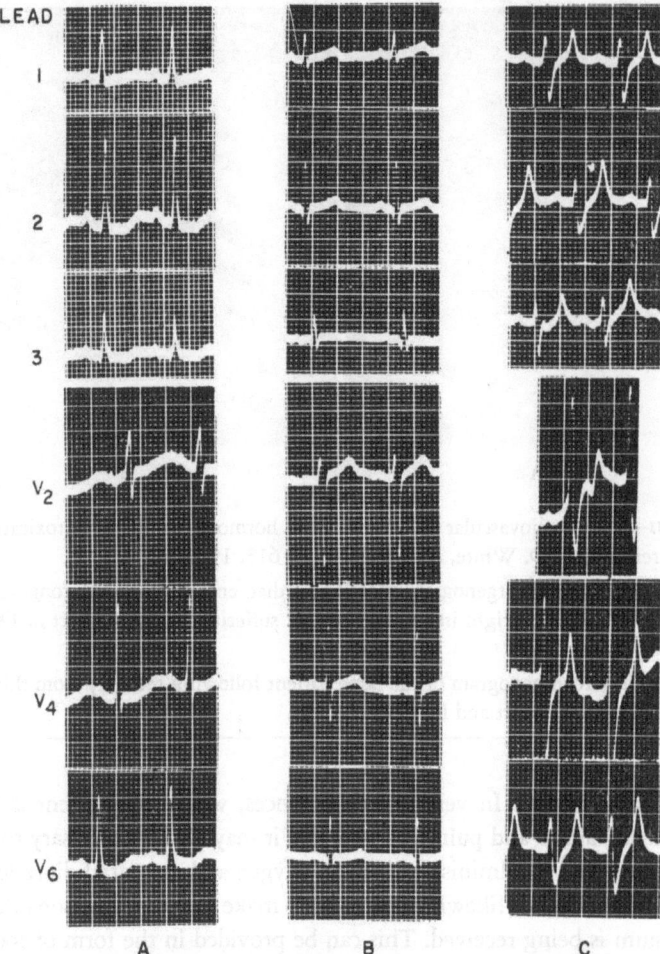

FIGURE III—35. Electrocardiographic tracings in a case of potassium depletion, a normal individual and a case of potassium intoxication. We are indebted to Dr. J. H. Currens for these tracings and for the accompanying descriptive comments.

SECTION A: In potassium deficiency, the RS-T segments are depressed and the T waves are low, iso-electric or inverted. When measurable, the Q-T interval is prolonged. Digitalis, marked tachycardia and fever may affect the RS-T segments and T waves in an approximately similar manner.

SECTION B: Normal individuals may show some differences in the height of their T waves, but the T waves of a given individual normally vary little from day to day. On this account serial electrocardiographic observations are usually more informative than an isolated observation.

SECTION C: In potassium intoxication the T waves become high and "peaked" and there is impairment of intraventricular conduction; the P waves widen and eventually disappear.

day usually suffices, especially if 2 or 3 gm. of sodium chloride per m^2 per day are added to the daily diet. During episodes of intercurrent infection or other unusual stress, the needs may be greater (i.e., doubled or tripled). However, under such circumstances it is preferable to meet the extra requirements by administering aqueous extract or cortisone. This provides other needed hormones and is much less likely to induce toxic effects. The same may be said of the therapy for hypoadrenocortical crisis.

When it is planned for chronic maintenance purposes to implant pellets of DOCA in lieu of daily intramuscular injections, the patient's DOCA requirements are first carefully appraised. This is done by (a) putting the patient on an ordinary, well-rounded diet, (b) prescribing 2 or 3 gm. per m^2 per day of extra sodium chloride, to be taken in the form of 1 gm. enteric-coated tablets* as divided doses with meals and (c) administering daily the patient's estimated optimal dose of DOCA intramuscularly in oily solution.

The patient is watched for signs of over- or underdosage, particularly the former. If either type of sign is observed, appropriate changes in the daily dose of DOCA are made. Once the apparently optimal dose has been found, it is continued for at least two and preferably three weeks in order to make sure that slowly accumulating manifestations of overdosage will not make their appearance. Experience has shown that headaches and other signs may not become evident until the three-week period is nearly terminated.

At the end of this appraisal period, DOCA therapy by pellet implantation may be substituted for intramuscular injections if the patient wishes. For each milligram of DOCA given daily by intramuscular injection in oil solution, two of the 125 mg. Ciba pellets or three or four of the 75 mg. Schering pellets should be substituted. The intramuscular doses are discontinued on the day the pellets are implanted. The Schering pellets† are implanted with sterile precautions at the end of individual subcutaneous pockets from 2 to 4 cm. deep; the Ciba pellets are implanted in pockets made by blunt dissection, through a small incision below a scapula, in the lateral subpectoral region or other reasonably protected site. Great care should be taken to avoid fragmenting the pellets in this operation.[19 d]

If the subject gains excess weight or develops other signs of DOCA poisoning following the implantation, the extra sodium chloride should be omitted. This usually suffices to eliminate the toxicity. Very occasionally it is also necessary to remove one or more pellets. Contrariwise, if the patient loses more than a

---

* If enteric-coated sodium chloride tablets are not well tolerated or pass through the intestinal tract unabsorbed, sodium chloride can be given as a 25 per cent solution in water.

† The H. Laurent Co., Inc., of Newark, N. J., makes a special instrument suitable for use with the cylindrical Schering pellets

small amount of weight or develops other manifestations of DOCA deficiency following pellet implantation, the sodium chloride therapy may be increased two- or threefold. This is likely to become indicated toward the end of the life of the pellets (i.e., about 300 days after implantation, see page 206).

About this time, new pellets should be implanted. Especially at the first reimplantation it is recommended that the patient's DOCA requirements be re-evaluated by two or three weeks of intramuscular DOCA dosage as outlined above. This is important because Na-K hormone requirements are apt to change as the disease progresses, usually downward but sometimes upward.

Cortisone (17-hydroxy-11-dehydrocorticosterone)[20 h, 91] is one of several compounds of the S-F-N hormone type which are being prepared synthetically. Until recently cortisone was available only for experimental purposes. It now is becoming generally obtainable for clinical use. The maintenance dose is between 10 and 20 mg. per m^2 per day. Patients receiving this hormone usually need small supplementary doses of DOCA (about 0.5 mg. per m^2 per day). Under severe stress, 60 to 120 mg. of cortisone per m^2 per day may be needed.

Cortisone may be given by mouth, intramuscularly or as pellets implanted subcutaneously. Doses taken orally are probably somewhat less effective than equal doses administered parenterally. Daily doses given by mouth are more effective if given in two to four divided doses during the course of the 24-hour period. A 50 mg. pellet of cortisone gives off about 0.5 mg. per day and lasts for about three or four months. Such a dose is two or three times more effective than a similar amount of cortisone given by injection. Twelve 50 mg. pellets per m^2, or approximately 600 mg., constitute the total dosage during a period of three or four months.

Chronic overdosage with cortisone is apt to result in clinical changes similar to those seen in patients with Cushing's syndrome (see pages 235 and 253). These untoward manifestations subside during the course of a few weeks following reduction or omission of the treatment.

Other supportive agents (isotonic saline, etc.). Intravenous infusions of fluids which provide needed electrolytes, water and dextrose are particularly valuable in the management of patients in hypoadrenocortical crisis. Requirements for fluids and substances are determined by two factors: (a) maintenance needs and (b) repair needs. The former are proportional to the surface area of the body; the latter are determined by loss of body substance or weight. Certain of the maintenance needs of normal persons receiving intravenous infusions are set forth in Table 7. These normal allotments should suffice also for the hypoadrenocortical patient receiving parenteral therapy, provided he is given adequate adrenocortical hormone substitution therapy. If he is not receiving such therapy,

TABLE III—7. Approximate normal minimum parenteral needs* per m² per day for temporary maintenance of water, electrolyte and caloric balances. Adapted from A. M. Butler, *Acta pædiat.* 38:59, 1949.

	\multicolumn{7}{c}{Substances needed}	
Obligatory losses	H_2O cc.	Na mEq.	Cl mEq.	K mEq.	Mg mEq.	P gm.	Glucose † gm.
(a) Insensible perspiration	500	5	5	1	—	—	—
(b) Renal excretion	220	6	6	12	3	0.1	—
(c) Energy production	—	—	—	—	—	—	60-250 (240 to 1,000 calories)
Total	720	11	11	13	3	0.1	(60-250)

* These values pertain only when the subject is receiving calories as glucose and no excessive protein or electrolytes.

† Glucose is listed as the only source of calories merely because it is suitable for parenteral administration. Fat is deposited in the body for the purpose of providing a source of calories under conditions of negative caloric balance. Accordingly, there is ordinarily no need to maintain caloric equilibrium by glucose therapy. Usually it suffices to give enough glucose to prevent ketosis (60 gm. per m² per 24 hours).

he will need severalfold more sodium and chloride and some additional water to prevent sodium depletion.

For reasons indicated earlier (see Figure 8) it is assumed that the dehydrated hypoadrenocortical patient is suffering almost exclusively from extracellular water loss. It is further assumed that this extracellular dehydration occurs in association with a tendency to intracellular edema. As shown in Table 8, this means that the hypoadrenocortical patient who has lost 5 per cent of his body weight has suffered approximately as much extracellular dehydration as the normal subject who has lost 10 per cent of his body weight in the form of water and electrolytes. Such losses are seen only in cases of marked dehydration. In milder cases the losses are not so large.

Table 9 combines the data of Tables 7 and 8 into a schedule which indicates approximately the total water, sodium, chloride and glucose needs of markedly dehydrated hypoadrenocortical patients during the first 24 hours of treatment. It is seen that these needs can be met with ordinary isotonic saline in 5 or 10 per cent glucose as shown in the right-hand pair of columns.* Actually, in most

* As discussed above, patients with Na-K hormone lack develop extracellular dehydration and intracellular edema because they suffer an abnormal loss of the extracellular osmoles, sodium and chloride. It follows that they are more in need of extracellular osmoles than of water. Moreover, patients with adrenal insufficiency have only a limited ability to excrete unneeded water loads (see Table 3, water test). Summation of these thoughts suggests that hypertonic saline should be better than isotonic (0.85 gm. per cent) saline in the therapy of Addisonian crisis. Approximately speaking, 1¼ normal (1.1 gm. per cent) saline would appear to be suitable. If used, the volumes indicated in Table 9 should be reduced by 20 per cent. We have not had an opportunity to test this thesis as yet.

TABLE III—8. *Approximate losses suffered during acute dehydration in moderately and markedly dehydrated normal persons and in a markedly dehydrated hypoadrenocortical patient.*

Type of subject	Degree of dehydration	Body wt. (water)		[H$_2$O]$_E$		[H$_2$O]$_I$		Na[H$_2$O]$_E$		Cl[H$_2$O]$_E$		K[H$_2$O]$_I$	
		gm. (cc.) per kg.	per cent of original	cc. per kg.	per cent of original	cc. per kg.	per cent of original	mEq. per kg.	per cent of original	mEq. per kg.	per cent of original	mEq. per kg.	per cent of original
Normal	moderate	50	5	25	12.5	25	5	3.5	12.5	2.5	12.5	3 to 3.5	5 —
Normal	marked	100	10	50	25.0	50	10	7	25.0	5	25.0	6 to 7	10 —
Hypo AC	marked	50	5	50	25.0	±0	±0	10	35.0	8	35.0	±0	±0

These data are based on the assumption that, in moderately acute dehydration, body weight loss is equal for practical purposes to water loss. Of the water lost, normally about half comes from extracellular fluid stores (which comprise about 20 per cent of normal body weight) and half is derived from intracellular fluids (which comprise about 50 per cent of normal body weight). It is also assumed on the basis of experience that approximately speaking (a) extracellular sodium and chloride are normally lost in such proportion to extracellular water that there is little alteration in extracellular electrolyte composition and (b) intracellular potassium is normally lost in somewhat less than normal proportion (150 mEq. per liter) to intracellular water (though in excess of normal with relation to protoplasmic catabolism) (1 gm. N to 3 mEq. K). Hence the "per cent of original" K[H$_2$O]$_I$ loss values are indicated to be somewhat less than those for [H$_2$O]$_I$ itself.

By contrast, in hypoadrenocorticism losses are believed to be almost exclusively of extracellular water and electrolytes. Moreover, in this condition sodium and chloride are apt to be lost in excess of extracellular water with a resultant tendency to marked hyponatremia and hypochloremia. In this table it has been assumed that extracellular sodium concentration has fallen from a normal level of 140 to 120 mEq. per liter and that extracellular chloride concentrations have similarly fallen from a normal value of 100 to the low value of 80 mEq. per liter. As indicated elsewhere in this chapter, the concentration values for the two extracellular electrolytes do not always fall to such low levels when patients develop hypoadrenocortical crisis. Hence the electrolyte losses described may be considered nearly maximal rather than average.

TABLE III—9. Approximate requirements for repair and maintenance of patients with moderate extracellular dehydration due to acute hypoadrenocorticism during the first 24 hours. This table combines the data of Tables 7 and 8. It assumes that the patient is receiving adequate amounts of Na-K hormone. It should be used only as a rough guide. The values listed may be found to be inadequate for small individuals, and somewhat overgenerous for larger individuals.

Weight of patient kg.	Repair needs			Maintenance needs					Total needs				Provided by physiologic saline with	
	H₂O cc.	Na mEq.	Cl mEq.	Surface area m²	H₂O cc.	Na mEq.	Cl mEq.	Glucose gm.	H₂O cc.	Na mEq.	Cl mEq.	Glucose gm.	5% D* cc.	10% D* cc.
5	250	50	40	0.3	220	3	3	20-75	470	53	43	20-75	—	500
10	500	100	80	0.5	360	5	5	30-125	860	105	85	30-125	—	850
20	1,000	200	160	0.75	540	8	8	45-180	1,540	208	168	45-180	—	1,500
30	1,500	300	240	1.0	720	11	11	60-250	2,220	311	251	60-250	—	2,000
40	2,000	400	320	1.2	860	13	13	70-280	2,860	413	333	70-280	2,700	—
50	2,500	500	400	1.3	940	14	14	80-320	3,440	514	414	80-320	3,300	—
60	3,000	600	480	1.5	1,080	16	16	90-360	4,080	616	496	90-360	4,000	—
70	3,500	700	560	1.7	1,220	19	19	100-400	4,720	719	579	100-400	4,500	—

D* = dextrose (glucose).

instances parenteral fluid therapy can be discontinued and oral fluids instituted within 12 hours after treatment is started. If the patient is still unable to take fluids by mouth at the end of the first day, repair needs as well as maintenance needs can usually be met during subsequent days by giving half-isotonic (0.43 gm. per cent) saline instead of isotonic (0.85 gm. per cent) saline in glucose. At least by the middle of the second day the patient should be able to begin a liquid diet. Soft solids and ordinary foods may be added as tolerated. From 2 to 3 gm. of sodium chloride per m^2 should also be given daily. The sodium salt can be given as enteric-coated tablets containing 1 gm. or as a solution containing 15 gm. of sodium chloride and 5 gm. of sodium citrate per 100 cc. Five cc. of this solution contain 1 gm. of sodium salt. Its palatability can be improved by diluting it to 1,000 cc. with 80 cc. of lemon juice, 160 gm. of sugar and about 800 cc. of water. Of this diluted solution 50 cc. must be given to yield 1 gm. of sodium salt.

For comments concerning the possibility that patients may develop a need for potassium salts after a day or two of adrenocortical hormone plus sodium salt treatment, see page 207. This need is not apt to develop in patients who begin to take milk and other complete foods by mouth within one or two days after treatment is started.

Other forms of therapy (antibiotics, sedatives). Since crises may be provoked by acute infections which greatly increase adrenocortical hormone requirements, it is important to make a careful search for infection and to give antibacterial therapy. Penicillin or chloromycetin may be given routinely in full therapeutic doses for prophylactic as well as for therapeutic purposes. Sulfa drugs should not be given before urine flow has become established.

Sedatives may also be needed. Barbiturates are reasonably safe to use. On the other hand, morphine and its homologues and derivatives are to be avoided because hypoadrenocortical patients are unusually sensitive to them.

Summary of approach to treatment. In instances of mild adrenocortical insufficiency, it usually suffices to add sodium chloride to the diet and to administer DOCA as outlined above.

In cases of severe insufficiency the patient must be placed in bed under constant nursing care. An intravenous infusion of saline-glucose solution (see Table 9) is started. The simplest sure means of providing adequate adrenocortical hormone treatment is to give full therapeutic doses of aqueous adrenocortical extract by way of the intravenous infusion. This is unfortunately an expensive method of treatment. When aqueous extract is used, there is no need to give DOCA, but in any case DOCA should be limited to average maintenance doses while full therapeutic doses of adrenocortical extract are being administered. Current experience suggests that cortisone plus DOCA in full therapeutic doses may prove to be an effective, but much less expensive means of treating Addisonian crisis.

The response to therapy is usually gratifying. Within a period of 2 to 36 hours the patient's water balance, circulation, strength and mental status should be markedly improved. Fever which cannot be attributed to infection occasionally develops. At times such fever appears to be related to signs of extra- or intracellular overhydration or other metabolic disturbance.

As the patient improves, he is gradually placed on a normal diet with additional sodium chloride. It is important to offer milk and other well-balanced foods as early as practicable because they make it possible for the patient to repair deficits of body substances which cannot be overcome with sodium chloride, glucose and water alone.

If the patient has been treated initially with aqueous adrenocortical extracts, he is given DOCA in maintenance doses. The aqueous extract is gradually diminished and finally discontinued altogether. If, on the other hand, he has been treated only with DOCA plus cortisone, then the doses of these hormones should be reduced to maintenance levels as the patient's condition returns toward normal. The oral administration of 5 to 10 mg. of cortisone per m^2 daily may add considerably to the patient's strength and sense of well being.

Intercurrent infections and other conditions encountered by patients receiving chronic maintenance therapy are managed in essentially the same way as are crises. Only relatively small quantities of adrenocortical hormone may be needed to prevent or abort an incipient crisis, although large quantities often are needed to bring about recovery once a crisis has developed. For this reason it is recommended that the patient's family keep a supply of aqueous adrenocortical extract and cortisone at home. The former should be stored in the refrigerator. The family should be instructed to call the attending physician at the first sign of a "cold" or other infection. If he is unable to see the patient promptly, or if he believes he may be difficult to reach at times, he may wish to leave a standing order that the patient be given about 4 cc. of aqueous extract per m^2 subcutaneously at intervals of four to eight hours pending his arrival.

Should a hypoadrenocortical patient develop a condition which requires surgical treatment, it is very desirable to use local rather than general anesthesia. Since surgery constitutes a predictable interval of stress, full therapeutic doses of aqueous adrenocortical extract should be administered before, during and as long as necessary after operation.

PROGNOSIS. Prior to the time when DOCA became available, the outlook for patients with chronic hypoadrenocorticism was dismal. Even when placed on a high sodium–low potassium dietary regimen patients succumbed to the disease within a few years. Today life expectancy with adequate but not excessive DOCA therapy is very good, particularly if adrenocortical extract is given during periods of stress. With the advent of cortisone and even more recently of corticosterone, which may control both Na-K and S-F-N needs, the outlook should be even better.

Children with chronic hypoadrenocorticism grow and mature in an essentially normal manner when their adrenocortical insufficiency is properly controlled. Though their exercise tolerance is apt to be less than normal, they are capable of leading active, useful lives. Unless encouraged to lead normal lives they are likely to develop the emotional attributes of chronic invalidism and to retain the childhood characteristic of dependency upon parents and guardians.

Overwhelming Sepsis or Other Illness and Acute Hypoadrenocorticism (Waterhouse-Friderichsen Syndrome—see Figure 36).[21] Patients suffering from bacteremia and metastatic sepsis may develop symptoms and signs which are quite suggestive of acute adrenocortical failure. In the typical case the child becomes suddenly ill. At first the picture corresponds to that seen in any acute infection but subsequently deviates rather abruptly from the expected. A septic type of fever with temperatures fluctuating to values as high as 108°F. develops. Diarrhea, non-localized abdominal pain and generalized convulsions may occur. A lethargic stupor supervenes and is associated with such evidences of circulatory collapse as cyanosis alternating with marked pallor, weak, rapid thready pulse and hypotension. The respirations become disproportionately rapid and shallow in comparison with those of clinically demonstrable pulmonary disease. A macular purpuric rash appears. Terminally the patient is likely to develop the same livid appearance that is commonly seen post mortem. Death usually takes place within two days of the onset of symptoms.

Blood cultures almost always are positive. The meningococcus is the offender in about three-quarters of the cases seen. In the remaining instances the disease usually is due to staphylococcal, streptococcal or pneumococcal septicemia. At post-mortem examination, bilateral adrenal hemorrhages are found in about 95 per cent of the cases. However, the hemorrhages vary markedly, some being very small and involving only a tiny fraction of the gland while others are massive. This observation, plus the fact that some patients of this type have been observed to respond well to ACTH treatment, suggests that at least some of these individuals may be suffering from primary pituitary rather than primary adrenocortical failure.

Until recently most of the evidence concerning the adrenocortical status of patients with overwhelming sepsis and possible adrenal hemorrhage was far from

The Adrenal Cortices

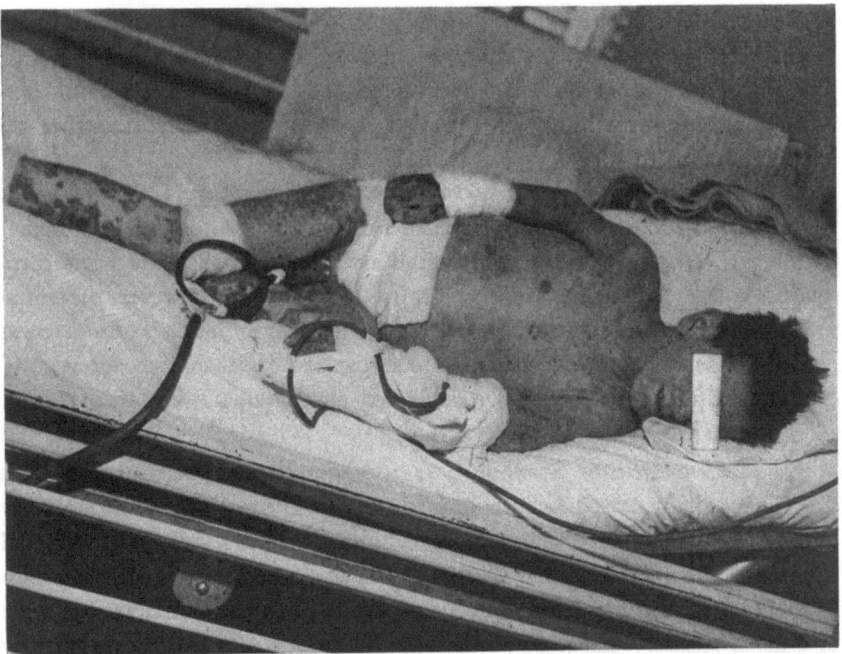

FIGURE III—36. Waterhouse-Friderichsen-like syndrome in a boy of 13 years.

CASE HISTORY

The patient developed an insidious condition characterized by vomiting, abdominal pain, obstipation and dehydration. Upon laparotomy the terminal ileum was found to be edematous and of purplish color. In addition there were petechial hemorrhages in other portions of the bowel and moderate quantities of sero-sanguinous fluid in the peritoneal cavity. Following the operation, increasing fever, tachycardia and hematuria developed. On the fifth postoperative day raised, purpuric lesions appeared on the skin over the patient's ankles, wrists and buttocks. As they became generalized, with bulla formation and necrosis, his condition became much worse. By the sixth day he was unresponsive, oliguric, unperistaltic and covered with coalescing ecchymoses. The eosinophil count had risen to 1,100 cells per mm^3, while the blood sugar had fallen to 40 mg. per cent. The serum potassium was slightly elevated at 6.1 mEq. per liter.

On the assumption that these changes reflected adrenocortical insufficiency in the presence of overwhelming disease, the patient was treated with aqueous adrenocortical extract in doses of 100 cc. per m^2 per 24 hours. Following institution of this therapy, he showed marked improvement. Within a few hours he became more responsive. The urine volume increased and the blood sugar rose and stabilized between 120 and 170 mg. per cent. The eosinophil count fell to a low of 430 cells per mm^3. Within 24 hours the patient could retain simple fluids given by mouth. Six days later, when adrenocortical extract therapy was discontinued, he held his gains. Six months later no residue of these disturbances was discernible.

objective. It now appears that fairly reliable information concerning this can be obtained by the relatively simple eosinophil count test (Table 3, Test 4). At present this test is being used as an index of the need for giving adrenocortical hormone therapy to severely sick patients. Our experience to date indicates that it is reliable in most instances.

Treatment of acute hypoadrenocorticism secondary to overwhelming sepsis is the same as for acute primary hypoadrenocorticism (see preceding section). Of the various adrenocortical preparations available, aqueous extract and cortisone are considered the agents of choice. It is to be stressed, however, that intravenous fluid, transfusion, oxygen and antibiotic therapy must also be given as needed. Patients who recover from episodes of apparent acute hypoadrenocorticism of the type under consideration here rarely have residual evidences of chronic adrenocortical insufficiency.

Hypoadrenocorticism Secondary to Hypopituitarism (ACTH Lack). This condition is characterized by adrenocortical underactivity which is due primarily to failure of the pituitary to produce ACTH rather than to a defect in the adrenal cortex (see Figure 29). It may be observed in any patient who is suffering from hypopituitarism of organic or functional origin. For a list of the various types of organic pituitary and juxta-pituitary lesions which can give rise to primary hypopituitarism, see Chapter VII.

It is unusual for patients suffering from hypoadrenocorticism secondary to hypopituitarism to present gross evidences of Na-K or S-F-N hormone insufficiency (see under primary hypoadrenocorticism). More commonly the clinical signs point only to deficiency in 17-KS-Gens (pubic and axillary alopecia). However, when the various tests for Na-K and S-F-N hormone deficiency listed in Table 3 are applied, some degree of adrenocortical hormone deficiency is usually demonstrable.

The fact that clinically silent hypoadrenocorticism can at times be demonstrated by specific tests suggests that adrenocortical hormone production rates, though low in relation to average normal, are not necessarily low in relation to the ordinary needs of the hypopituitary individual. A possible explanation for this lies in the fact that patients with panhypopituitarism may be hypothyroid as well as hypoadrenocortical (see Figure 37).

Another situation of potential clinical importance is met with in patients who have unilateral adrenocortical cancers (see Figure 38).[18, 22] Such cancers* often produce large amounts of adrenocortical hormones. These in turn inhibit pituitary

---

* These comments apply particularly to patients with clinical signs of Cushing's syndrome, including chronic eosinopenia. They are less apt to be of importance in patients showing only pathologic masculinization.

ACTH production and hence prompt functional involution of the contralateral, potentially normal adrenal cortex. Because of the hyperproductive adrenocortical tumor, the patient does not show signs of adrenal insufficiency during the life of the tumor. However, when such a tumor is removed surgically, the patient is likely to experience an acute episode of severe hypoadrenocorticism in the immediate postoperative period. Unless this state is anticipated and appropriate therapeutic measures are instituted, the outcome may be fatal.

Such disaster has been avoided successfully by the following pre-, intra- and postoperative measures. Just before operation, an intravenous infusion made up of equal parts of isotonic saline and 5 per cent glucose solution is started and allowed to run at a rate of about 1.0 cc. per m^2 per minute. This makes it easy to transfuse blood or to administer aqueous adrenocortical extract during the operation should need arise. An inlying urethral catheter is also inserted in order that urine flow can be measured accurately. A generous supply of aqueous extract is sent to the operating room with the patient.

If an adrenocortical tumor is found at operation, aqueous adrenocortical extract therapy is started as soon as circulation to the tumor is clamped off. The doses used have ranged between 5 and 7 cc. per m^2 per hour. The extract is added to the saline in glucose infusion in suitable proportion or is administered intramuscularly or subcutaneously at hourly intervals.

During the first 24 hours of the postoperative period the following observations are made at the intervals stated in order that undesirable changes can be recognized early: q. ½ hour–pulse; q. 1 hour–blood pressure, temperature, fluid intake and urine output; q. 2 hours–eosinophil count; q. 4 hours–electrocardiogram, percussion of precordium for heart size. During subsequent days, depending upon the condition of the patient, these measurements may be spaced at increasingly long intervals. The inlying urethral catheter is removed at the end of 24 hours unless the patient has developed oliguria or edema. In the case of older children who are able to void into a receptacle the catheter may be removed sooner.

If signs of adrenocortical insufficiency develop (tachycardia, fever, hypotension, elevated eosinophil count, microcardia, loss of tissue elasticity, dry mucous membranes) isotonic saline in 5 per cent glucose may be substituted for the half-isotonic saline solution and adrenocortical extract therapy may be increased. This change has not been necessary in our experience. If, contrariwise, signs of Na-K hormone intoxication with excess sodium retention and potassium depletion develop (edema, macrocardia, pulmonary rales, flattening of the T waves in the electrocardiogram; see Figure 35), the potassium ion solution no. 2 given

Continued on page 223

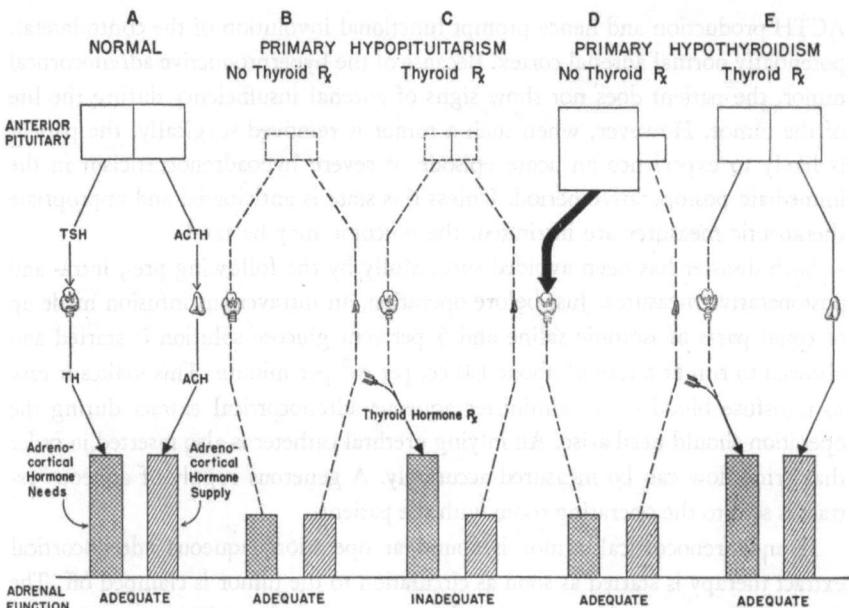

FIGURE III—37. Diagrammatic representation of probable relations between pituitary, thyroid and adrenal status in patients with primary hypopituitarism and in patients with hypopituitarism secondary to hypothyroidism. TSH=thyroid-stimulating hormone; ACTH =adrenocorticotropic hormone; TH=thyroid hormone; ACH=adrenocortical hormones.

SECTION A: In normal persons the anterior pituitary stimulates both the thyroid and the adrenal cortices to produce their respective hormones. Adrenal hormone requirements, which are determined in part by the thyroid activity, are met satisfactorily.

SECTION B: In primary panhypopituitarism with secondary hypothyroidism and secondary hypoadrenocorticism the tissue requirements for and the supply of adrenocortical hormones are apt to be proportionately decreased. As a result, gross clinical evidences of hypoadrenocorticism with respect to Na-K or S-F-N hormones are unlikely.

SECTION C: When B type patients are treated with thyroid hormone, tissue requirements for adrenocortical hormones are increased, but because of the primary pituitary deficiency there cannot be any spontaneous increase in adrenocortical hormone production. As a consequence, clinical evidences of hypoadrenocorticism may develop.

SECTION D: Patients with primary hypothyroidism are apt to have secondary hypopituitarism and tertiary hypoadrenocorticism. Note that type D patients have approximately the same status as type B, even though the primary defect is different.

SECTION E: Note that type D patients do not develop hypoadrenocorticism when given thyroid therapy, because pituitary and hence adrenocortical function are restored to normal by thyroid hormone treatment.

The Adrenal Cortices

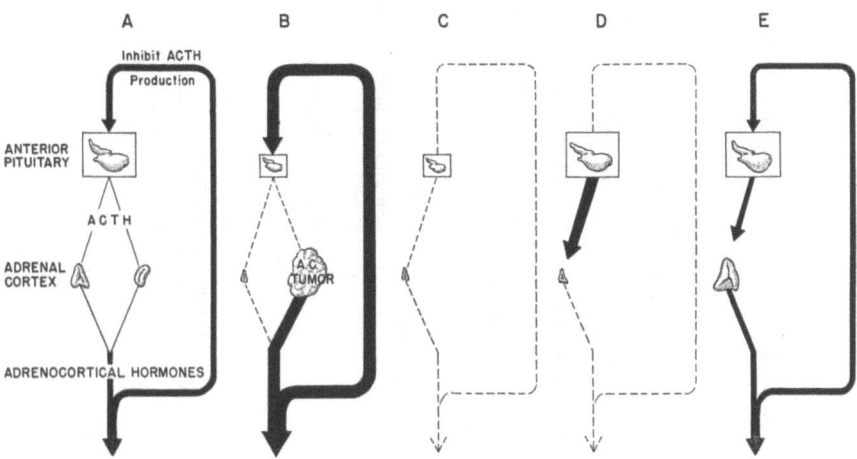

FIGURE III—38. Diagrammatic representation of relations pertaining before and after removal of a unilateral adrenocortical cancer.

SECTION A: In normal persons note that both adrenal cortices are producing adrenocortical hormone under the stimulus of adrenocorticotropic hormone (ACTH) and that the adrenocortical hormones partially inhibit ACTH production.

SECTION B: As shown by the heavy arrow, unilateral adrenocortical cancer produces excessive amounts of adrenocortical hormones, which inhibit ACTH production. As a consequence, the normal, contralateral adrenal cortex involutes. However, these relations are observed much more commonly in patients showing signs of S-F-N hormone excess (i.e., Cushing's syndrome) than in those showing only signs of virilism.

SECTION C: This is the situation which exists immediately following surgical removal of the cancer indicated in Section B. Observe that the patient momentarily is left with a pituitary which is not secreting ACTH and with an adrenal cortex which is involuted and functionally inactive. As a consequence, this type of patient is very apt to develop marked hypoadrenocorticism as soon as hormones produced by the adrenal tumor have been eliminated.

SECTION D: Under the conditions of adrenocortical hormone lack indicated in Section C, the pituitary resumes production of ACTH, which in turn stimulates the remaining adrenal cortex to develop and to secrete its hormones. This recovery phase may take several days.

SECTION E: Finally, the one remaining adrenal gland produced as much hormone as is ordinarily produced by two healthy glands (Section A). However, to accomplish this, the single remaining gland may become somewhat hypertrophied in relation to average normal size.

TABLE III—10. Theoretically expected characteristics of syndromes due to excess production of the various major types of adrenocortical hormone. See text for comments.

Na-K hormones	S-F-N hormones	17-KS-Gens	
MANIFESTATIONS	MANIFESTATIONS	MANIFESTATIONS	
		Normal mixture	Abnormal mixture
Extracellular hyperhydration with edema, hypertension, cardiac enlargement	Diabetic glucose tolerance, glycosuria	Precocious sex hair growth, acne	Excess hair, acne
Intracellular potassium depletion with muscle weakness	Wasting of muscles, bones, involution of lymphoid tissues, eosinopenia	Abnormally high output of urinary 17-KS	Penile or clitoral enlargement, deepening of voice, heavy musculature, accelerated skeletal development
Low sweat sodium chloride concentration	Disturbance in fat metabolism?	Urinary 17-KS pattern normal?	Abnormally high output of urinary 17-KS
Hypochloremia	Abnormally elevated urinary 11-17-OCS		Urinary 17-KS pattern abnormal
Hypokalemia			
Alkalosis			
CLINICAL CONDITION	CLINICAL CONDITION	CLINICAL CONDITION	
Essential hypertension?	Diabetes mellitus?	?	Adrenocortical virilism
	Cushing's syndrome		

in Chapter IX, Table 8, may be substituted for the half-isotonic saline in glucose infusion fluid.

On the second or third postoperative day oral feedings of skim milk, bread, jelly and other simple foods are given in small amounts as tolerated at four hourly intervals. As soon thereafter as it becomes certain that food is well tolerated, an ordinary diet for age can be offered.

Starting also on the third postoperative day, if no complications have arisen, the original dosage of aqueous adrenocortical extract is reduced each day by 15 or 20 per cent. The amount is reduced more rapidly if signs of overdosage have arisen and more gradually if signs of adrenocortical insufficiency have become apparent. Adrenocortical hormone therapy can usually be discontinued altogether by the ninth postoperative day.

We have avoided using ACTH preoperatively for fear of inducing spread of an adrenocortical cancer. Postoperatively administration of ACTH to hasten regeneration of atrophic adrenocortical tissue is usually not necessary. On the other hand, it might be of value in patients with severe postoperative adrenocortical insufficiency.

HYPERADRENOCORTICISM

As was the case for hypoadrenocorticism, the present condition can be divided into groups and subgroups according to the nature and location of the primary defect. Thus hyperadrenocorticism occurring as a consequence of an adrenocortical carcinoma or adenoma is considered primary hyperadrenocorticism. Contrariwise, hyperadrenocorticism seen in association with bilateral adrenocortical hyperplasia is considered to be probably secondary to increased ACTH production. If this thesis is correct, it follows that the primary defect may lie either in the anterior pituitary or in those hypothalamic centers which presumably determine ACTH production. Alternatively there is a possibility that the real fault lies in the adrenal cortices in the sense that they are abnormally responsive to ACTH stimulation or are producing abnormal hormones which act in some way to upset the normal balanced relationship between the pituitary and the adrenal glands. In this connection it is noteworthy that the zonæ reticularis of patients with masculinization due to bilateral adrenocortical hyperplasia contain cells with abnormal staining qualities.[14 d]

Patients with adrenocortical hyperactivity also can be separated approximately according to the type or types of adrenal hormone produced in excess. Table 10 sets forth in brief the types of clinical cases which one might theoretically expect to see on this basis. In reality, the picture suggested under the Na-K hormone heading has not been recognized as a clinical entity as yet, though it may exist in modified form in certain patients with essential hypertension. Only one case presenting a virtually uncomplicated picture of diabetes mellitus caused by primary adrenocortical overactivity has been encountered to date.[23 a] Some patients have shown abnormal masculinization and an abnormal mixture of 17-KS in their urine, but no gross evidences of excess Na-K or S-F-N hormone production. In other words, the theoretically pure pictures may occur from time to time but they are not commonly recognized at present.

As a rule the picture seen clinically is not suggestive of pure hyperadrenocorticism with respect to one or another of the adrenocortical hormones. Rather, it suggests that the patient is suffering from the effects of mixed hyperadrenocorticism. Thus Cushing's syndrome in its purest form appears to be due to excess Na-K and S-F-N hormone production. Patients sometimes seem also to have an excess of the normal, non-androgenic 17-KS-precursors. Occasionally as evidenced by masculinization, they appear to be suffering from the effects of abnormal, androgenic 17-KS-precursors and thus to have both Cushing's syndrome and adrenocortical virilism. At the other end of the spectrum, some patients with pronounced masculinization have some manifestations of Cushing's syndrome, while others appear to be suffering either from Na-K hormone deficiency or from a hormonal disturbance which produces its metabolic equivalent.

These considerations indicate that the following subdivision of clinical hyperadrenocorticism into adrenocortical virilism, Cushing's syndrome and masculinization plus electrolyte disturbances similar to those of Addison's disease is both arbitrary and somewhat inaccurate. However, the subdivision does facilitate a systematic presentation of the clinical features of various types of hyperadrenocorticism. The outstanding clinical manifestations of these conditions as observed in young children are listed in Table 11. Descriptive comments and qualifying remarks are given in the following text.

Adrenocortical Virilism.[14 b-d, 23] This is an uncommon, but not a rare condition. About 100 cases due to congenital, bilateral hyperplasia of the adrenal cortices have been reported to date.[23 b] Of these about 80 per cent were females and 20 per cent males. In addition, about 40 children with masculinization caused by an adrenocortical tumor have been listed. About two-thirds of these were girls. All instances of masculinization developing postnatally and before the age of 10 years were due to adrenal tumor; with only a few exceptions, cases of masculinization which appeared to date back to birth were caused by benign bilateral hyperplasia.*

---

* This condition sometimes is familial.[23 c] We have seen three cases in a single family.

TABLE III—11. Some manifestations of Cushing's syndrome, adrenocortical virilism, adrenocortical feminism and mixed hyper-hypoadrenocorticism as observed clinically in pure form in children. Mixtures of (A) and (B) often seen; mixtures of (A) and (D) occasionally seen.

Manifestations	Cushing's syndrome	Adrenocortical virilism	(B) plus hypoadrenocorticism	Adrenocortical feminism
	(A)	(B)	(C)	(D)
Obesity	+	0	0	0
Plethoric appearance	+	0	0	0
Striæ atrophicæ	+	0	0	0
Diabetes	±+	0	0	0
Elevated urinary 11-17-OCS	+	±0	±0	0
Eosinopenia	+	0?	0?	0
Weakness	+	0	±+	0
Stunted growth	+	early 0	±	0
Abnormal hirsutism	+	+	+	0
Acne	+	late +	+	0
Masculinization	0	+	+	0
Congenital genital tract defects	0	±+♀;0♂	+♀	0
Accelerated growth	0	early +	±+	0
Accelerated skeletal maturity	0	+	+	+
Elevated urinary 17-KS	±0	+	+	+
Signs of Na-K hormone lack	0	0	+	0
Abnormal feminization	0	0	±0	+
Elevated urinary estrogens	±+	±+	±+	+

For reasons outlined earlier (page 156), it is thought that the clinical signs of this disease are due to the production of qualitatively abnormal adrenocortical hormones rather than to a simple overproduction of one of the normal adrenocortical hormones.

CLINICAL MANIFESTATIONS. The homologous masculine structures of males and females respond to the abnormal adrenal androgens in a similar manner. The response is modified, however, by the age of the patient at the onset of the condition. If adrenocortical virilism starts in the female during early intrauterine life, pseudo-hermaphroditic changes occur. These are usually characterized by congenital malformations of the lower genital tract. For example, the vagina may fail to develop or a urogenital sinus may form with the urethra delivering into the anterior wall of the vagina rather than into the perineum (see Figures 39 to 41).

No such phenomena are observed if the disease starts postnatally. As might be expected, male patients with this disease do not develop congenital malformations of the genital tract. Hence, in contrast to girls, they are usually of essentially normal appearance at birth.

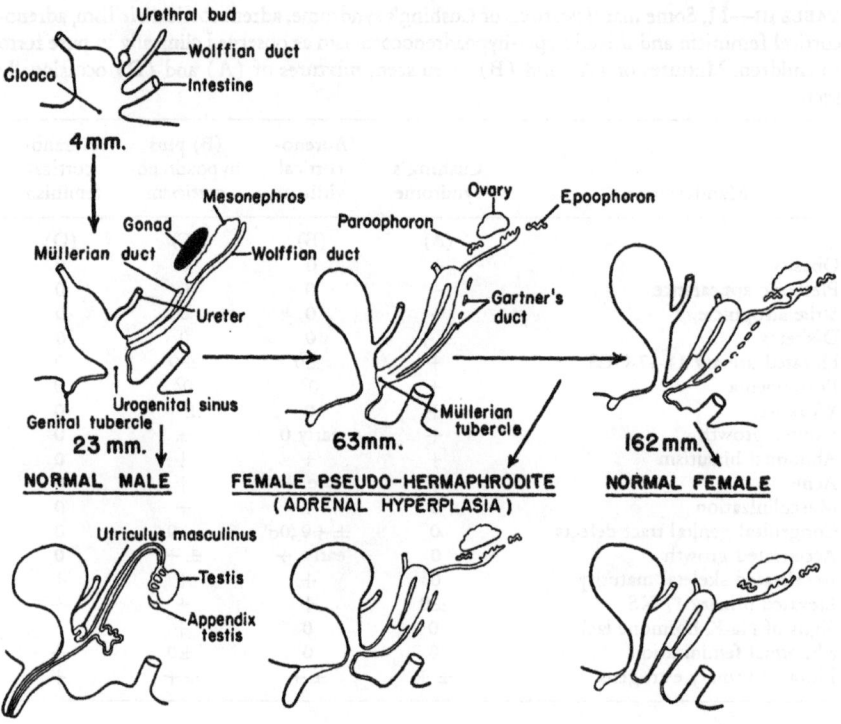

FIGURE III—39. Embryologic development of the urogenital sinus. At the 23 mm. stage the embryo is ambisexual, with both Müllerian and Wolffian ducts. By the 63 mm. stage the Müllerian duct shows complete development in the female, while the Wolffian duct has disappeared. The vagina is joined to the urogenital sinus by the Müllerian tubercle, which is not yet patent. Later, there is a communication between the vagina and the urogenital sinus, but by the 162 mm. stage the separation of the vagina and the urethra is completed by the growth of the anterior vaginal wall. Masculinizing effects of congenital adrenal hyperplasia are probably manifested between the 63 mm. and the 162 mm. stage (12 to 20 weeks). From L. Wilkins, *Pediatrics* 3:533, 1949.

Following birth, the adrenal androgens continue to exert an abnormal influence upon the growth and development of the child. The changes induced occur not only in the genital structures but also in muscles, bones, skin and larynx.

In the female the clitoris continues to hypertrophy and may attain considerable size (see Figure 42). Though the ovaries and uterus are usually present, breast development and menstruation fail to occur when the patient reaches adolescent age. Instead, the breasts remain flat and the individual tends to have a masculine body habitus. Gross and microscopic examination of the ovaries may reveal

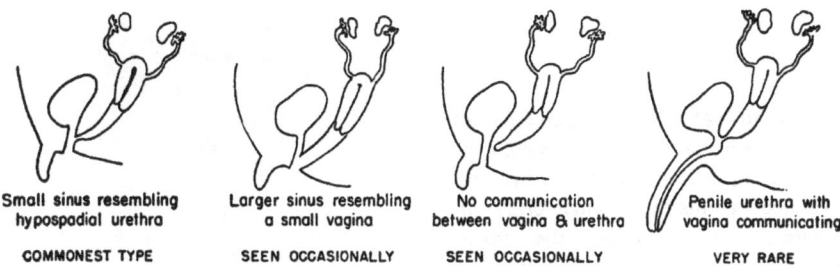

FIGURE III—40. Variations in the type of urogenital sinus seen in female pseudo-hermaphrodites with adrenocortical hyperplasia. From L. Wilkins, *Pediatrics* 3:533, 1949.

various abnormalities. At times they are abnormally elongated and of vermiform, immature appearance. Occasionally cells resembling those seen in the adrenal cortex (hyperplastic cell rests?) are found within the substance of the ovary.[23 d, e] At times also, the tunica may be abnormally thickened in a manner reminiscent of the Stein-Leventhal syndrome (see Chapter V, page 351).

In the male the penis grows to adult proportions at an early age (see Figures 43, 44), but the testes usually remain of normal size for age. Biopsy examination during the preadolescent age period may reveal essentially normal, immature-appearing testicular tissue (see Figure 45, left), but these patients may subsequently undergo apparently normal testicular adolescence (see Figure 45, right). In association with the penile growth, there is premature development of the scrotum, prostate and seminal vesicles.

In children of either sex the adrenal androgens cause accelerated growth in stature, accelerated skeletal maturation, muscular hypertrophy, pubic and axillary hair growth, acne, recession of the temporal hair line and deepening of the voice. The accelerated growth rate usually leads to a period of relative gigantism. This, however, is of only temporary duration, because precocious closure of the skeletal epiphyses brings statural growth to a stop even before normal adult stature has been attained (see Figure 46). Consequently, these patients tend as adults to be short and stocky in appearance. The age at which sex hair appears is somewhat variable ($\pm$ 1 to 5 years). Acne usually develops before the fifth year. Recession of temporal hair and deepening of the voice are late phenomena and usually do not occur before adolescent age. Baldness may develop subsequently.

Local signs of an adrenal lesion are universally absent in patients with bilateral adrenocortical hyperplasia. In cases of adrenal tumor there may be no signs until the lesion attains considerable size. When a tumor mass becomes palpable

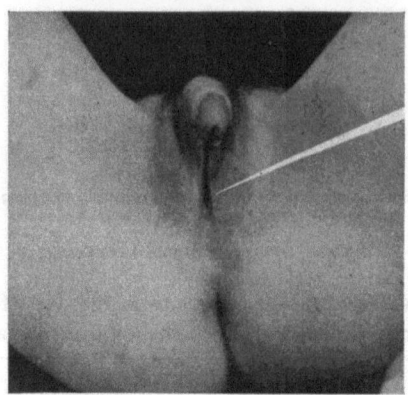

FIGURE III—41. External genitalia of a pseudo-hermaphrodite with masculinization due to congenital adrenocortical hyperplasia. The arrow points to the single orifice of the urogenital sinus. Note, also, the clitoral hypertrophy and the hypospadiac crease on the ventral aspect of the clitoris.

in the region of the kidneys, evidences of spread of a malignant adrenocortical cancer to the renal veins, vena cava, liver and lungs may be noted. In the absence of local clinical signs of an adrenal tumor, helpful information may be obtained by pyelography or by roentgenographic examination following perirenal air insufflation.[23, f] Opinion is divided concerning the latter procedure. In experienced hands it probably can be considered reasonably safe and of some diagnostic value. In inexperienced hands it has led to collapse and death. Negative results obtained by this method are not necessarily conclusive. Because of this and because it usually is important to visualize both adrenals before removing an adrenal tumor, we have not utilized this procedure on our patients.

LABORATORY STUDIES. Additional information is provided by laboratory studies. Quantitative and qualitative measurements of the urinary 17-KS usually give abnormal values (high 17-KS output, abnormal pattern by chromatographic fractionation). In cases of pure adrenocortical virilism, the urinary 11-17-OCS output is normal or only slightly elevated. Tests designed to reveal disturbances in Na-K and S-F-N hormone metabolism give essentially normal results. For a discussion of the application and interpretation of these tests, see the foregoing section on diagnostic procedures and Table 3.

DIAGNOSIS. Penile or clitoral enlargement, congenital malformations of the lower genital tract in the female, hirsutism, and precocious acne suggest adrenocortical virilism. Congenital hypertrophy of the clitoris is occasionally seen as an isolated malformation. In the absence of other signs of precocious masculinization enlargement of this organ may be indicative of non-endocrine partial hermaphroditism (see Chapter v).

A good presumptive diagnosis of adrenocortical virilism can usually be made with the aid of the information outlined above, especially the urinary 17-KS measurements. A positive diagnosis can be made only by direct exploratory inspection of the adrenal glands. This is, of course, imperative where there is reason to suspect a neoplasm. On the other hand, exploratory operation may be considered an elective procedure in patients with no particular manifestations of adrenocortical cancer and with a history of masculinization dating back to intrauterine life as evidenced by congenital malformations of the lower genital tract in the female. The vast majority of such patients have bilateral adrenocortical hyperplasia rather than cancer. A new and interesting observation suggests that cortisone administration may aid in the differential diagnosis of adrenocortical hyperplasia versus adrenocortical adenoma or carcinoma. The administration of 50 to 75 mg. of cortisone per m^2 per day is usually more than sufficient to inhibit pituitary ACTH production and hence to cause a marked fall in the urinary 17-KS excretion of patients with bilateral adrenocortical hyperplasia. By contrast, in a patient with an adrenocortical adenoma no significant decrease in 17-KS output was observed during a period of cortisone treatment.[23 h]

Cushing's syndrome is also to be distinguished (see below). It has a number of clinical characteristics not shown by patients with straightforward adrenocortical virilism. Also, it is characterized by an elevation in the urinary 11-17-OCS rather than in the urinary 17-KS values and by chronic eosinopenia. Certain patients may show evidences of both adrenocortical virilism and Cushing's syndrome.

Finally, there is another type of mixed adrenocortical disease, with signs of virilism and of hypoadrenocorticism with respect to the water and electrolyte hormone. This condition is discussed briefly in a later section. To rule this condition and Cushing's syndrome in or out, it is suggested that one or more tests for Na-K and for S-F-N deficiency or excess be run. These are particularly important if major operative procedures are to be undertaken, because they may reveal clinically silent disturbances in adrenocortical function. Following surgical exploration of the adrenals with or without removal of adrenal tissue, signs of acute hypoadrenocorticism may develop in a patient who has never had any spontaneous manifestations of this condition previously.

TREATMENT. Prompt surgical intervention is indicated for adrenocortical cancer. Attention should be given to the possibility that acute adrenocortical insufficiency will develop following operative removal of such a tumor or of adrenocortical or ovarian tissue for biopsy purposes. These manifestations can be most distressing and of fatal outcome unless vigorously combatted. The chances that this type of difficulty will arise are less in patients with straightforward adrenocortical virilism than they are in patients with Cushing's syndrome or in patients with mixed adrenocortical disease. Methods for preventing and overcoming this

Continued on page 233

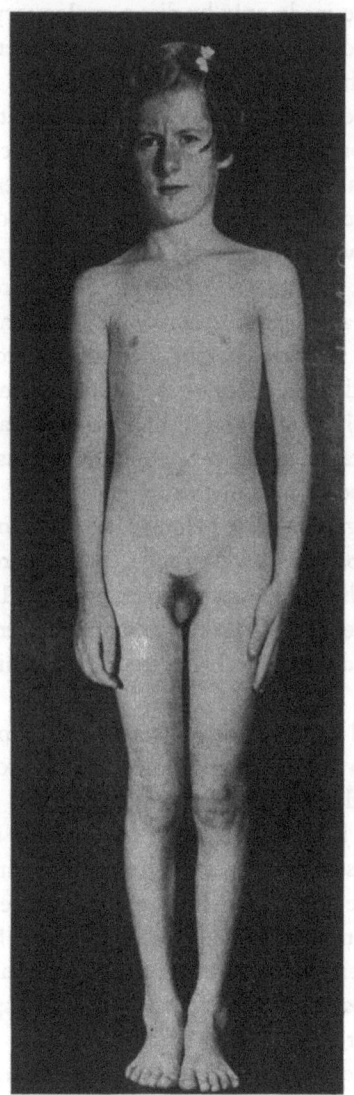 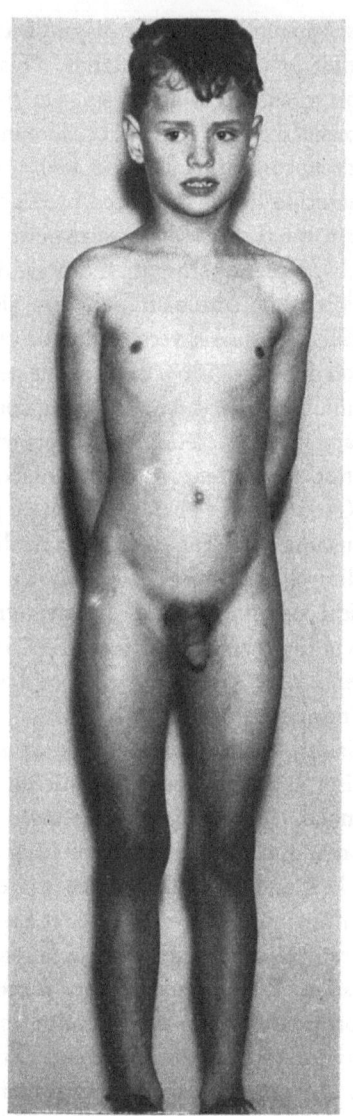

(Left)
FIGURE III—42. Adrenocortical virilism with pseudo-hermaphroditism due to bilateral adrenocortical hyperplasia in an 11-year-old girl. From N. B. Talbot, A. M. Butler and R. A. Berman, *J. Clin. Investigation* 21:559, 1942.

(Right)
FIGURE III—43. Probable congenital adrenocortical virilism (pseudo-precocious puberty) due to bilateral adrenocortical hyperplasia in a boy of five years (see also Figure 45, left).

CASE HISTORY (FIGURE 43)

The parents of this patient felt certain that he was of normal appearance at birth. Starting at about one year of age, penile development, pubic hair growth and a rapid increase in stature gradually became evident, together with mild facial acne and a tendency to deepening of the voice. He had no other noteworthy symptoms or signs.

On physical examination at 5 years of age, he measured 132 cm. in height and weighed 23 kg. Thus he corresponded in height to an average normal boy of nine years and in weight to an average boy of seven years. Generally speaking, he was a tall, slim, slightly apprehensive boy, with a rather low, hoarse voice. Pubic but no axillary hair was present. The penis and scrotum were of approximately adult size. On the other hand, the testes were of approximately normal size, shape and consistency for a boy of his age. If anything, they were slightly enlarged. A detailed neurologic examination revealed no definite abnormality.

Routine blood and urine tests revealed no abnormalities. Electroencephalograms gave normal results. The lumbar puncture yielded spinal fluid containing 25 mg. of total protein and 75 mg. of sugar per 100 cc. Roentgenograms of the skeleton, including the skull, revealed only that his bone age was 10 years. The urinary 17-KS output ranged between 19 and 20 mg. per 24 hours. Dr. O. Cope explored the adrenals through a wide transverse anterior abdominal incision. Both glands were thought to be unusually large and consistent with a diagnosis of bilateral adrenocortical hyperplasia. A small adrenal biopsy, which included the three layers of the cortex but not the medulla, failed to reveal any definite abnormality. A testicular biopsy failed to show any development of Leydig's interstitial cells but did show some increase in the caliber of the tubular lumina (see Figure 45, left). The patient's postoperative course was uneventful.

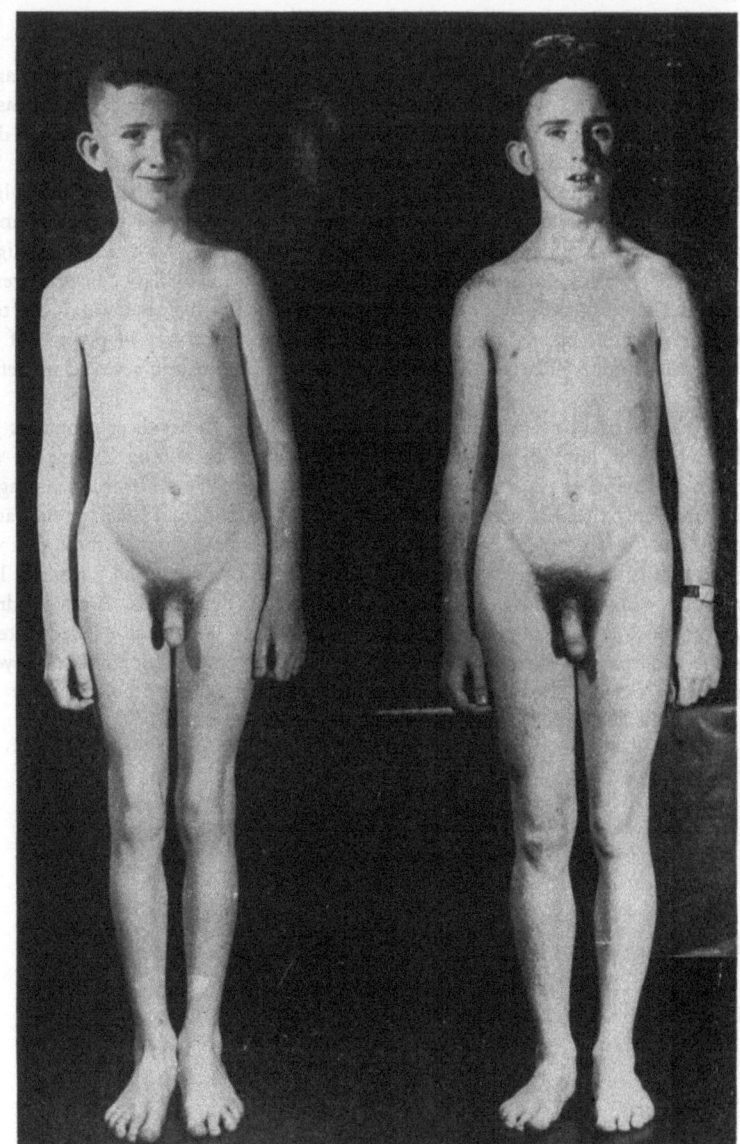

FIGURE III—44. Adrenocortical virilism due to bilateral adrenocortical hyperplasia.
LEFT: Appearance of the patient at 7½ years. Note that his penis was enlarged but his testes were of essentially normal size for age.
RIGHT: His appearance at 11½ years, when his testes had grown to adult size and had developed early evidences of spermatogenesis (see also Figure 45, right). From N. B. Talbot, A. M. Butler and R. A. Berman, *J. Clin. Investigation* 21:559, 1942.

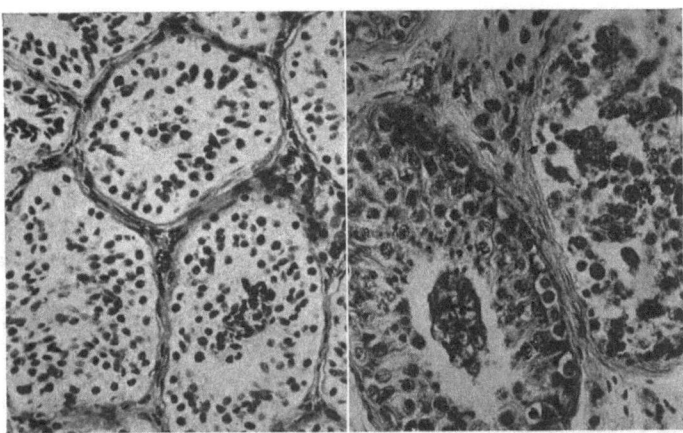

FIGURE III—45. Testicular biopsies on two patients with congenital adrenocortical virilism. Magnification x 100.
LEFT: Biopsy on the patient of Figure 43, a boy of 5 years, whose secondary sex characters were well developed but whose testes were of essentially normal size for age. Note that there is no evidence of spermatogenesis or of Leydig cell development. The tubules, however, were of larger than normal diameter for age.
RIGHT: Biopsy on the patient of Figure 44 when he was 12½ years of age. Note that the tubules are well developed and show active spermatocytogenesis.

---

complication have been outlined above in the section dealing with hypoadrenocorticism secondary to hypopituitarism (page 218).

For patients with bilateral adrenocortical hyperplasia no clearly beneficial therapy has been available until lately. Unilateral adrenalectomy is not helpful, because the cortex of the remaining gland tends promptly to undergo a compensatory hypertrophy. As a result, 17-KS production (which may fall temporarily following unilateral adrenalectomy) is not fundamentally altered by this procedure. More drastic subtotal adrenalectomy places the patient in a precarious position with respect to hypoadrenocorticism, from which he may die if he develops a severe infection. That is, if one removes enough adrenal cortex to eliminate the abnormal adrenal androgens, there is a high probability that one also will have removed enough tissue to deprive the individual of life-sustaining Na-K and S-F-N hormones.

In girls of adolescent age breast development can be induced by the administration of estrogenic hormones. Stilbesterol in oral doses of 4 to 6 mg. per day usually is satisfactory (see Chapter V, page 343). Such feminization is only for cosmetic and psychological purposes. It has no beneficial influence on the adreno-

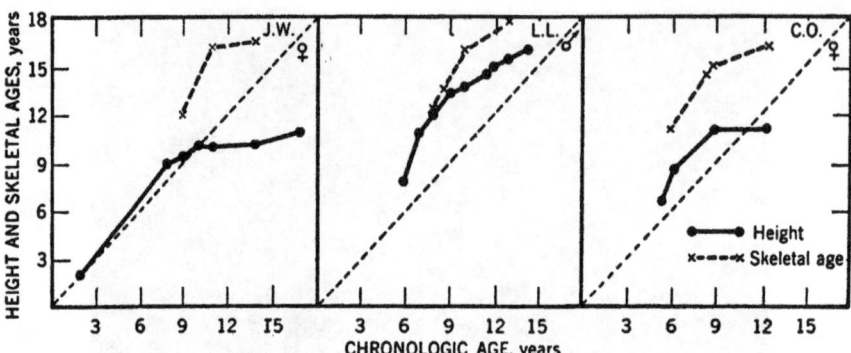

FIGURE III—46. Height and skeletal ages of three children with congenital adrenocortical virilism due to adrenocortical hyperplasia plotted against chronologic age. Height ages and skeletal ages were established on the basis of the average for normal children of the same height and sex. The broken lines show where the plots would fall if the height and skeletal ages corresponded exactly to the chronologic age. Note that skeletal age advances with abnormal rapidity. After skeletal epiphyseal fusion has occurred (skeletal age 16 years in girls, 18 years in boys) growth in height ceases. Thus, though such patients may be tall for their age while very young, as in the case of Subject C. O., they are apt to stop growing before they have attained a normal adult stature. From N. B. Talbot and E. H. Sobel, *Advances Pediat.* 2:238, 1947.

cortical dysfunction. Amputation of the clitoris may also be considered if the enlargement of the organ embarrasses the patient. We prefer to postpone this procedure until the patient is old enough to take part in the decision. Plastic surgery to the perineum also may be undertaken if circumstances warrant.

As mentioned above, recent studies indicate that cortisone is capable of inhibiting the hyper-17-ketosteroiduria characteristic of this form of the disease.[23, g, h] Maintenance dosage schedules currently are being worked out. It now looks as if as little as 20 or 30 mg. of cortisone per m^2 per day may suffice to abolish the excessive 17-ketosteroiduria. However, unless the dose is kept at minimum effective levels, signs of Cushing's syndrome begin to appear. There is reasonable hope that dose schedules can be devised which will exert the desired beneficial influence without prompting undesirable effects.

PROGNOSIS. The outlook for patients with adrenocortical carcinomas varies, since some of these tumors are highly malignant and metastasize widely. In such cases the prognosis is bad. On the other hand, surgical removal of less malignant, encapsulated tumors may result in survival for several years and lead to disappearance of many of the symptoms and signs of masculinization. The completeness of the cure can be judged from serial measurements of the urinary 17-KS output. After successful removal of a masculinizing adrenocortical carcinoma, 17-KS values fall to and remain at normal levels. If the 17-KS fail to fall to normal levels or if they fall and then rise again to abnormal heights, it means that removal of the tumor was incomplete or that metastases have developed.

The prognosis for patients with congenital adrenocortical hyperplasia depends in part on the sex. Limited observations suggest that as boys grow older they may become indistinguishable from normal adult men, except for an abnormally elevated urinary 17-KS output. The testes may undergo normal adolescence and show evidence of normal spermatogenesis (see Figure 45, right). In girls the outlook has been much more serious for, at least prior to the advent of cortisone treatment, patients all failed to undergo normal feminine changes during the adolescent age period. They have remained amenorrheic and have had a chronic tendency to shows signs of masculinization. Results from cortisone treatment are still of a preliminary nature. One girl of almost adolescent age spontaneously underwent the menarche after a few months of treatment. It is too soon to say what the long-term results will be.

Cushing's Syndrome.[23 a, 24] This is one of the most distressing of all diseases. Fortunately it is relatively rare, only about 18 reasonably authentic pediatric cases having been recorded in the literature during the past 25 years. Of these about half were males and half females. The youngest patient was only a few months old.

All available evidence indicates that this condition is caused by hyperadrenocorticism. It is not known, however, whether all its manifestations are due to the effects of a single S-F-N type of hormone, such as cortisone, or, as suggested in Table 10, certain of the symptoms and signs are referable to an excess of a type of potent Na-K hormone similar to 11-desoxycorticosterone.

In about 40 per cent of the cases reported the disease was due to a unilateral adrenocortical carcinoma. These are assumed to be examples of primary hyperadrenocorticism. In most of the others there was bilateral adrenocortical hyperplasia. In a few the adrenals appeared to be normal in structure. In practically all cases of Cushing's syndrome there are hyaline changes in the basophilic cells of the anterior pituitary.[24 f] It is not clear whether these reflect retrograde effects of adrenocortical hormones acting on the pituitary or indicate primary pituitary pathology. About 40 per cent of the patients who had adrenocortical hyperplasia also had a basophilic adenoma of the pituitary.

CLINICAL MANIFESTATIONS. These patients present a strikingly abnormal appearance (Figures 47 to 49). One of the most outstanding clinical manifestations is obesity of a special sort. This may be characterized more by a peculiar distribution of subcutaneous tissue than by an absolute excess weight gain; occasional

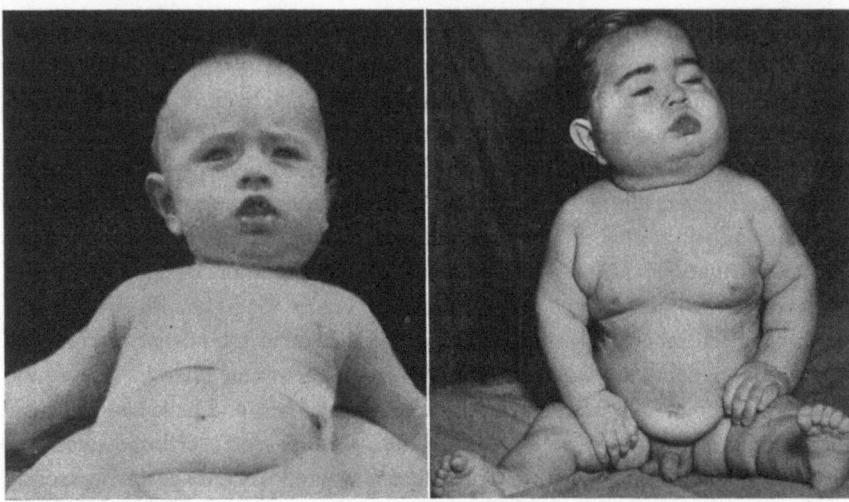

FIGURE III—47. Cushing's syndrome and masculinization due to adrenocortical carcinoma.
LEFT: Appearance of the patient at 3½ months. Signs of masculinization were noted first at 6½ months.
RIGHT: His appearance at eight months. He now showed obesity, especially of the head, neck and shoulders; marked fullness of the cheeks; plethoric skin; facial acne; hirsutism of the face, back and pubis; enlargement of the penis and scrotum, but not of the testes; hypertension (150/90); and eosinopenia (0 to 5 cells per mm^3). Serum electrolytes and glucose tolerance were normal. The skeleton was normal. Urinary 17-KS output was about 15 mg. per 24 hours. The right-sided adrenocortical tumor was removed successfully. The non-tumorous adrenal cortex was found to be markedly atrophied. The patient's course following operation has been satisfactory.

patients actually appear to be emaciated when considered as a whole. The face, trunk and abdomen are seemingly obese, while the extremities are not. The cheeks may be so full that it is difficult to see the ears of the patient when he faces the observer squarely, and often there is a pad of excess subcutaneous tissue located on the back at the base of the neck. This heavy accumulation of tissue about the head and neck has led to the descriptive terms "buffalo distribution of obesity" and "moon face."

Another characteristic seen in nearly all patients with this condition is plethora of the face. Other parts of the body may appear mottled and of dusky, purplish hue. Especially over the abdomen, thighs, arms and breasts there may be purplish striæ atrophicæ, which are as much as 1 cm. wide and 10 cm. long. They tend to run a parallel course and to be depressed below the level of the surrounding skin. In addition, ecchymoses and petechial hemorrhagic areas will be found on the skin in some cases. Acneiform infection also is common. It may appear as a few comedones or as an eruption involving a major portion of the body. The abdomen and extremities usually are spared. The skin lesions occasionally resemble keratosis pilaris. In one instance, the acne had a linear, segmental distribution over the back suggestive of herpes.

There usually is an abnormal growth of hair over the pubis, face and thighs. But in contrast to patients with straightforward adrenocortical virilism, patients with pure Cushing's syndrome show no signs of abnormal clitoral or penile development (see Figure 49). The syndrome may, however, be complicated by either abnormal masculinization (Figures 47 and 48)[24 d, g] or feminization (see page 247).

Muscular weakness is observed in over 90 per cent of patients with pure Cushing's syndrome and may be quite distressing to them. It may be manifested by inability to climb stairs or walk uphill without frequent periods of rest.

Hypertension also is noted in about 9 out of 10 patients. The systolic pressure usually exceeds 150 and the diastolic pressure 100 mm. Hg; recorded blood pressures average about 170/130 mm. Hg; maximum recorded levels for children are 250/180 mm. Hg.

Osteoporosis is found in at least three out of four adult cases; its incidence in children is not known exactly. It is particularly apt to be present in the spine (see Figure 50). The phosphatase level is normal in contrast to osteitis fibrosa generalisata and to osteomalacia, in which secondary hyperparathyroidism occurs with elevated serum alkaline phosphatase levels (see Chapter II, page 82). There is, however, a tendency to hypercalcuria, renal calcinosis, nephrolithiasis, bacilluria and pyuria. Also in association with the osteoporosis, there may be back pains and nerve root pains as well as actual shrinkage of stature due to collapse of vertebræ.

In adolescent girls and women amenorrhea is the rule. Adult male patients complain of impotence.

Diabetes is demonstrable in some form in about half the cases studied. Frank diabetes with fasting hyperglycemia, glycosuria and acetonuria is uncommon. More frequently impaired carbohydrate tolerance is revealed only by application of the glucose tolerance test. When present, diabetes is of the insulin-resistant type.

Emotionally patients may become severely depressed. It is not known whether their reaction constitutes a psychologic response to this distressing disease or is a direct result of hormonal action.

A patient with a long-standing history or with a rapidly growing and metastasizing tumor of the adrenal cortex may also have a palpable mass in the upper

Continued on page 243

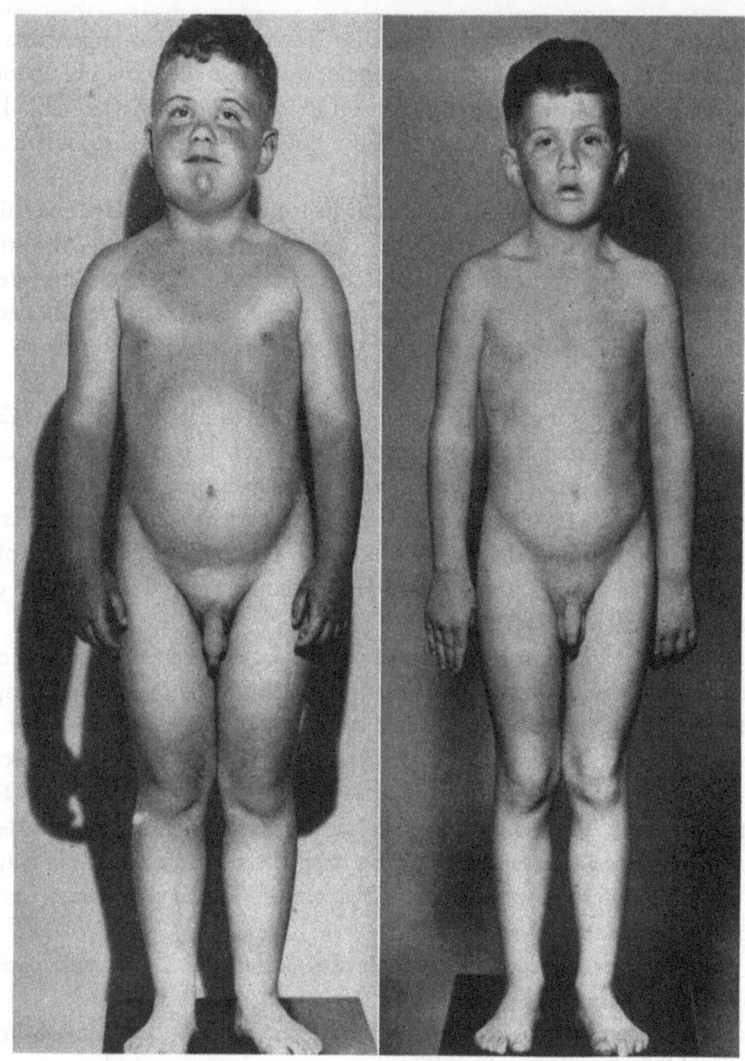

FIGURE III—48. Pseudo-precocious puberty with partial Cushing's syndrome due to adrenocortical carcinoma.
LEFT: Appearance of the patient at 6½ years.
RIGHT: His appearance at 7 years.

CASE HISTORY

This boy was apparently healthy until the age of six, when he suddenly commenced to gain weight at a markedly accelerated rate (6 years, 20 kg.; 6½ years, 29 kg.). Growth of pubic hair and development of penis and scrotum took place concomitantly.

On physical examination the patient measured 121 cm. and was found to be of husky, somewhat plethoric appearance. While his penis was of late adolescent size, his testes were of approximately normal size for age. His heart was slightly enlarged in transverse diameter on both physical and roentgenographic examination. His blood pressure was 130/100. His bone age corresponded to his chronologic age. Laboratory studies revealed that the serum sodium, chloride and bicarbonate concentrations were normal. The serum potassium was slightly low (3.9 mEq. per liter). The sweat chloride concentration (10 mEq. per liter) was lower than average normal. Tests of carbohydrate metabolism yielded normal results. The eosinophil count was 112 cells per mm^3. The urinary 11-17-OCS output was normal (0.2 mg. per 24 hours); the 17-KS output was 6.6 mg. per 24 hours.

An adrenocortical carcinoma weighing 14 gm. was removed from the right side by Dr. O. Cope. The patient's postoperative course has been satisfactory. As shown by the right-hand photograph he has lost his body obesity, facial puffiness and high cheek and chin color. The hypertension has subsided, and the urinary 17-KS output has fallen to about 0.9 mg. per 24 hours.

[240]   CHAPTER III:

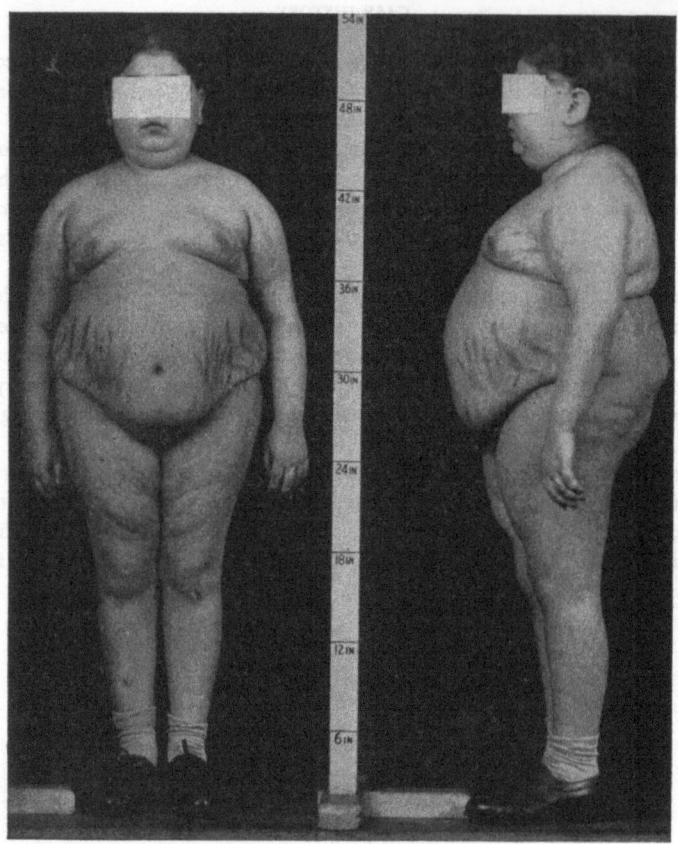

FIGURE III—49. Cushing's syndrome in a girl of 11 years. Left-hand photograph from F. Albright, in *The Harvey Lectures, 1942-43*, Series 38:127, Lancaster, Science Press, 1943.

CASE HISTORY

The patient was admitted to the hospital with the chief complaints of obesity and low back pain. She had been essentially well and of normal appearance until three years previously, when she commenced to gain weight at an increasing rate. She commented that her face and abdomen had become big and fat but that her arms and legs remained all right. Shortly after the onset of these difficulties a physician placed her on a reduction diet and prescribed thyroid pills, which she took intermittently up to the time of admission. Though she did not gain weight while following her diet, the slightest deviations resulted in gains. She was able to run and play with other children and continued at school.

Eleven months prior to admission, she fell on her buttocks while playing tennis. She felt momentary pain and discomfort but was able to go home without difficulty. A few days later, however, she commenced to have rather severe pain in her back and found that it hurt if she moved about. In association with this there were some dysuria and

CASE HISTORY (continued)

urgency. In consequence, she went to bed for a period of about six weeks. At the end of this time she was able to walk but could not bend over. Her condition remained about the same until a month before she came to this hospital, when she noticed a tendency to edema of the ankles, especially upon walking. She found, though, that her obesity had increased in the last month or so and had also noticed the presence of hair on her face, arms and legs. The family history and the patient's own history gave no pertinent information. A review of the various systems also failed to reveal additional points of interest.

On physical examination the patient weighed 62 kg. and measured 132 cm. in height. It was estimated that she had gained about 20 kg. in weight and lost about 5 cm. in height during the preceding three years. Her general appearance is well represented in the accompanying photographs. It was noted that her face was fat, especially about the jaw, and that her chest and abdomen were protuberant and flabby; the "puffy" obesity extending about a third of the way down the humerus, at which point it ceased abruptly. There was a large and prominent fat pad at the base of the neck. Her legs and lower arms were small in relation to her trunk. On both flanks and axillæ there were many bright, cherry red striæ running in an approximately vertical plane. In the areas of the striæ the skin was loose and easily wrinkled. On her spine and back there was a considerable amount of hair. Her eyes, ears, nose, throat and teeth were normal. Her neck was free from lymphadenopathy. Her thyroid was not remarkable. Her chest was clear and resonant. Her breasts were prominent but contained no glandular tissue. Her heart was approximately within normal limits in respect to size. There were no murmurs and the sounds were of good quality, the rate being about 120 per minute. The blood pressure in her arms was 164/100 mm. Hg. Her abdomen was free from palpable masses. There was nothing remarkable about her extremities, and her reflexes were physiologic. Her clitoris was normal.

Laboratory studies revealed the urine to be normal, the specific gravity ranging between 1.008 and 1.030. The Sulkowitch test for calcium gave a 2+ positive response. The red cell count was 5,800,000 and the white cell count was 16,000, with a differential of P 78, L 18, M 4 and E 0. Examination of the blood smear revealed the red cells to be normochromic and normocytic. The hematocrit was 45 per cent. Stool examination revealed no blood or other abnormalities. A series of basal metabolism rate determinations gave an average value of about ±0 by the height standard and −34 per cent by the weight standard. Fasting blood sugar values ranged between 60 and 85 mg. per cent. The serum sodium was 140, total base 153, chloride 100 and the carbon dioxide content 28 mEq. per liter, respectively. The serum NPN was 15 mg. per cent, the serum protein was 5.5 gm. per cent. A glucose tolerance test (100 gm. PO) was as follows: F—85, ½ hour—162, 1½—193, 2—156, 3—132, 4—108 mg. per cent. An insulin tolerance test (0.1 unit per kg.) F—76, 1/3 hour—55, ½—45, ¾—48, 1—94, 1½—74, 2—76. The serum cholesterol was 111 mg. per cent. The serum calcium ranged between 10.5 and 10.8 mg. per cent, the serum phosphorus between 3.2 and 4 mg. per cent, and the serum alkaline phosphatase between 2.4 and 4.1 B.U. per cent. The urinary creatine ranged between 0 and about 600 mg. per 24 hours. The urinary creatinine ranged between about 580 and 680 mg. per 24 hours; this was an abnormally low output for an 11-year-old girl (normal ±20 mg. per kg.) and can be considered indicative of decreased protoplasmic or muscle mass. There were less than 3 mouse units of gonadotropic hormone (FSH) per

CASE HISTORY (continued)

24-hour urine specimen, a normal situation for an 11-year-old girl. The urinary 17-KS output was abnormally high, ranging between 15 and 20 mg. per 24 hours. At this first admission no urinary 11-17-OCS measurements were made. However, values ranging between .34 and 4.4 mg. per 24 hours were obtained when the patient was between 14 and 16 years of age. The higher values, of which there were several and which were definitely abnormal, occurred at times when the disease was clinically active; the lower values were obtained when the disease was in clinical remission. Roentgenograms showed the skull, chest, hands and feet to be essentially normal. There was, however, decalcification of the pelvis as well as the spinal changes shown in Figure 50. Air injection of the perirenal spaces on both sides indicated slightly enlarged adrenal glands.

On the basis of the foregoing information a tentative diagnosis of Cushing's syndrome due to bilateral adrenocortical hyperplasia was made. Accordingly, the effects of a series of therapeutic agents including testosterone and various related steroids, insulin, potassium salt and radiation of the pituitary were studied. While it cannot be stated with certainty, the most effective agent appears to have been pituitary irradiation. The patient was given a total of approximately 3,600 roentgens to the pituitary through four channels, using 1,200 KV therapy. Following this treatment, the disease appeared to undergo a remission, as evidenced by loss of striæ and hirsutism, thickening of the skin, increase in physical strength, increase of 10 cm. in stature within a period of about two years and marked improvement in calcification of the spine (Figure 50). Moreover, when the patient was about 13 years old she began to have regular, natural menstrual periods and true breast development occurred. At this time gonadotropic hormone (FSH) appeared in the urine in amounts up to 52 mouse units per 24 hours.

Unfortunately, about four years later, when the patient was 17 years of age, there was an exacerbation of Cushing's syndrome, with acne, hirsutism, excess weight gain, and irregularity and eventual cessation of menstruation. At this time the urinary 11-17-OCS rose to levels about 4 mg. per 24 hours and the 17-KS output to 13 mg. per 24 hours. Because of these changes and because of the fact that she was considerably incapacitated by weakness, particularly of the legs, the patient was again subjected to perirenal air insufflation. While the roentgenograms obtained following this procedure were difficult to interpret, there appeared to be a suspicious shadow in the region of the left adrenal gland.

Exploratory operations, at which both the adrenals and the pelvis were explored, were then performed by Dr. E. Churchill. The ovaries were small and atrophic and the adrenal glands appeared to be normal, but microscopic examinations of adrenal tissue revealed cortical hyperplasia. The patient tolerated this surgery without difficulty and appeared to be unchanged as a consequence of it. For 14 days prior to the operation she was given 25 mg. of testosterone propionate daily, and for 8 days preoperatively and 12 days postoperatively she was given between 4 and 6 gm. of potassium chloride daily. Whether this therapy had any influence upon the adrenal findings at operation or any bearing on the fact that she did not have any serious difficulties postoperatively it is hard to say. In these connections, though adrenal therapy was not used, it is important to note that large amounts of both lypo-adrenal extract and aqueous adrenal extract were kept on hand during the intra- and postoperative periods. The patient was once again subjected to radiation of the pituitary. The total dose and the method used were the same as indicated above. It is too early to judge the effects.

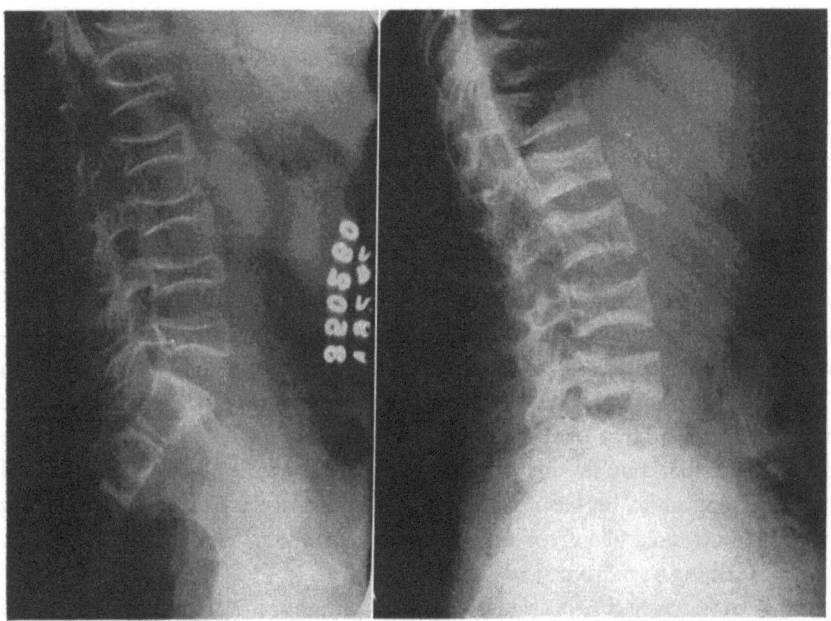

FIGURE III—50. Osteoporosis of the spine due to Cushing's syndrome in the patient of Figure 49.
LEFT: Note that none of the vertebræ except the end plates are denser than the intervertebral discs; note also that the intervertebral discs have expanded at the expense of the vertebræ, so that they are now wider than the vertebræ themselves.
RIGHT: Partial healing.

---

abdomen in which roentgenograms disclose the presence of calcification. In association with this the patient may show evidences of cachexia and anemia. Local signs of an expanding lesion in the region of the pituitary are but rarely encountered.

Blood count measurements show eosinopenia in the vast majority of patients who are in an active phase of Cushing's syndrome (see Figure 21). About a third of such patients also have polycythemia. Hypochloremic, hypokalemic alkalosis is found occasionally.[24 l, j] Urine steroid assays consistently yield abnormally elevated urinary 11-17-OCS values (see Figure 27). The urinary 17-KS values are apt to be within normal limits or slightly elevated in patients with pure Cushing's syndrome. In patients with evidences both of Cushing's syndrome and adrenocortical virilism or feminization, the 17-KS values may be grossly elevated (see Table 6).

DIAGNOSIS. The combination of buffalo-type obesity, plethora, striæ atrophicæ, acne, hirsutism, weakness, hypertension, slowing of growth and osteoporosis is almost uniquely characteristic of Cushing's syndrome. Eosinopenia and increased urinary 11-17-OCS output are other important findings. Some tendency to decreased glucose tolerance may be present. This, however, is not considered essential to the diagnosis.

DIFFERENTIAL DIAGNOSIS. There should be little difficulty in distinguishing between Cushing's syndrome and such conditions as simple dietary obesity, adolescent acne, non-endocrine hirsutism, essential hypertension, ordinary diabetes mellitus or bony demineralization due to hyperparathyroidism, renal disease or poor calcium absorption. Adrenocortical virilism may be associated with Cushing's syndrome. Hyper-11-17-oxycorticosteroiduria and eosinopenia are observed frequently in endocrinologically normal persons when they become severely stressed. But in this type of patient the extra 11-17-OCS or S-F-N hormones appear to be serving the helpful and necessary purpose of meeting increased hormonal requirements with the result that signs of toxicity (i.e., signs of Cushing's syndrome) are absent.

For a consideration of various means of demonstrating the presence of an adrenal tumor, see the preceding section on adrenocortical virilism.

TREATMENT AND PROGNOSIS. There are few more difficult conditions to treat than Cushing's syndrome. This is reflected in part by the fact that those working with the problem have no fixed opinion concerning the optimal method of approach. It also is indicated by the fact that most patients with this disease have died within about three years of the onset of symptoms despite all attempts at therapy. Some of these deaths were caused by metastatic spread of adrenocortical cancer cells. Others were due to the metabolic effects of excess adrenocortical hormones.

There are at present three chief methods of approach to therapy. One is surgical and consists in the detection and eradication of an adrenocortical tumor if one is present. Alternatively, when bilateral hyperplasia of the adrenal cortices rather than a tumor is found, some surgeons attempt to perform extensive subtotal adrenalectomy.

Concerning these therapeutic manœuvres the following may be said. First, any surgery on the adrenals of patients with Cushing's syndrome is hazardous, for the individual tends to develop acute hypoadrenocorticism postoperatively unless extensive precautions are taken (Figure 38 and page 229). Even when such measures are taken, the patient may go through a long period when he is exceedingly weak, anorexic and in severe abdominal pain and when he suffers from persistent disturbances involving water and electrolyte metabolism. Second, the surgeon has to be prepared to decide at the operating table what steps to take. Experience indicates that a second operation on the adrenals of these patients may be tolerated poorly. Thus, if the surgeon finds a hyperplastic gland on one side, he must decide immediately whether to leave it untouched or to undertake a subtotal resection. Then he must decide whether to explore the opposite side and do the same. Contrariwise, if an atrophic gland is found on one side, he must recognize it as such and realize that there is probably a tumor on the opposite side.

A second method of approach is to undertake heavy radiation of the pituitary. From 2,000 to 3,000 roentgens given in divided doses has effected apparent remissions in a few cases. While this method of treatment may be considered favorably for patients who are known to have bilateral adrenocortical hyperplasia, it is not appropriate when there is a malignant lesion of the adrenal cortex; this type of therapy should, therefore, be used only after adrenal tumor has been ruled out by surgical exploration.

The third method of approach should likewise be reserved for patients with hyperplasia rather than carcinoma of the adrenal cortex. It consists in attempts either to inhibit ACTH production by administering a steroid hormone such as testosterone[11 b] or to counterbalance the metabolic disturbances of Cushing's syndrome by administering testosterone[24 e, h] and prescribing diets of low sodium and high potassium content (see Table 4). Incidentally, there is a possibility that chemical agents capable of selectively destroying the adrenal cortex in whole or in part may become available for clinical use. It is already known that 2,2-Bis (parachlorophenyl) -1, 1-dichloroethane (DDD or TDE), an insecticide agent, causes severe adrenocortical atrophy in dogs.[24 k, l] The atrophy occurs chiefly in the zonæ fasciculata and reticularis; the zona glomerulosa is largely spared. This substance also prompts fatty degeneration of the liver and fatty infiltration of the kidneys. On these accounts it may never be considered suitable for human use except under most extremely desperate circumstances.

Physicians who are particularly interested in the management of this disease are constantly trying new combinations of therapy in an effort to better the therapeutic score. It is therefore suggested that patients with Cushing's syndrome be referred for treatment to one of the medical centers known to have special experience with this condition.

Adrenocortical Virilism Complicated by Signs Suggestive of Na-K Hormone Lack.[14 c, 23 b, 25] This heading refers to a type of patient who in early infancy develops (a) symptoms and signs of a major disturbance in water and electrolyte metabolism* which clinically resemble those seen consequential to Na-K hormone lack in patients with ordinary hypoadrenocorticism and (b) signs of masculinization† similar to those seen in patients with ordinary congenital adrenocortical virilism. Clear signs of excess or deficient S-F-N hormone production are absent. Since genital tract anomalies call attention to this condition at the time of birth in girls, the possibility that gastrointestinal and circulatory disturbances may be due to this disease should not escape attention. However, since boys are unlikely to show gross genital pathology during the first months of life, it may not be recognized that nutritional and circulatory disturbances are due to adrenocortical disease unless careful search is made for abnormal skin pigmentation, for precocious masculinization and for chemical evidences of Na-K hormone deficiency. The methods used for the latter purpose are the same as for ordinary primary hypoadrenocorticism (see above).

The foregoing implies, perhaps too strongly, that the disturbances in sodium, potassium, chloride and water metabolism observed in these patients are due to an absolute lack or deficiency of Na-K hormone. The thesis may be questioned because it has been found recently that administration of ACTH in such cases may result not only in an increased output of urinary 17-KS and 11-17-OCS but also in a marked sodium diuresis.[25 d] This suggests that ACTH may have stimulated the abnormal adrenal cortices to secrete an anti-Na-K hormone. The result would, of course, be equivalent to withdrawing Na-K hormone. Doses of DOCA as large as 20 mg. per m^2 per day have failed in these patients to correct tendencies to hyponatremia, hyperkalemia and extracellular dehydration even when given for several weeks in association with a diet of ordinary sodium and potassium content. Such a regimen would cause marked manifestations of Na-K hormone toxicity (see Figure 4) in normal persons and in patients with ordinary hypoadrenocorticism.

The clinical picture presented by a patient with congenital adrenocortical virilism is illustrated in Figure 51, and a testicular biopsy on this patient is shown in Figure 52. Experience with this and similar patients has shown that signs of adrenocortical insufficiency can usually be controlled satisfactorily by adding sodium chloride to the diet and by administering DOCA. About 6 gm. of sodium chloride per m^2 per day and from 2 to 4 mg. of DOCA per m^2 per day

---

* Nausea, vomiting (which may be very suggestive of pyloric stenosis), dehydration and circulatory collapse. Skin pigmentation is often seen in association with these. In addition, there may be gross disturbances in cardiac rate and rhythm suggestive of congenital heart disease. The fact that the cardiac disturbances are in actuality due to potassium intoxication may be recognized by electrocardiography.[25 e]

† Penile or clitoral enlargement, genital tract malformation, abnormal urinary 17-KS excretion and so forth.

usually suffice. Provided sufficient doses of DOCA are given, aqueous adrenocortical extract can usually be omitted.

The prognosis in this condition is, with two exceptions, about the same as for patients with simple masculinization due to bilateral adrenocortical hyperplasia. The first exception concerns the metabolic disturbance which may be fatal to the patient if left untreated. The second concerns the tendency to develop testicular tumors apparently comprised of hyperplastic adrenocortical cell rest tissue.

Abnormal Feminization and Other Changes Due to Adrenocortical Tumor. Although rare, abnormal feminization can occur as a result of adrenocortical tumor.[26]

Precocious Adrenarche. This is a physiologic condition in which normal adrenocortical 17-KS-Gens secretion occurs at an unusually early age and before the gonads have been stimulated to adolescent activity. It is noted clinically most often in girls (see Figure 53, left). On physical examination they show pubic and sometimes axillary hair growth but fail to show such signs of ovarian estrogen production as breast development, vaginal cornification and so forth, or such signs of masculinization as clitoral hypertrophy or urogenital malformations. The condition is entirely benign. In due course true sexual development occurs in a normal manner. If not, the patient may be found to have signs of congenital ovarian agenesis (see Chapter v, page 344).

Precocious adrenarche may be contrasted with precocious gonadarche (Figure 53, right) in which the gonads become activated before the adrenals.* Girls with this condition show breast and vaginal changes but no pubic or axillary hair growth. Like children having the adrenarche first, they develop eventually into normal adults.

In the average child the adrenarche and gonadarche occur simultaneously.

Therapeutic Hyperadrenocorticism Produced by Means of ACTH or Cortisone. The discovery that ACTH and cortisone treatment can cause marked temporary improvement in patients with certain conditions (see Table 12) has led to extensive experimental use of these agents.[27, 91] But since the studies carried out to date must still be considered preliminary in nature, only limited comments will be offered here.

General comments. In the first place, the adrenocortical status of patients with the various conditions listed in Table 12 is not thoroughly understood. Some are presumably euadrenocortical (see Figure 28, left), some may be suffering stress-induced hypoadrenocorticism (right-hand columns of middle section), while others may have developed functional, adaptative hyperadrenocorticism

---

* The term "gonadarche" is used to signify the time when adolescent gonadal activity starts.

[248]   CHAPTER III:

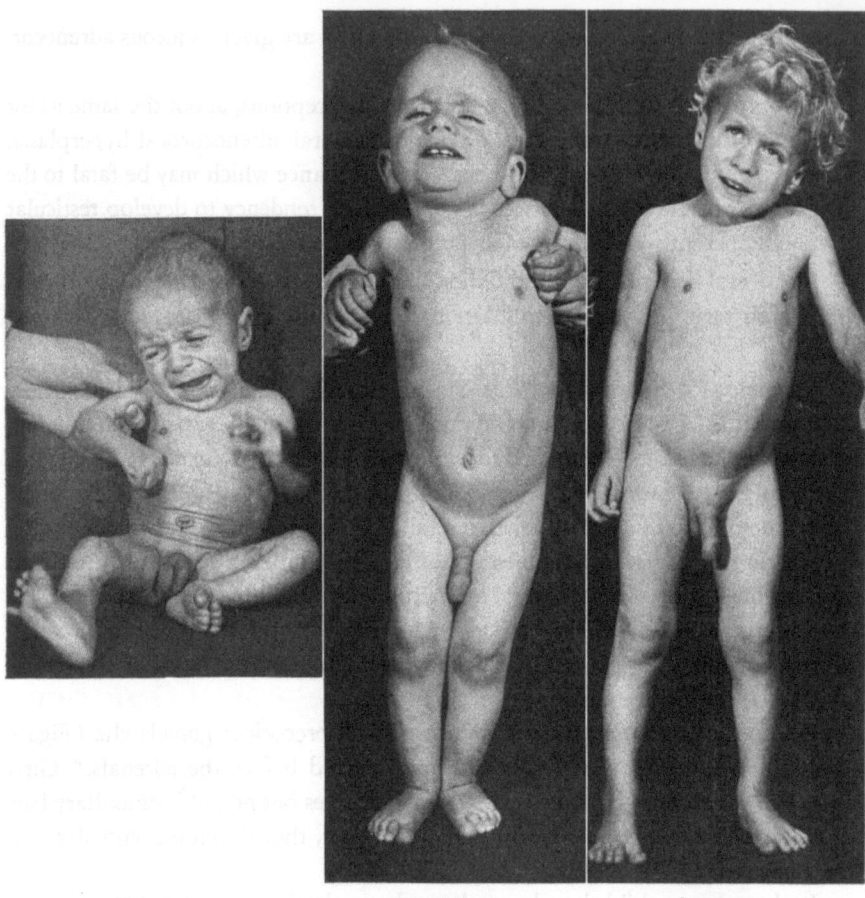

7 WEEKS   18 MONTHS   3 YEARS

FIGURE III—51. Appearance at various ages of a boy with congenital adrenocortical virilism and disturbances in sodium, potassium and chloride metabolism secondary to proved bilateral adrenocortical hyperplasia.

CASE HISTORY

At seven weeks the patient showed penile enlargement, hyperpigmentation of the genitalia and nipples and mottling of the skin indicative of circulatory inefficiency. Pubic hair appeared at about three years. His head and face had assumed oblong adult male proportions by the age of four. His testes became markedly enlarged because of hyperplastic adrenocortical cell-rest tumor masses at about nine years. At about the same time his musculature became herculean, his voice deep bass. Tendencies towards hyponatremia,

The Adrenal Cortices

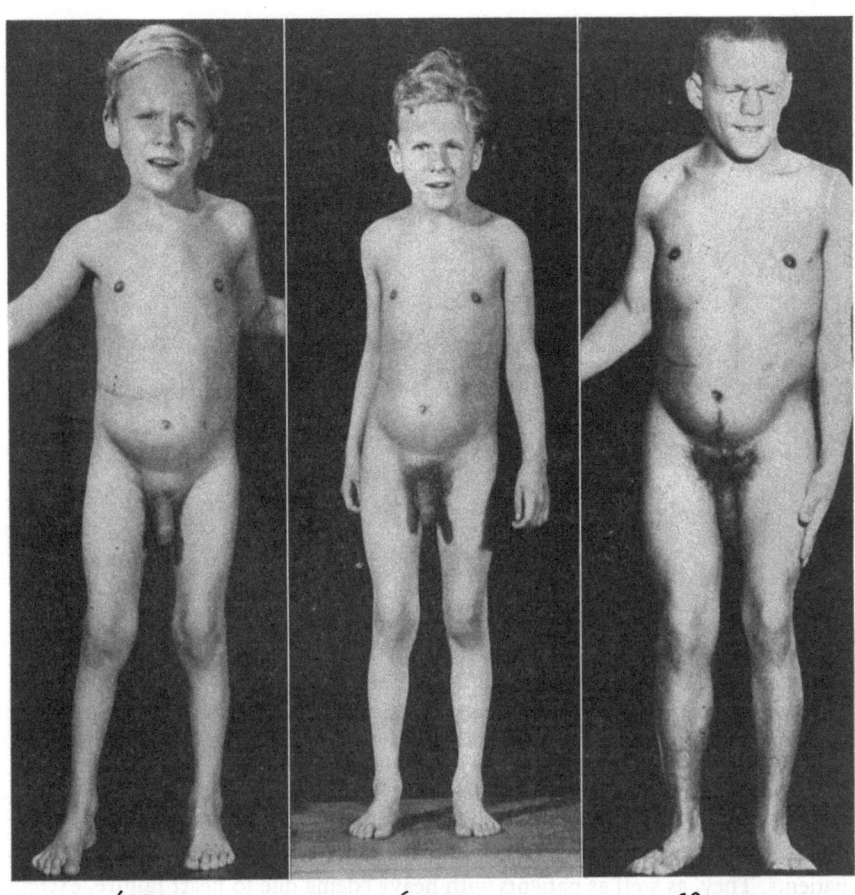

4 YEARS   6 YEARS   10 YEARS

CASE HISTORY (continued)

hypochloremia, hyperkalemia and circulatory collapse, first noted shortly after birth, have persisted. They have been controlled satisfactorily by the addition of sodium chloride to his diet and by administration of DOCA. He has shown essentially no signs of excessive or deficient S-F-N hormone production. The urinary 17-KS output has always been abnormally elevated—the level at two years being about 10 mg., at five years about 25 mg. and since the age of eight about 150 mg. per 24 hours. Chromatography of these steroids indicated an abnormal pattern similar to those shown in Figure 15.

From A. M. Butler, R. A. Ross and N. B. Talbot, *J. Pediat.* 15:831, 1939; and L. I. Gardner, R. C. Sniffen, A. S. Zygmuntowicz and N. B. Talbot, *Pediatrics* 5:808, 1950.

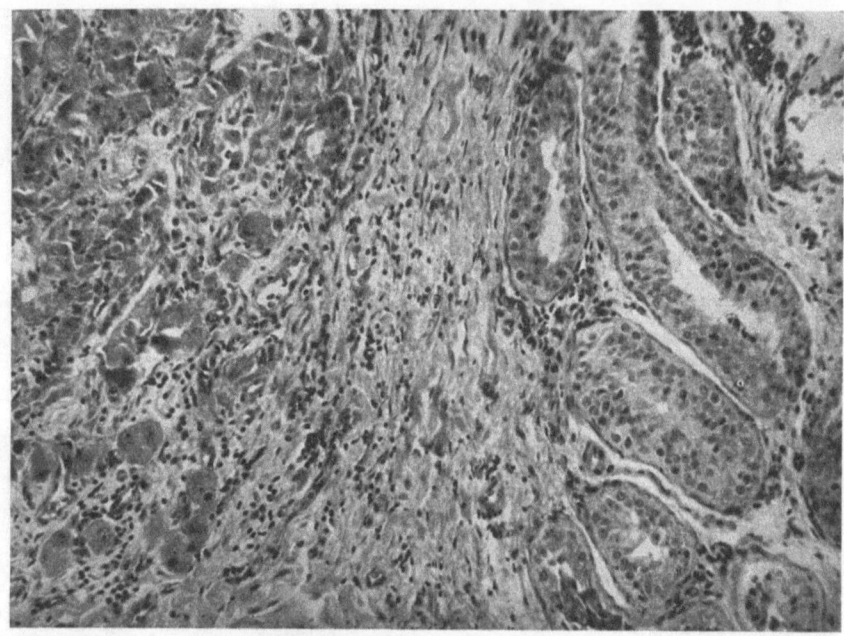

FIGURE III—52. Hyperplastic adrenocortical cell rest in the testis of the patient of Figure 51. On the left is the hyperplastic adrenocortical rest tissue. On the right are relatively immature testicular tubules and apparently inactive interstitial tissue. Magnification x 80.

which paradoxically aggravates rather than ameliorates the primary disease condition. The latter possibility comes to mind especially with regard to nephrosis patients. They, as well as patients with heavy edema due to heart failure, excrete in the urine abnormally large amounts of lipid-soluble substances which by bioassay have sodium-retaining activity.[27 f] These substances are presumed to be of adrenocortical origin. Stated in other words, our purpose in administering ACTH or one of the various adrenocortical steroids to one type of patient may be quite different from that obtaining in another type of patient. In some we may wish to augment adrenocortical activity, in others to suppress it in certain respects.

ACTH tends to induce adrenocortical hypertrophy and an increase in the secretion of all types of adrenocortical hormone. Consequently, it causes signs of increased Na-K, S-F-N and 17-KS-Gens production. Among the activities of these hormones is suppression of endogenous ACTH production. While this phenomenon is minimal and of little clinical importance in subjects to whom ACTH is given only for a few days, it may become worthy of attention in subjects given heavy doses of ACTH for long periods of time. Under the latter circum-

The Adrenal Cortices   [251]

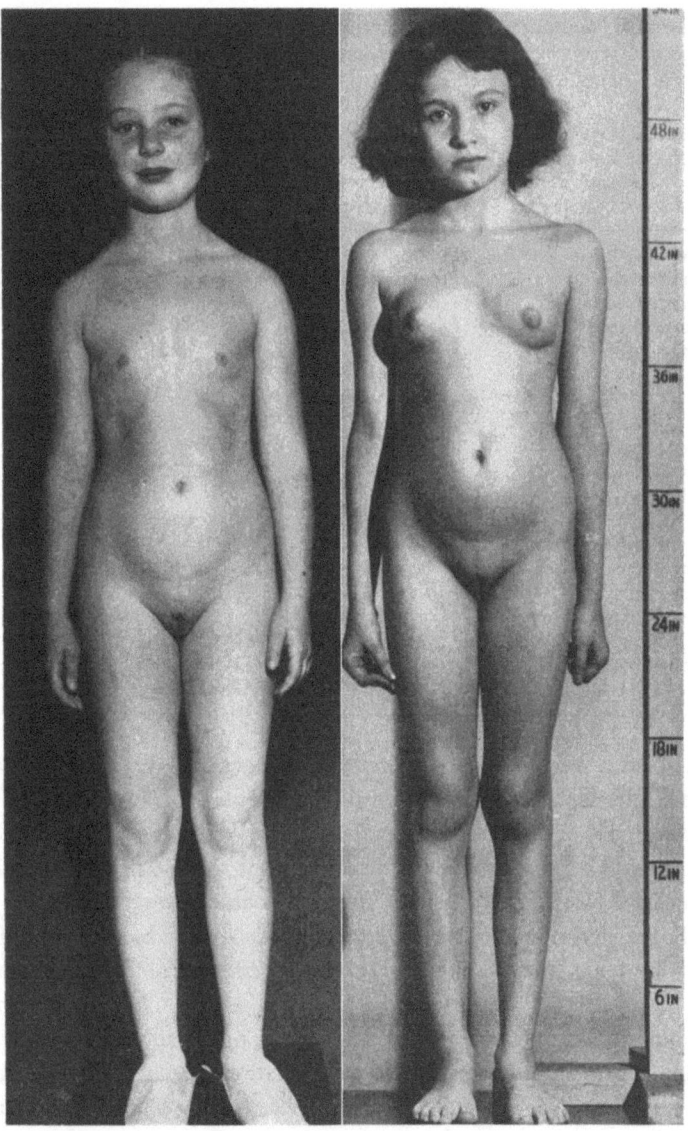

FIGURE III—53. These patients illustrate the fact that adolescent changes are under the control of separate endocrine factors and can occur unevenly.
LEFT: "Precocious adrenarche" in a girl of seven years. Note the growth of pubic hair in the absence of breast development.
RIGHT: "Precocious gonadarche" in a girl of eight years. Note that there is breast development but no pubic or axillary hair growth. This appeared subsequently.

TABLE III—12. Preliminary grouping of diseases other than ordinary hypoadrenocorticism and hypopituitarism on the basis of response to ACTH and cortisone therapy. Adapted from G. W. Thorn et al., New Eng. J. Med. 242:783, 1950.

Pediatric conditions in which ACTH or cortisone therapy has induced at least temporary improvement	Conditions in which no benefit has been obtained	Conditions in which these hormones are detrimental
Rheumatoid arthritis	Poliomyelitis	Diabetes mellitus
Rheumatic fever	Progressive muscular dystrophy	Congestive heart failure
Lupus erythematosis		Hypertension (ACTH)
Dermatomyositis	Cystic fibrosis of the pancreas	Acne
Periarteritis nodosa		Hirsutism
	Herpes simplex	Cushing's syndrome
Asthma		
Eczema		
Vasomotor rhinitis		
Urticaria		
Serum sickness		
Anorexia nervosa		
Idiopathic hypoglycemia		
Nephrosis		
Ulcerative colitis		
Acute inflammatory diseases of the eye		

stance, about a week may be required for endogenous ACTH production to be resumed, following abrupt cessation of exogenous ACTH treatment. From the third to fifth day of this period the patient may show mild signs of adrenocortical insufficiency. This reaction, which usually is not worrisome, can be minimized by reducing ACTH doses gradually over the course of several days.

Cortisone, in contrast to ACTH, augments the level of but one type of adrenocortical hormone. In so doing it acts to suppress natural ACTH secretion and hence to lower the concentration of ACTH in the circulation. This leads to a diminution in the size and secretory activity of the adrenal cortices. If heavy cortisone treatment is continued for more than a few days, marked functional and anatomic atrophy of the glands takes place. This involution is fundamentally very similar to that observed in patients having Cushing's syndrome due to a unilateral adrenocortical cancer (see Figure 38). As is the case following removal of an adrenocortical cancer, up to 10 days may be needed for resumption of endogenous ACTH production, regeneration of adrenocortical tissue and restoration of adequate adrenocortical secretory activity when cortisone therapy is stopped abruptly. During this interval patients must be observed carefully for symptoms and signs of adrenocortical insufficiency. Recovery from cortisone-induced adrenocortical atrophy can be determined by application of the ACTH-eosinophil test (see Table 3, Test 3).[27g]

The likelihood of encountering such signs probably can be decreased considerably by discontinuing cortisone gradually (i.e., over a period of about 10 days, the dose being reduced by one-fifth at two-day intervals). It also may be possible to minimize this problem by administering ACTH for several days prior to or during the interval of cortisone withdrawal. The value of the latter therapeutic manœuvre remains to be established.

Undesirable effects. Many of the clinically undesirable effects of cortisone and ACTH treatment can be predicted from the physiologic actions outlined in earlier sections of this chapter. Electrolyte and water disturbances are common. Cortisone is much less apt to induce these particular changes because its Na-K action is weak, but with ACTH therapy there is a strong tendency to water, sodium and chloride retention and to excessive loss of potassium. These changes lead within a week to weight gain, and later to edema. Eventually they can also result in the development of intracellular potassium deficiency, hypokalemic-hypochloremic alkalosis, electrocardiographic changes and muscle weakness, as discussed under Na-K hormone excess, page 139. The sodium and water retention can be prevented in part at least by restricting the sodium chloride and water intake. The tendency to potassium depletion, which can develop apart from obvious sodium and water retention, can be minimized by administering potassium chloride in doses of 2 to 3.5 gm. per m^2 per day. This total dose should be divided into three or more parts and given in aqueous solution or in the form of enteric-coated tablets. Caution should be exercised in the administration of potassium to patients with marked renal insufficiency of the type that sometimes results in azotemia and grossly diminished urea clearance. These patients may retain the potassium in lethal amounts. Such toxicity can be recognized by electrocardiographic studies (see Figure 35).

Both ACTH and cortisone are likely to induce a rise in blood sugar values under conditions of fasting and in a few cases they have caused frank diabetes mellitus.[91] Restriction of carbohydrate intake may be of some value in limiting these effects. When diabetes develops, insulin should be given if adrenocortical hormone therapy is to be continued. Diabetes ordinarily subsides when the adrenocortical therapy is discontinued. However, there is a possibility of inducing permanent diabetes of the type seen in dogs following pituitary glycotropic hormone treatment (see Chapter IX, page 543). It has been suggested that the development of diabetes in patients receiving ACTH or cortisone represents the unmasking of inadequate pancreatic islet cell reserve (i.e., latent diabetes mellitus).[91]

Within a matter of days, most patients receiving ACTH or cortisone in full doses develop the full-cheeked, plethoric, rounded faces seen in spontaneous Cushing's syndrome (see Figures 47-49). If the treatment is prolonged, cervical and supraclavicular "fat" pads, large abdomen, acne, marked oiliness of the scalp and hair, abdominal striæ and hirsutism also may appear. Recession of the hairline over the temporal regions is seen as another manifestation. These changes regress quite soon after cessation of therapy.

A distressing and sometimes frightening complication which probably is seen more often in adults than in children is psychic change. This usually consists in a sense of well-being verging on hypomania; sometimes it takes the form of a severe depression. Generally speaking, these psychic changes are rare and are most apt to occur in patients with organic, central nervous system disease or with markedly unstable personalities.[91] The euphoria seen in mentally healthy patients may simply reflect the fact that they are enjoying relief from a chronically disabling or painful condition. In the case of patients known to be emotionally unstable, the advice of a psychiatrist should be sought before chronic treatment with ACTH or adrenocortical hormones is undertaken.

Hormonal therapy also may cause trouble by masking symptoms and signs of important illness. Thus perforations of the gastrointestinal tract can occur without the development of abdominal pain, fever or other localizing signs. Similarly patients can have widespread pneumonia, yet be afebrile, feel fine and have few if any gross manifestations of this condition.[27 n] In other words, adrenocortical hormones are antipyretic and to some extent analgesic. Moreover, by minimizing tissue reaction to toxic bodies, they may lessen the body's ability to wall off bacterial foci. These facts must be borne closely in mind both in the selection of patients for ACTH or adrenocortical hormone therapy and in the administration of either type of hormone.

Dosages of ACTH and cortisone in conditions other than ordinary hypoadrenocorticism and ordinary hypopituitarism. This is a new and rapidly developing area in medical therapeutics. The following comments should therefore be considered of a preliminary and tentative nature.

Quantitatively, the effectiveness of ACTH and cortisone varies somewhat from individual to individual and from condition to condition. Roughly speaking, between 12 and 60 mg. per m^2 per day of Armour Standard ACTH equivalent* are needed to produce a satisfactory therapeutic effect under most circum-

* Armour ACTH Standard is of such a strength that 4 micrograms given intravenously to an hypophysectomized rat will cause a 20 to 40 per cent fall in adrenal ascorbic acid. As other manufacturers develop and market ACTH, it is to be expected that their units of potency will differ markedly from those produced by the Armour Laboratories.

stances. This daily dose usually is divided into four parts, which are given intramuscularly at six-hour intervals. This timing is suggested by the fact that a single dose of presently available ACTH preparations is active for 8 to 12 hours, exerting its maximum effect in about four hours. In certain instances heavier doses may be needed; in at least one condition, namely idiopathic spontaneous hypoglycemia, small doses of 10 to 18 mg. of Armour ACTH given at 48-hour intervals to patients between six months and five years of age have sufficed to prevent recurrence of hypoglycemic episodes.[27 h] It is anticipated that longer-acting ACTH preparations may become available in the near future.

As regards cortisone, clinical experience suggests that children suffering from rheumatoid arthritis need almost as much of this hormone as adult arthritics to obtain relief.[27 l] It is not yet known whether this finding will be duplicated in children with various other conditions. Roughly speaking, when the adrenal cortices are normally active or hyperactive, the daily requirement is between 100 and 200 mg. of cortisone given orally or by intramuscular injection. The dose is usually divided into three or four parts, administered every six or eight hours.

The effectiveness with which a given dose of ACTH or cortisone has induced a state of hyperadrenocorticism may be judged approximately by the clinical response (see below under various conditions) and by application of certain of the indices listed in Table 3. The absolute eosinophil count is of some value, though this measurement appears to be too sensitive an index of increased adrenocortical hormone activity in some patients and too insensitive in others. Induction of absolute eosinopenia usually indicates adequate dosage; failure to produce or sustain this change does not necessarily mean that hormonal dosages are inadequate. Production of definite hyper-11-17-oxycorticosteroiduria and of hyper-17-ketosteroiduria can probably be considered a reasonably reliable indication of adequate ACTH therapy. The value of these indices with respect to adequacy of cortisone treatment remains to be determined.

In judging the effectiveness of ACTH, it is to be remembered that a few hours of treatment will produce a much greater degree of hyperadrenocorticism in patients with normally developed and active adrenal cortices than in patients having atrophic, functionally quiescent glands. In the latter instance, as following removal of an adrenocortical tumor or cessation of cortisone therapy (see above), up to 10 days of ACTH stimulation may be needed for full regeneration and reactivation of the adrenal cortices.

Therapeutic use of ACTH, cortisone and allied substances in non-endocrine conditions.[9 l, m, 27 a-e] Table 12 gives a tentative listing of pediatric conditions in which ACTH or cortisone have induced at least temporary improvement, and also mentions some of the diseases in which these substances have been found to be of little or no value or to be grossly detrimental.

In most of the diseases where improvement in clinical symptoms and signs is obtained, the tendency is for the pathological manifestations to recur when hormonal treatment is discontinued. Thus, it appears that ACTH and cortisone do not necessarily eliminate or cure the basic disease process even though they may momentarily make the patient feel much better. Neither do they seem to halt immunologic defense reactions. On the other hand, it would appear that they temporarily prevent such reactions from causing the clinical symptoms and signs characteristic of the particular condition. Brief remarks on selected diseases follow. These are intended only to indicate the types of effect which may be obtained with ACTH and cortisone.

Conditions "Benefited" by ACTH or Cortisone

Rheumatoid arthritis.[27 a, b, d, e] Administration of either ACTH or cortisone to patients with this disease causes marked symptomatic improvement within a day. Fever, fatigability and lassitude subside. Joint stiffness, swelling, soreness, redness, warmth and tenderness diminish markedly. Subcutaneous nodules vanish within a period of ten days to two weeks. Lymphadenopathy and splenomegaly also subside, as do vasomotor symptoms and paresthesias. There is a great increase in appetite and a tendency to rapid weight gain. Joint motion improves somewhat, although it may not become restored to normal. The erythrocyte sedimentation rate gradually falls toward normal; the blood hemoglobin level rises.

When treatment is stopped all the foregoing manifestations of disease usually reappear within a few days or within a few weeks. This underscores the thought that ACTH and cortisone do not "put out the fire." The possibility of devising schedules of therapy which serve to keep clinical manifestations of rheumatoid arthritis in abeyance without at the same time causing serious signs of hyperadrenocorticism is currently under active study in a number of clinics.

Acute rheumatic fever.[27 c, j, k] In over half the patients with this condition thus far treated, administration either of ACTH or cortisone has produced marked improvement within one or two days. The fever and signs of toxicity subside, pathologic cardiac manifestations diminish, joint symptoms disappear and the appetite and strength improve. Within two or three weeks of treatment the sedimentation rate falls to normal and rheumatic nodules disappear. Reports concerning the progress of cardiac murmurs vary. It is not yet known whether ACTH and cortisone are capable of preventing the tissue changes of rheumatic fever that ordinarily lead to permanent valvular damage.

Following discontinuation of treatment, there is a variable tendency to exacerbation of the rheumatic manifestations. In some patients treated for a few weeks, the exacerbation is brief, transient and of mild degree. In others it is intense and prolonged. This information suggests that hormonal therapy does not eliminate or cure the basic rheumatic process, at least when given after clinical signs of the disease have appeared.

In view of the fact that cortisone is much less apt than ACTH to cause water and salt retention, cortisone would appear to be the drug of choice for rheumatic patients suffering cardiac decompensation. The tendency of ACTH to induce water retention can be counteracted fairly successfully by feeding a low sodium diet. In an emergency, mercurial diuretics also may be employed.

Lupus erythematosus, dermatomyositis and periarteritis nodosa.[9 l, 27 e] In patients with lupus erythematosus disappearance of fever and of the skin lesions after several days of therapy has been noted. Joint symptoms, when present, tend to subside. Marked reticulocytosis, mild polymorphonuclear leucocytosis and increased hemoglobin values also are seen. There is reason to hope that significant remissions may be obtainable after prolonged, intensive ACTH therapy. Unfortunately, it appears that hormonal therapy is without beneficial effect upon the renal disturbances seen in patients with lupus erythematosus.

A number of children with dermatomyositis have been treated with somewhat variable results. It appears that ACTH can favorably influence the skin changes and the inflammatory and destructive processes which characterize the myositis component of this disease. This may be accompanied by some slight-to-moderate improvement in muscle strength. Testosterone also appears to be of value in this respect. Methyl testosterone has been used in doses of 5 to 50 mg. by mouth daily, by itself as well as in conjunction with ACTH or cortisone.

ACTH and cortisone can inhibit the acute process of periarteritis nodosa, but appear incapable of preventing progressive fibrous obliteration of affected blood vessels.

In none of these conditions has permanent remission been observed following cessation of hormonal therapy.

Bronchial asthma and other allergic conditions.[9 l, 27 e, 1] ACTH treatment usually produces a marked improvement in asthmatic symptoms within a period of 4 to 36 hours. If continued for five to seven days, this therapy often causes disappearance of all rhonchi and wheezes and marked increase in vital capacity. Following cessation of treatment, the patient may enjoy a remission of several weeks' duration. This type of treatment is worthy of consideration, particularly in patients found resistant to standard forms of treatment.

Infantile atopic eczema has also been found to respond very well to ACTH administration. Redness and roughness of the skin and itching may subside almost completely within a period of two to four days. Vasomotor rhinitis, urticaria and serum sickness are reported to respond in a correspondingly satisfactory manner.

Anorexia nervosa.[91] One of the remarkable effects of ACTH and cortisone treatment is to prompt a great increase in appetite. The mechanism whereby it induces this effect is unknown. In patients with severe anorexia nervosa, as well as in patients with rheumatoid arthritis, ulcerative colitis and other debilitating diseases, hormonal therapy can yield striking results. The effect is noticeable within a day or two and can lead to rapid weight gain, which is presumed to be due in the main to an improvement in caloric balance resulting from the increased dietary intake. The usefulness of this form of treatment as an adjunct to psychotherapy in the management of patients with anorexia nervosa deserves further study.

Idiopathic hypoglycemia.[27 h] The fact that ACTH has been used successfully in the management of infants and young children with idiopathic hypoglycemia has already been mentioned. After an initial course of treatment with ordinary doses of ACTH, these patients may be maintained successfully on very small doses given at intervals of two days. Incidentally, this is one of the few conditions wherein presently available knowledge concerning the physiologic effects of adrenocortical hormones provides a reasonably clear explanation for their therapeutic effectiveness (see discussion under S-F-N hormones, page 148).

Nephrosis.[9 l, 27 e, m] Experience with children suffering nephrotic edema indicates that administration of ACTH will produce diuresis in the majority of patients treated. Initially there is apt to be a decrease in urine volume and a gain in weight. These changes can be minimized by feeding a salt-poor diet and by restricting the water intake. It also is advisable to make certain that the patient has a reasonably adequate potassium intake (± 50 mEq. per m^2 per day). Diuresis may develop after 5 to 10 days of treatment. Alternately, diuresis may develop within one to three days, if ACTH treatment of five to seven days' duration is abruptly discontinued. The diuresis may result in the loss of most of the edema fluid. Occasional patients who fail to develop polyuria and to shed their edema after one course of treatment do so during or after a second course. At present there is no way of predicting which patients will respond favorably.

ACTH does not cure nephrosis. As in the case of spontaneous or measles-induced diuresis, patients treated with ACTH tend sooner or later to re-accumulate edema fluid. In treating nephrotic patients with ACTH or cortisone it is important to bear in mind that these hormones may, by their analgesic, antipyretic and other actions, make it very difficult to recognize the development of peritonitis or other hidden lesion in the patient. This fact should act as a deterrent to the use of these hormones in a routine or carefree manner.

In speculating on the mechanisms involved in ACTH-produced diuresis, one possibility is suggested by the fact that ACTH stimulates increased S-F-N hormone production. S-F-N hormones are known to negate or cancel the sodium-retaining effect of Na-K hormone at the kidney tubule and to inhibit the production or action of posterior pituitary anti-diuretic hormone. Another possibility is suggested by the fact that individuals treated with ACTH may undergo a temporary period of relative hypoadrenocorticism following cessation of therapy. This may result in a transient tendency toward sodium and water diuresis similar to that seen in patients with Addison's disease. These speculations are inserted to indicate the variety of interesting clues concerning possible factors involved in edema formation and dissipation provided by ACTH and cortisone studies.

Ulcerative colitis.[9 1, 27 e] Striking effects have been noted following institution of ACTH treatment to patients with this condition. Within one or two weeks there may be cessation of bloody diarrhea, disappearance of abdominal distress, marked increase in appetite and appreciable weight gain. Proctoscopic findings also may improve. The remission may be sustained for a considerable period following discontinuation of therapy. On the other hand, some patients with ulcerative colitis not only have failed to improve markedly while under ACTH treatment, but also have developed serious complications of their disease which went unrecognized apparently because of the aforementioned analgesic and other effects of hormonal therapy. For example, a few patients have suffered perforation of the intestine without developing symptoms indicative of this lesion.

Concluding theoretical comments. It is well known that infantile eczema often improves markedly during periods of bacteremia, pneumonia or other severe stress. Under such circumstances a marked eosinopenia is also shown. This suggests that eczematous infants, if subjected to appropriate stress, can develop a vigorous pituitary–adrenocortical alarm reaction. As a corollary to this, it may be postulated that (a) patients with eczematous, rheumatoid and certain allied conditions require a larger than normal stimulus to develop this reaction, (b) the alarm reaction mechanism becomes fatigued after prolonged stimulation by certain chronic conditions,[10 c] (c) eczema, rheumatism and allied conditions do not constitute a proper stimulus to the alarm reaction system or (d) the tissues of patients suffering from these conditions have an unusually high threshold of response to adrenocortical hormone.

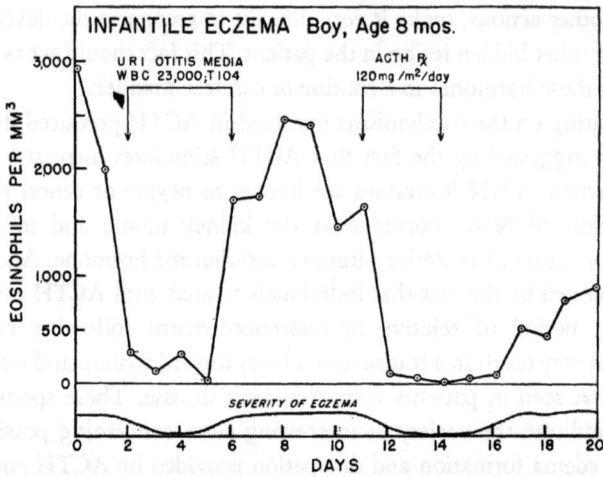

FIGURE III—54. Transient alleviation of infantile eczema by stress-induced (physiologic) and by ACTH-induced (pathologic) hyperadrenocorticism. Note that both conditions caused an equal fall in eosinophil count and improvement in eczema.

A point of interest with relation to these possibilities is suggested by current observations on the clinical and metabolic changes seen upon administration of ACTH or cortisone to patients suffering from one or another of these chronic diseases. As mentioned previously almost without exception patients develop clinical and metabolic signs of Cushing's syndrome when given ACTH and cortisone for long periods. In other words this type of therapy results in the production of hormones in excess of certain physiologic needs (see Figure 28, right-hand columns). It remains to be determined whether the undesirable side effects are totally separable from the beneficial effects of adrenocortical hormone therapy. Observations on eczematous patients are encouraging in these respects. As shown by Figure 54, stress-induced physiologic hyperadrenocorticism is just as effective as ACTH- or cortisone-induced (pathologic?) hyperadrenocorticism in causing a temporary subsidence of infantile eczema. Similar clinical observations indicate that the stress of measles or peritonitis may bring about a transient remission (diuresis) in juvenile nephrotic patients as successfully as ACTH or cortisone. Studies on chronically ill patients (such as the burned patient of Figure 16, who had spontaneous hyperadrenocorticism for almost 60 days) indicate that stress-induced, physiologic hyperadrenocorticism does not necessarily lead to the development of Cushing's syndrome. In other words, it does not appear that adrenocortical hormones must be present in excess of **ordinary body needs** in order to effect the therapeutic benefits under consideration here.

These agents usually cannot be considered curative in the same sense as the antibiotics. In most instances they merely give temporary relief from the underlying condition. In the ultimate analysis, therefore, it may be found that their greatest value has been to point the way to the development of therapy which is both non-toxic and permanent.

REFERENCES

1 (a) KENDALL, E. C. The function of the adrenal cortex. *Proc. Staff Meet., Mayo Clin.* 15:297, 1940.
   (b) REICHSTEIN, T. and SHOPPEE, C. W. The hormones of the adrenal cortex. In *Vitamins and Hormones.* Vol. I. Edited by R. S. Harris and K. V. Thimann. New York, Academic Press, 1943.

2 (a) MASON, H. L. Urinary steroids in adrenal disease and the metabolism of adrenal hormones. In *Recent Progress in Hormone Research.* Vol. III. Edited by G. Pincus. New York, Academic Press, 1948.
   (b) SPRAGUE, R. G., POWER, M. H., MASON, H. L., ALBERT, A., MATHIESON, D. R., HENCH, P. S., KENDALL, E. C., SLOCUMB, C. H. and POLLEY, H. F. Observations on the physiologic effects of cortisone and ACTH in man. *Arch. Int. Med.* 85:199, 1950.

3 (a) LOEB, R. F., ATCHLEY, D. W., BENEDICT, E. M. and LELAND, J. Electrolyte balance studies in adrenalectomized dogs with particular reference to the excretion of sodium. *J. Exper. Med.* 57:775, 1933.
   (b) LOEB, R. F. Adrenal cortex and electrolyte behavior. In *The Harvey Lectures, 1941-42.* Series 17:100. Lancaster, Science Press, 1942.
   (c) SWINGLE, W. W. and REMINGTON, J. W. The role of the adrenal cortex in physiological processes. *Physiol. Rev.* 24:89, 1944.
   (d) INGLE, D. J. The physiological action of the adrenal hormones. In *The Chemistry and Physiology of Hormones.* Washington, D. C., Amer. Assn. for the Advancement of Science, 1944.

4 (a) CONN, J. W. Electrolyte composition of sweat; clinical implications as an index of adrenal cortical function. *Arch. Int. Med.* 83:416, 1949.
   (b) CONN, J. W. The mechanism of acclimatization to heat. In *Advances in Internal Medicine.* Vol. III. Edited by W. Dock and I. Snapper. New York, Interscience Publishers, 1949.
   (c) LOCKE, W., TALBOT, N. B., JONES, H. S. and WORCESTER, J. Studies on the combined use of measurements of sweat electrolyte composition and rate of sweating as an index of adrenal cortical activity. *J. Clin. Invest.* 30:325, 1951.
   (d) FRAWLEY, T. F. and THORN, G. W. The salivary sodium potassium concentration in varying states of adrenal cortical activity. In *Proceedings of the Second Clinical ACTH Conference.* Edited by J. R. Mote. Philadelphia, Blakiston, 1951.

5 (a) LOEB, R. F., ATCHLEY, D. W., FERREBEE, J. W. and RAGAN, C. Observations on the effect of desoxycorticosterone esters and progesterone in patients with Addison's disease. *Tr. A. Am. Physicians* 54:285, 1939.
   (b) DARROW, D. C. and MILLER, H. C. The production of cardiac lesions by repeated injections of desoxycorticosterone acetate. *J. Clin. Invest.* 21:601, 1942.

6 (a) DARROW, D. C., SCHWARTZ, R., IANNUCCI, J. F. and COVILLE, F. The relation of serum bicarbonate concentration to muscle composition. *J. Clin. Invest.* 27:198, 1948.
   (b) DANOWSKI, T. S., ELKINTON, J. R., BURROWS, B. A. and WINKLER, A. W. Exchanges of sodium and potassium in familial periodic paralysis. *J. Clin. Invest.* 27:65, 1948.
   (c) GARDNER, L. I., TALBOT, N. B., COOK, C. D. and BERMAN, H. Effect of potassium deficiency on carbohydrate metabolism. *J. Lab. & Clin. Med.* 35:592, 1950.

(d) BROWN, M. R., CURRENS, J. H. and MARCHAND, J. F. Muscular paralysis and electrocardiographic abnormalities resulting from potassium loss in chronic nephritis. *J. A. M. A.* 124:545, 1944.
(e) WINKLER, A. W., SMITH, P. K. and HOFF, H. E. Absence of beneficial effects from injections of desoxycorticosterone acetate and of cortical adrenal extract in experimental anuria. *J. Clin. Invest.* 21:419, 1942.
(f) SELDIN, D. W., WELT, L. G. and CORT, J. H. The effects of pituitary and adrenal hormones on the metabolism and excretions of water and electrolytes; potassium. Read before the Interurban Clinical Club, New Haven, December 1, 1950.
(g) ELIEL, L. P., PEARSON, O. H. and RAWSON, R. W. Postoperative potassium deficit and metabolic alkalosis. *New Eng. J. Med.* 243:471, 1950, and *ibid* 518.
(h) CURRENS, J. H. and CRAWFORD, J. D. The electrocardiogram and disturbances of potassium metabolism. *New Eng. J. Med.* 243:843, 1950.
(i) CORSA, L., JR., OLNEY, J. M., JR., STEENBURG, R. W., BALL, M. R. and MOORE, F. D. The measurement of exchangeable potassium in man by isotopic dilution. *J. Clin. Invest.* 29:1280, 1950.
(j) STERN, T. V., COLE, V. V., BASS, A. C. and OVERMAN, R. R. Dynamic aspects of sodium metabolism in experimental adrenal insufficiency using radioactive sodium. *Am. J. Physiol.* 2:437, 1951.
(k) FORBES, G. B. and PIRLEY, A. Estimation of total body sodium by isotopic dilution; studies on young adults. *J. Clin. Invest.* (In press.)
(l) CORSA, L., JR., COOK, C. D. and TALBOT, N. B. Unpublished data.
(m) SHOHL, A. T. *Mineral Metabolism.* New York, Reinhold, 1939.

7 (a) LOEB, R. F. Effect of sodium chloride in treatment of patient with Addison's disease. *Proc. Soc. Exper. Biol. & Med.* 30:808, 1933.
(b) HARROP, G. A., WEINSTEIN, A., SOFFER, L. J. and TRESCHER, J. H. Diagnosis and treatment of Addison's disease. *J. A. M. A.* 100:1850, 1933.
(c) TRUSKOWSKI, R. and ZWEMER, R. Cortico-adrenal insufficiency and potassium metabolism. *Biochem. J.* 30:1345, 1936.

8 (a) SILVETTE, H. and BRITTON, S. W. Effects of adrenalectomy and cortico-adrenal extract on renal excretion and tissue fluids. *Am. J. Physiol.* 104:399, 1933.
(b) HARRISON, H. E. and DARROW, D. C. The distribution of body water and electrolytes in adrenal insufficiency. *J. Clin. Invest.* 17:77, 1938.
(c) MUNTWYLOR, E. R., MELLORS, R. C. and MAUTZ, F. R. Electrolyte and water equilibria in the dog; electrolyte and water exchange between skeletal muscle and blood in adrenal insufficiency. *J. Biol. Chem.* 134:367, 1940.
(d) HARROP, G. A. The influence of the adrenal cortex upon the distribution of body water. *Bull. Johns Hopkins Hosp.* 59:11, 1936.
(e) GUADINO, M. and LEVITT, N. F. Influence of the adrenal cortex on body water distribution and renal function. *J. Clin. Invest.* 28:1487, 1949.

9 (a) LONG, C. N. H., KATZIN, B. and FRY, E. G. The adrenal cortex and carbohydrate metabolism. *Endocrinology* 26:309, 1940.
(b) THORN, G. W., KOEPF, G. F., LEWIS, R. A. and OLSEN, E. F. Carbohydrate metabolism in Addison's disease. *J. Clin. Invest.* 19:813, 1940.
(c) LEWIS, R. A., KUHLMAN, D., DELBRIE, C., KOEPF, G. F. and THORN, G. W. The effect of adrenal cortex on carbohydrate metabolism. *Endocrinology* 27:971, 1940.
(d) KENDALL, E. C. The adrenal cortex. *Arch. Path.* 32:474, 1941.
(e) PFIFFNER, J. J. The adrenal cortical hormones. *Advances Enzymol.* 2:325, 1942.
(f) INGLE, D. J. Problems relating to the adrenal cortex. *Endocrinology* 31:419, 1942.
(g) WHITE, A. Integration of the effects of adrenal cortical, thyroid and growth hormones in fasting metabolism. In *Recent Progress in Hormone Research.* Vol. IV. Edited by G. Pincus. New York, Academic Press, 1949.

- (h) THORN, G. W. and FORSHAM, P. H. Metabolic changes in man following adrenal and pituitary hormone administration. In *Recent Progress in Hormone Research.* Vol. IV. Edited by G. Pincus. New York, Academic Press, 1949.
- (i) KINSELL, L., MARGEN, S., MICHAELS, G., REISS, R., FRANTZ, R. and CARBONE, J. The effects of ACTH, of cortisone and of other steroid compounds upon fat metabolism in diabetic and non-diabetic human subjects. *J. Clin. Endocrinol.* 10:815, 1950.
- (j) ADLERSBERG, D., SCHAEFER, L. E. and DRITCH, R. Effect of cortisone, ACTH and DOCA on serum lipids. *J. Clin. Invest.* 29:795, 1950.
- (k) RAGAN, C., HOWES, E. L., PLOTZ, C. M., MEYER, K. and BLUNT, J. W. Effect of cortisone on production of granulation tissue in rabbit. *Proc. Soc. Exper. Biol. & Med.* 72:718, 1949.
- (l) THORN, G. W., FORSHAM, P. H., FRAWLEY, T. F., HILL, S. R., JR., ROCHE, M., STAEHELIN, D. and WILSON, D. L. Medical progress: the clinical usefulness of ACTH and cortisone. *New Eng. J. Med.* 242:783, 1950, and *ibid* 824 and 865.
- (m) HEILMAN, D. H. Effect of 11-dehydro-17-hydroxycorticosterone and 11-dehydrocorticosterone on migration of macrophages in tissue culture. *Proc. Staff Meet., Mayo Clin.* 20:318, 1945.

10 (a) INGLE, D. J. The work performance of adrenalectomized rats treated with corticosterone and chemically related compounds. *Endocrinology* 26:472, 1940.
- (b) INGLE, D. J. and LUKENS, F. D. W. Reversal of fatigue in the adrenalectomized rat by glucose and other agents. *Endocrinology* 29:443, 1941.
- (c) SELYE, H. The general adaptation syndrome and the diseases of adaptation. *J. Clin. Endocrinol.* 6:117, 1946.
- (d) INGLE, D. J. Optimal requirements for adrenal cortical hormones as observed in adrenalectomized animals. *J. Clin. Endocrinol.* 4:208, 1944.
- (e) TEPPERMAN, J., ENGLE, F. L. and LONG, C. N. H. A review of adrenal cortical hypertrophy. *Endocrinology* 32:373, 1943.
- (f) FORSHAM, P. H., THORN, G. W., PRUNTY, F. T. G. and HILLS, H. G. Clinical studies with pituitary adrenocorticotropin. *J. Clin. Endocrinol.* 8:15, 1948.
- (g) HOFFMAN, W. C., LEWIS, R. A. and THORN, G. W. Electro-encephalogram in Addison's disease. *Bull. Johns Hopkins Hosp.* 70:335, 1942.
- (h) MIRICK, G. S. The effect of adrenocorticotropic hormone and cortisone on antibody production in human beings. *J. Clin. Invest.* 29:836, 1950.
- (i) STOERK, H. C. Inhibition of tuberculin reaction by cortisone in vaccinated guinea pigs. *Federation Proc.* 9:345, 1950.
- (j) TOMPSETT, R., LE MAISTRE, C., MUSCHENHEIM, C. and MC DERMOTT, W. Effects of ACTH on tuberculosis in humans. *J. Clin. Invest.* 29:849, 1950.
- (k) ROSE, B. and BROWNE, J. S. L. The effect of adrenalectomy on the histamine content of the tissues of the rat. *Am. J. Physiol.* 131:589, 1941.
- (l) KARADY, S., ROSE, B. and BROWNE, J. S. L. Decrease of histaminase in tissue by adrenalectomy and its restoration by cortico-adrenal extract. *Am. J. Physiol.* 130:539, 1940.
- (m) BANTING, F. G. and GAIRNS, S. Suprarenal insufficiency. *Am. J. Physiol.* 77:100, 1926.
- (n) WYMAN, L. C. Studies on suprarenal insufficiency; anaphylaxis in suprarenalectomized rats. *Am. J. Physiol.* 89:356, 1929.
- (o) ROSE, B., PARE, J. A. P., PUMP, K., STANFORD, R. and JOHNSON, L. G. Influence of ACTH on the excretion of histamine and histidine in patients with allergic states or rheumatoid arthritis. *J. Clin. Invest.* 29:841, 1950.
- (p) INGBAR, S. H., RELMAN, A. S., BURROWS, B. A., KASS, E. H., SISSON, J. H. and BURNETT, C. H. Changes in normal renal function resulting from ACTH and cortisone. *J. Clin. Invest.* 29:824, 1950.
- (q) CONN, J. W., LOUIS, L. H. and JOHNSTON, M. W. Alleviation of experimental diabetes in man by administration of reduced glutathione (GSH): metabolic implications. *Science* 109:279, 1949.
- (r) TALBOT, N. B. Unpublished observations.

11 (a) WEIL, P. G. and BROWNE, J. S. L. The excretion of cortin under conditions of damage. *J. Clin. Invest.* 19:772, 1940.
   (b) TALBOT, N. B., ALBRIGHT, F., SALTZMAN, A. H., ZYGMUNTOWICZ, A. and WIXOM, R. The excretion of 11-oxycorticosteroid-like substances by normal and abnormal subjects. *J. Clin. Endocrinol.* 77:331, 1947.
   (c) TALBOT, N. B., ZYGMUNTOWICZ, A., WOOD, M. and CHRISTO, E. Observations on adrenal cortical "sugar-fat-nitrogen" hormone ("11-17-OCS") and "17-ketosteroid precursor" production by normal and abnormal individuals of various ages with comments on the fact that (a) there may be two ACTH's and (b) the normal adrenal cortex may not produce true androgens. In *Proceedings of the First Clinical ACTH Conference.* Edited by J. R. Mote. Philadelphia, Blakiston, 1950.
   (d) SPRECHLER, M. The corticosteroids, with special reference to the urinary excretion in normal and pathological cases; a survey. *Acta endocrinol.* 2:70, 1949.
   (e) VENNING, E. H. The effect of ACTH during the neonatal period. In *Proceedings of the First Clinical ACTH Conference.* Edited by J. R. Mote. Philadelphia, Blakiston, 1950.

12 (a) BRUCH, H. and MC CUNE, D. J. Involution of the adrenal glands in newly born infants; a biochemical inquiry into its physiologic significance. *Am. J. Dis. Child.* 52:863, 1936.
   (b) JAILER, J. Adrenal function during pregnancy and the effect of ACTH during pregnancy. In *Proceedings of the Second Clinical ACTH Conference.* Edited by J. R. Mote. Philadelphia, Blakiston, 1951.

13 (a) TALBOT, N. B. and BUTLER, A. M. Urinary 17-ketosteroid assays in clinical medicine. *J. Clin. Endocrinol.* 2:724, 1942.
   (b) LIBERMAN, S. and DOBRINER, K. Steroid excretion in health and disease; chemistry. In *Recent Progress in Hormone Research.* Vol. III. Edited by G. Pincus. New York, Academic Press, 1948.
   (c) ENGSTROM, W. W., MASON, H. L. and KEPLER, E. J. Excretion of neutral 17-ketosteroids in adrenal cortical tumor and feminine pseudohermaphroditism with adrenal cortical hyperplasia. *J. Clin. Endocrinol.* 4:152, 1944.

14 (a) TALBOT, N. B. and SOBEL, E. H. Endocrine and other factors determining the growth of children. In *Advances in Pediatrics.* Vol. II. Edited by S. Z. Levine, *et al.* New York, Interscience Publishers, 1947.
   (b) TALBOT, N. B., BUTLER, A. M. and BERMAN, R. A. Adrenal cortical hyperplasia with virilism: diagnosis, course and treatment. *J. Clin. Invest.* 21:559, 1942.
   (c) GARDNER, L. I., SNIFFEN, R. C., ZYGMUNTOWICZ, A. S. and TALBOT, N. B. Follow-up studies in a boy with mixed adrenal cortical disease. *Pediatrics* 5:808, 1950.
   (d) BLACKMAN, S. S., JR. Concerning function and origin of reticular zone of adrenal cortex; hyperplasia in adrenogenital syndrome. *Bull. Johns Hopkins Hosp.* 78:180, 1946.
   (e) SAYERS, G. The adrenal cortex and homeostasis. *Physiol. Rev.* 30:241, 1950.

15 (a) EVANS, H. M. The function of the anterior hypophysis. In *The Harvey Lectures, 1923-24.* Series 19:212. Lancaster, Science Press, 1924.
   (b) SMITH, P. E. Hypophysectomy and replacement therapy in the rat. *Am. J. Anat.* 45:205, 1930.
   (c) COLLIP, J. B., ANDERSON, E. M. and THOMSON, D. L. Adrenotropic hormone of anterior pituitary lobe. *Lancet* 2:347, 1933.
   (d) SWANN, H. G. The pituitary-adrenocortical relationship. *Physiol. Rev.* 20:493, 1940.
   (e) SAYERS, G. and SAYERS, N. The pituitary-adrenal system. In *Recent Progress in Hormone Research.* Vol. II. Edited by G. Pincus. New York, Academic Press, 1948.
   (f) LI, C. H. Relative size of adrenocorticotrophically active peptide fragments. *Federation Proc.* 8:461, 1949.
   (g) KINSELL, L. W., LI, C. H., MARGEN, S., MICHAELS, G. D. and HEDGES, R. N. Metabolic effects of peptide mixture derived from ACTH (Li) in comparison with those resulting from whole ACTH administration in a human subject. In *Proceedings of the First Clinical ACTH Conference.* Edited by J. R. Mote. Philadelphia, Blakiston, 1950.

(h) TALBOT, N. B., WOOD, M., CAMPBELL, A. M., CHRISTO, E. and ZYGMUNTOWICZ, A. S. Concerning the probability that there are at least two adrenocorticotropic hormones in the human. In *Proceedings of the Second Clinical ACTH Conference.* Edited by J. R. Mote. Philadelphia, Blakiston, 1951.

16 (a) DEANE, H. W., SHAW, J. H. and GREEP, R. O. The effect of altered sodium or potassium intake on the width and cytochemistry of the zona glomerulosa of the rat's adrenal cortex. *Endocrinology* 43:133, 1948.

(b) BERGNER, G. E. and DEANE, H. W. Effects of pituitary adrenocorticotropic hormone on the intact rat with special reference to cytochemical changes in the adrenal cortex. *Endocrinology* 43:240, 1948.

17 MC DERMOTT, W. V., FRY, E. G., BROBECK, J. R. and LONG, C. N. H. Mechanism of control of adrenocorticotropic hormone. *Yale J. Biol. & Med.* 23:53, 1950.

18 (a) INGLE, D. J. and KENDALL, E. C. Atrophy of adrenal cortex of rat produced by administration of large amounts of cortin. *Science* 86:245, 1937.

(b) SELYE, H. Compensatory atrophy of the adrenals. *J. A. M. A.* 115:2246, 1940.

(c) WELLS, B. B. and KENDALL, E. C. A qualitative difference in the effect of compounds separated from the adrenal cortex on distribution of electrolytes and on atrophy of the adrenal and thymus glands of rats. *Proc. Staff Meet., Mayo Clin.* 15:133, 1940.

(d) SELYE, H. and DOSNE, C. Physiological significance of compensatory adrenal atrophy. *Endocrinology* 30:581, 1942.

19 (a) LEVY, M. S., POWER, M. H. and KEPLER, E. J. The specificity of the "water test" as a diagnostic procedure in Addison's disease. *J. Clin. Endocrinol.* 6:607, 1946.

(b) FORSHAM, P. H., THORN, G. W., PRUNTY, F. T. G. and HILLS, A. G. Clinical studies with pituitary adrenocorticotropin. *J. Clin. Endocrinol.* 8:15, 1948.

(c) THORN, G. W., FORSHAM, P. H., PRUNTY, F. T. G. and HILLS, A. G. A test for adrenal cortical insufficiency; the response to pituitary adrenocorticotropic hormone. *J. A. M. A.* 137:1005, 1948. Correction *ibid* 137:1544, 1948.

(d) THORN, G. W., FORSHAM, P. H. and EMERSON, K., JR. *The Diagnosis and Treatment of Adrenal Insufficiency.* Springfield, Ill., C. C. Thomas, 1949.

(e) RECANT, L., HUME, D. M., FORSHAM, P. H. and THORN, G. W. Studies on the effect of epinephrine on the pituitary adrenocortical system. *J. Clin. Endocrinol.* (In press.)

(f) THORN, G. W. and CLINTON, M., JR. Metabolic changes in a patient with Addison's disease following onset of diabetes mellitus. *J. Clin. Endocrinol.* 3:335, 1943.

(g) FRASER, R. W., ALBRIGHT, F. and SMITH, P. H. Value of the glucose tolerance test, insulin tolerance test and glucose-insulin tolerance test in the diagnosis of endocrinologic disorders of glucose metabolism. *J. Clin. Endocrinol.* 1:297, 1941.

(h) HIMSWORTH, H. P. Syndrome of diabetes mellitus and its causes. *Lancet* 1:465, 1949.

(i) TALBOT, N. B., SALTZMAN, A. H., WIXOM, R. L. and WOLFE, J. K. Colorimetric assay of urinary corticosteroid-like substances. *J. Biol. Chem.* 160:535, 1945.

(j) HEARD, R. D. H., SOBEL, H. and VENNING, E. H. The neutral lipide-soluble reducing substances of urine as an index of adrenal cortical function. *J. Biol. Chem.* 165:699, 1946.

(k) CUTLER, H. H., POWER, M. H. and WILDER, R. M. Concentrations of chloride sodium and potassium in urine and blood; their diagnostic significance in adrenal insufficiency. *J. A. M. A.* 111:117, 1938.

(l) WINKLER, A. W. and CRANKSHAW, O. F. Chloride depletion in conditions other than Addison's disease. *J. Clin. Invest.* 17:1, 1938.

(m) THORN, G. W., HOWARD, R. P. and DAYMAN, H. Electrolyte changes in pulmonary tuberculosis with special reference to adrenal cortical function. *Bull. Johns Hopkins Hosp.* 67:345, 1940.

(n) WILLSON, D. M., ROBINSON, F. J., POWER, M. H. and WILDER, R. M. Diagnosis of Addison's disease; further experience with the Cutler-Power-Wilder sodium chloride restriction test. *Arch. Int. Med.* 69:460, 1942.

(o) BUTLER, A. M., GAMBLE, J. L., TALBOT, N. B., MAC LACHLAN, E. A., APPLETON, J., FAHEY, K. and LINTON, M. A., JR. Studies on a life raft ration: prevention of excessive water loss and dehydration of castaways; the parenteral provision of caloric, nitrogen and electrolyte requirements. In *Final Report of Office of Emergency Management, Committee on Medical Research,* contract 364, June 11, 1946, and *ibid,* contract 478, June 5, 1946.
(p) THORN, G. W., KOEPF, G. F. and CLINTON, M., JR. Renal failure simulating adrenocortical insufficiency. *New Eng. J. Med.* 231:76, 1944.
(q) FRASER, R. W., FORBES, A. P., ALBRIGHT, F., SULKOWITCH, A. and REIFENSTEIN, E. C., JR. Colorimetric assay of 17-ketosteroids in urine; survey of use of this test in endocrine investigation, diagnosis and therapy. *J. Clin. Endocrinol.* 1:234, 1941.
(r) TALBOT, N. B., BUTLER, A. M. and MAC LACHLAN, E. A. Alpha and beta neutral ketosteroids (androgens); preliminary observations on their normal urinary excretion and the clinical usefulness of their assay in differential diagnosis. *New Eng. J. Med.* 223: 369, 1940.
(s) TAUSSKY, H., SWAN, R. and SHORR, E. An inquiry into the specificity of the uric acid creatinine ratio as a measure of adrenal cortical responsiveness. In *Proceedings of the Second Clinical ACTH Conference.* Edited by J. R. Mote. Philadelphia, Blakiston, 1951.

20 (a) ATKINSON, F. R. B. Addison's disease in children. *Brit. J. Child. Dis.* 35:96, 1938.
(b) MC GAVAK, T. H. Some pitfalls in the treatment of Addison's disease. *J. Clin. Endocrinol.* 1:68, 1941.
(c) THORN, G. W. Treatment of Addison's disease. *J. Clin. Endocrinol.* 1:76, 1941.
(d) CURRENS, J. H. and WHITE, P. D. Congestive heart failure and electrocardiographic abnormalities resulting from excessive desoxycorticosterone acetate therapy in the treatment of Addison's disease. *Am. Heart J.* 28:611, 1944.
(e) HAMPTON, H. P. and KEPLER, E. J. Addison's disease: treatment and prognosis. *Am. J. M. Sc.* 202:264, 1941.
(f) LUKENS, F. D. W. Diagnosis and treatment of disorders of the adrenal glands. *M. Clin. North America* 26:1803, 1942.
(g) THORN, G. W., DORRANCE, S. S. and DAY, E. Addison's disease; evaluation of synthetic desoxycorticosterone acetate therapy in 158 patients. *Ann. Int. Med.* 16:1053, 1942.
(h) THORN, G. W., FORSHAM, P.H., BENNETT, L. L., ROCHE, M., REISS, R. S., SLESSOR, A., FLINK, E. B. and SOMERVILLE, W. Clinical and metabolic changes in Addison's disease following administration of compound E acetate. *Tr. A. Am. Physicians* 62:233, 1949.

21 (a) SNELLING, C. E. and ERB, I. H. Hemorrhage and subsequent calcification of the suprarenal. *J. Pediat.* 6:22, 1935.
(b) KUNSTADTER, R. H. The Waterhouse-Friderichsen syndrome. *Arch. Pediat.* 56:489, 1939.

22 (a) CAHILL, G. F. Hormonal tumors of the adrenal. *Surgery* 16:233, 1944.
(b) SOFFER, L. J. Clinical and experimental studies of adrenal cortical hyperfunction. *Bull. New York Acad. Med.* 24:32, 1948.

23 (a) KEPLER, E. J. and KEATING, F. R. Diseases of the adrenal glands; tumors of the adrenal cortex, diseases of the adrenal medulla and allied disturbances. *Arch. Int. Med.* 68:1010, 1941.
(b) BRATRUD, T. E. and THOMPSON, W. H. Congenital hyperplasia of the adrenals. *Staff Meet., Bull. Hosp. Univ. Minnesota* 15:25, 1943.
(c) JACOBZINER, H. and GORFINKEL, A. Familial congenital adrenal cortical syndrome. *Am. J. Dis. Child.* 52:308, 1936.
(d) NELSON, A. A. Accessory adrenal cortical tissue. *Arch. Path.* 27:955, 1939.
(e) KEPLER, E. J., DOCKERTY, M. B. and PRIESTLEY, J. T. Adrenal-like tumor associated with Cushing's syndrome (so-called masculinovoblastoma, luteoma, hypernephroma, adrenal cortical carcinoma of the ovary). *Am. J. Obst. & Gynec.* 47:43, 1944.

(f) COPE, O. and SCHATZKI, R. Tumors of the adrenal glands; a modified air injection roentgen technic for demonstrating cortical and medullary tumors. *Arch. Int. Med.* 64:1222, 1939.
(g) WILKINS, L., LEWIS, R. A., KLEIN, R., GARDNER, L. I., CRIGLER, J. F., JR., ROSENBERG, E. and MIGEON, C. J. Cortisone therapy in congenital adrenal hyperplasia. *J. Clin. Endocrinol.* 11:1, 1951.
(h) VENNING, E. H. Observations on the metabolic changes resulting from the administration of ACTH to patients with asthma and allied conditions. In *Proceedings of the Second Clinical ACTH Conference.* Edited by J. R. Mote. Philadelphia, Blakiston, 1951.
(i) WILKINS, L. *The Diagnosis and Treatment of Endocrine Disorders in Childhood and Adolescence.* Springfield, Ill., C. C. Thomas, 1950.

24 (a) CUSHING, H. *Pituitary Body and Its Disorders.* Philadelphia, J. B. Lippincott, 1912.
(b) HEINBECKER, P. The pathogenesis of Cushing's syndrome. *Medicine* 23:225, 1944.
(c) MARKS, T. M., THOMAS, J. M. and WARKANY, J. Adrenocortical obesity in children. *Am. J. Dis. Child.* 60:923, 1940.
(d) FARBER, J. E., GUSTINA, F. J. and POSTOLOFF, A. V. Cushing's syndrome in children. *Am. J. Dis. Child.* 65:593, 1943.
(e) ALBRIGHT, F. Cushing's syndrome; its pathological physiology, its relationship to the adreno-genital syndrome, and its connection with the problem of the reaction of the body to injurious agents. ("Alarm Reaction" of Selye.) In *The Harvey Lectures, 1942-43.* Series 38:123. Lancaster, Science Press, 1943.
(f) CROOKE, A. C. A change in the basophil cells of the pituitary gland common to conditions which exhibit the syndrome attributed to basophil adenoma. *J. Path. & Bact.* 41:339, 1935.
(g) WALTERS, W., WILDER, R. M. and KEPLER, E. J. Suprarenal cortical syndrome with presentation of ten cases. *Ann. Surg.* 100:670, 1934.
(h) DEAKINS, M. L., FRIEDGOOD, H. B. and FERREBEE, J. W. Some effects of testosterone, testosterone propionate, methyl testosterone, stilbestrol and x-ray therapy in a patient with Cushing's syndrome. *J. Clin. Endocrinol.* 4:376, 1944.
(i) WILLSON, D. M., POWER, M. H. and KEPLER, E. J. Alkalosis and low plasma potassium in a case of Cushing's syndrome. *J. Clin. Invest.* 19:701, 1940.
(j) MC QUARRIE, I. The experiments of nature and other essays. In *The Porter Lectures, Series 12.* Lawrence, Univ. Kansas, Extension Division, 1944.
(k) NELSON, A. A. and WOODARD, G. Severe adrenal cortical atrophy (cytotoxia) and hepatic damage produced in dogs by feeding 2, 2-Bis (parachlorophenyl) -1, 1-dichloroethane (DDD or TDE). *Arch. Path.* 48:387, 1949.
(l) NICHOLS, J. and GARDNER, L. I. Studies with 2, 2-Bis (parachlorophenyl) -1, 1-dichloroethane, a new adrenocorticolytic agent. *Trans. Soc. for Ped. Research*, May, 1950.

25 (a) BUTLER, A. M., ROSS, R. A. and TALBOT, N. B. Probable adrenal insufficiency in an infant. *J. Pediat.* 15:831, 1939.
(b) DIJKHUIZEN, R. K. and BEHR, E. Adrenal hypertrophy in infants: a new clinical entity of the neonatal period. *Acta pædiat.* 27:279, 1940.
(c) WILKINS, L. and RICHTER, C. P. A great craving for salt by a child with corticoadrenal insufficiency. *J. A. M. A.* 114:866, 1940.
(d) WILKINS, L. Hyperadrenocorticism. *Pediatrics* 3:533, 1949.
(e) KYLE, L. H. and KNOP, C. Q. Simulation of cardiac disease by adrenocortical failure in infants. *New Eng. J. Med.* 243:681, 1950.

26 (a) KEPLER, E. J., WALTERS, W. and DIXON, R. K. Menstruation in a child aged nineteen months as a result of a tumor of the left adrenal cortex; successful surgical treatment. *Proc. Staff Meet., Mayo Clin.* 13:362, 1938.
(b) NEFF, F. C., TICE, G. M., WALKER, G. A. and OCKERBLAD, N. Adrenal tumor in a female infant with hypertrichosis, hypertension, overdevelopment of external genitalia, obesity, but absence of breast enlargement. *J. Clin. Endocrinol.* 2:125, 1942.

(c) WILKINS, L. A feminizing adrenal tumor causing gynecomastia in a boy of five years contrasted with a virilizing tumor in a five-year-old girl; classification of seventy cases of adrenal tumor in children according to their hormonal manifestations and a review of eleven cases of feminizing adrenal tumor in adults. *J. Clin. Endocrinol.* 8:111, 1948.

27 (a) HENCH, P. S., KENDALL, E. C., SLOCUMB, C. H. and POLLEY, H. F. The effect of a hormone of the adrenal cortex (17-hydroxy-11-dehydrocorticosterone: compound E) and of pituitary adrenocorticotropic hormone on rheumatoid arthritis; preliminary report. *Ann. Rheumat. Dis.* 8:97, 1949.

(b) BAUER, W., BOLAND, E. W., FREYBERG, R. H., HOLBROOK, W. P. and ROSENBERG, E. F. *Proceedings of the Seventh International Congress on Rheumatic Disease.* New York, May 30-June 3, 1949.

(c) HENCH, P. S., SLOCUMB, C. H., BARNES, A. R., SMITH, H. L., POLLEY, H. F. and KENDALL, E. C. The effects of the adrenal cortical hormone 17-hydroxy-11-dehydrocorticosterone (compound E) on the acute phase of rheumatic fever; preliminary report. *Proc. Staff Meet., Mayo Clin.* 24:277, 1949.

(d) BOLAND, E. W. and HEADLEY, N. H. Effects of cortisone acetate on rheumatoid arthritis. *J. A. M. A.* 141:301, 1949.

(e) *Proceedings of the First Clinical ACTH Conference.* Edited by J. R. Mote. Philadelphia, Blakiston, 1950.

(f) DEMING, Q. B. and LUETSCHER, J. A., JR. Increased sodium-retaining corticoid excretion in edema with some observations on the effects of cortisone in nephrosis. *J. Clin. Invest.* 29:808, 1950.

(g) FORSHAM, P. H., THORN, G. W., FRAWLEY, T. F. and WILSON, L. W. Studies on the functional state of the adrenal cortex during and following ACTH and cortisone therapy. *Proc. Am. Soc. for Clin. Invest.* May, 1950.

(h) MC QUARRIE, I., BAUER, E. G., ZIEGLER, M. R. and WRIGHT, W. S. The metabolic and clinical effects of pituitary adrenocorticotrophic hormone in spontaneous hypoglycemosis. In *Proceedings of the First Clinical ACTH Conference.* Edited by J. R. Mote. Philadelphia, Blakiston, 1950.

(i) CLARKE, W. Personal communication.

(j) MC EWEN, C., BUNIM, J. J., BALDWIN, J. S., KUTTNER, A. G., APPEL, S. B. and KALTMAN, A. J. Effect of cortisone and ACTH on rheumatic fever. *Bull. New York Acad. Med.* 26:212, 1950.

(k) MASSELL, B. F., WARREN, J. E., STURGIS, G. P., HALL, B. and CRAIGE, E. The clinical response of rheumatic fever and acute carditis to ACTH. *New Eng. J. Med.* 242:641, 1950.

(l) BORDLEY, J. E., CAREY, R. A., HARVEY, A. M., HOWARD, J. E., KATTUS, A. A., NEWMAN, E. V. and WINKENWERDER, W. L. Preliminary observations on effect of adrenocorticotrophic hormone (ACTH) in allergic disease. *Bull. Johns Hopkins Hosp.* 85:396, 1949.

(m) BARNETT, H. L., MC NAMARA, H., MC CRORY, W., FORMAN, C., RAPOPORT, M., MICHIE, A. and BARBERO, G. The effects of ACTH and cortisone on the nephrotic syndrome. *Pediatrics* (In press.)

(n) KASS, E. H. and FINLAND, M. Effect of ACTH on induced fever. *New Eng. J. Med.* 243: 693, 1950.

(o) INGLE, D. J. The biologic properties of cortisone: a review. *J. Clin. Endocrinol.* 10:312, 1950.

(p) *Proceedings of the Second Clinical ACTH Conference.* Edited by J. R. Mote. Philadelphia, Blakiston, 1951.

THE ADRENAL MEDULLÆ

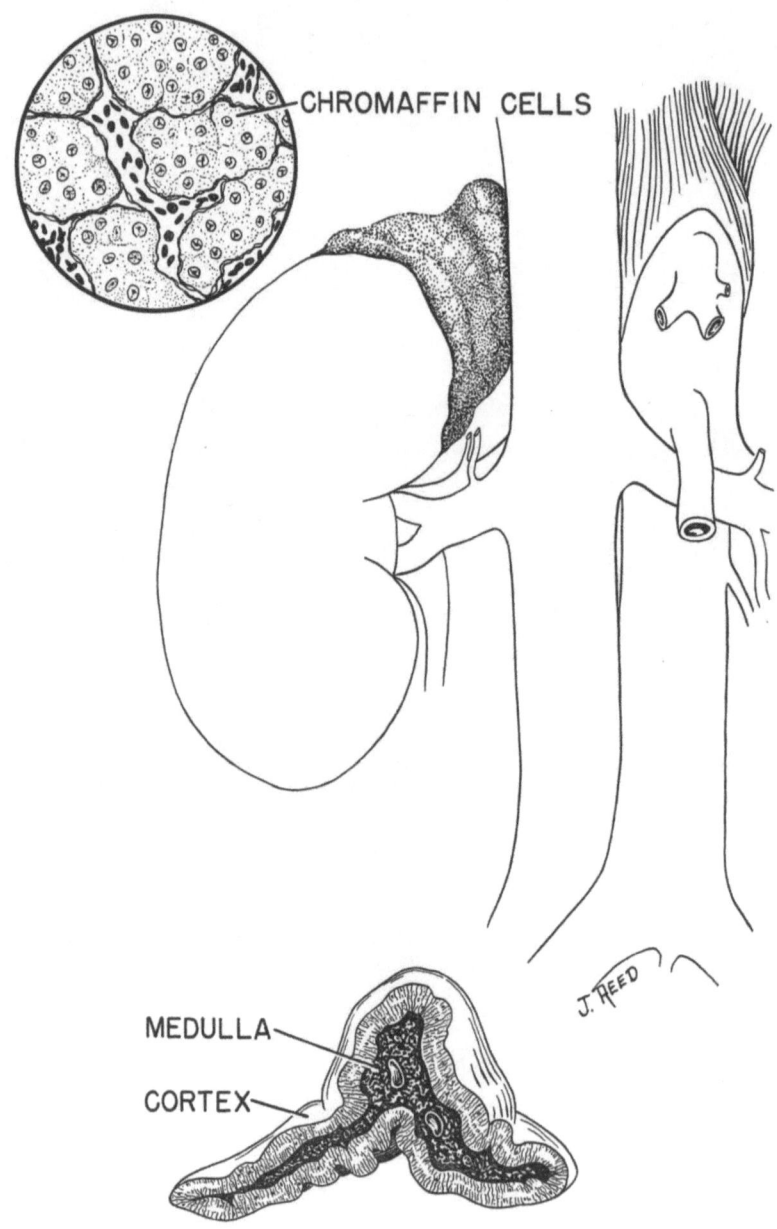

CHAPTER IV

THE ADRENAL MEDULLÆ

BASIC CONSIDERATIONS

ORIGIN

The adrenal medullæ like the ganglia of the sympathetic nervous system originate from ectoderm of the neural crest. The cells forming the medullæ are modified neuroblasts and are distinguished by their brown staining reaction to chrome salts. For this reason they are called "chromaffin" cells. Accessory paraganglia containing cells of similar staining reaction and function may occur anywhere along the paravertebral sympathetic chain or in association with a sympathetic plexus. The term "adrenal medulla," as used hereafter parenthetically includes such structures.

ADRENOMEDULLARY AND RELATED SYMPATHETIC HORMONES

Two closely related substances, epinephrine and nor-epinephrine, have been extracted from the adrenal medullæ of cattle.[1] Epinephrine, in contrast to nor-epinephrine, contains a methyl group. This suggests that nor-epinephrine may be a precursor of epinephrine. Both are chemically similar to tyrosine and are probably derivatives of this amino acid in the body.

Epinephrine is defined in the United States Pharmacopia as the levorotatory form of methyl-aminoethanolcatechol. The epinephrine contained in pharmaceutical preparations intended for clinical use may have been extracted from animal adrenal medullæ prepared synthetically. Synthetic epinephrine conforms to the foregoing chemical definition. Preparations of biologic origin contain between 12 and 18 per cent of the non-methylated nor-epinephrine.

The literature[2] contains extensive discussions concerning the presence in the body of two additional substances, sympathin E and sympathin I which, it is postulated, are produced by the sympathetic nerve endings. Sympathin E is thought to effect the excitatory stimuli and sympathin I the inhibitory stimuli of the postganglionic adrenergic nerves.

CONTROL OF ADRENOMEDULLARY ACTIVITY

The adrenal medullæ are actually specialized sympathetic ganglia. Like these ganglia, they are stimulated to activity when sympathetic nerve impulses, which may originate at the base of the brain, cause acetylcholine to be formed at the preganglionic nerve endings. The ganglia respond by activating postganglionic nerves which prompt sympathin production in various tissues; the adrenal medullæ respond by secreting epinephrine (and possibly also nor-epinephrine) into the circulation (see Figure 1).

The secretion of epinephrine is decreased as a result of denervation of the adrenal medullæ. However, in the absence of nervous stimuli it can be induced by such substances as histamine and potassium.[2, 3]

FACTORS WHICH INFLUENCE ADRENOMEDULLARY ACTIVITY

The classic experiments of Walter Cannon have shown that numerous types of acute stress including pain, hunger, rage and fear prompt an immediate outpouring of epinephrine.[4] Hypoglycemia also incites this reaction. Consideration of the multiple effects of epinephrine enumerated below suggests strongly that this acute alarm reaction mechanism has the purpose of protecting the organism from certain types of threat. In other words, it constitutes one of the homeostatic systems of the body. Unlike other such bodily systems, it is largely dispensable.

ACTIONS OF EPINEPHRINE AND RELATED SUBSTANCES

Epinephrine apparently acts directly on all structures which are innervated by postganglionic adrenergic nerves of the sympathetic nervous system. In all cases

The Adrenal Medullæ

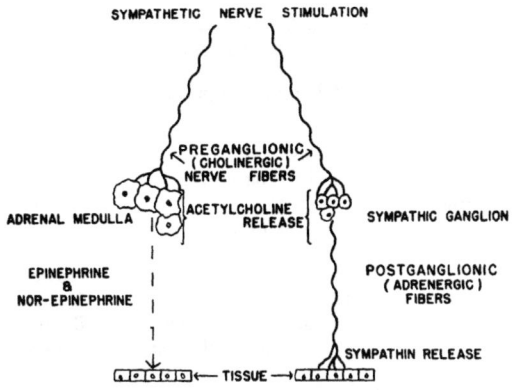

FIGURE IV—1. Effects of sympathetic nerve stimulation.

it has the same effect as does stimulation of these nerves, regardless of whether this effect is excitatory or inhibitory. Nor-epinephrine appears to act only on structures with excitatory innervation.[5]

Table 1 summarizes many of the effects of epinephrine. These may be commented upon briefly as follows.

Cardiovascular Effects. Administration of true epinephrine causes a rise in blood pressure by means of direct stimulation of cardiac output. In most areas, it causes vasodilatation though in the blood vessels of the skin it causes constriction. By contrast, nor-epinephrine appears to be predominantly an intensely vasoconstricting agent. It can thus intensify the hypertensive effects of true epinephrine. By itself it can also produce an elevation in blood pressure.

Epinephrine is apt to cause an acceleration in cardiac rate. Subsequently the rate may be slowed by reflexes set in motion by hypertension. Epinephrine may also cause cardiac arrhythmia, especially ventricular tachycardia. This may be followed by ventricular fibrillation and death. Light chloroform anesthesia favors the development of ventricular fibrillation in the presence of even small amounts of epinephrine.

Metabolic Effects. Important among these is the tendency of epinephrine to prompt hepatic glycogenolysis, with resultant elevation in blood glucose and potassium concentrations.* This reaction is of course contingent upon the presence of an adequate supply of glycogen in liver cells (see also under epinephrine tolerance test, Chapter IX). It can result either in a rise in blood sugar concentration from normal to supranormal levels or from subnormal to normal levels. The latter phenomenon may be in the nature of a bodily defense or homeostatic reaction, for it will be remembered that hypoglycemia is one of the con-

* Nor-epinephrine has only about one-eighth the hyperglycemic action of epinephrine.[1]

TABLE IV—1. Responses of effector organs to autonomic nerve impulses. From L. Goodman and A. Gilman, *The Pharmacological Basis of Therapeutics*, New York, Macmillan, 1941.

	Adrenergic impulses	Cholinergic impulses
Eye		
Iris	Mydriasis	Miosis
Ciliary muscle	Relaxed for far vision	Accommodated for near vision
Smooth muscle of orbit	Constricted; exophthalmos	—
Heart		
Rate	Accelerated	Slowed
Output	Increased	Decreased
Rhythm	Ventricular extrasystoles; tachycardia; fibrillation	Bradycardia; A-V block; vagal arrest
Blood vessels		
Coronary	Dilated	Constricted
Skin and mucosa	Constricted	Dilated
Muscle	Dilated	Dilated
Cerebral	Constricted	Dilated
Pulmonary	Constricted	Dilated
Abdominal viscera	Constricted	—
Lung		
Bronchial muscle	Dilated	Constricted
Bronchial glands	Inhibited?	Secretion increased
Stomach		
Motility and tone	Decreased	Increased
Sphincters	Contracted as a rule	Relaxed as a rule
Secretion	Inhibited?	Increased, particularly the organic constituents
Intestine		
Motility and tone	Decreased	Increased
Sphincters	Contracted as a rule	Relaxed as a rule
Secretions	Inhibited?	Increased
Gall bladder and ducts	Relaxed?	Contracted
Urinary bladder		
Detrusor	Relaxed	Contracted
Trigone and sphincter	Contracted	Relaxed
Ureter		
Motility and tone	Decreased	Increased
Uterus (human)		
Pregnant	Stimulated	Stimulated
Nonpregnant	Stimulated?	Variable
Skin		
Pilomotor muscles	Contracted	—
Sweat glands	Secretion (restricted)	Secretion (general) increased
Spleen capsule	Constricted	
Adrenal medulla	—	Secretion of epinephrine
Liver	Glycogenolysis	—
Pancreatic islets and acini	—	Secretion?
Salivary glands	Secretions (sparse, thick, mucinous)	Secretion (profuse, watery)
Lacrimal glands	—	Secretion increased
Nasopharyngeal glands	—	Secretion increased
Skeletal muscle	—	Stimulated
Autonomic ganglion cells	—	Stimulated

ditions which prompts endogenous liberation of epinephrine by the adrenal medullæ (see also Chapter III, Figures 22 and 23).

In addition to its effect upon hepatic glycogenolysis, epinephrine prompts a breakdown of muscle glycogen with formation and liberation into the blood stream of lactic acid. The circulating lactic acid in turn is converted into hepatic glycogen under the influence of insulin and possibly also adrenocortical S-F-N hormone.[6] Thus epinephrine prompts glycogenesis as well as glycogenolysis; the former may predominate over the latter action. When it does, it results in an over-all increase in hepatic glycogen stores.

Finally, epinephrine prompts a 20 to 80 per cent increase in oxygen consumption. This is not due to an increase in the rate of utilization of glucose, for epinephrine inhibits the oxidation of glucose.[2, 7] On the other hand, it may be explained by transformation of lactic acid to glycogen.

Effects on Other Endocrine Glands. As discussed in Chapter III, epinephrine causes release of adrenocorticotropic hormone (ACTH) by the anterior pituitary gland. Preliminary observations indicate that nor-epinephrine does not have this action.[8] Epinephrine also may prompt release of thyroid-stimulating hormone (TSH) by the anterior pituitary.[9]

ANTI-EPINEPHRINE OR ADRENOLYTIC SUBSTANCES

Histamine has many effects which are exactly contrary to those of epinephrine. Histamine, however, also stimulates the release of epinephrine from the medullæ. Ergotoxine, ergotamine and dibenamine directly prevent the excitatory but not the inhibitory effects of epinephrine upon body cells. They also prevent the effects of sympathetic nerve stimulation.[10, 11] Certain benzodioxane derivatives, including 2-piperidylmethyl-1, 4-benzodioxane (compound 933F)[10] appear to accelerate destruction of circulating epinephrine and thus to prevent epinephrine from reaching reactive end organs. They do not, however, prevent response of tissues to postganglionic adrenergic nerves (i.e., sympathin).

CLINICAL CONSIDERATIONS

HYPOEPINEPHRINISM DUE TO ADRENOMEDULLARY FAILURE

There is no clinical syndrome known to be due specifically to adrenomedullary failure. Possibly, the hypoglycemic unresponsiveness seen in certain patients with Addison's disease is due in part to destruction of the medullæ as well as the cortices of the adrenal glands (see Chapter III, Figure 25).

HYPEREPINEPHRINISM DUE TO ADRENOMEDULLARY TUMOR (PHEOCHROMOCYTOMA AND RELATED TUMORS)

Tumors of the adrenal medullæ or of paraganglia may be made up of any of the cell forms from which mature pheochromocytes develop. The more embryonal sympathogonioma and neuroblastoma are highly malignant and usually do not produce epinephrine. The commonest epinephrine-producing tumor is the pheochromocytoma. This is composed of relatively mature chromaffin cells. Approximately 10 per cent of such tumors are found to be malignant on histologic examination. Though local recurrence of pheochromocytoma has been described,[12] instances of death due to metastatic spread are rare. A somewhat less mature tumor, the pheochromoblastoma, also may produce epinephrine. This type of tumor is more malignant than the pheochromocytoma.

Approximately 10 per cent of pheochromocytomas arise outside the adrenal medullæ in one of the other collections of chromaffin tissue situated along the abdominal aorta or paravertebrally in the abdominal or pleural cavity.[13-15] Those tumors which occur in the adrenal medullæ are more often right- than left-sided. In approximately 10 per cent of such cases two tumors are found, either or both of which may be intra- or extra-adrenal. The pheochromocytomas have a wide range in size (10 to 2,000 gm.).[15]

Extracts of pheochromocytomas have been shown to contain an epinephrine-like substance by bio-assay, and epinephrine has been obtained from some tumors in pure crystalline form. By such means it has been estimated that pheochromocytomas may contain from 1 to 40 mg. of epinephrine per gm. of wet tissue weight. By contrast, the normal adrenal medullæ contain only about 0.4 mg. per gm. wet tissue weight.[15, 16] One tumor yielded 682 mg. of crystalline epinephrine[16] compared with the normal adult content of 8 to 10 mg. for both glands.

Recent studies on three pheochromocytomas have shown that 50 to 90 per cent of their epinephrine content was nor-epinephrine,[1] compared with 12 to 18 per cent nor-epinephrine obtained from extracts of cattle medullæ.[1] The relative amounts of these two substances produced by normal human adrenal medullæ is not known. This variability in the types of epinephrine produced by individual tumors may help to explain the pleomorphism of the clinical picture shown by individual patients.

CLINICAL MANIFESTATIONS. There are some excellent reviews of the classical manifestations of pheochromocytoma.[17, 18] Figure 2 summarizes the history and course of the disease in a child with pheochromocytoma. Table 2 lists most of the clinical manifestations of acute and chronic hyperepinephrinism as it has been observed in patients of all ages. It will be noted that for purposes of organ-

Continued on page 280

TABLE IV—2. Composite listing of various clinical manifestations of hyperepinephrinism which may be observed in patients of all ages.

		Per cent of incidence in patients of Table 3
A. *Factors initiating attacks:*	B. *Attack aura:*	
1. Emotional stress	1. Sensation of fear	—
2. Pain	2. Pain in heart	—
3. Exertion	3. Nausea	—
4. Meals	4. Usually none recorded	—
5. Changes in position		—
6. Usually none evident		—
C. *Ordinary manifestations of attack:*		
I. Central nervous system group:		
1. Severe pounding headache		50
3. Dilatation of pupils		9
3. Dizziness		9
4. Anxiety, nervousness, anxious appearance		45
5. Weakness or exhaustion		9
6. Somnolence		18
7. Cerebral hemorrhage		—
8. Manic episodes		9
II. Cardiovascular and vasomotor group:		
9. Hypertension (intermittent; normal between attacks)		36
10. Heart pounding		27
11. Heart pains; precordial oppression		27
12. Tachycardia (occasionally, bradycardia)		27
13. Dyspnea		27
14. Sweating (occasionally also polydipsia)		27
15. Pallor (sometimes acro cyanosis)		45
16. Cold extremities		36
17. Pain or tingling of fingers or toes		9
18. Pulmonary edema		9
19. Shock with or without death		9
III. Gastrointestinal group:		
20. Nausea, vomiting		36
21. Abdominal pain or distress		18
D. *Characteristics of termination of attack:*		
1. Subsidence of foregoing symptoms and signs		—
2. Flushing		—
3. Sweating		—
4. Sense of weakness or exhaustion		—
E. *Complications which may develop in the course of the disease:*		
1. Sustained hypertension		45
2. Eye changes		100
3. Cardiac enlargement, murmurs, failure		55
4. Renal function changes (usually mild to moderate)		9
5. Thyroid enlargement		36
6. Weight loss or failure to gain despite large appetite		27
7. Fever		18
F. *Conditions most commonly confused with hyperepinephrinism:*		
1. Anxiety neurosis or behavior problem	4. Thyrotoxicosis	—
	5. Rheumatic fever with heart disease	—
2. Essential hypertension		—
3. Primary chronic nephritis	6. Diabetes mellitus	—

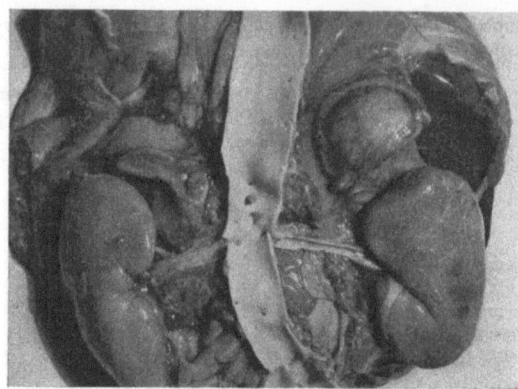

FIGURE IV—2. Pheochromocytoma in a child of six years.

CASE HISTORY

The patient was essentially well until he was 5½ years of age, when he developed a sore throat from which he failed to make a prompt recovery. His appetite decreased, and he appeared to be listless and irritable. At about the same time he began to have intermittent headaches and afternoon fever. During the ensuing three months he lost 12 pounds in weight and began to vomit, at first only after meals but later at other times. He also began to complain of cramp-like periumbilical pains. Laboratory studies revealed a trace of albumin in the urine and malrotation of the colon. His abdominal pain subsequently became so severe that he was given codein. A short time later he developed visual disturbances.

Upon admission to the Boston Children's Hospital at six years of age, he was found to be an emaciated child, measuring 112 cm. in height and weighing 13.5 kg. He appeared to have almost no subcutaneous fat. He perspired freely and complained of feeling hot and tired. The pupils of his eyes were moderately dilated. Examination of the optic fundi revealed papilledema, narrowing of the arterioles and nicking of the retinal veins. No hemorrhages or exudates were seen. The heart appeared to be of normal size, but the pulse rate was increased to 112 beats per minute and the blood pressure was elevated to 250/140 mm. Hg. The peripheral pulses were forceful, and the peripheral blood vessels appeared to be thickened. Upon examination of the abdomen, it was thought that the lower pole of the right kidney could be felt. The rest of the physical examination was not remarkable.

Routine examination of the blood and urine, as well as measurements of the serum sodium, chloride, phosphorus and protein yielded normal results. The urea clearance was found to be 148 per cent of normal. The erythrocyte sedimentation rate was 85 mm. per hour. Roentgenograms of the skull indicated separation of the sutures. Lumbar puncture yielded normal spinal fluid under an initial pressure of 275 mm. of water. Intravenous pyelograms showed the right kidney to be lower than the left. It was suspected that there might be an overlying right adrenal tumor.

Through an abdominal incision, bilateral adrenal exploration was carried out. The left gland was considered to be normal, and the surgeon was unable to make out any definite tumor in the right gland. However, in his operative notes, he remarked that exposure of

CASE HISTORY (continued)

the right gland had not been complete and that exploration of the adrenal glands through posterior incision would have been more satisfactory. Microscopic inspection of the appendix, which was removed at this operation, revealed extensive degenerative changes in the blood vessels. Postoperatively the patient's pulse rose to 170 and then gradually fell to about 120 beats per minute. His blood pressure, however, remained elevated at levels ranging from 180/145 to 160/125 mm. Hg. Great difficulty was encountered in the maintenance of a satisfactory state of hydration and nutrition. Abdominal pain of sufficient severity to require morphine medication continued. Within a few days the patient began to pass bloody stools and to show increased weakness, dehydration and cachexia. Death occurred two weeks after the operation. The clinical diagnosis was malignant hypertension.

At post-mortem examination no abnormalities of the adrenals could definitely be made out until a posterior incision was made. It was then evident that the right gland contained an abnormal mass and that it was of firmer texture than the left gland. Upon dissection the right gland was found to weigh 12 gm. and the left to weigh 3 gm., an approximately normal value. Further inspection revealed a sizable tumor nodule in the right medulla and another much smaller nodule measuring only 5 mm. in diameter in the left medulla. The tumors were chiefly composed of chromophilic adrenomedullary cells. A few cells resembling those seen in the cortices were also found. No mitotic figures were evident. The cortices were intact, though that on the right was considerably thinned as a result of the adjacent tumor. Other pathologic findings included cardiac enlargement with left ventricular hypertrophy and extensive degenerative vascular disease. This was of pronounced degree in the spleen and also in the ilium, where it had led to marked ulceration and suppuration of the mucosa. The kidneys showed only minimal vascular changes. No evidence of true arteriolar sclerosis was found. The microscopic diagnoses were therefore (a) pheochromocytoma and (b) necrotizing obliterating endarteritis.

We are indebted to Dr. S. Farber for the opportunity to reproduce the photograph and summary of this case.

ization this table has been divided arbitrarily into various sections and subsections. Tables 3 and 4 set forth the findings obtained on a series of 11 children with hyperepinephrinism as recorded in the recent literature. These children, taken as a group, showed most of the symptoms and signs listed in Table 2 but individual children had individually characteristic symptom-sign patterns (see Table 3, column 6).

All patients with epinephrine-producing adrenomedullary tumors have hypertension. In some the hypertension is more or less evenly sustained from the onset of the disease. In others, during the early stages attacks of hypertension alternate with normotensive periods. The incidence of such hypertensive episodes is quite variable, ranging from once a month to several times a day. Even in individual patients there may be no regular periodicity in the rate of occurrence. However, attacks are apt to increase in frequency as the disease progresses until sustained hypertension with or without superimposed attacks develops.

About 50 per cent of the patients of Table 3 had severe headaches, excess perspiration (especially over the upper half of the body) and a sense of apprehension or nervousness. One-third of them complained of nausea and vomiting. Another third failed to gain weight or lost weight despite a ravenous appetite. Coldness and pallor or bluish discoloration of the extremities were noted occasionally. During attacks heart action was described as being very forceful and either rapid or slow. Extra systoles were sometimes noted. Electrocardiograms yielded abnormal, but non-specific results. About half the patients had either cardiac enlargement, with a loud, usually systolic murmur or other evidence of cardiac embarrassment. Table 4 summarizes the findings in the optic fundus and shows that all the children had some retinal manifestations of the disease.

The various recorded laboratory studies are of interest in several respects. Tests of renal function indicated that the kidneys were less markedly involved than is often the case in patients with hypertension primarily renal in origin. There was a tendency to marked elevation in the basal metabolic rate (BMR). The serum protein-bound iodine (PBI) concentration was low normal in the one instance so studied, and the radio-active iodine uptake (RaI) by the thyroid gland was normal rather than increased in another. In the former patient potassium iodide (KI) therapy had no beneficial effect. These observations suggest that the hypermetabolism was not associated with or due to hyperthyroidism.

While hyperglycemia was sometimes present during attacks, this was not a common finding. Blood sugar values were usually normal or only slightly elevated between attacks. On the other hand, patients having a diabetic type of glucose tolerance curve and a clinical picture suggestive of diabetes mellitus are described in the literature.[19, 20]

DIAGNOSIS. This condition is suggested particularly when hypertension, excess sweating in association with sporadic evidences of vasoconstriction, fever, tachycardia and eyeground changes occur together. The occurrence of even a slight fall in systolic and diastolic blood pressure when the patient assumes an erect position is suggestive of pheochromocytoma. Excess sweating is not noted in patients with essential or malignant hypertension. Vasoconstriction is evidenced by coldness of the hands and feet, blanching of the fingers and bluish red mottling of the legs or hands. In severe and prolonged attacks the peripheral pulse may disappear entirely. Fever of 1°F. or more is observable in over 70 per cent of all patients with this disease.* In some the temperature rises to levels as high as 105°F. In suspicious cases frequent rectal temperature recordings over a period of 48 hours may be of considerable diagnostic value. The fever is not necessarily related to paroxysmal symptoms. The eyeground pathology is most commonly manifested by blood vessel changes.

As Table 3, column 3, suggests, the significance of these manifestations was not suspected early, since the majority of these patients had had the disease for two or more years before definitive action was taken.

DIFFERENTIAL DIAGNOSIS. This condition may be confused easily with malignant hypertension of renal, adrenocortical or unknown origin. It also may be confused with episodes of transient hypertension occurring in healthy hyperreactive individuals under circumstances of emotional stress and strain. Like other fundamentally normal persons, they do not have cardiac abnormalities or eyeground changes.

Other conditions to be differentiated are thyrotoxicosis, rheumatic fever with heart disease and diabetes mellitus. Patients with thyrotoxicosis can present a difficult diagnostic problem, for they, like patients with chronic hyperepinephrinism, have markedly elevated basal metabolic rates, tendency to weight loss despite large dietary intake and nervous dispositions. However, in contrast to patients with adrenomedullary tumors, thyrotoxic patients rarely have eyeground changes suggestive of hypertensive retinopathy and usually have a warm and flushed rather than a cold, cyanotic, sweaty type of skin. The differentiation is made by applying such a specific test of thyroid status as the serum proteinbound iodine measurement or by giving potassium iodide therapy. A definitely favorable response to such therapy is strong evidence in favor of a diagnosis of thyrotoxicosis and against a diagnosis of hyperepinephrinism.

An erroneous diagnosis of rheumatic fever with heart disease has been made

* The value indicated here is higher than that shown in Table 2. The discrepancy may be due to the fact that fever is not always recognized unless the temperature is taken frequently.

TABLE IV—3. Summary of observations on 11 patients with adrenomedullary tumors.

Case no.	Age, years	Duration of symptoms, years	Sex	Intermittent attacks	Signs and symptoms (See Table 2)	Blood pressure, mm. Hg
1	10	½	M	none	C 1, 5, 6, 14 E 1, 2	210 to 265 systolic
See T. Esperson et al., Acta chir. Scandinav. 94: 271, 1946						
2	11	1½?	M	daily	C 1, 4, 8, 14, 15, 16 E 1, 2, 3	260/210 With attacks Systolic > 300
See C. H. Snyder et al., Am. J. Dis. Child. 73: 581, 1947 (Case 1)						
3	11	3	F	yes	C 1, 4, 9, 14, 16, 20 E 1, 2, 3	200/140
See C. H. Snyder et al., op. cit. (Case 3)						
4	11	3	M	yes	C 1, 9, 10, 14, 15, 20, 21 E 2, 7	260/190
See M. Goldenberg et al., J. A. M. A. 135: 971, 1947 (Case 8); and G. F. Cahill, ibid. 138: 180, 1948 (Case 3)						
5	12	2	F	none	C 4, 12, 14 E 1, 2, 5 Thought to have thyrotoxicosis	180/120 to 240/170
See C. H. Snyder, op. cit. (Case 2); Goldenberg, op. cit. (Case 11); Cahill, op. cit. (Case 11)						
6	12	4?	F	daily	C 2, 3, 11, 12, 14, 15, 19; E 1, 2, 5	285/230
See V. L. Evans, J. Lab. and Clin. Med. 22: 1117, 1936-37						
7	14	6?	F	none	C 10, 11, 13 E 1, 2, 3, 4, 6	at 8 yr. 95/60 at 11 yr. 130/100 at 13 yr. 170/100 at 14 yr. 200/150
See D. N. Kremer, Arch. Int. Med. 57: 999, 1936						
8	16	½	M	yes	C 1, 6, 9, 11, 13, 14, 15, 16, 18, 20, 21; E 2, 3	200/100 to 300/140
See F. A. Coller, et al., Arch. Surg. 28: 1136, 1934						
9	17	¼ ?	F	frequent	C1, 4, 10, 15, 17 E 1, 2, 3, 6	220/125
See A. Hyman, et al., J. Urol. 49: 755, 1943						
10	17	2	F	yes	C 9, 20 E 2, 5, 6	300/200
See E. J. Holst, Acta Med. Scandinav. 94: 510, 1938						
11	17	short	F	none	C 4, 12, 13, 14, 16 E 1, 2, 3, 5, 7	190/140
See New Eng. J. Med., 235: 906, 1946 (Cabot case, MGH)						

TABLE IV—3 (continued)

Laboratory studies	Special tests	Operations	End result	Adrenomedullary tumors
Urea clearance normal	IVP normal	Left adrenal explored; no tumor found	Died 6 mo. postoperatively	Malignant left, invading veins
Urea clearance 56% Urine normal; BMR +9, −1%	IVP: tumor above right kidney	Removal of right tumor	Died 2½ hr. postoperatively	1 on right
Urine normal; BMR +67, +48% RaI uptake normal	IVP normal 933 F. test positive	Attempted removal of right tumors	Died during operation	2 on right
Urine normal	IVP: right kidney small, poor funct. 933 F. test positive	Removal of right tumor	Successful	1 on right?
Albuminuria; BMR +47, +67% X-ray: calcification of left adrenal; PBI 4.8 = μg.% No response to KI therapy	933 F. test positive	Removal of left tumor; later of pre-aortic tumor	Successful	2
Blood urea N 50 mg.% Albuminuria PSP 65% in 2 hr. BMR +60%	None	None	Died in shock during attack	1 on left
Albuminuria; cylindruria PSP 35% in 2 hr. BMR +34 at 8 yr.	None	None	Died of acute heart failure	Bilateral
Albuminuria; cylindruria PSP 52% in 2 hr.	Amyl nitrate caused marked fall B P	Removal at second attempt	Successful	1 on left
BMR −1%	No B P response to cold pressor test	Removal of left tumor	Successful	1 on left
Glycosuria; albuminuria BMR +30%	IVP: abnormal left kidney	Attempted removal	Died when tumor blood vessel was clamped	Weight, 280 gm. ?
BMR +69, +79% RaI uptake normal PBI normal NPN normal	None		Died during cecostomy	1 on left Weight, 420 gm.

TABLE IV—4. Eye manifestations of children of Table 3.

Case no.	Blood vessel changes	Exudates	Hemorrhages	Papilledema	Atrophy of optic discs	Comments
1						Hypertensive retinopathy
2	+?	+	+	bilateral +		Large blind spots, scotomata, eyes prominent
3	+			0		Pupils not dilated
4	+	+	+	+		—
5				+		Vision decreased
6	+	+		+		—
7			+	+	+	Nephritic retinitis, atrophy of retina
8	+		+			—
9	+					—
10						Moderate retinal changes
11	+					—

more than once in patients with adrenomedullary tumor. Actually, though there may be fever, cardiac enlargement and cardiac murmurs in both conditions, it should not be difficult to distinguish between them when their respective characteristics are considered as a whole.

Diabetes mellitus may present a rare, but interesting differential diagnostic problem, for in this condition, also, renal impairment, hypertension and eyeground changes can occur as late complications. On the other hand, it is most uncommon to see episodes of hypertension, tachycardia and sweating early in the course of juvenile diabetes. This combination, plus widely fluctuating insulin requirements, should suggest the possibility of adrenomedullary tumor.

DIAGNOSTIC PROCEDURES. There is no entirely reliable and safe diagnostic test for determining the presence of an epinephrine-producing adrenomedullary tumor. As often is the case under such circumstances, the literature is replete with papers suggesting various methods of approach. Of the tests reported, the following appear most worthy of specific mention:

*The histamine test.** This test is used to induce an attack in patients who give a history suggestive of previous episodes of acute hyperepinephrinism, but who

---

* This test is performed as follows: The patient is placed in a bed. A slow intravenous infusion of saline is administered by means of an apparatus of the ordinary "drip bulb" type which has a three-way stopcock incorporated into the rubber tubing between the "drip bulb" and intravenous needle. With the drip running, the patient's pulse and blood pressure are measured at five-minute intervals for 30 minutes or until they have become reasonably steady. A test dose of histamine base (0.015 to 0.030 mg. per m^2) in a small volume of saline is then given through the three-way stopcock. The pulse and blood pressure are now measured at one-minute intervals and the patient's subjective sensations are noted. The action of histamine on the blood pressure is prompt and of short duration (i.e., ±10 minutes).[21]

are found at the time of examination to be normotensive and free from definite signs of adrenomedullary tumor.* Histamine is used because it directly stimulates release of epinephrine from adrenomedullary tissue.

When pheochromocytoma is present, the epinephrine thus released is apt to induce a marked and at times alarming increase in blood pressure. This is accompanied by various other of the manifestations of epinephrine action. Consequently, the patient is likely to say that he is having an "attack." Very occasionally, as in spontaneous episodes, the artificially induced attack is complicated by the occurrence of cerebral hemorrhage or pulmonary edema.

Hypertension caused by a sudden, excessive release of epinephrine in response to histamine can usually be controlled promptly by the administration of benzodioxane (see next section). This fact has both therapeutic and diagnostic importance.

In contrast to the foregoing, individuals who do not have an adrenomedullary tumor are apt to show a fall in blood pressure. There also may be such other evidences of histamine action as generalized vasodilatation with flushing of the skin, headache (due to transitory intracranial hypertension), visual disturbances, bronchial constriction and dyspnea and, in cases of severe toxic reaction, shock. Fortunately, serious toxic reactions to histamine are rare. They can be counteracted by the prompt administration of epinephrine (0.3 mg. per m^2 intramuscularly).

The benzodioxane test. This test is employed in patients who have sustained hypertension and symptoms suggestive of hyperepinephrinism. It is based on the fact that drugs with adrenolytic properties are apt to prompt a fall in the blood pressure of hypertensive patients when the hypertension is due to hyperepinephrinism. This agent has been used successfully to prevent and to eliminate hypertension secondary to the administration of histamine in patients with pheochromocytoma.

Piperidylmethyl benzodioxane (933F) is the most widely used member of this group of drugs.[22] This drug is administered intravenously as described above for histamine. The dose used is about 10 mg. per m^2, an amount considerably below that tolerated by normal individuals; the material is made up in a 1 or 2 per cent solution in saline. Administration of the dose requires about two minutes. A considerable fall (i.e., 50 to 70 mm. Hg) in systolic and diastolic pressures within about 15 minutes is considered suggestive of hyperepinephrinism. For a more detailed discussion of this test and of ways to evaluate blood pressure changes, the reader is urged to read the references.[22, 23]

* Histamine also may prompt an attack in patients with chronic hypertension due to pheochromocytoma.

Unfortunately, this test is neither entirely reliable nor free from danger. There have been failures to obtain a positive response in patients who subsequently were shown at operation to have an adrenomedullary tumor. Moreover, occasional patients with essential hypertension suffer to an alarming degree from central nervous system stimulation when given the drug. This is manifested by extreme agitation and a tendency to increased hypertension. Other possible manifestations are tachycardia, flushing, headache and dizziness.[22, 24] There is no specific treatment for such episodes. The untoward manifestations subside spontaneously.

Other diagnostic procedures. The presence of a tumor along the vertebral column or in the region of the adrenals is sometimes demonstrable in appropriate roentgenograms. Intravenous pyelography may aid in this regard by indicating displacement of one or both kidneys by an adjacent tumor mass. Insufflation of air into the perirenal spaces has been tried without altogether satisfactory results as regards diagnosis and with accidental fatality in at least one case.[25] Thorough surgical exposure of the adrenals still constitutes the most reliable diagnostic procedure. It is essential that a diagnostic exploration be as complete as possible, for adrenomedullary tumors have been missed at operation. The previously mentioned possibility of extra-adrenal pheochromocytomas also should be borne in mind.

TREATMENT. The condition is treated by surgical extirpation of the tumor (or tumors). A variety of steps have been taken by various surgeons in an attempt to lessen the intra- and postoperative hazards of this procedure. Development of marked hypertension during the induction of anesthesia or while manipulating the tumor constitutes one of the most common hazards. Contrariwise, when the tumor is removed, there may be a sharp fall in blood pressure, collapse and shock. Unfortunately, the factors responsible for the latter phenomena are not well understood. Consequently, they must be treated largely on an empirical, symptomatic basis. Attempts to sustain the circulation and blood pressure by administering true epinephrine intravenously have not always been successful. Possibly, the administration of nor-epinephrine will be more effective.* Adrenocortical extract therapy has been of equivocal value.[26, 27]

PROGNOSIS. Unfortunately, the operative hazards discussed above often interfere with the successful removal of a pheochromocytoma. Of the 11 children considered in Table 3, the correct diagnosis was made in the case of nine. One of the nine was so ill that she died before surgical intervention could be carried out. An operation was performed in the case of eight of the children. Of these

* Nor-epinephrine is available on a study basis under the name "Levophen."

four died during the procedure or during the immediate postoperative period. Successful removal of the tumor in the other four cases was followed by marked improvement. With complete elimination of hyperepinephrinism, the hypertension, optic fundus and other changes tend to disappear or to be considerably ameliorated.

In cases where hyperepinephrinism persists, the prognosis is very poor. Death may occur during an acute episode of epinephrine discharge as a consequence of cardiovascular failure, acute cerebral hemorrhage or other major vascular accident. Pending such fatal complications the patient tends to show progressive arteriosclerotic or degenerative changes in the eyes, heart, kidneys and other organs.

THE PHARMACOLOGY OF EPINEPHRINE[10]

USP PREPARATIONS

The USP does not specify which proportion of epinephrine (the levorotatory form of methyl-aminoethanolcatechol) may be obtained from the adrenal medullæ of domestic animals and which may be prepared synthetically. The most commonly used preparation is a 1:1,000 aqueous solution of epinephrine hydrochloride prepared for parenteral administration. This material gradually turns dark on exposure to air and light and deteriorates in a few hours when diluted. Accordingly, when a preparation of reasonably standard potency is desired, it is well to open a hermetically sealed vial containing 1 cc. of the concentrate. Epinephrine is also obtainable in an oily solution (0.2 per cent concentration) for intramuscular injection when prolonged systemic effects are desired. Finally, epinephrine is obtainable as a solution of epinephrine hydrochloride 1:100 (NNR). This is not intended for a parenteral injection but for inhalation in asthma.

COMMENTS ON THE THERAPEUTIC USE OF EPINEPHRINE[10]

When epinephrine is given parenterally, the usual route is subcutaneous. If the aqueous solution is used, the dose per m^2 ranges from 0.1 to 0.3 mg. (0.1 to 0.3 cc.); if the oily solution is used, from 0.9 to 1.8 mg. (0.45 to 0.9 cc.). Thus administered the drug is destroyed in the body within a few minutes after it reaches the blood stream. The site of destruction is not known.

Epinephrine is not effective when given orally.

In Control of Hemorrhage. The drug is used in concentrations of 1:2,000 to 1:50,000 and applied directly to accessible bleeding surfaces. It is effective only against bleeding from smaller arterioles and capillaries.

For Congestion of Nasal Mucosa and Conjunctiva. Epinephrine causes marked vasoconstriction and blanching when its solutions are applied to the nasal mucosa and conjunctiva.

For Bronchial Asthma. Epinephrine is found of great value in the symptomatic treatment of bronchial asthma. It should, however, be reserved for the relief of acute paroxysms, because a patient may develop tolerance for the substance if it is given frequently. During an acute attack a dose may have to be repeated at 10 or 15 minute intervals until relief is obtained.

In Miscellaneous Disorders. Epinephrine often affords symptomatic relief in patients with violent urticarial serum reaction, serum sickness, angioneurotic edema and hay fever.

It is of doubtful value in the treatment of shock and in the management of patients suffering from heart block or acute cardiac failure. In the case of patients suffering from hypertension or other organic cardiovascular lesions it should be used with caution. When dealing with syncopal attacks, it is important to make sure that they are due to periods of asystole or marked bradycardia rather than to short runs of abnormal ventricular rhythms, since, in the latter instance, epinephrine may precipitate fatal ventricular fibrillation.

Epinephrine is rarely effective in reviving patients who appear to be dead as a result of drowning, electric shock, anesthesia or the like. The explanation may be that the arrested heart is beyond resuscitation or that intravenously or intracardially administered epinephrine precipitates ventricular fibrillation.

REFERENCES

1. GOLDENBERG, M., FABER, M., ALSTON, E. J. and CHARGAFF, E. C. Evidence for the occurrence of nor-epinephrine in the adrenal medulla. *Science* 109:534, 1949.
2. CORI, C. F. and WELCH, A. D. The adrenal medulla. In *Glandular Physiology and Therapy*. Chicago, A. M. A., 1942.
3. CAMP, W. J. R. and HIGGINS, J. A. The role of potassium in epinephrine action. *J. Pharmacol. & Exper. Therap.* 57:376, 1936.
4. CANNON, W. B. *Bodily Changes in Pain, Hunger, Fear and Rage*. New York, Appleton, 1915.
5. GOLDENBERG, M., PINES, K. L., BALDWIN, E. DE F., GREENE, D. G. and ROH, C. F. The hemodynamic response of man to nor-epinephrine and epinephrine and its relation to the problem of hypertension. *Am. J. Med.* 5:792, 1948.
6. LONG, C. N. H., KATZIN, B. and FRY, E. G. The adrenal cortex and carbohydrate metabolism. *Endocrinology* 26:309, 1940.
7. CORI, C. F. Mammalian carbohydrate metabolism. *Physiol. Rev.* 11:143, 1931.

8   THORN, G. W., BOYLES, T. B., MASSELL, B. F., FORSHAM, P. H., HILL, S. R., JR., SMITH, S., III and WARREN, J. E. Medical progress: studies on the relation of pituitary-adrenal function to rheumatic disease. *New Eng. J. Med.* 241:529, 1949.

9   SOFFER, L. J., VOLTERRA, M., GABRILOVE, L., POLLACK, A. and JACOBS, M. The effect of iodine and adrenalin administration on circulating thyrotropic factor. *J. Clin. Invest.* 26:1197, 1947.

10 GOODMAN, L. S. and GILMAN, A. *The Pharmacological Basis of Therapeutics.* New York, Macmillan, 1941.

11 NICKERSON, M. and GOODMAN, L. S. Pharmacological properties of a new adrenergic blocking agent; N, N-dibenzyl-B-chlorothylamine (dibenamine). *J. Pharmacol. & Exper. Therap.* 89:167, 1947.

12 CALKINS, E. and HOWARD, J. E. Bilateral familial pheochromocytomata with paroxysmal hypertension; successful surgical removal of tumors in two cases, with discussion of certain diagnostic procedures and physiological considerations. *J. Clin. Endocrinol.* 7:475, 1947.

13 BISKIND, G. R., MEYER, M. A. and BEADNER, S. A. Adrenal medullary tumor. *J. Clin. Endocrinol.* 1:113, 1941.

14 PHILIPS, B. Intrathoracic pheochromocytoma. *Arch. Path.* 30:916, 1940.

15 KIRSHBAUM, J. D. and BALKIN, R. B. Adrenalin-producing pheochromocytoma of the adrenal associated with hypertension. *Ann. Surg.* 116:54, 1942.

16 KVALE, W. F., ROTH, G. M., CLAGETT, O. T. and DOCKERTY, M. B. Headache and paroxysmal hypertension; observations before and after the surgical removal of pheochromocytoma. *S. Clin. North America* 24:922, 1944.

17 HOWARD, J. E. and BARKER, W. H. Paroxysmal hypertension and other clinical manifestations associated with benign chromaffin cell tumors (pheochromocytomata). *Bull. Johns Hopkins Hosp.* 61:371, 1937.

18 (a) MAC KEITH, R. Adrenal sympathetic syndrome. *Brit. Heart J.* 6:1, 1944.
   (b) SMITHWICK, R. H., GREER, W. E. R., ROBERTSON, C. W. and WILKINS, R. W. Pheochromocytoma: a discussion of symptoms, signs and procedures of diagnostic value. *New Eng. J. Med.* 242:252, 1950.

19 DUNCAN, L. E., JR., SEMANS, J. H. and HOWARD, J. E. Adrenal medullary tumor (pheochromocytoma) and diabetes mellitus; disappearance of diabetes after removal of the tumor. *Ann. Int. Med.* 20:815, 1944.

20 GOLDNER, M. G. Pheochromocytoma with diabetes. *J. Clin. Endocrinol.* 7:716, 1947.

21 ROTH, G. M. and KVALE, W. F. A tentative test for pheochromocytoma. *Am. J. M. Sc.* 210:653, 1940.

22 GOLDENBERG, M., SNYDER, C. H. and ARANOW, H. New test for hypertension due to circulating epinephrine. *J. A. M. A.* 135:971, 1947.

23 ROTH, G. M. and KVALE, W. F. Pharmacologic tests as an aid in diagnosis of pheochromocytoma. *Mod. Concepts Cardiovas. Dis.* 18:41, 1949.

24 DRILL, V. A. Reactions from the use of benzodioxone (933F) in diagnosis of pheochromocytoma. *New Eng. J. Med.* 241:777, 1949.

25 WEYRAUCH, H. M., JR. Death from air embolism following perirenal insufflation. *J. A. M. A.* 114:652, 1940.

26 THORN, G. W., HINDLE, J. A. and SANDEMEYER, J. A. Pheochromocytoma of the adrenal associated with persistent hypertension. *Ann. Int. Med.* 21:122, 1944.

27 HATCH, F. N., RICHARDS, V. and SPIEGL, R. J. Adrenal medullary tumor (pheochromocytoma). *Am. J. Med.* 6:633, 1949.

THE OVARIES

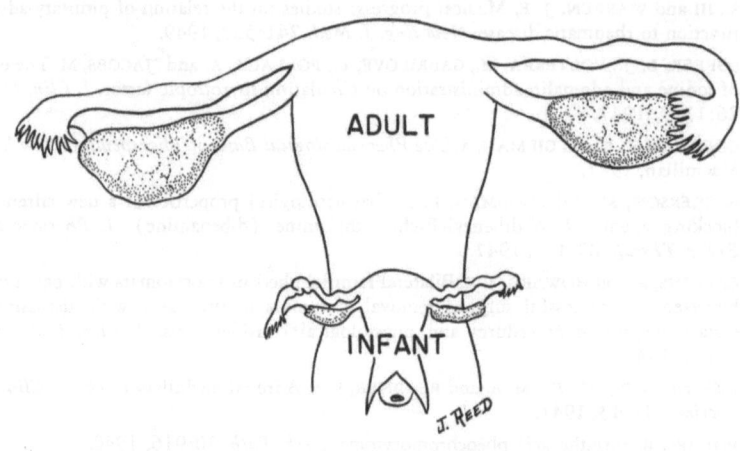

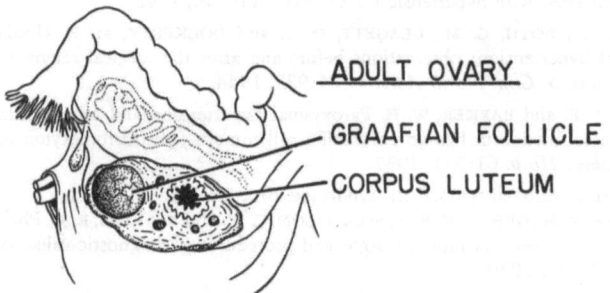

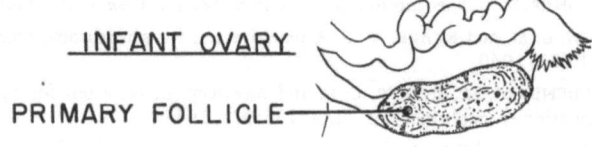

CHAPTER V

THE OVARIES

BASIC CONSIDERATIONS

GENERAL FUNCTIONS OF THE OVARIES

The ovaries perform two separate but interrelated functions: (1) the production and release of ova and (2) the elaboration of hormones concerned with (a) the development and maintenance of the accessory genital organs and secondary sex characters and (b) the provision of an environment suitable for the growth of ova which have been fertilized.

GENETIC AND HORMONAL INFLUENCES IN SEX DETERMINATION

The type of gonad, and therefore the ultimate sex, of the individual is determined primarily by the sex chromosomes at the instant of conjugation of the parental ovum and spermatozoon. However, genetic influences alone cannot bring the infantile sex organs to full anatomic and physiologic maturity. This is only accomplished by the end of puberty, under the influence of the gonadal hormones.[1a] In the case of the female, these hormones are estrogen and progesterone.[1b-f] They are produced in the ovary by definite anatomic structures, the follicle and the corpus luteum.

EMBRYOLOGY, ANATOMY AND GENERAL PHYSIOLOGY OF THE OVARIES

Embryology. The ovaries arise from strips of thickened cœlomic epithelium, the genital ridges, on the ventro-mesial aspect of the mesonephros. The female genital ducts develop from the embryonic Müllerian ducts, which grow backward to parallel the nearby mesonephric ducts. Caudally, the two Müllerian ducts fuse to form a terminal unpaired tube, which ends in the urogenital sinus. The paired upper portions become the Fallopian tubes, while the fused terminal portion becomes the uterus and upper vagina. The lowermost portion of the vagina is derived from the urogenital sinus.

Anatomy and General Physiology. Structurally, each ovary consists of a collection of germ cells embedded in a connective tissue framework. In late fetal life each germ cell has become inclosed in an ovisac composed of one or more layers of cells. The entire mass of ovum plus ovisac is called a follicle and constitutes the unit of organization of the ovary. Estimates of the number of ova present in the ovaries at birth vary from 70,000 to 400,000. In the 30 years which constitute the period of active sexual life of the human female, only about 400 ova undergo full maturation and expulsion from the ovary. The remainder of the original follicles degenerate and disappear by a process known as atresia. Atresia begins during intra-uterine life, becomes very rapid during childhood, continues at a lessened rate during the period of active sexual life and is completed after the menopause. The postmenopausal ovary is totally devoid of follicles, consisting merely of follicular remnants and fibrous scars.

Oogenesis and follicular growth. As a primitive follicle develops, it migrates from its original position beneath the tunica albuginea toward the interior of the ovary. Cells surrounding the ovum, the so-called granulosa cells, undergo proliferation, and later a crescentic cavity, or antrum, is created on one side of the follicle by liquefaction of a portion of the granulosa cells. A clear serous fluid, the liquor folliculi, accumulates in the antrum and slowly distends the follicle to preovulatory size. The ovum undergoes partial maturation with reduction in the number of chromosomes and extrusion of the first polar body. Concomitantly, the connective tissue surrounding the follicle becomes differentiated into the so-called theca interna and theca externa. The theca interna, which is contiguous to the granulosa layer, becomes rich in epithelioid cells and capillaries. These epithelioid cells are thought to be the source of the estrogenic hormone, which is slowly secreted into the liquor folliculi after the follicle has achieved the requisite development. The theca externa becomes a fibrous supporting structure.

Ovulation and corpus luteum formation. When the follicle has attained a diameter of 0.5 cm., it alters the direction of its migration and begins to move toward the periphery. By the time the follicle has enlarged to a diameter of 1.0 to 1.5 cm., it has reached the surface of the ovary and has begun to protrude. Rupture of the wall follows, and the ovum is discharged into the abdominal cavity for conveyance to the uterus via the Fallopian tube. In the meantime, the collapsed follicle undergoes rapid transformation into the corpus luteum. Thus,

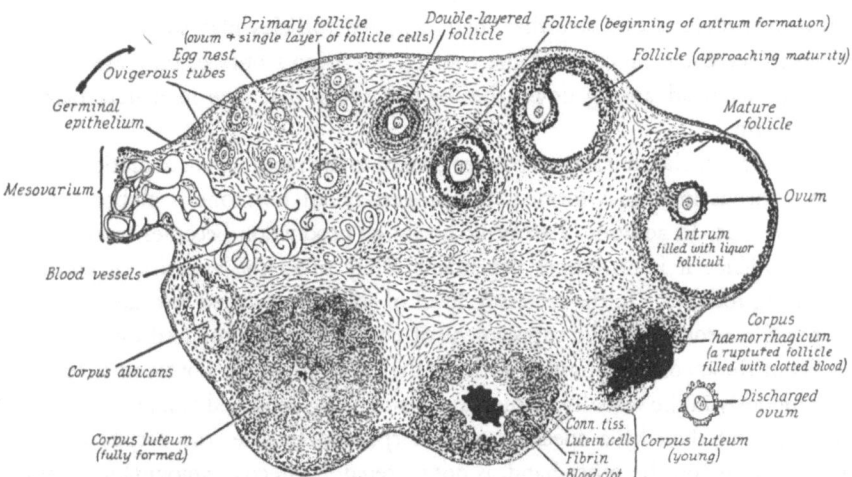

FIGURE V—1. Schematic diagram of a mammalian ovary showing, in a clockwise direction, the sequence of events in the origin, growth and rupture of the ovarian follicle and the formation and retrogression of a corpus luteum. From B. M. Patton, *Embryology of the Pig*. Philadelphia, Blakiston, 1927.

the corpus luteum is not an entirely new structure, but simply an altered follicle which has entered a new phase of its life. The theca interna undergoes rapid proliferation and furnishes a rich blood supply to the granulosa cells, which are transformed into granulosa lutein cells. These cells enlarge and acquire fat and pigment. If properly stimulated (see below), the granulosa lutein cells elaborate the estrogenic hormone and, in addition, the characteristic corpus luteum hormone, progesterone. The subsequent course of the corpus luteum depends upon the fate of the ovum. If the ovum is fertilized, the corpus luteum persists until approximately the fourth month of gestation as the corpus luteum of pregnancy. If conception does not occur, the corpus luteum begins to regress between the eighth and the tenth day after follicular rupture. Hyalinization ultimately reduces the corpus luteum to the scarlike corpus albicans. The normal sequence of these physiological processes is shown diagrammatically in Figure 1.

Partial follicular maturation may precede atresia even in the immature organism; sporadic follicles may develop sufficiently to produce small quantities of estrogen. As the individual matures, crops of follicles begin to undergo more advanced development and to manifest this development at increasingly regular intervals. Normally, all of the follicles in a given group except the one destined to ovulate undergo atresia at some point in their development. The physiological contribution made by the follicles which undergo atresia is poorly understood.

However, there is evidence that these blighted follicles play some part in the internal secretory function of the ovaries. In Allen's phrase, they are "like a football team advancing down the field in order that one man may make a touchdown."

When follicular maturation has progressed to the point where ovulation occurs and a corpus luteum is formed, the progestational hormone is elaborated for the first time. In addition, estrogenic hormone production becomes more nearly cyclical, since it is no longer dependent solely upon the vagaries of partially maturing follicles. On the teetering level of follicle-produced estrogen is superimposed a strong periodic supplement of corpus-luteum-produced estrogen.

From these considerations it follows that the estrogenic hormone is formed continuously in the sexually mature organism, being produced first by developing follicles and then by a specially metamorphosed follicle, the corpus luteum. Progesterone, on the other hand, is not secreted in effective amounts until after ovulation. While there is evidence to suggest that a small quantity is produced by the luteinized theca, the corpus luteum is ordinarily the only significant source.

Estrus and menstrual cycles. The intervals determined by the ovarian changes of the mature organism are called estrus cycles in subprimate mammalian species and menstrual cycles in primates. In subprimate species, the most obvious indication of a reproductive cycle is a recurrent increase in sexual desire, called heat or estrus. Estrus reflects the attainment of maximal proliferation of the epithelium of the accessory sexual organs and occurs when the rate of hormone production by the maturing follicle is also maximal. Hence, the follicular hormone is called the estrogenic hormone. In both estrus and menstrual cycles proliferation and regression of the epithelium of the accessory sexual organs occur as consequences of alternately increasing and decreasing stimulation by the ovarian hormones. In primates proliferation is not signalized by a clearly recognizable period of heat; the most conspicuous phenomenon, menstruation, is a dramatic accentuation of the stage of regression. The differences between the various components of the estrus and menstrual cycles are more quantitative than qualitative, and if both types of cycles be divided into pre- and postovulatory phases, their fundamental similarity becomes apparent.

Pituitary control of the ovary. From the foregoing it should not be inferred that the ovaries enjoy any large measure of physiologic autonomy. For both the initiation and regulation of their varied functional activities, the gonads are almost completely dependent upon hormones secreted by the anterior lobe of the pituitary gland. Primordial ovarian follicles are capable of progressing to the antrum stage without pituitary assistance. However, for complete maturation of the follicle, ovulation, formation of the corpus luteum and elaboration of the follicular and luteal hormones, stimulation by the pituitary gonadotropic hormones is essential.

The pituitary gonadotropins. Three distinct protein hormones possessing gonadotropic activity are thought to be secreted by the hypophysis: follicle-stimulating hormone (FSH), luteinizing hormone.(LH)* and luteotropin, a factor which, in all probability, is identical with the lactogenic hormone. All three of these hormones have been isolated from animal pituitaries in essentially pure form. Gross gonadotropic activity can also be demonstrated in human body fluids, although clinical assay methods capable of distinguishing between the various gonadotropic hormones do not yet exist. Gonadotropins are continuously detectable in the urine of adult men and women.† In women, cyclic variations occur in the levels of gonadotropin excretion, the greatest amounts usually appearing during midcycle, just before or contemporaneous with the peak of estrogen production.

Physiologic effects of the gonadotropins. The effects of the various gonadotropic hormones upon the human ovary cannot be stated with precision. However, the action of the gonadotropic factors upon the ovaries of rodents has been studied in great detail. It is presumed that similar hypophyseal-ovarian relationships obtain in the human being. In rodents, administration of FSH causes the follicle to progress from the antrum to the preovulatory stage without producing hormones. If a small amount of LH is injected in addition to FSH, the follicle is stimulated to further growth and to the production of the estrogenic hormone. If larger amounts of LH are given together with FSH, ovulation is induced and the formation of a non-functioning corpus luteum occurs. If luteotropin is administered, the corpus luteum can be maintained for a time and caused to secrete the progestational hormone.

Reciprocal effects of the ovarian hormones upon the pituitary. The estrogenic and progestational hormones exert reciprocal effects upon the release of the pituitary gonadotropic hormones. The estrogenic hormone inhibits the further release of FSH from the pituitary, but stimulates the liberation of LH and perhaps of luteotropin. The progestational hormone, conversely, inhibits release of LH from the pituitary.** The lag in these reciprocal responses gives time for successive waves of activity; without a lag, the ovary and the pituitary

---

* In the male this pituitary hormone stimulates development of the interstitial cells of the testes, the so-called Leydig cells. Hence, when dealing with males, one refers to this hormone as the interstitial-cell-stimulating hormone (ICSH).

† It is the gonad, not the pituitary, which fails at the climacteric.

** The rigorous check exerted upon the pituitary by the ovarian hormones is well illustrated in the syndrome of agenesis of the follicular elements of the ovary. Free from ovarian restraint under these conditions (the rudimentary ovaries elaborate no hormones whatever), the pituitary releases large amounts of gonadotropic hormones into the circulation.

would presumably come into equilibrium and the periodicity would disappear.

Other factors affecting pituitary gonadotropic activity. Many factors besides the titer of the estrogenic and progestational hormones are thought to influence pituitary gonadotropic activity. Hormones from other target glands, such as the thyroid, doubtless affect gonadotropic function. Dietary factors are also important in sustaining gonadotropin production. During chronic starvation, the sexual cycles recur less and less frequently and finally cease altogether. Finally, pituitary gonadotropic function may be susceptible to modification by nervous or neurohormonal mechanisms (see page 303).

OVARIAN HORMONES

Definitions of "Estrogen" and "Progestin." In response to proper sequential stimulation by the various pituitary gonadotropins, the ovary normally elaborates two types of hormones: (a) the estrogenic and (b) the progestational hormones. By definition of the American Medical Association committee on the nomenclature of hormones, the term "estrogen" refers collectively to all substances producing estrus growth in the vagina, uterus and mammary glands of castrate or immature female animals and the term "progestin" to compounds having the common action of producing progestational changes in the female genital tract.

While there is experimental and clinical evidence to indicate that the ovary may secrete androgens under certain special conditions, the conclusion that androgen production is a normal ovarian function is not at present warranted.

Estrogen

Chemistry of natural and synthetic compounds.[1b] Chemically, the natural forms of both the estrogenic and the progestational hormones possess the carbon skeleton of 1.2 cyclopentanophenanthrene and are therefore classed as steroids. The estrogenic steroids which have so far been isolated from human tissues and body fluids are estradiol, estrone and estriol. It has been shown experimentally that the physiologic potency of estradiol greatly exceeds that of estrone, and that the potency of estrone, in turn, exceeds that of estriol. Estradiol is therefore regarded as the true estrogenic hormone, estrone and estriol as break-down products.

Included among the substances physiologically defined as estrogens are a number of synthetic compounds which bear no structural resemblance to the cyclopentenophenanthrene hormonal steroids. Representative compounds in this group include diethylstilbestrol, hexestrol and triphenylchlorethylene. The structural formulas of these substances are shown as follows:

REPRESENTATIVE ESTROGENS, NATURAL AND SYNTHETIC

ESTRADIOL   ESTRONE   ESTRIOL

DIETHYLSTILBESTROL   HEXESTROL

TRIPHENYLCHLORETHYLENE

PROGESTERONE AND RELATED COMPOUNDS

PROGESTERONE   PREGNANDIOL   PREGNENINOLONE

Although the chemical nature of the estrogen in human ovaries has not been established, both estradiol and estrone have been isolated in chemically pure form from the ovaries of the sow. Estrone is present in small quantities in male urine, and all three natural estrogens are demonstrable in the urine of adult females during some phase of the menstrual cycle. The total quantity of estrogenic material excreted varies according to the stage of the cycle, and the ratios of the various compounds to one another also vary. One peak in total estrogen excretion is demonstrable about the middle of the cycle coincident with maximal growth of the follicle, and another peak during the early part of the week preceding menstruation, when corpus luteum function is at its height.

Extra-ovarian sources. Besides the ovaries, the human placenta almost certainly produces estrogenic compounds. Likewise, there is considerable evidence pointing to the secretion of estrogen by the adrenal cortices, at least under certain conditions. Production of estrogen by stallion testes is well established but analogous function by human testes has not been demonstrated.

Intermediary metabolism. There is little or no storage of either estrogens or progestin in the body. They are utilized, inactivated or excreted almost as rapidly as they are formed.

From experiments performed by administering estrogens and studying the recovery products, it has been deduced that the following reactions can occur in the human organism:
$$\left.\begin{array}{c}\text{estradiol}\\\uparrow\quad\downarrow\\\text{estrone}\end{array}\right\} \rightarrow \text{estriol}$$

It is not known whether the formation of estrone is a necessary step in the conversion of estradiol to estriol. These transformations are thought to be effected by the liver and perhaps, to a lesser extent, by other non-endocrine organs; the ovaries and uterus do not seem to be essential. It therefore appears that these transformations are not related to the utilization of estrogens in the body but rather to modes of inactivation.

Like the majority of steroid hormones, estrogen undergoes partial inactivation in the body. Comparatively small amounts are eliminated, through the urine or bile, in an active form. Inactivation is thought to depend upon enzymic processes which effect oxidative degradation of the steroid nucleus, reduction or conjugation. Little is known concerning the details of any of these mechanisms except conjugation, which clearly occurs in the liver. The urinary estrogens consist of traces of estradiol and larger amounts of estrone and estriol. The two latter compounds are present largely in esterified form, estrone as a sulfate and estriol as a monoglucuronide. Unlike the free steroids, the conjugates are water soluble, and perhaps this facilitates their excretion in the urine.

Physiologic actions.[15] The physiologic actions of estrogen are complex and diverse. While many estrogenic effects seem clearly designed to prepare the genital tract for possible pregnancy, others have little or no apparent connection with sexual function. In considering the actions of estrogen upon the genital organs, one must distinguish between those which are exerted directly and those which are mediated via the anterior lobe of the pituitary gland.

Direct genital actions. In its simplest genital actions estrogen appears in the role of a growth hormone with the specific capacity to stimulate the derivatives of the Müllerian ducts, the vagina, uterus and Fallopian tubes. The slowly increasing production of estrogenic hormone during adolescence brings about growth of the accessory sexual organs from infantile to adult proportions; the continuous secretion of estrogens by the developing follicles and the corpus luteum sustains the mature proportions of these organs throughout the period of active sexual life. In response to the oscillating titer of estrogenic hormone in adult life, the epithelial linings of these organs undergo periodic proliferation and regression.

During the follicular phase of the menstrual cycle the vaginal epithelium increases in height and the surface layers tend to lose their nuclei and to become cornified. Glycogen is deposited in the epithelial cells, and the vaginal secretion becomes more acid in reaction. The cervical epithelium proliferates and a thin watery mucus is secreted by the cervical glands. The surface epithelium, glands and stromal tissues of the endometrium grow and acquire an increased capacity to respond to progesterone stimulation. Vasodilatation of the vascular tree of the endometrium occurs as a result of the liberation of acetylcholine. Both the ciliated and the non-ciliated cells of the tubal epithelium increase in height and reach their maximal secretory activity just before or immediately after ovulation. Changes also take place in the rhythmical contractility of the uterine and tubal musculature. In the human being the character of the hormone-induced changes in myometrial contractility has not been fully defined. In lower animals, however, uterine motility is characterized by low amplitude, high frequency waves and a tonic type of spontaneous contraction during the follicular phase.

Genital actions mediated by the pituitary. In addition, the genital organs are affected indirectly by various actions of the estrogenic hormone upon anterior pituitary function. The manner in which estrogen influences the release of the various gonadotropins from the pituitary has been described earlier. Estrogen stimulates the release of adrenocorticotropin, resulting in the growth of pubic and axillary hair during adolescence (see under 17-KS-Gens, Chapter III). Estrogen inhibits the release of lactogenic hormone from the pituitary. When the blood estrogen concentration falls after parturition, lactation occurs; if estrogen is then administered, lactation is suppressed. Estrogen appears to be capable of inducing both ductal and lobulo-alveolar development in the primate breast, although the manner in which this action is exerted is still controversial. While estrogen has some capacity to stimulate the breast directly, this stimulus seems to be more completely expressed in the presence of a normally functioning anterior pituitary.

Extra-genital actions. The extra-genital actions of estrogen are numerous and important. The hormone causes thickening of the skin, and under its influence the sebaceous glands undergo partial involution. The skin responds with increased pigmentation, particularly in the region of the mammary areolæ and the linea abdominalis. The buccal and gingival mucous membranes manifest increased proliferation. Estrogen induces a number of peripheral vascular reactions reminiscent of those seen in the vascular tree of the uterus; there is visible engorgement of the blood vessels of the nasal mucosa, dilatation and decreased pressure in the capillary vessels of the nail bed and a fall in the venous pressure of the hand. Lineal bone growth is inhibited (apparently by suppression of pituitary growth hormone production) and epiphyseal closure accelerated by estrogenic action. The hormone induces a slight retention of nitrogen, calcium, phosphorus, sodium, chloride and water and a minimal rise in blood volume. Urinary citric acid excretion is increased by estrogen.

Progesterone. Besides the estrogenic hormone, the ovaries elaborate a steroid principle, progesterone, which has the specific function of preparing the uterus for the reception and nourishment of the embryo.

Chemistry of natural and synthetic compounds.[1b] The chemical nature of the progestin of human ovaries has not yet been determined. However, it is commonly assumed to be very similar to, if not identical with, progesterone which has been isolated from sow ovaries in chemically pure form. Inasmuch as this hormone is the product of the corpus luteum, a transformed follicle, its structural similarity to the estrogenic steroids is not surprising. A synthetic progestational steroid, anhydro-hydroxy-progesterone (pregneninolone or ethinyl testosterone)* has been prepared from estradiol. Unlike progesterone, this compound is effective when administered orally, from 5 to 10 mg. by mouth being roughly equivalent to 1 mg. of progesterone given intramuscularly. The structural formulas of progesterone and important related compounds are shown below.

Ovarian and extra-ovarian sources. Progesterone is not demonstrable as such in the urine. However, a number of other steroid compounds, of which the chief is pregnandiol, appear in the urine after the administration of progesterone and are thought to represent its reduction products. Pregnandiol does not occur in free form in urine, but in conjugation with glucuronic acid. Since the presence or absence of pregnandiol in the urine correlates well with the finding of a proliferative or a secretory endometrium, respectively, it is inferred that pregnandiol represents a major excretion product of the corpus luteum hormone in the human being. The case for placental production of progesterone rests on circumstantial, but convincing, evidence. Finally, human adrenal cortices appear to be capable of secreting progesterone. It is not clear, however, whether progesterone is ever elaborated by the adrenals under normal conditions.

Intermediary metabolism. The site of conversion of progesterone to pregnandiol in human beings is not known, although the recovery of progesterone metabolites from bile strongly suggests the liver. Conjugation of pregnandiol with glucuronic acid is also thought to occur in the liver.

* Known commercially as Pranone.

Physiologic actions.[1g]   Physiologically speaking, progesterone is a highly specialized hormone compared to estrogen.

Direct genital actions.   Its principal target is the proliferative endometrium, which it prepares for the nidation and nourishment of the fertilized ovum. In physiologic doses progesterone exerts little, if any, effect upon an endometrium not primed with estrogen. This is doubtless a consequence of the fact that in nature follicular secretion invariably precedes luteal secretion. The myometrium is also affected, as is evidenced by a change in the character of uterine contractions. The effects of progesterone upon the motility of the human uterus have not yet been fully elucidated. It appears, however, that the responsiveness of the uterus to posterior pituitary extract is heightened during the luteal phase and that the contractions are accompanied by cramps. Cramps do not occur during menstruation following an anovulatory cycle, when no progesterone has been produced. The lobules of the breast become distended during the premenstrual phase of ovulatory menstrual cycles, presumably as a result of progesterone stimulation.

Indirect genital actions.   Besides exerting these primary effects upon the genital tract, progesterone exerts secondary effects through its participation in the intermediary metabolism of estrogen and through its influence upon anterior pituitary function. Progesterone decreases the rate of estrogen degradation, increasing the proportion of circulating estriol. As stated earlier, progesterone inhibits the release of LH from the pituitary and perhaps thereby prevents multiple ovulation and potential superfetation.

Extra-genital actions.   Progesterone promotes a slight-to-moderate retention of sodium, chloride and water and facilitates the renal excretion of potassium. These actions are reminiscent of those produced by the Na-K hormone of the adrenal cortices. In all probability, progesterone is more important than estrogen in the production of premenstrual edema.

THE SEXUAL DEVELOPMENT OF THE CHILD AND ADOLESCENT

Pseudo-Precocity of the Newborn.   The genital tissues of the majority of newborn female infants manifest a transient sexual precocity.[2a] The labia majora and minora undergo considerable hypertrophy during the last weeks of intrauterine life and are relatively large at delivery. The vaginal epithelium is thickened and contains glycogen for the first three or four weeks after birth. A glairy, whitish vaginal discharge, which is acid in reaction and which contains

Döderlein bacilli, is also present. About the seventh day after birth, slight vaginal bleeding from the temporarily hyperplastic endometrium occurs in about 1 per cent of infants. The uterus of the newborn is congested and approximately 40 per cent heavier than that of the year-old child (see Figure 2). Breast enlargement, associated with the secretion of "witch's milk," is observed in the majority of newborn infants of both sexes.

There is a gradual recession of these changes over a period of three or four months. By the second month, glycogen has disappeared from the vaginal epithelium. Associated with its disappearance is an alteration of the vaginal pH toward neutrality and replacement of the Döderlein bacilli with Gram-positive cocci and diplococci. The uterus slowly shrinks, and its birth weight is not regained until the end of the fifth year. Secretion of "witch's milk" ceases, and by the end of the fourth month the breasts have reverted to the infantile type.

This temporary precocity is attributed largely to stimulation by estrogens of maternal origin. The estrogen concentration of the newborn child's blood corresponds closely to the estrogen concentration of maternal blood. An excretory tide of estrogens appears in the infant's urine during the first week after birth and diminishes toward the end of this period. Prolactin, which is demonstrable in the urine of infants before and during the period of lactation, probably plays a role in the secretion of milk by the infant's breast. Whether this hormone is fetal or maternal in origin is unknown. It has been suggested that release of prolactin from the infant's pituitary may be stimulated by the rapid fall in blood estrogen concentration after birth.

Genital Status during the Preadolescent and Adolescent Years. From the third or fourth month of life (by which time the last of the precocious changes, hyperplasia of the breasts, has disappeared) until the eighth to the eleventh year, sexual development is largely in abeyance.*

The central nervous system. The factors which regulate the timing of normal sexual development are poorly understood. Since puberal changes can be induced in the secondary sex organs of immature girls and even of infants by estrogen administration, gross insensitivity of the target organs cannot be responsible for the lack of sexual maturation in childhood. Moreover, even the fetal hypophysis

---

* It is important to distinguish between the various terms which are used in the discussion of sexual differentiation. The term "adolescence" properly denotes the whole period of childhood during which sexual differentiation occurs. The period extends over many years and is not terminated until the organism attains full capacity to reproduce its kind and has also completed bodily growth and maturation. The term "menarche" refers to the first menstrual period, which is usually anovulatory and therefore not indicative of the attainment of full reproductive maturity. The term "puberty" has been involved in much ambiguity. It correctly refers to the moment at which reproduction becomes possible, i.e., in the female, the first ovulation. Thus it may be considered a milestone along the adolescent path to maturity.

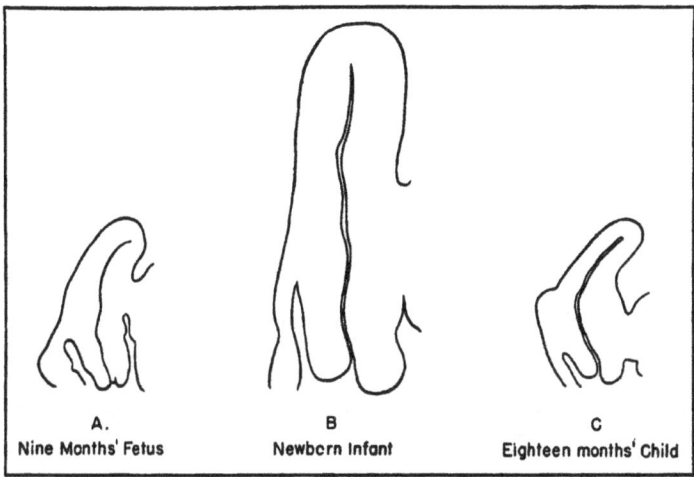

FIGURE V—2. Scale drawings of the fetal, neonatal and infantile uterus showing the transient enlargement of the neonatal uterus produced by maternal estrogens. From H. Bayer, *Vorlesungen über allgemeine Geburtshülfe*, I: 1. Strassburg, Schlesier and Schweikhardt, 1908.

is proven to contain gonadotropins and the gland of the child is potentially capable of stimulating the sex organs at any time. It is believed, therefore, that the release of gonadotropins at the onset of adolescence is dependent upon some neural or neuro-hormonal mechanism which is inhibited during childhood. Removal of the inhibition is thought to be dependent upon the maturation of certain centers in the nervous system, which ordinarily occurs about the turn of the first decade. In lower animals which ovulate only at the climax of a long series of love antics, it seems clear that sexual centers are located in the hypothalamic area of the midbrain and that an intact hypothalamic-hypophyseal connection is essential for the release of LH. In man, the existence of sexual centers is less certain. However, the occurrence of sexual precocity and of sexual infantilism in boys and girls with hypothalamic lesions suggests that similar centers are present in the human central nervous system.

The ovaries. At birth the ovaries are long, slender and flat (see Figures 3 and 27). Their size and weight increase very slowly from birth until the menarche and more rapidly between the menarche and puberty. Approximately 90 per cent of postnatal ovarian growth is accomplished during the second decade. By the time puberty is reached, the ovaries have lost their primitive, ribbonlike appearance and have become almond-shaped. However, their surface is strikingly smooth as compared with that of adult ovaries, which are pitted and

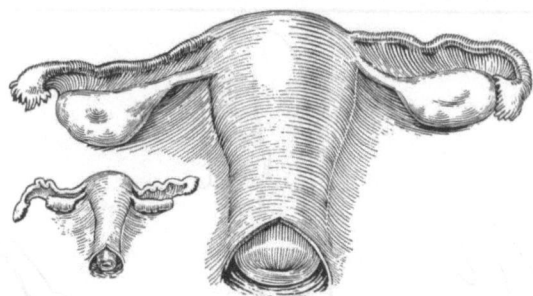

FIGURE V—3. Scale drawings of the uterus and adnexa of the newborn infant and of the girl at puberty. Note the thinness and elongation of the infant's ovaries and the convolution of its Fallopian tubes. The surface of the pubertal ovary differs from that of the mature ovary in that it is smooth, lacking the pits and scars which result from ovulation.

scarred as a consequence of repeated ovulations. Between the ages of 8 and 10 occasional follicles attain sufficient development to secrete estrogens before undergoing atresia, and the ovary begins to function tentatively as a gland of internal secretion.

The genitalia. After completing its postnatal involution, the uterus exhibits little growth until the eighth year of life. However, once ovarian follicular development has progressed sufficiently to permit estrogen secretion, uterine growth becomes rapid. It is the corpus that is mainly affected. Although the cervix was longer than the corpus during the preadolescent period, it now becomes less responsive, with the result that the corpus ultimately exceeds it in length by a ratio of 2:1. The endometrium retains its infantile structure of simple tubular glands until just before the menarche, when it undergoes a rapid metamorphosis.

The Fallopian tubes, which are convoluted in infancy and childhood, straighten as they mature. They increase both in width and length and their mucosal plicæ acquire complex convolutions. Ciliated cells appear in the lining epithelium and the muscular walls of the tube become capable of sluggish peristalsis.

The vagina widens and deepens, and its walls acquire transverse folds. The vaginal epithelium again becomes stratified squamous in type and glycogen is deposited in its cells. There is a reappearance of the Döderlein flora and secretional acidity. From its rudimentary infantile state Bartholin's gland is gradually transformed into a complex racemose structure capable of secretory activity.

Appearance of Secondary Sex Characters during Adolescence. Concomitant with the changes in the primary and secondary sex organs just described, there are visible manifestations of increasing sexual development due to the

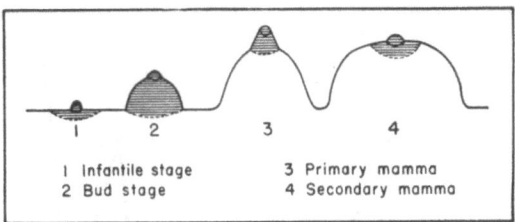

FIGURE V—4. Stages in the sexual differentiation of the human breast. Adapted from E. C. Hamblen, *Endocrine Gynecology*, Springfield, Thomas, 1939.

appearance of the secondary sexual characteristics.[2 b-h] Of these, breast development is the most obvious (see Figure 4). The infantile breast is characterized by a papilla only slightly elevated above a disc-shaped areola. Under hormonal stimulation, the infantile breast progresses to the bud stage, in which the areola becomes elevated and forms with the papilla a small, conical protuberance. This stage is reached by most girls in the tenth or eleventh year. As the amount of fat in the region underlying and immediately surrounding the areola increases, the bud is rapidly transformed into the so-called primary mamma. At this stage the areola is raised still higher above the general level of the chest wall and resembles a "truncated cone situated on the summit of a flattened hillock." The secondary mamma or mature breast usually characterizes adult women, although some women never achieve this degree of mammary development. Only the papilla projects from the completely mature breast, the areola having receded to the level of the hillock.

Appearance of hair* on the labia is ordinarily the next visible indication of premenarcheal sexual development. Growing first on the labia majora, the hair spreads medially and upward to the mons pubis, then laterally to complete the characteristic feminine inverted triangle. At about this same time, remolding of the bony pelvis commonly begins. The pelves of prepuberal girls are long-oval in shape and are characterized by an acetabular constriction, which is formed by an inward projection of the pelvic walls into the pelvic canal medial to each acetabulum. During childhood the superior pelvic aperture grows slowly and symmetrically. However, as the menarche approaches the pelvis widens more rapidly than it increases in the antero-posterior diameter, the forepart widens and the acetabular constriction begins to disappear. Remolding requires about 18 months for completion. Increase in subcutaneous fat accentuates the widen-

* The physical characteristics of both axillary and pubic hair change as maturation proceeds. Unpigmented down is succeeded by short, straight pigmented hair, then by a sparse growth of long, curly pigmented hair and finally by a dense growth of tightly coiled mature hair.

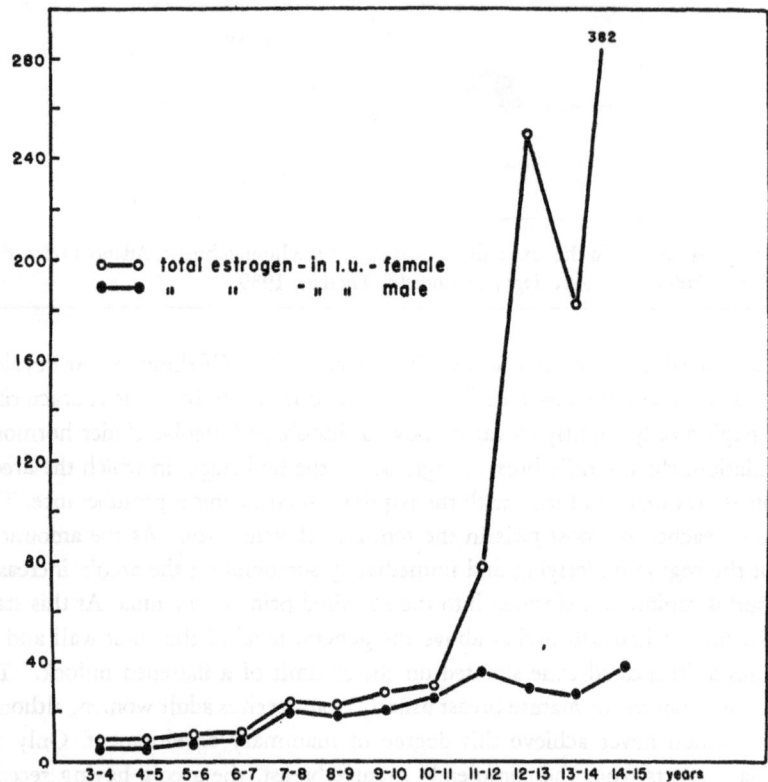

FIGURE V—5. The urinary excretion of total estrogens in international units by boys and girls of different ages. From I. T. Nathanson, L. E. Towne and J. C. Aub, *Endocrinology*, 28:851, 1941.

---

ing of the hips. After a considerable interval, hair appears in the axillary fossæ. The menarche generally follows this development; occasionally it precedes it.

Hormone Production at Various Ages.[21,3] Estrogens in small, constant and equal amounts become demonstrable in the urine of both boys and girls between the ages of three and seven (see Figure 5). Since only rare Graafian follicles undergo appreciable enlargement before the age of eight, it is thought that the adrenal cortices are the source of these urinary steroids. When the girl is approximately eight years of age, estrogen excretion begins to increase; between the ages of 8 and 11 there is a steeper increase in the rate of estrogen excretion. About the age of 11, estrogen excretion in girls becomes enormously accelerated and cyclic in character. The development of cyclic estrogen excretion

TABLE V—1. The relation between the chronologic ages of 14 girls and the presence of gonadotropic hormone in their urine. From I. T. Nathanson et al., Endocrinology 28:851, 1941.

Patient	Chronologic age		Gonadotropin assay *	Menarcheal age	
	yr.	mo.		yr.	mo.
A	9	1	−		
B	9	8	−		
C	10	0	−		
D	10	4	−		
	12	11	+	13	0
E	10	3	−		
	10	9	−		
	11	3	−		
	11	8	+	12	7
F	10	9	−		
	11	3	+	11	8
G	11	6	−		
	11	9	−	14	5
H	11	6	−		
I	11	9	+	11	6
	12	3	+		
J	11	6	+	12	5
	13	11	+		
K	12	0	−	13	7
L	12	5	+	13	3
	12	9	+		
M	13	3	+	13	6
	13	9	+		
N	14	8	+		
	14	11	+	14	11

* The material to be assayed is concentrated in such a manner that a positive reaction indicates the presence of a minimum of 20 mouse units per 24 hours. One mouse unit is arbitrarily defined as the amount of material which, when injected in five equal parts over a period of 48 hours, produces follicle stimulation in the ovaries of the animal 96 hours after the first injection.

is generally contemporaneous with the early visible indications of secondary sexual development.

Gonadotropins first become demonstrable* in the urine of girls† about the age of 11. In Table 1 is set forth the relation between the chronologic ages of

* A methodological artefact is undoubtedly responsible for the fact that gonadotropins are not demonstrable in the urine until long after the upsurge in urinary estrogen excretion, which is presumably due to the supplementation of adrenal by ovarian estrogens. Gonadotropins are, in all probability, secreted in childhood in concentrations too low to be detected by current assay techniques. Hypophysectomy in immature animals causes involution of the ovaries below their normal weight; gonadectomy results in some degree of accessory organ involution.

† In companion studies Nathanson and his coworkers found that urinary gonadotropic activity is first demonstrable in males during the thirteenth year of life (see also Chapter VI, Table 1). These data are consonant with the observation that the female matures earlier than the male.

14 girls and the presence of gonadotropins in their urine. Whenever possible, the ages at which these girls ultimately experienced the menarche is also indicated. From these and other[21] studies, it appears that sexual immaturity is associated with an absence of gonadotropic hormones. The menarche is associated with progressive increases in the amounts of gonadotropins and in the frequency with which they can be detected in the urine.

Pregnandiol appears in the urine during the luteal phase of the menstrual cycle a year or two later than gonadotropins.

Correlation between Hormone Production and Sexual Differentiation. A correlation between the data on hormone excretion and the physical evidences of sexual differentiation may now be attempted. Childhood is characterized by low-grade estrogen elaboration by the ovaries. About the age of 11, gonadotropic hormone release from the pituitary increases significantly and results in elaboration by the ovaries of sufficient estrogen to stimulate genital growth. The secretion of gonadotropins is sporadic. Consequently, the production of estrogen is sporadic. As the endometrium develops, it exhibits proliferative phases paralleling the ovarian estrogen cycles. Eventually, the oscillations in the estrogen level become sufficiently pronounced to induce a vascular crisis in the endometrium, and the first menstrual period occurs.

AGE	SEXUAL CHARACTERISTICS	STATUS OF HORMONE PRODUCTION
3–7	Infantile.	Very small amounts of estrogens and 17-KS in urine.
	ADOLESCENCE	
8	Ovarian follicles display more advanced development. Uterus begins to grow.	Urinary excretion of estrogens and 17-KS begins to increase.
10–11	Budding of breasts. *Adrenarche* (appearance of pubic hair).	Estrogen excretion greatly accelerated.
11–12	Remolding of bony pelvis. Vaginal changes. Breasts advance to primary mamma stage. Growth of external and internal genitalia greatly accelerated.	Gonadotropins become demonstrable in the urine. Estrogen excretion further augmented, becomes cyclic in character.
13–14	Appearance of axillary hair. *Menarche* (first menstrual period, average age 13.5).	
14–15	*Puberty* (earliest normal pregnancies).	Pregnandiol appears in the urine during the luteal phase.
16–17	End of skeletal growth.	

Finally, the rising peaks of estrogen production reach a level adequate to stimulate the release of appreciable quantities of LH from the pituitary. Ovulation takes place, initiating the luteal phase of the menstrual cycle. The endometrium, which proliferated under the influence of estrogen, is now subjected to the additive and qualitatively different action of progesterone. Conception having become possible, puberty is established and the organism enters into the later stage of adolescence.

Summary and Comments. The approximate ages and order of appearance of the female sexual characteristics and their relation to the changes in hormone production are conveniently summarized in the preceding table.

It should be appreciated that many normal girls fail to conform precisely to this developmental pattern. There is a wide range in the age at which given characteristics may appear and in the tempo with which they succeed one another. Moreover, reversals in the sequence are common.

THE MENSTRUAL CYCLE

To visualize the phenomenon of menstruation[3 a-c] in correct perspective, it is important to appreciate the fact that periodic uterine bleeding is of comparatively recent evolutionary origin. A process peculiar to primates, menstruation represents a by-product of the anatomical changes imposed upon mammals as viviparity became an evolutionary goal. The longer the retention of the embryo in the uterus, the more complex became the endometrial preparation for the implantation and nutrition of the fertilized ovum. If, during a given cycle, fertilization did not occur, this succulent and elaborately vascularized lining was "aborted" and the entire structure reconstituted during the succeeding cycle.

A clinical corollary of the recent evolutionary origin of menstruation is its functional instability. Less firmly grounded than many other hormonally induced phenomena, it is established with difficulty and readily disordered. The adolescent must experience approximately 40 menstrual cycles before the periodicity characteristic of the mature woman is achieved; literally, the adolescent must "learn" how to menstruate. A lenient view of adolescent irregularities should therefore be adopted, and hormone therapy employed with the utmost restraint. Unwise interference may jeopardize the establishment of the mature pituitary–ovarian–uterine cyclic relationships upon which normal menstruation depends.

The manner in which the pituitary and ovarian hormones interact to produce the menstrual cycle has already been described (page 308). There remains to be considered the way in which the uterus responds to the stimuli thus provided (see Figure 6).

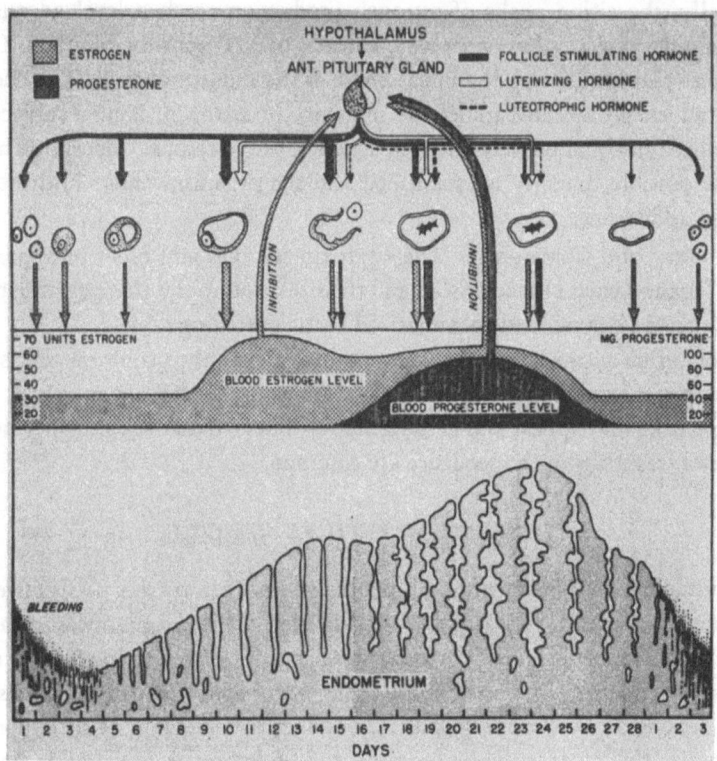

FIGURE V—6. Simplified diagram showing the relations of the hypothalamus, anterior pituitary gland, ovaries and endometrium in the normal sexually mature female during a 28-day menstrual cycle. On the highest level of the figure, the hypothalamus is represented as stimulating the anterior pituitary to discharge the gonadotropic hormones into the circulation. Thus activated, the anterior pituitary releases varying ratios of follicle-stimulating hormone, luteinizing hormones and luteotropin during the different phases of the cycle. These hormones act upon the ovaries to induce follicular development, ovulation, corpus luteum formation and the production of the estrogenic and progestational hormones. The estrogen level per liter of blood as determined in international units and the progesterone level in milligrams as calculated from the pregnandiol content of the urine are shown in their relation to the menstrual cycle. The inhibitory actions of the ovarian hormones upon the anterior pituitary are also indicated.

The changes in the endometrium brought about by the ovarian hormones are represented on the lowest level of the figure. The growth, regression and desquamation of the endometrium are indicated by its varying heights. The alteration of the endometrial glands from tubular to saccular structure under the influence of progesterone is shown diagrammatically.

The mature endometrial cycle consists of a relatively long period of growth and differentiation and a short period of regression, manifested externally by menstrual bleeding. Although the state of the uterine mucosa is continually changing, it is convenient to divide the cycle into phases of proliferation, secretion, premenstrual regression and menstruation.

Proliferative Phase. Re-epithelialization of the raw surface of the endometrium begins while menstrual bleeding is still in progress. The cells lining the gland stumps multiply and migrate outward so rapidly that within 48 hours after menstruation has ceased the bare stroma has been re-covered. Thereafter, a period of quiescence ensues. During this period, which is quite variable in length, there is an almost complete absence of mitotic activity; the endometrium consists of a dense and poorly vascularized stroma surrounding the basal stumps of the endometrial glands.

As the follicle which is destined to ovulate during the next cycle matures, the rate of estrogen secretion rises rapidly. Consequently, the endometrium proliferates at an increasing rate until ovulation occurs. All elements of the endometrium participate in this growth. The glands widen and elongate and, by the end of the proliferative phase, may exhibit slight tortuosity. The stroma loses its dense appearance, becoming looser in texture and slightly edematous. The blood vessels grow steadily longer and branch in the subepithelial zone to form a capillary network. A slight regression in many endometria at the termination of the proliferative phase has been observed in transplants. This is probably ascribable to the temporary disruption in follicular function produced by ovulation.

Secretory Phase. As soon as the corpus luteum has begun actively to secrete, the endometrium is subjected to the influence of progesterone as well as that of estrogen. Mitotic activity gradually ceases and differentiation begins. The glands widen and become increasingly tortuous. When luteal activity is at its height, the functional layer of the mucosa becomes distinguishable from its parent basal layer. Three layers in all can now be made out: (a) the zona compacta, which lies directly beneath the surface epithelium and which is composed chiefly of the edematous stroma surrounding the relatively narrow terminal portions of the uterine glands, (b) the middle zona spongiosa, which derives its name from the extreme sacculation of the mid-portions of the glands therein and (c) the innermost zona basalis. This layer participates very little in the cyclic changes and consists of a dense cellular stroma containing the narrow basal ends of the glands.

The stromal cells, especially those of the zona compacta, enlarge and become rounded and epithelioid in type, so that they resemble the decidual cells of pregnancy. Proliferation of arterioles continues for a longer time than does that of the other structural elements of the mucosa; pronounced spiraling is the result, particularly in the zona spongiosa. More delicate capillary proliferation occurs just beneath the endometrial surface.

Phases of Regression and Menstruation. The stage of premenstrual regression reflects the withdrawal of growth stimuli from the endometrium: in ovulatory cycles it occurs after corpus luteum activity has begun to decline; in anovulatory cycles it follows the degeneration of a follicle. Blood flow decreases and the stromal fluid is re-absorbed, reducing the thickness of the endometrium. To accommodate themselves to the restricted space, the spiral arterioles necessarily become more tortuous. The stasis thus induced is thought to be responsible for the necrosis of the endometrium and the weakening of the vessels that culminates in hemorrhage. In addition, tissue degeneration apparently releases some substance which brings about constriction of the spiral arterioles. The straight arterioles in the basal layer remain unaffected, so that the integrity of the basalis circulation is not compromised.

Except for brief periods, vasoconstriction of the coiled arterioles continues throughout menstruation. It is during these periods of relaxation that menstrual bleeding occurs. Fragmentation of the entire functionalis ordinarily occurs in ovulatory cycles; in anovulatory cycles there is usually less tissue loss. Bleeding ceases when an adequate circulation is re-established in sound vessels.

The preponderance of evidence supports the concept that endometrial growth is due almost entirely to estrogenic stimulation. Regression, and hence the sequence of events that leads to menstruation, appears to be initiated by a reduction in the level of the blood estrogen circulation or by an alteration in estrogen metabolism brought about by the production and subsequent withdrawal of progesterone.

METHODS OF DIAGNOSIS

The extent of development of the primary and secondary sexual organs provides a direct, if rough, index of the state of ovarian function in the preadolescent and adolescent patient. Moreover, a detailed history and physical examination often reveal the presence of systemic disease to which the gonadal disturbance is clearly secondary. However, for the recognition of many of the abnormalities in this field special diagnostic procedures are essential.[4a]

Indices of Estrogen Production. Adequacy of ovarian function with respect to estrogen production can be gauged in a number of different ways, each of which provides somewhat different information.

Urinary estrogen excretion. When available, biologic or chemical assays of the urine provide an excellent means of quantitating estrogen production. Estrogens are present in the urine chiefly in a conjugated form and must be freed by acid hydrolysis, extracted with a steroid solvent and partially purified before being assayed. Most of the biologic tests utilize the assay method of Allen and Doisy, based on the ability of the injected material to induce estrus growth of the vaginal epithelium of the castrate rat or mouse. A number of chemical methods are now becoming available for the quantitative determination of estrogens. While these methods are less cumbersome than bio-assay methods, they share the difficulty that numerous determinations are required to quantitate the fluctuations in estrogen excretion known to occur in normal adolescent and adult females. Fortunately, there are a number of simpler techniques which enable one to infer the rate of estrogen production indirectly.

Cytology of urinary sediment and vaginal pH. In preadolescent children suspected of sexual precocity, microscopic examination of the unstained urinary sediment and determination of the vaginal pH with nitrazine paper are valuable methods for detecting the presence of physiologically significant amounts of estrogen in the circulation. Prior to the advent of effective amounts of estrogens, the sediment contains only rounded basal cells (see below) and the pH of the vaginal secretions is alkaline. Contrary to what one might suppose, these are not all vaginal cells washed out by the urinary stream. The majority are cells shed from the stratified squamous epithelial lining of the lower two-thirds of the urethra.[4 b] This portion of the urethra, like the lowermost portion of the vagina, is a derivative of the urogenital sinus. It is therefore responsive to estrogenic stimulation and exhibits cyclic epithelial growth and cornification. After the advent of estrogens, the sediment contains cornified epithelial cells and the pH is acid (see Figure 7).

Vaginal smear.[4 c] More detailed information concerning the level of circulating estrogen and the mode of estrogen production (i.e., whether continuous or cyclic) can be gained by study of the stained vaginal smear. The ovarian cycle is reflected in the vagina, just as it is in the uterus. When stimulated by the estrogenic hormone, the vaginal mucous membrane increases in thickness. As this occurs, superficial cells grow farther and farther away from their blood supply and undergo the same essentially degenerative process (cornification) that occurs in the skin. Consequently, in smears made from the superficial vaginal lining the extent of the proliferative process may be established by the degree of cornification seen in the smears.

The manner of obtaining and preparing the smears is extremely simple. A dry curved-glass pipette is inserted about three inches into the vagina with the

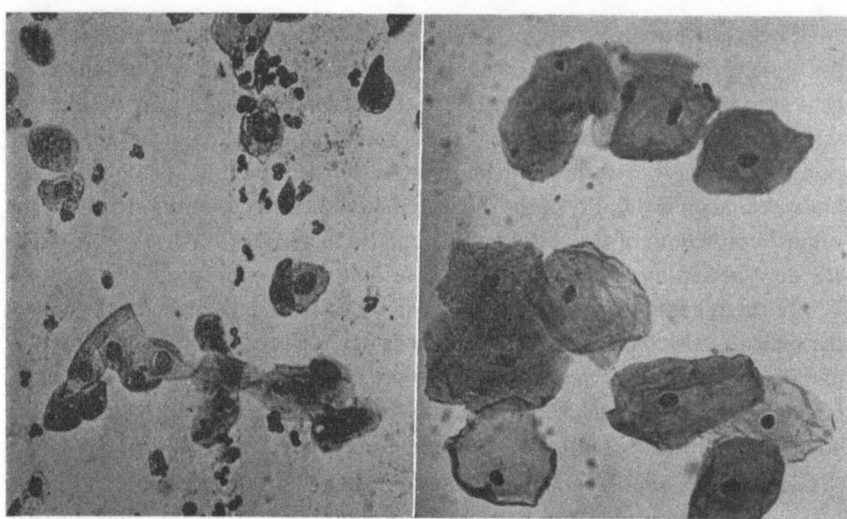

FIGURE V—7. Vaginal smears of childhood and maturity.
LEFT: During normal childhood the basal cells are rounded and numerous leukocytes are characteristic.
RIGHT: On sexual maturity the epithelial cells become large and cornified and their nuclei pyknotic as a result of stimulation by estrogenic hormone.

---

bulb compressed (see Figure 8). Vaginal secretions are then aspirated by releasing the bulb while the pipette is slowly withdrawn. The material thus collected is blown on the surface of a clean microscope slide and further spread with the convex side of the pipette. The slide carrying the wet smear is immediately dropped into a Coplin jar containing equal parts of 95 per cent alcohol and ether. After becoming fixed in this solution, the smear is treated with a differential stain such as that devised by Shorr* and examined.

Severe estrogen deficiency is characterized by the presence of small bluish-staining atrophic cells of rounded shape from the basal layer of the vagina. Under estrogenic influence larger green-staining squamous epithelial cells appear (see Figure 7). With full cornification the squamous cells assume a brilliant orange-red hue. By observing the day-to-day changes in the vaginal smear, one can detect fluctuations in estrogenic activity.

The prognostic value of the vaginal smear in adolescent amenorrhea has been pointed out by Shorr (see Figure 9). The demonstration of cyclic ovarian activity in a patient showing development of the secondary sexual characteristics warrants a good prognosis for the eventual establishment of normal menstrual

* Single Differential Stain (Shorr) can be obtained from Wyeth, Inc., Philadelphia.

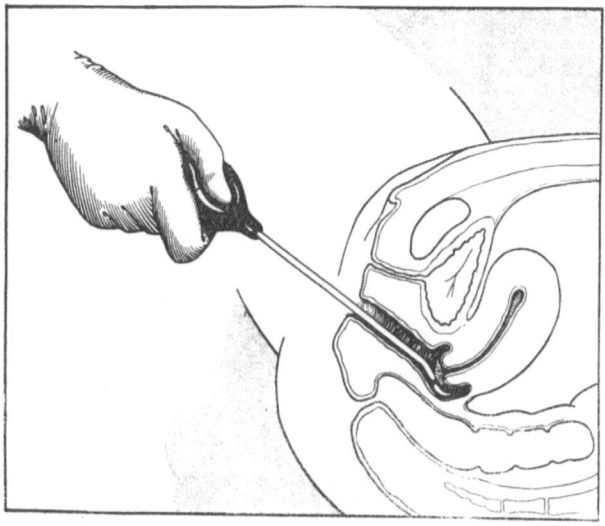

FIGURE V—8. The technique of aspirating vaginal secretion for making smears. The tip of the pipette should dip into the pool of secretions which collects in the posterior fornix.

function. On the other hand, the occurrence of vaginal smears which are persistently of the atrophic type in a sexually undeveloped girl of 15 or 16 years favors the diagnosis of true sexual infantilism rather than of simple delayed puberty. Postmenarcheal amenorrhea is likely to be less significant if the vaginal smears show some degree of ovarian activity than if the smear picture is consistently atrophic in type. In the case of patients of the former type, menstruation is often resumed spontaneously when general health is improved; in that of patients with atrophic vaginal smears, spontaneous termination of the amenorrhea is much less likely.

"Medical" dilatation and curettage. Another simple test for estrogen effect is the "medical" dilatation and curettage of Albright. It will be recalled that progesterone is physiologically almost inert in the absence of estrogen. If, however, the endometrium has been "primed" by the action of estrogen, the intramuscular administration of an adequate amount of progesterone (i.e., 5 mg. daily, for five days) will cause further growth of the proliferated endometrium. More importantly, once this temporary growth stimulus has been withdrawn, uterine bleeding will occur unless the progesterone level is being sustained by an endogenous source, the corpus luteum. The corpus luteum may be either the short-lived structure which forms after ovulation or the longer-lived corpus luteum of pregnancy. A corpus luteum of the former type is recognized by the

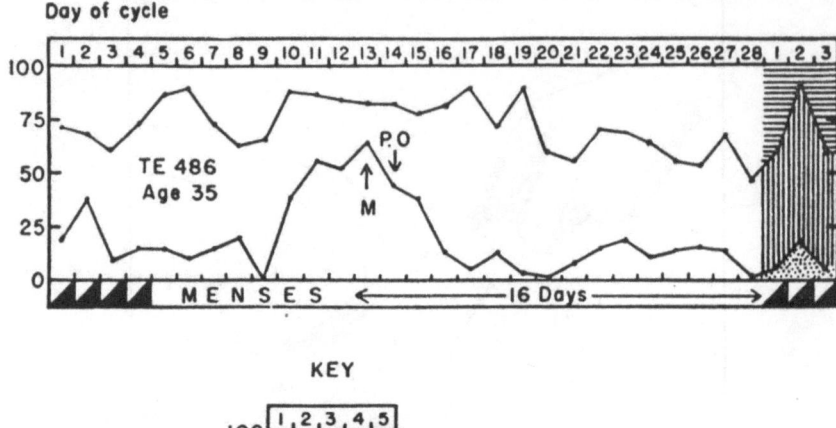

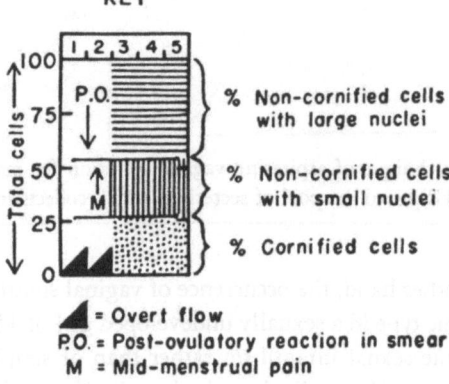

▲ = Overt flow
P.O. = Post-ovulatory reaction in smear
M = Mid-menstrual pain

FIGURE V—9. Graph representing the cytological changes occurring in the vaginal smear during a normal ovulatory cycle. The classification is based on an evaluation of 200 epithelial cells in each smear. Menstrual phase, days 1-4; postmenstrual phase, days 5-9; preovulatory phase, days 10-12; ovulatory peak, day 13; postovulatory reaction, day 14; early luteal phase, days 15-16; late luteal phase, days 17-27; premenstrual phase, day 28. From I. L. C. de Allende, E. Schorr and C. G. Hartman, *Contributions to Embryology* 31:1, 1945, as adapted by E. Schorr, *J. Mt. Sinai Hosp.* 12:667, 1945.

occurrence of menstrual bleeding within 10 days after the last injection; that of the latter by characteristic physical signs and by the presence of chorionic gonadotropin in the urine. In the absence of either of these sources of endogenous progesterone, failure to bleed following cessation of progesterone treatment implies severe estrogenic insufficiency.

Endometrial biopsy.[4 d] Since the endometrium reflects the physiologic actions of both of the ovarian hormones, histologic examination of properly timed biopsy specimens of the tissue provides considerable information. In general, if an endometrium is well developed, one can assume that it is receiving an adequate supply of its selective growth hormone, estrogen, and that the anterior pituitary is releasing considerable amounts of follicle-stimulating hormone and small amounts, at least, of luteinizing hormone. If, in an endometrial specimen taken just before the expected date of menstruation, or better still, on the first day of the menstrual flow definite secretory changes are noted, there can be no question that the endometrium is being supplied with the corpus luteum hormone, progesterone. The presence of progesterone, in turn, implies that the pituitary has secreted enough luteinizing hormone to cause ovulation and enough luteotropin to sustain progesterone production.

In adolescent patients recourse need rarely be had to endometrial biopsy to gauge estrogen effect; this information can be gained more easily by study of the vaginal smear. On the other hand, the fact that an endometrial biopsy enables one to determine whether or not ovulation has occurred makes it of value in the management of cases of menorrhagia. In many instances a complete curettage under anesthesia is necessary to terminate an episode of prolonged bleeding: this provides an opportunity for the study of endometrial histology and also, incidentally, for thorough bimanual palpation of the pelvic organs. Subsequent biopsies may be needed to evaluate the patient's response to treatment, particularly if facilities for urinary pregnandiol determinations (see below) are not available. Such biopsies can frequently be secured by an experienced physician as an office procedure. If the hymeneal ring is sufficiently elastic to allow the insertion of a small bivalve speculum into the vagina and if the cervical canal is of a caliber to accommodate a biopsy curette without preliminary dilatation, anesthesia as a rule is not necessary.

Indices of Progesterone Production. Since estrogen is the basic growth hormone of the female genital tract and progesterone is a specialized hormone whose only function is to prepare the uterus for pregnancy, the clinical effects of ovarian insufficiency with respect to progesterone production are less conspicuous than those with respect to estrogen production. Physical examination of the patient does not enable one to recognize progesterone deficiency and in suspected cases recourse must be had to special diagnostic procedures.

Endometrial biopsy. Use of this procedure as a source of information concerning progesterone production has been considered above. Since biopsies are sometimes difficult, if not impossible, to obtain in unanesthetized patients, less traumatic procedures of the types described below are employed whenever possible.

Urinary pregnandiol excretion. Chemical methods, both gravimetric[4,e] and colorimetric[4,f] have been developed for the quantitative determination of pregnandiol in the urine. Fortunately, these procedures are much simpler to carry out than are the chemical methods for assaying urinary estrogen.

Pregnandiol is absent from the urine of normal children and adult males and from that of adult females during the follicular phase of the menstrual cycle. It appears suddenly in the urine about 12 or 13 days before the onset of the next menstrual period (i.e., within a day or so after ovulation). The amount excreted daily in the urine varies from 1 to 6 mg.; the total quantity excreted during the luteal phase is approximately 40 mg. Since pregnandiol excretion attains its peak about the twenty-first day of the menstrual cycle and falls sharply to zero two or three days before the onset of bleeding, urine collections must be carefully timed. Basal body temperatures (see below) are distinctly helpful in this connection.

Absence of pregnandiol from the urine during the two weeks preceding menstruation indicates the absence of a functionally active corpus luteum (i.e., an anovulatory cycle).

Basal body temperature curve.[4,5] Basal body temperature curves provide valuable information concerning the occurrence of ovulation and progesterone formation. Rhythmic variations in body temperature during the menstrual cycle were noted many years ago, but it was not until recently that the role of the ovarian hormones in these fluctuations was clearly elucidated. During the follicular phase of an ovulatory cycle the temperature varies moderately, usually by less than five-tenths of a degree. Approximately 14 days before the onset of the next menstrual period there is a distinct drop in temperature of one-half a degree or more, followed on the next day by a rise to a level higher than that maintained during the follicular phase. During the luteal phase of the cycle this new level is sustained, with minor fluctuations, until the beginning of menstruation, when another drop occurs. During anovulatory cycles the temperature fluctuates erratically and no orderly pattern is discernible (see Figure 10).

Reliable curves are not obtained unless the patient has been carefully instructed in the details of taking and recording the temperature. The temperature should be taken rectally with a clinical thermometer each morning immediately upon awakening—before rising, drinking, eating or smoking. The thermometer should be kept at the bedside and shaken down directly after each reading, so that no muscular effort need be expended on awakening. Precision in reading the thermometer is important. Convenient forms on which to chart temperature readings are obtainable from the Planned Parenthood Federation* and from a number of pharmaceutical firms, although ordinary graph paper can be em-

* Planned Parenthood Federation of America, Inc., 501 Madison Avenue, New York 22, New York.

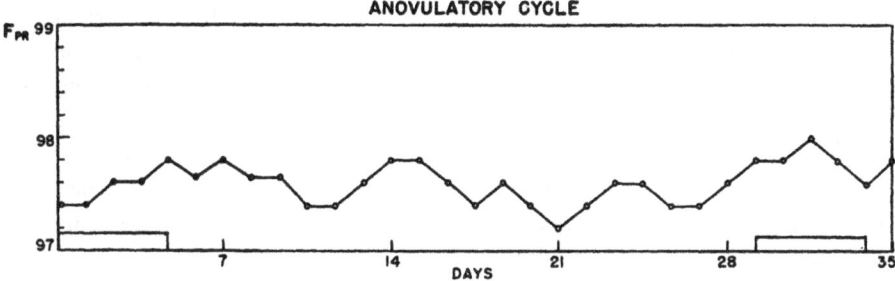

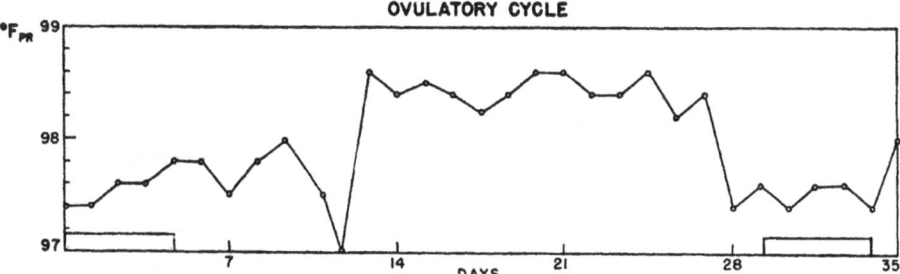

FIGURE V—10. Representative basal body temperature records.
ABOVE: Monophasic curve characteristic of an anovulatory menstrual cycle.
BELOW: Biphasic curve characteristic of an ovulatory cycle. A sharp fall in temperature (occurring on day 11 of the ovulatory cycle shown) followed by a prompt rise to a level higher than that maintained during the first half of the cycle is thought to signalize ovulation.

ployed, if desired. Patients are instructed to note on the chart obvious causes for temperature variations, such as colds or other intercurrent illnesses. Unusually high or low readings are always suspect, and should be retaken before being plotted on the chart.

High-strung patients who lead erratic lives and who suffer from insomnia may exhibit such violent temperature fluctuations that the influence of ovarian function upon body temperature is completely obscured. For most people, however, satisfactory curves can be obtained. These curves are especially helpful in confirming a diagnosis of primary dysmenorrhea (cramps are a feature of ovulatory cycles only) and in following the progress of patients with metropathia hemorrhagica.

Indices of Gonadotropin Production. The diagnostic procedures just described are of material aid in recognizing the existence of ovarian insufficiency and in roughly quantitating its extent. However, they shed no light on the origin of the insufficiency. In clinical practice it is particularly important to determine whether ovarian failure is primarily pituitary or primarily ovarian in origin. This can be accomplished by examining the urine for the presence of the pituitary gonadotropic hormones.[4 h] Ovarian failure due to pituitary insufficiency is characterized by the absence of gonadotropins from the urine; that due to primary ovarian inadequacy, by the presence of the gonadotropic hormones in the urine in amounts greatly in excess of normal.*

Numerous techniques for the bio-assay of urinary gonadotropins have been devised. All consist in the preparation of concentrated and partially purified extracts of urine and their administration to immature rodents. The sex organs of the rodents are subsequently examined for signs of gonadotropic stimulation. Many different end-points are employed: ovarian enlargement, the appearance of follicles and corpora lutea in the ovaries, uterine weight increase and opening of the vaginal orifice. Standards of normal vary from method to method and from laboratory to laboratory.

In view of the wide fluctuations in gonadotropin excretion which occur during various phases of the menstrual cycle, caution must be exercised in interpreting the results of individual assays. The diagnosis of pituitary insufficiency with respect to gonadotropic function should not be made until repeated determinations have shown an absence of gonadotropin.

CLINICAL CONSIDERATIONS

TYPES OF SEXUAL PRECOCITY

Sexual precocity is considered to be present in the female child when indications of genital maturation become apparent before the age of eight.[5 a-d] Precocity is conventionally subdivided into: (a) the isosexual type, in which development conforms to the true sex of the individual and (b) the heterosexual type, in which development is wholly or in part characteristic of the opposite sex. The only causes of heterosexual precocity in females are tumors and hyperplasia of the adrenal cortex. These are discussed in Chapter III. Except for passing mention of those exceedingly rare adrenocortical lesions in which there is a mixture of iso- and heterosexual precocity, the subsequent discussion will be devoted entirely to isosexual precocity, the causes of which may be classified as follows:

* Patients with primary ovarian insufficiency do not have gonadotropins in the urine until they reach adolescent age (i.e., 8 to 13 years).

A. True precocious puberty
  1. Hypothalamic
    (a) Destructive lesions
      (1) Tumors and cysts
      (2) Post-meningitic and post-encephalitic lesions
    (b) Idiopathic
      (1) "Constitutional" precocity
      (2) Polyostotic fibrous dysplasia
B. Pseudo-precocious puberty
  1. Ovarian
    (a) Granulosa cell tumors
    (b) Follicle cysts
    (c) Miscellaneous tumors—teratoma, chorionepithelioma, etc.
  2. Adrenal
    (a) Tumors of the adrenal cortex proper
    (b) Adrenal rest cell tumors
  3. End organ
    (a) Mammoplasia of infancy
  4. Medicational
    (a) Estrogen
    (b) Promizole

The incidence of the various types of isosexual precocity cannot be stated with precision, because the verification of many of the reported cases is incomplete. Estimation of the frequency with which "constitutional" precocity, in particular, occurs is fraught with inaccuracy since the diagnosis depends upon the exclusion of known causes of precocity. It is believed, however, that constitutional precocity accounts for 80 or 90 per cent of all female precocity, although there is only one negative autopsy on record and in only a few instances have ovarian and adrenal lesions been excluded by laparatomy. Despite this reservation, it can be said that the order of frequency of the commoner causes of sexual precocity in the female is approximately as follows: (a) hypothalamic "constitutional" precocity, (b) ovarian tumor or follicle cyst and (c) polyostotic fibrous dysplasia. The salient characteristics of the various types of isosexual precocity are set forth in Table 2.

True Precocious Puberty. Because of the clinical importance of the distinction, it should be pointed out that the terms "precocious puberty" and "sexual precocity" are not synonymous. Often loosely employed, "precocious puberty" correctly refers only to those cases of isosexual precocity in which maturation

TABLE V—2. Clinical characteristics of various types of isosexual precocity in the female.

Type of precocity	Alternative name	Cause	Development of breasts, vagina and uterus; menstruation	Ovulation	Excretion Estrogen	Excretion Gonadotropin	Sexual hair and 17-KS	Other features often associated
I. True precocious puberty								
A. Hypothalamic								
1. Destructive lesions		Tumors, cysts; encephalitic and meningitic lesions	+	+	+	+	+	Increased cranial pressure and neurologic signs
2. Constitutional		Idiopathic; in rare instances, familial	+	+	+	+	+	
3. Polyostotic fibrous dysplasia	Albright's syndrome; ost. fibr. dissem.	Idiopathic	+	+	+	?	+	Bony lesions, patchy cut. pigm.
B. Pituitary	(Not yet seen clinically)							
II. Pseudo-precocious puberty								
A. Ovarian		Granulosa cell tumors, follicle cysts, misc. tumors	+	0	++	0	+ or 0	Abdomen may be enlarged and tumor palpable
B. Adrenal		Tumors (adrenal and adr. rest cell)	+	0	?	0	++	Viril. generally accompanies fem.
C. End organ	Mammoplasia of infancy and childhood	Unknown	Breasts hypertrophied; others immature	0	0?	0?	0	
D. Medicational		Ingestion of: (a) Estrogen (b) Promizole?	+ Breasts hypertrophied	0 0	++ ?	0 ?	+	

The various symbols have the following meanings: + denotes precocious occurrence or abnormally increased for patient of this age but within normal adult limits; ++, an increase in hormone excretion which exceeds normal adult limits; N, normal for age; 0, absent.

The Ovaries

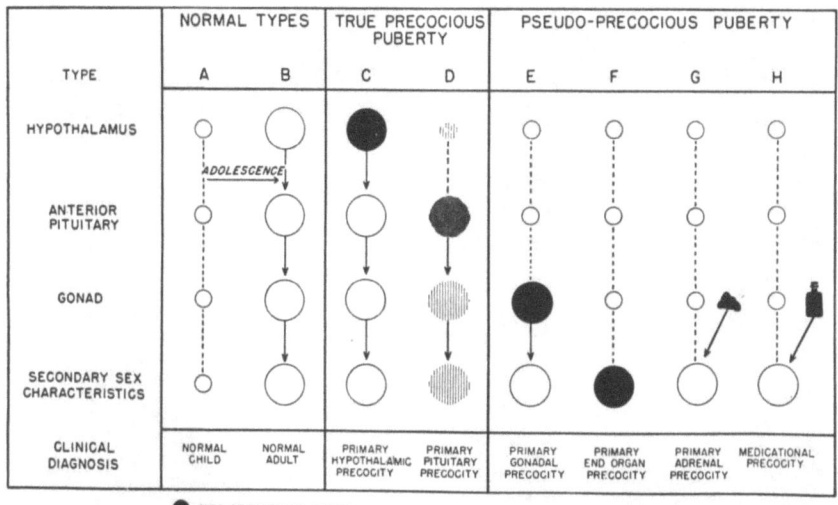

FIGURE V—11. Diagrammatic representation of the relations of the hypothalamus, anterior pituitary gland, gonads and secondary sexual characteristics in the normal child, the normal adult and in patients with sexual precocity of various types.

has occurred in a normal manner but at an abnormally early age. In these cases gonadotropin release has occurred prematurely, and childhood has thereby been skipped or greatly foreshortened. Since the ovaries attain mature size and function, true ovulatory menstrual cycles eventually become established, and pregnancy can occur. Gonadotropic hormones have been demonstrated in the urine in only a few cases, probably owing to methodological inadequacy; gonadal hormones are excreted in amounts somewhat less than, or equal to, those excreted by normal adult females.

Primary hypothalamic precocity (Figure 11, Type C). In all conditions grouped under this heading, the primary disturbance lies in the hypothalamus, which causes the anterior pituitary gland to release gonadotropic hormones into the circulation at an abnormally early age. The ovaries respond with the production of both estrogen and progesterone, and as a result the secondary sexual organs attain adult form and function.

Precocity Due to Destructive Lesions

Precocious puberty associated with hypothalamic lesions occurs almost exclusively in males. However, at least 10 well-authenticated instances of such precocity have occured in females. Six of these cases were attributed to tumors or cysts arising in the tuber cinereum, the floor of the third ventricle or the mammil-

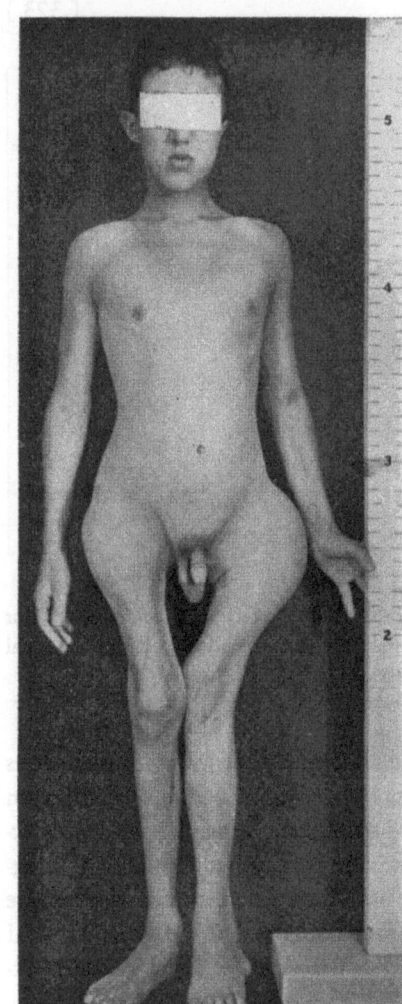
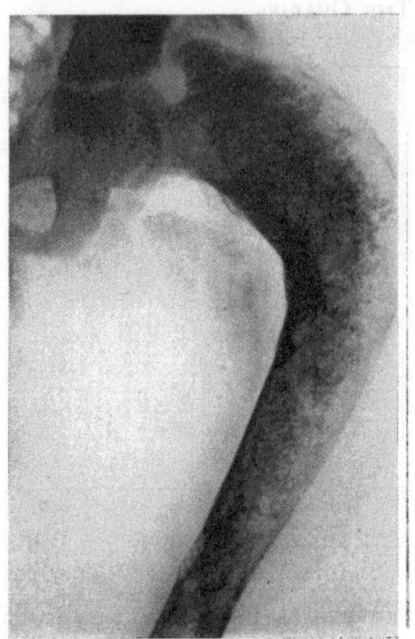

lary bodies, two were associated with post-meningitic hydrocephalus and two appeared to represent sequelæ of measles encephalitis (see Figures 18-20).

For details in regard to neurologic diagnosis of hypothalamic lesions the appropriate texts should be consulted.[16 a-c] Temporary misclassification of the disorder as "constitutional" precocity is likely to occur for two reasons: (a) the primary manifestations are sometimes endocrine rather than neurologic and (b) pneumo-encephalography occasionally fails to disclose abnormalities in patients later proved to have hypothalamic lesions. The prognosis of patients with this type of precocity is serious. Indications for treatment depend upon the nature of the lesion in the brain.

Idiopathic Precocity

"Constitutional" precocity.[7] No cause for this condition has so far been discovered. The precocity is attributed to an abnormality in the genetic factors which govern the time of maturation of the hypothalamic sex center. The order of appearance of sex characters is identical with that enumerated for normal adolescence; the abnormality consists entirely in the age at which sexual maturation is initiated. Maturation may begin at an astonishingly early age as in a patient reported by Novak, in whom the menarche occurred at 15 months and in whom a corpus luteum was demonstrated at 22 months (see Figures 12 and 13). With the onset of precocity, the growth rate of such children is accelerated, so that initially they are often abnormally tall. However, premature epiphyseal closure may occur and shorten the duration of the growth period. As a result, growth often stops before normal adult stature is attained.

The etiologic diagnosis must be made by exclusion. The immediate clinical findings may permit a direct diagnosis of polyostotic fibrous dysplasia, hypothalamic precocity due to a destructive lesion, ovarian tumor or adrenal tumor. If not, hormone assays may provide material assistance. Gonadotropins may be demonstrable in the urine in small amounts; estrogen, likewise, may be present but not in amounts excessive for the child's physiologic age. In addition, pregnandiol may eventually appear in the urine and endometrial biopsy disclose secretory changes in the premenstrual endometrium. If the case is one of pseudoprecocity due to ovarian tumor, estrogen excretion will generally exceed the norm for adult women; if due to an adrenal tumor, the excretion of both estrogens and 17-KS may be excessive. If doubt concerning the normality of the ovaries persists after a careful pelvic examination under anesthesia, exploratory laparotomy is warranted. Once made, the diagnosis of idiopathic precocity must be reviewed periodically.

Except for the hazard of precocious pregnancy and the possibility of subnormal stature, the prognosis of girls with idiopathic sexual precocity is good.

[326]

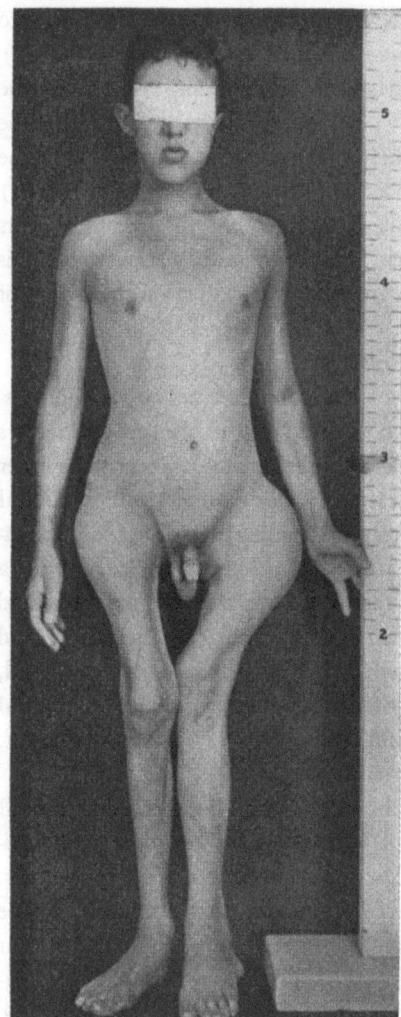

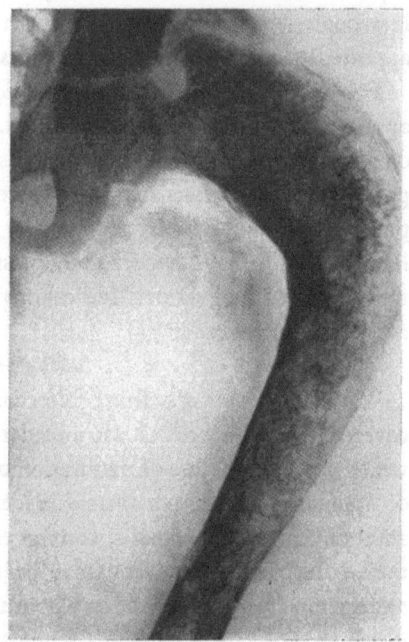

(Right)

FIGURE V—15. Roentgenogram of the left femur of the patient in Figure 14. Expansion and distortion of the shaft is evident. No cysts are actually present in such bones; their mottled appearance is due to irregular dense trabeculæ which cross in all directions. From M. A. Falconer, C. L. Cope and A. H. T. Robb-Smith, *Quart. J. Med.* 11:121, 1942.

(Left)

FIGURE V—14. Osteitis fibrosa disseminata in a boy of 11 years. The photograph illustrates extraordinarily well the typical facial asymmetry and the forward and outward bowing of the upper halves of both femora which produces bilateral coxa vara.

This patient also has somatic and sexual precocity.

From M. A. Falconer, C. L. Cope and A. H. T. Robb-Smith, *Quart. J. Med.* 11:121, 1942.

From such meager information as is available, it does not appear that the menopause is accelerated or that premature senility occurs. Steps should be taken to protect these patients from sex violation. Perhaps because of the psychological defenselessness of the child, such acts occur not infrequently. For example, 83 cases of pregnancy were found in a group of 310 cases of female sexual precocity.[5c] To lessen the child's vulnerability without engendering morbidity obviously requires discretion. There is no specific treatment for "constitutional" precocity.

Polyostotic fibrous dysplasia.[8 a-d] The characteristic features of this syndrome in its complete form are (a) a disseminated osteitis fibrosa (both hyper- and hypo-ostotic) with a segmental distribution, (b) areas of cutaneous pigmentation which are so distributed as to suggest a connection with bone lesions and (c) sexual and somatic precocity. Approximately 40 cases exhibiting these classic features have been reported. If cases of fibrous dysplasia of the skeleton with or without the other abnormalities be considered instances of the syndrome, approximately 90 cases (39 male and 51 female) are on record.

The cause of the condition is totally obscure. It is thought that an embryologic defect or an underlying neurologic disturbance may be at fault. There is no evidence that the disease is hereditary. Only two females with the disease have so far come to autopsy. In one case, there was a considerable diminution in the size of one mammillary body and an accessory nucleus in the adjacent tissue. In the other, no hypothalamic lesion was demonstrable but the fact that the basophil cells of the pituitary were hyperplastic suggests that these cells were being stimulated, possibly by a disturbance originating in the hypothalamus.

The disease is most frequently manifest in early childhood, and its active phase seems to terminate when adult life is reached. Usually symptoms referable to the bony lesions, such as pathologic fractures or skeletal deformities, call attention to the disorder (see Figure 14).

The bone lesions, which are thought to be due to an embryonic defect in the conversion of mesenchyme to bone, consist mainly of masses of fibrous tissue which replace the medullary structures of the involved bone. In the absence of trauma, the skeletal lesions are painless. The femur is the commonest site for fractures, and coxa vara is the commonest deformity. Lesions of the skull are seen frequently. The changes in the vault, occiput and mandible closely resemble those seen elsewhere in the skeleton. The lesions affecting the basal portions of the frontal bone, and the sphenoid, ethmoid and maxillary bones, on the other hand, differ from the lesions of fibrous dysplasia seen elsewhere. In these locations a sclerotic overgrowth of bone occurs. Deformity of the orbit with ocular proptosis, obstruction of the nasal passages and complete or partial obliteration of the paranasal sinuses may occur. Bony pressure may impair the function of the cranial nerves, especially the optic nerve. Roentgenologically, the osseous lesions appear as focal, disseminated zones of osteoporosis (see Figure 15) except at the base of the skull, where the affected bones may exhibit such greatly increased density as to obscure the normal landmarks (see Figure 16). Regions of severe involvement often lie adjacent to areas which are perfectly normal in appearance, a condition which stands in marked contrast to that observed in hyperparathyroidism.

The areas of skin pigmentation vary in size from small, inconspicuous lesions which are easily overlooked (in one of Albright's cases the spots became visible only when the back of the head was shaved) to large, disfiguring blotches. The affected areas are light brown, normal in texture and not elevated. The edges of the lesions tend to be wavy and irregular. Any region may be affected, but probably the most frequent sites are the lower lumbar region, the buttocks and the thighs. There is no correlation between the extent of pigmentation and that of the bony dystrophy, but when the bony lesions are predominantly unilateral, the pigmented areas tend to be on the same side and to show a similar distribution (see Figure 17).

Precocious puberty was present in 20 of the 51 female subjects reported. That is, it occurred in 39 per cent of these subjects and in 22 per cent of the entire series of 90 cases. The menarcheal ages reported have ranged from three months to 10 years, the average age being three years. It is not yet known whether there is a tendency for the menopause to occur prematurely in these patients. Corpora lutea were not demonstrable in the ovaries of the two patients who came to autopsy. However, the benign clinical course, the absence of ovarian and adrenal lesions in the cases which have come to laparotomy or autopsy and the failure to demonstrate excessive estrogen excretion in the few instances in which assays have been performed argue for a central origin of the precocity.

In seven patients, nodular or diffuse enlargement of the thyroid was noted; and in two of them hyperthyroidism as well.

Laboratory studies do not contribute materially to the diagnosis except to aid in the exclusion of hyperparathyroidism. While hypercalcuria is found occasionally, the levels of serum calcium and phosphorus are normal. The serum phosphatase is often moderately increased, presumably in proportion to the activity of the osseous lesions.

The prognosis of these patients as regards life is good. There is no tendency for the bony lesions to undergo malignant degeneration. However, deformities resulting from repeated pathologic fractures may give rise to severe disability,

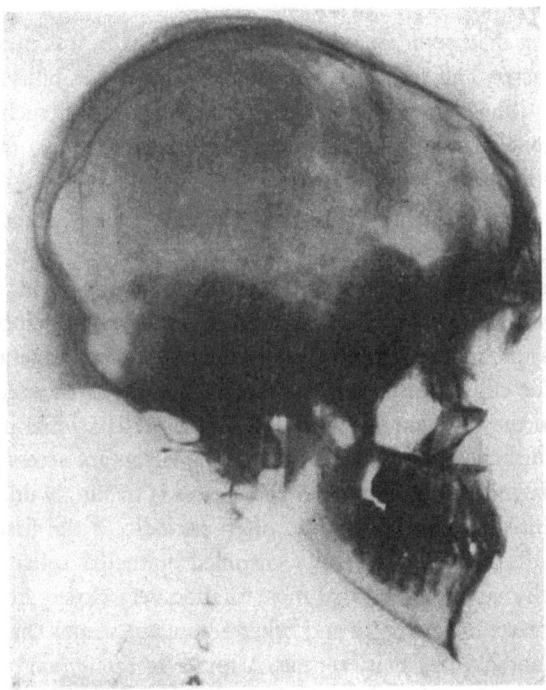

FIGURE V—16. Roentgenogram of the skull of an 18-year-old patient with osteitis fibrosa disseminata. The base of the skull shows a diffuse bony overgrowth, particularly involving the sphenoid bone, petrous temporal bone and the bones of the roof and lateral wall of the nose. Because of the large hemispherical bony swelling in front of the sella turcica, its outlines can be traced only vaguely. The right frontal sinus is occluded by bony overgrowth, and in the occipital region there is marked subpericranial deposition of new bone. From M. A. Falconer, C. L. Cope and A. H. T. Robb-Smith, *Quart. J. Med.* 11:121, 1942.

especially when the "shepherd's crook deformity" results from repeated fractures of the upper end of the femur. There is no specific treatment.

Primary pituitary precocity (Figure 11, Type D). Though theoretically possible, this type of precocious puberty has not yet been observed clinically.

Pseudo-Precocious Puberty. The term "pseudo-precocious puberty" is properly applicable to cases of isosexual precocity in which premature development of the secondary sexual organs has occurred due to: (a) an ovarian or adrenocortical tumor, (b) unusual sensitivity of end organs to normal hormonal stimulation and (c) sex hormones or other compounds supplied exogenously. In all of these instances there is no central activation of the pituitary with the release of gonadotropic hormones, and the gonads therefore remain immature. Although uterine bleeding may occur, sometimes in pseudo-cycles, it is necessarily anovulatory in character, and therefore pregnancy is not a possibility. Gonadotropic hormones are almost invariably absent from the urine in such cases; on the other hand, gonadal hormones are often excreted in amounts far greater than those excreted by normal adult females.

Primary ovarian precocity (Figure 11, Type E). Pseudo-precocious puberty develops most frequently as a result of ovarian tumors and cysts which produce a premature supply of estrogen and hence precocious secondary sexual phenomena. The well-known granulosa cell tumor is the commonest cause, although follicular cysts and, in rare instances, chorionepitheliomas and teratomas are also responsible. The clinical history of patients having one of these tumors depends primarily upon the fact that endocrine activity is present while mechanical and circulatory disturbances, and occasionally malignancy, are accessory factors.

The clinical syndrome presented in these cases is strikingly uniform. In most instances a whitish vaginal discharge, often periodic, is the first symptom. A smear of this discharge reveals fully cornified epithelial cells. Later, vaginal bleeding, which may mimic normal menstruation very closely in its periodicity, occurs. The breasts hypertrophy and other secondary sexual characteristics, including pubic and axillary hair, appear. A tumor in the region of an ovary can usually be made out by either abdominal* or rectal examination. Finally, skeletal growth is likely to display rapid acceleration.

Sixteen well-authenticated cases of granulosa cell tumor have been reported in children ranging in age from 14 weeks to 12 years. In a few instances, attention was attracted to the condition by swelling of the abdomen, failure to gain weight and pain associated with torsion of the tumor or intestinal obstruction. In most cases, however, endocrine phenomena dominated the clinical picture (see Figure 19). Accurate hormonal studies were relatively infrequent, but those which were performed generally showed an excretion of estrogen far in excess of normal adult levels.

Most such tumors are unilateral, although a few bilateral ones have been found. In size they vary from microscopic nodules to masses as large as a human head. They are encapsulated and lobular. While they may contain cystic areas, they are generally solid and their surface is smooth. The degree of malignancy in granulosa cell tumors is still a matter of dispute. In different series of cases, the recurrence rate has varied from 4.5 to 33 per cent.

In the cases in which complete removal of a granulosa cell tumor was possible the clinical course has been extremely benign. Uterine bleeding ceased, and com-

---

* In children the uterus and adnexa are abdominal rather than pelvic organs. Therefore, the presence of a tumor in the abdominal cavity is not inconsistent with the diagnosis.

Continued on page 334

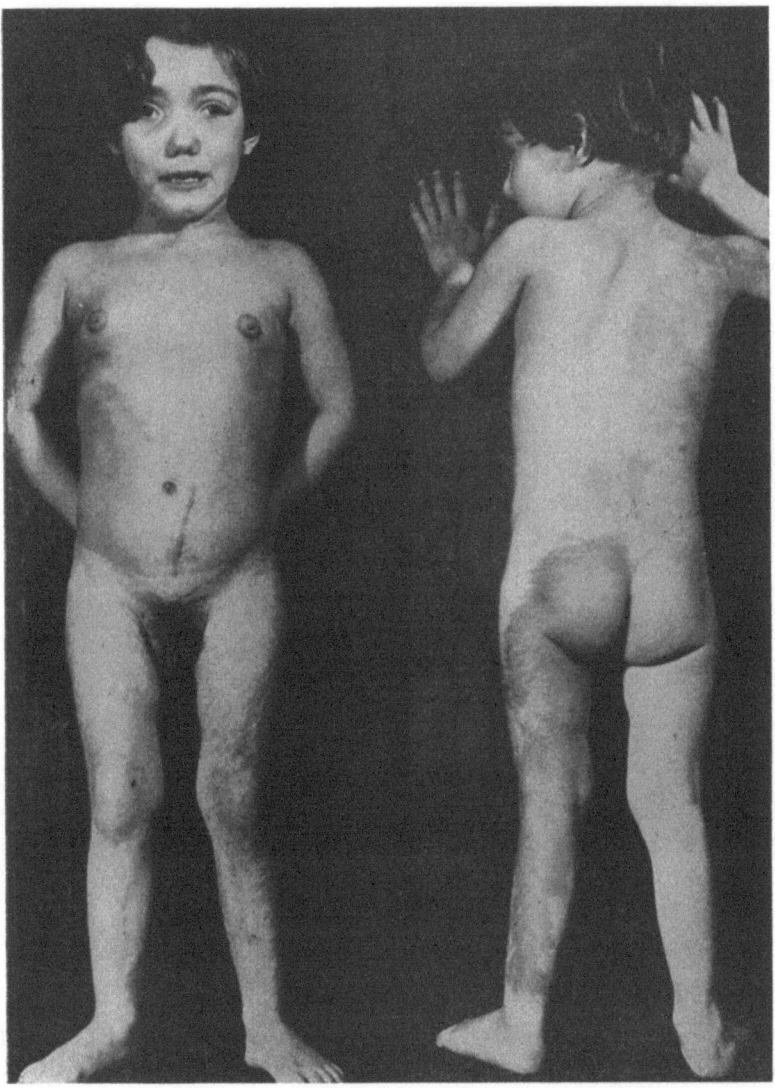

FIGURE V—17. Osteitis fibrosa disseminata in a child of 3³/₁₂ years. The pigmented areas on the face, trunk, buttock, thigh and leg have the characteristic serrated "coast of Maine" edges. Note also the breast development, areolar pigmentation, enlarged labia and pubic hair growth. Periodic vaginal bleeding had commenced at the age of 4½ months. From F. Albright, A. M. Butler, A. O. Hampton and P. Smith. *New Eng. J. Med.* 216:727, 1937.

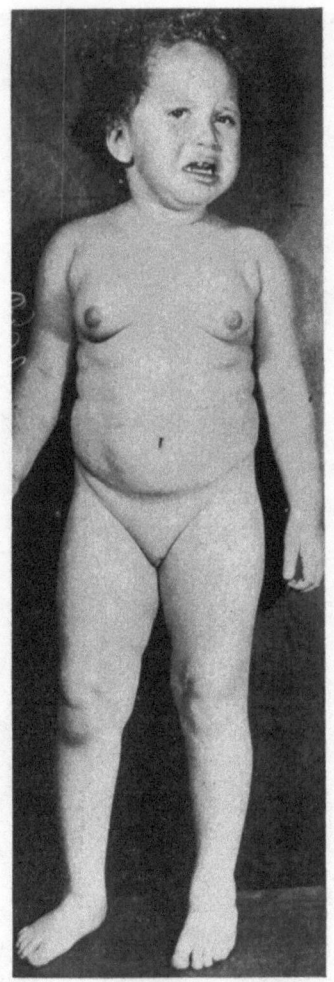
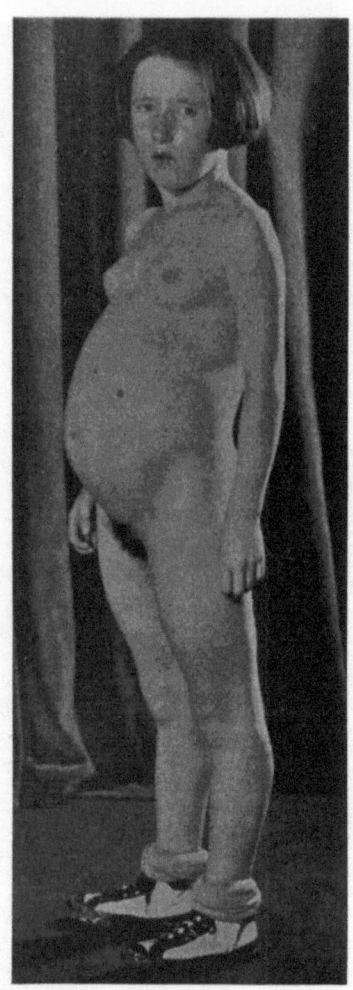

(Left)

FIGURE V—18. True precocious puberty due to an astrocytic hamartoma in the hypothalamus and the floor of the third ventricle. The patient is shown at two years. Vaginal bleeding and breast enlargement were first noted seven months previously. From R. E. Gross, *Am. J. Dis. Child.* 59:579, 1940.

(Right)

FIGURE V—19. Pseudo-precocious puberty and abdominal distension due to a huge granulosa cell carcinoma of the left ovary. The patient is shown at seven years. Vaginal bleeding, breast enlargement and a luxuriant growth of axillary and pubic hair were first noted four months previously. "Menstrual periods" recurred monthly until hospital admission. From P. B. Bland and L. Goldstein, *Surg., Gynec. & Obst.* 61:250, 1935.

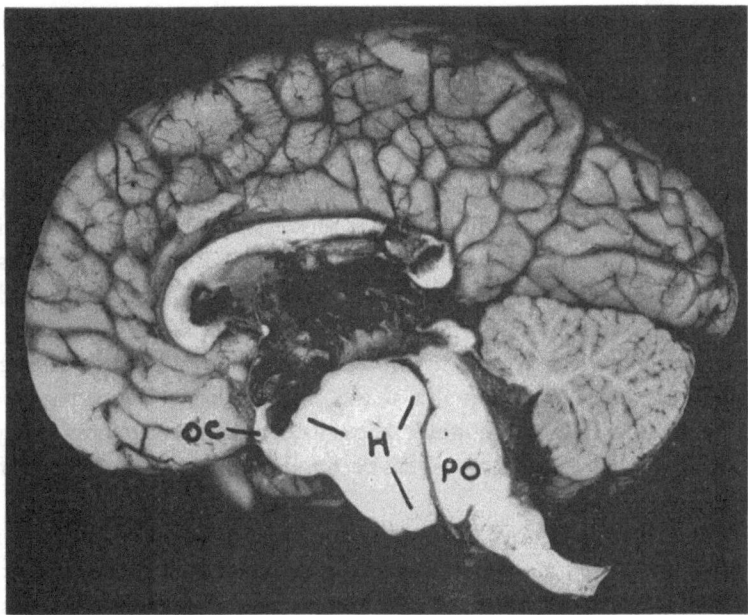

FIGURE V—20. Sagittal section of the brain of a sexually precocious child of two years (see Figure 18). Bulging below the inferior surface of the brain is an encapsulated astrocytic hamartoma which extends from the optic chiasm to the pons. H, hamartoma; OC, optic chiasm; PO, pons. From R. E. Gross, *Am. J. Dis. Child.* 59:579, 1940.

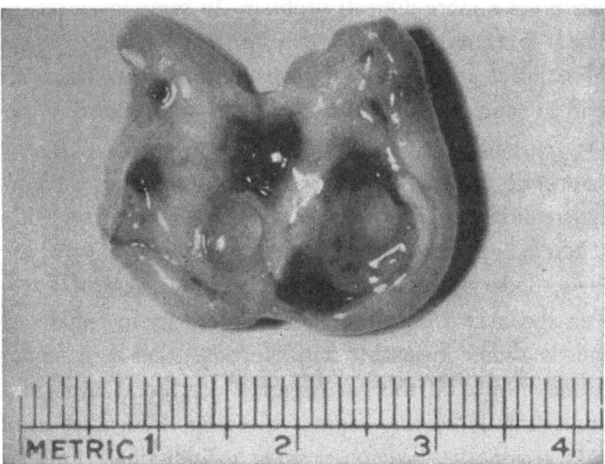

FIGURE V—21. Sagittal section of an ovary of the same patient. Note the developing and regressing follicles and the follicular cyst in the lower left central portion of the ovary and also the darker staining corpora hemorrhagica. Courtesy of Dr. S. Farber.

plete or partial regression of the hypertrophied secondary sexual organs occurred, demonstrating the endocrine activity of the tumor to be the cause of the precocity. In the few instances in which follow-up of the patients was adequate, puberty "recurred" at the expected time and appeared to be normal in all respects.

Next to granulosa cell tumors, follicular cysts are the commonest ovarian cause of sexual precocity. In some instances such cysts are bilateral and multiple, suggesting that the primary disturbance is central.[9 f] Adequate hormonal assays have rarely been carried out, but in one two-year-old patient described by Geschichter[5 b] gonadotropic hormone was demonstrable in the urine. This fact and the persistence of sex precocity following the removal of the cysts suggest that such cases are really examples of the "constitutional" idiopathic type of precocity. In other instances, however, the cysts have appeared to possess physiologic autonomy, since their removal has been followed by a disappearance of the precocity.[9 d]

Teratomas have produced the syndrome of pseudo-precocious puberty in a few instances.[9 e] Even more rare is precocity due to chorionepithelioma of the ovary.[9 c] In one such case chorionic gonadotropin as well as estrogen was demonstrated in the urine. Chorionepitheliomas are extremely malignant tumors and have led to death with metastases within a year and a half.

Oophorectomy is indicated for granulosa cell tumors, teratomas, chorionepitheliomas and single ovarian cysts. The management of patients with multiple follicular cysts poses a more difficult problem. In some instances castration has been performed. It seems to us preferable to treat the case conservatively and to regard the child as an instance of "constitutional" precocity, accepting the abnormality in somatic growth which may occur and protecting the child from sex violation.

Primary adrenal precocity (adrenocortical feminism) (Figure 11, Type G).[10] In this condition estrogen production, either by tumors of the adrenal proper or by adrenal cell rest tumors, is the fundamental cause of the precocious growth of the secondary sexual organs.

As has been shown in Chapter III, sexual precocity in females with adrenocortical lesions is almost invariably heterologous—that is, it tends to progress along masculine lines with the development of clitoral hypertrophy, a deep voice and hirsutism. However, vaginal bleeding, sometimes associated with mammary enlargement, has been observed as an additional feature in 15 reasonably well-authenticated cases. Only in exceptional instances have signs of isosexual precocity preceded those of heterosexual precocity. In the few cases in which hormone assays have been carried out the results have been paradoxical, due partly, perhaps, to methodological difficulties. However, because of the mixture of iso- and heterosexual precocity, the adrenals have usually come promptly under suspicion. The adrenal lesion responsible for this syndrome has been a tumor in the majority of cases, and usually it has been malignant. In two instances isosexual precocity resulted from activity of an "adrenal rest" in the vicinity of the ovary.

Primary end organ precocity (Figure 11, Type F). In this condition unusual sensitivity of the secondary sexual organs to hormonal stimulation is the fundamental cause of the sexual precocity. Although the entire hypothalamic–pituitary–ovarian chain remains in the dormant infantile state, certain end organs exhibit growth in response to the minute quantities of estrogens circulating in childhood.

Thus, breast development or pubic hair growth may be observed without other evidences of sexual maturation. The authors have noted minimal mammary enlargement as an isolated finding in a number of females approximately two years of age (see Figures 22 and 23). Such patients show no other signs of sexual maturation. The size of the ovaries and uterus is consistent with the child's chronologic age, the vaginal smear contains no cornified cells, and assays of the urine for estrogen, gonadotropin and 17-KS yield essentially zero values.* In the case of one patient who was followed for a considerable length of time the mammoplasia ultimately disappeared, suggesting that the condition may be transitory in some instances. Such patients require careful study and prolonged observation to exclude the possibility of incipient hyperhormonal precocity.

Primary medicational precocity (Figure 11, Type H). In this condition premature growth of the secondary sexual organs occurs in response to stimulation by sex hormones or other compounds supplied exogenously. We have seen one instance of pseudo-precocity resulting from accidental ingestion of estrogen. In this case the intense pigmentation of the child's nipples suggested that the sexual development was not endogenous in origin. Stilbestrol was later found to be the responsible agent. Instances of pseudo-precocity in patients undergoing promizole therapy have also been reported,[11] but the laboratory documentation of the cases in question is inadequate to permit an analysis of the mechanism involved. Precocity is not a universal occurrence in promizole treatment.

* Caution must be used in interpreting such assay values; they do not provide unequivocal evidence that the hormone excretion of the patient is within normal limits. They indicate only that the quantities of hormone appearing in a 24-hour urine sample are small compared with those found in adolescent and adult females. It would seem desirable to run urine assays on a two- or three-day collection of urine from a two-year-old child in order to procure results comparable to those obtained on the adolescent or adult. (The two-year-old child has a surface area of approximately 0.5 m^2, which is one-half or one-third that of the adolescent or adult female.)

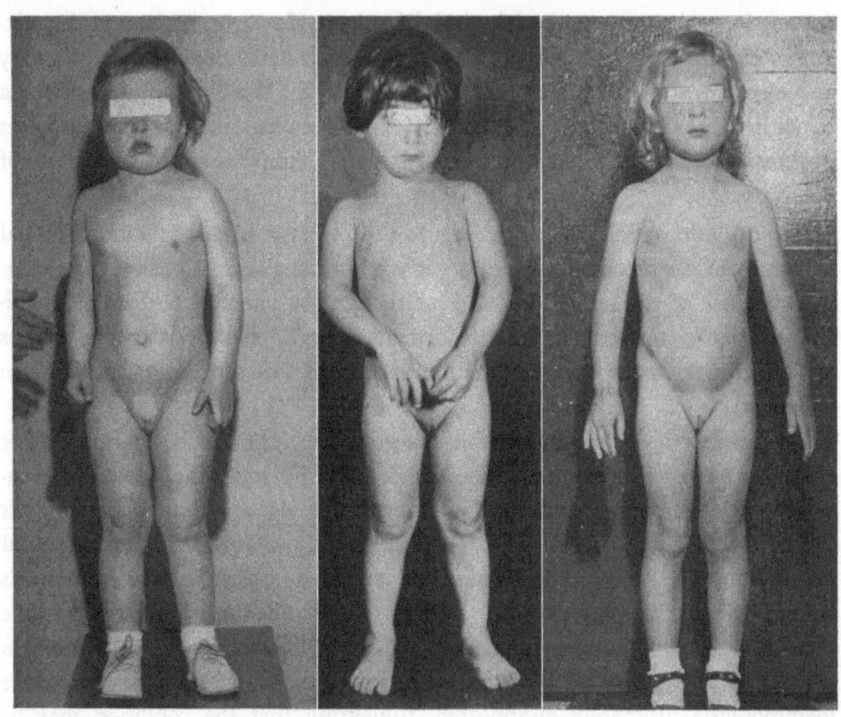

FIGURE V—22. Mammoplasia in girls of two, three and four years. Note the sexual immaturity of these patients in all other respects.

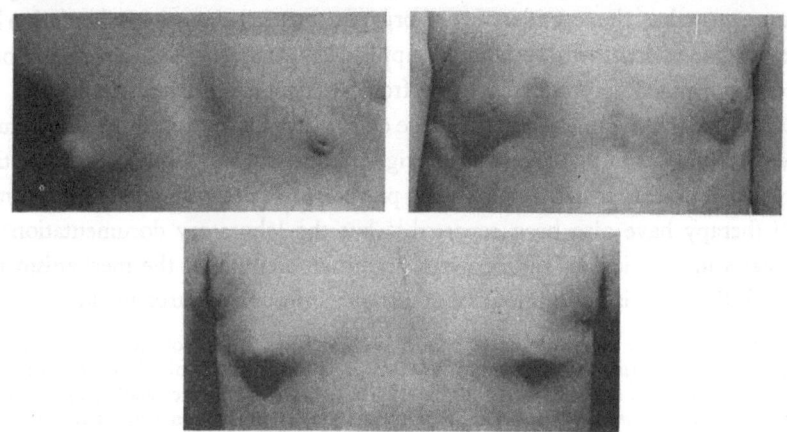

FIGURE V—23. Close-up views of the breasts of the three patients shown in Figure 22.

TYPES OF SEXUAL INFANTILISM

Sexual infantilism, the retention of the infantile state as regards sexual development, is considered to be present in the female when indications of genital maturation have not become apparent by the age of 16 years.[12]

Wide variations obtain in the time of initiation of normal sexual development and in its rate of progression. Accordingly, it may be difficult to distinguish adolescence which is merely delayed from that resulting from a true defect in the neuro-hormonal mechanism which initiates and sustains sexual development. Thus, in 100 normal girls it was found[2h] that budding of the breasts, the first sign of genital maturation, occurred at various ages between 10.7 and 14.7 years. The range for other indices of sexual maturation is equally wide.

Genetic factors appear to be of great importance in the timing of genital development. Thus, there is a strong positive correlation between the age of menarche in mothers and daughters; likewise, the mean difference in months between the age of menarche in sisters is less than that of unrelated groups. Moreover, the type of body build, which reflects at least in part the operation of genetic factors, and the age at which the menses appear are intimately related to one another. Broad-built, stocky girls menstruate earlier than slender-built girls. Climate appears to exert an influence upon the timing of sexual maturation, although socio-economic and racial differences may participate in the operation of this factor. The menarche consistently occurs earlier in temperate than torrid or frigid zones. Caution is therefore indicated in evaluating the status and prognosis of patients presenting the problem of sexual infantilism.

Any lesion impairing the integrity of the hypothalamic–pituitary–ovarian mechanism which initiates sexual development is potentially capable of causing true sexual infantilism (see Figure 24). Three major categories of such disorders exist in accordance with this schema, and the causes of sexual infantilism in the female may, therefore, be classified as follows:

A. Primary hypothalamic infantilism
   1. Destructive lesions (Froehlich's syndrome)
   2. Congenital defect (Laurence-Moon-Biedl syndrome)

B. Primary pituitary infantilism
   1. Pituitary lesions
      (a) Generalized pituitary deficiency
      (b) Fractional pituitary deficiency
   2. Factors inducing functional hypopituitarism
      (a) Thyroid: hyper- and hypothyroidism

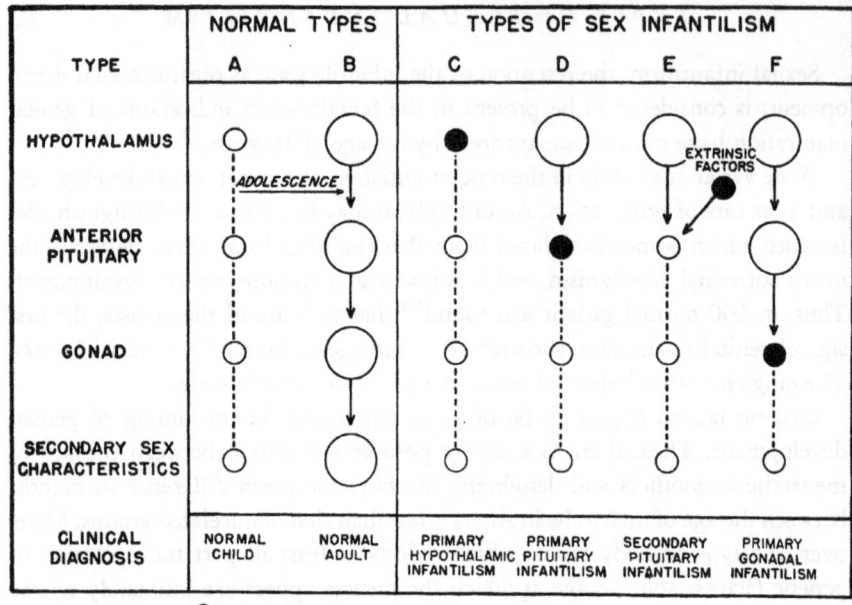

FIGURE V—24. Diagrammatic representation of the relations of the hypothalamus, anterior pituitary gland, gonads and secondary sexual characteristics in normal children and adults and in patients with sexual infantilism of various types.

    (b) Pancreas: diabetes mellitus
    (c) Adrenal cortex: insufficiency and hyperfunctioning lesions
    (d) Chronic infectious and debilitating diseases
    (e) Nutritional disturbances: obesity and undernutrition

  c. Primary ovarian infantilism
    1. Agenesis of the follicular elements of the ovary
    2. Castration (disease, radiation and surgery)

The outstanding clinical manifestations of these conditions are indicated in Table 3.

True infantilism is a comparatively rare phenomenon and the available data is inadequate to permit more than a broad generalization regarding the incidence of the various types. The miscellaneous diseases leading to functional hypopituitarism and the syndrome of agenesis of the follicular elements of the ovary probably account for the largest proportion of cases. All other causes of infantilism approach the status of clinical rarities.

TABLE V—3. Clinical characteristics of various types of sexual infantilism in the female.

Type of infantilism	Alternate name	Cause	Development of breasts, vagina and uterus; menstruation	Gonadotropin excretion	Sexual hair; 17-KS output	Height	Defects which may be associated
1. Hypothalamic							
(a) Destructive lesions	Froehlich's syndrome	Supra-sellar cyst (craniopharyngioma)	0	0	0 or −	Variable	Diabetes insipidus; obesity
(b) Congenital defect	Laurence-Moon-Biedl syndrome	Genetic defects	0 or −	?	?	Variable	Obesity; retinitis pigmentosa; polydactylism; mental deficiency
2. Pituitary							
(a) Generalized deficiency	Pituitary dwarfism; panhypopituitarism	Usually idiopathic. Rarely tumor, infarction, infection or trauma to pituitary	0	0	0 or −	Short	Hypothyroidism; adrenal insufficiency
(b) Specific gonadotropin deficiency	Idiopathic lack of follicle-stimulating hormone	Idiopathic pituitary or CNS lesion or disturbance	0	0	N or −	Normal	
3. Ovarian							
(a) Agenesis of follicular elements	Turner's syndrome; ovarian dwarfism	Multiple genetic defects	0	Usually ++	−	Usually short	Sphinx neck; coarctation of aorta; eye defects; congenital deafness; bony defects; hypertension, etc.
(b) Castration		Destruction of ovaries by x-ray, disease or surgery	0	Usually ++	N or −	Normal	

The various symbols have the following meanings: + denotes precocious occurrence or abnormally increased for patient of this age, but within normal adult limits; ++, an increase in hormone excretion which exceeds normal adult limits; N, normal for age; 0, absent; −, subnormal.

Primary Hypothalamic Infantilism (Figure 24, Type C). In this condition destruction or hypoplasia of certain specific areas in the hypothalamus is the fundamental cause of the sexual infantilism. Though both the anterior pituitary gland and the ovaries are normal in form and potential function, the appropriate neural stimulus for gonadotropin release is never delivered to the pituitary. The ovaries, in consequence, remain in the dormant infantile state.

Infantilism due to destructive lesions (Froehlich's syndrome).[13a,b] Froehlich's syndrome is a very rare disorder which, if it begins in childhood, produces sexual infantilism. Frequently attached to girls with simple dietary obesity and delayed menstruation, this diagnosis should be reserved for patients in whom the existence of a hypothalamic lesion can be demonstrated by x-ray or can be inferred from definite neuro-endocrine manifestations (see also Chapter VII). The syndrome is due to a lesion in the hypothalamus (commonly a cystic craniopharyngioma lying above the sella turcica) rather than to primary pituitary disease. In the majority of patients in this age group endocrine rather than neurologic manifestations predominate; signs of increased intracranial pressure are uncommon. Growth is often greatly retarded and sexual development absent. The bodily habitus is variable. In most instances the child is rotund, with a heavy deposition of fat about the abdomen, buttocks and thighs; occasionally the child is gracile and slender. But regardless of the type of habitus, the scalp hair tends to be fine and silky and body hair to be absent. The skin is fine in texture and of a pasty color. The breasts remain infantile, and menstruation fails to occur. Body temperature is often subnormal, and the basal metabolic rate, likewise, tends to be low. Diabetes insipidus is sometimes observed. Roentgenograms of the sella turcica reveal destruction of the clinoid processes in a large percentage of the cases. Inasmuch as the cysts usually exert pressure from above, they tend to flatten the sella rather than to balloon it. In about 75 per cent of the cases abnormal areas of increased density, due to areas of calcification in the wall of the cyst, can be visualized above the sella (see Chapter VII, Figure 5).

As one would predict, gonadotropins are absent from the urine or are demonstrable only in minimal amounts. The 17-KS excretion may also be abnormally low, implying interference with the release of adrenocorticotropic hormone (see Chapter III, page 158).

Surgical intervention is contraindicated in Froehlich's syndrome unless there are alterations in the visual fields or signs of increased intracranial pressure. Barring such indications, one should initiate a program of therapy designed to replace all endocrine functions which are demonstrably deficient. For the nongonadal components of such a medical program, see Chapter VII. The gonadal deficiency should be treated by estrogen replacement, which must be continued indefinitely. Deprived of estrogen, such patients are prone to become prematurely senile. Atrophy of the skin and osteoporosis occur; the latter may lead eventually to much suffering. Estrogen replacement, by bringing about pseudomenstruation and breast development, has a valuable effect upon the morale of these patients. After approximately two years of estrogen therapy the breast enlargement becomes semi-permanent. In addition, the vagina gradually achieves adult dimensions and its mucosa becomes pink and succulent.

A convenient method for feminizing patients with estrogen is to administer diethylstilbestrol continuously in a dosage of 1 mg. daily until the uterus has attained adult proportions or until bleeding occurs from the hyperplastic endometrium. The time required to induce this degree of development is highly variable; a year or more is needed in some instances. Once uterine growth has reached this point, it is desirable to administer estrogen cyclically. It is our custom to give 1 mg. of diethylstilbestrol daily for six weeks, omit it for two weeks, then resume stilbestrol for six weeks. Estrogen-withdrawal bleeding will usually occur during the two-week rest period. Some clinicians prefer to supplement this therapy with a progestin in order to simulate normal menstruation more closely. However, the cost of the therapy is substantially increased and normal ovarian-pituitary reciprocity is not restored by the addition of progesterone to the program. Therefore, combined therapy seems to have little to commend it except when there is inadequate endometrial desquamation following estrogen withdrawal and metropathic bleeding must be prevented.

Infantilism due to congenital defect (Laurence-Moon-Biedl syndrome).[14 a-c] Sexual infantilism is a frequent, though not invariable, feature of this syndrome. Linkage of a number of genetic defects is thought to be responsible for the condition and a congenital hypothalamic defect is postulated as the cause of the hypogonadism. The sexual retardation is generally overshadowed by other features of the syndrome, which in classic cases comprise: (a) obesity, (b) retinitis pigmentosa, (c) mental deficiency, (d) polydactylism and (e) familial occurrence. Few patients with Laurence-Moon-Biedl syndrome have been adequately studied from the endocrine point of view.

In view of the frequent occurrence of mental deficiency in patients with this syndrome, it seems preferable not to attempt to modify their sexual infantilism.

Primary Pituitary Infantilism (Figure 24, Type D). In this condition, anatomic or physiologic disturbances affecting the function of the anterior pituitary gland are the fundamental cause of the sexual infantilism. The hypothalamus delivers the appropriate neural stimulus to the pituitary when the child reaches the proper developmental age. However, because of hypoplasia or destruction the pituitary is unable to respond with the release of gonadotropic hormones and the ovaries, though normal in form and in potential function, remain in the quiescent infantile state.

Infantilism due to pituitary lesions. In dealing with patients of this type, it is important to distinguish between abnormalities which lead to deficiency with respect to all anterior–pituitary–tropic functions (generalized pituitary deficiency) and abnormalities which lead to deficiency only with respect to pituitary gonadotropic factors (fractional pituitary deficiency).

Generalized pituitary deficiency.[15 a, b] Absence of sexual development is one of the consequences of hypoplasia or atrophy of the anterior lobe of the pituitary gland. While tumor pressure is a common cause of pituitary atrophy in adult life, it is a rare cause of atrophy in childhood. The etiology of the majority of cases of so-called "pituitary dwarfism" is totally obscure; it is thought that acute infectious diseases and hereditary factors may play a role. The primary and secondary sexual organs of such patients are infantile and gonadotropins are absent from their urine. For other clinical features of this syndrome, see Chapter VII.

Fractional pituitary deficiency.[4 h, 12] In rare instances an idiopathic impairment of pituitary gonadotropic activity occurs without demonstrable defects in any of the other pituitary functions. The sex organs of such patients are completely undeveloped, and gonadotropins are absent from their urine. But they are not dwarfed, although their body proportions may be eunuchoid and their bone age somewhat retarded. Adrenal 17-ketosteroid-precursor production is fairly normal, as evidenced by the presence of axillary and pubic hair and by urinary 17-KS excretion levels, which are only slightly reduced.

Stimulative therapy with gonadotropins would appear to be ideal for patients with either generalized pituitary deficiency or specific gonadotropic deficiency. However, therapy with currently available gonadotropin preparations has proved disappointing. Replacement therapy with estrogens, as outlined under the treatment of hypothalamic infantilism, should be given.

Infantilism due to factors inducing functional hypopituitarism (Figure 24, Type E). Physiologic disturbances in an anatomically normal pituitary gland are equally capable of producing sexual infantilism. These disturbances may be produced by thyroid, pancreatic, adrenal, infectious and nutritional disorders.

Thyroid disorders. Hypothyroidism and, less commonly, hyperthyroidism may delay the appearance of mature sexual characteristics. Sexual maturity is often achieved eventually even by untreated cretins, but while some cretins have carried pregnancies to term, many are sterile and have scanty, irregular menstrual flow, presumably from a proliferative endometrium. Gonadotropins are likely to be absent from the urine, or present only in small amounts. In this condition, the genital component of the clinical picture is incidental (see also Chapter I, page 14).

Diabetes mellitus.[15c] Retarded sexual development, amounting in some instances to actual infantilism, occurs occasionally in patients with juvenile diabetes. It is thought that the retardation is nutritional in origin, since adequate control of the diabetes with diet and insulin usually allows for the normal progress of somatic and sexual maturation (see also Chapter IX, page 454).

Adrenal disorders. Adrenal insufficiency is an exceedingly rare cause of sexual infantilism; more commonly, hyperfunctioning adrenal lesions are responsible. Hyperplasia of abnormal androgenic elements of the adrenal cortex in embryonic life or in infancy can lead to failure of normal feminine development and to masculinization. The condition may pass unrecognized until virilization becomes unmistakable. When Cushing's syndrome has its onset before puberty, sexual retardation may be one of the clinical features. For further comments on these diseases, see Chapter III.

Chronic infectious and debilitating diseases and nutritional disturbances. There are good reasons for suspecting that these disorders delay maturation by inducing functional pituitary insufficiency. Normal sexual development is largely dependent upon normal infantile and preadolescent development. However, there may be no postponement in the maturation of very badly handicapped individuals and prolonged delay in the maturation of individuals whose general health has suffered minimal impairment (see also Chapter VII).

Infantilism due to functional hypopituitarism resulting from thyroid, pancreatic, adrenal, infectious and nutritional disturbances needs no treatment other than that directed at the primary disorder. One condition, hyperplasia of the androgenic elements of the adrenal cortices, constitutes an exception to this statement. Replacement therapy with estrogen is sometimes moderately successful in feminizing these patients and should be attempted. Larger doses of diethylstilbestrol (4 to 6 mg. per day) may be necessary to feminize patients in this category. From preliminary studies it appears that cortisone may indirectly exert a feminizing influence on girls with adrenal hyperplasia. For additional information concerning this type of therapy, see Chapter III.

Primary ovarian infantilism (Figure 24, Type F). This condition results from congenital absence of the hormone-producing structures of the ovary or from postnatal castration, either by surgery or disease. When the child reaches the proper developmental age, the hypothalamus activates the pituitary and the gonadotropic hormones are released, but the ovary is unable to respond with the production of sex hormones.

Agenesis of the Follicular Elements of the Ovary.[16 a-f] Approximately 100 instances of this condition, known variously as Turner's syndrome, "ovarian agenesis" and "ovarian dwarfism," have now been reported. In classic cases the following features are observed: (a) sexual infantilism, due to the presence of rudimentary ovaries, which are totally devoid of germinal elements, (b) short, but not actually dwarfed, stature, (c) diminished, and sometimes absent, pubic and axillary hair and (d) late union of the epiphyses and diffuse osteoporosis. The associated hormonal pattern in typical patients comprises: (a) subnormal levels of urinary estrogen, (b) diminished excretion of 17-KS and (c) high levels of urinary gonadotropins. The short stature and the rudimentary condition of the ovaries are thought to be due to linked genetic defects. Consonant with this hypothesis is the large number of additional congenital anomalies which occasionally accompany the syndrome. These comprise: (a) webbing of the neck, or "sphinx neck," as Castillo[16 f] aptly describes it (see Figure 26), (b) mental retardation, (c) ocular abnormalities, such as bilateral cataracts, bilateral ptosis, colobama, mild exophthalmos, retinal albinism, strabismus and "tubular vision," (d) congenital deafness, (e) vascular abnormalities, such as coarctation of the aorta and hemangioma of the intestine, (f) bony abnormalities, such as cubitus valgus, pes cavus, Madelung's deformity (distortion of the radius at its lower end, with ulnar displacement backward), spina bifida, fusion of cervical vertebræ, shortened phalanges, abnormal development of ribs and osteogenesis imperfecta tarda, (g) renal anomalies, such as horseshoe kidney, and (h) hypertension, which may be of unexplained origin.

The primary ovarian origin of the sexual infantilism was initially inferred from the high levels of gonadotropins in the urine. This finding differentiated the condition from failure of normal sexual development due to pituitary deficiency. Exploratory laparotomies have subsequently established the correctness of the original deduction. No structure resembling a mature ovary is discernible in such patients; on the posterior surface of each broad ligament there is a glistening white streak approximately 3 mm. in width, which runs parallel to the Fallopian tube from the uterine cornu to the fimbriated end (see Figure 27). On microscopic examination, this streak is found to consist entirely of tissue resembling ovarian stroma. No germinal epithelium or follicles can be found (see Figure 28). It appears that such gonads have failed to develop beyond the stage of the primitive genital ridge. The internal and external genitalia, while small owing to the lack of estrogen stimulation, are seldom deformed (occasionally there is malformation of the uterus).

Except for the defect in statural growth and for the other congenital anomalies which may be associated, it seems reasonable to ascribe all the cardinal features of the syndrome to estrogen lack. Such sparse axillary and pubic hair growth as may occur in these patients is probably due to stimulation from adrenal 17-ketosteroid precursors. However, there is evidence to suggest that for adequate 17-KS production, estrogen stimulation of the pituitary is essential. This interpretation is supported by the fact that increased growth of axillary and pubic hair and increased 17-KS excretion follow estrogen therapy in such patients. Estrogens do not prompt pubic and axillary hair growth in patients with Addison's disease. The osteoporosis, which resembles that occurring after the menopause, and the late union of the epiphyses seem directly attributable to estrogen deficiency.

Certain patients conform to the syndrome in all respects except for normal stature; presumably the genetic factors controlling growth are not implicated in these individuals. Other patients, for reasons which are totally obscure, excrete gonadotropins in normal rather than in increased amounts. Thus, gonadotropin assays, while of great value in distinguishing primary ovarian from primary pituitary or hypothalamic deficiencies, cannot be relied upon completely.

Castration. Very few preadolescent castrates have been subjected to careful study. But such individuals appear to attain to normal stature; some exhibit normal body proportions (see Figure 25) and others are eunuchoid. While estrogen excretion is uniformly low in such patients, the available data are not adequate to warrant dogmatic statements concerning the levels of gonadotropin excretion to be anticipated. However, it is known that certain castrates, surprisingly, do not excrete large quantities of urinary gonadotropins.

Replacement therapy with estrogen, as outlined under the treatment of hypothalamic infantilism, is indicated.

ADOLESCENT MENSTRUAL DISORDERS

Physiologic Considerations. In view of the complexity of the neuro-hormonal factors whose synchrony is required for mature sexual function, the occurrence of menstrual disorders during adolescence is not surprising.[17 a-c] From experimental studies it appears that the hypophysis, although physiologically neuter at birth, acquires important functional differences in the two sexes by the time the organism achieves sexual maturity. The rate of gonadotropin secretion by the male pituitary is sufficient to maintain the integrity of the male genital organs, but is never sufficient to induce luteinization of ovarian follicles if this be tested by grafting an ovary into an adult male animal. What is apparently demanded of the male pituitary is that it secrete the gonadotropic hormones at a low and relatively constant rate; what is demanded of the female is a rhythmic

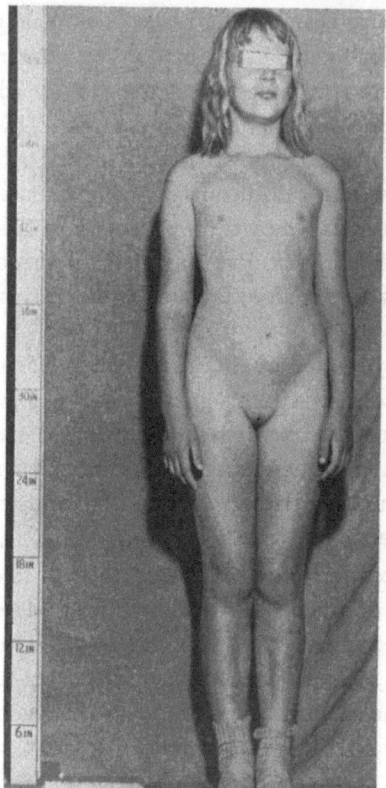 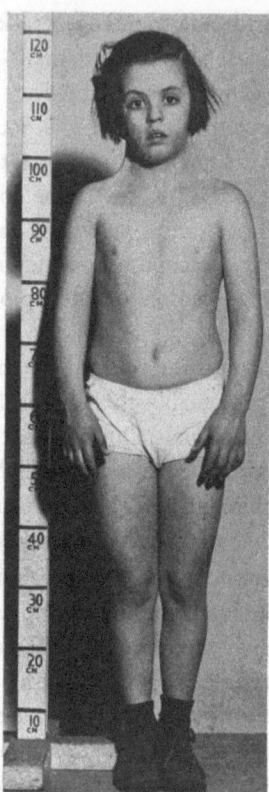

(Left)

FIGURE V—25. Appearance of a girl of 10 8/12 years who was subjected to a panhysterectomy at the age of three months because of hydrometrocalpas. Note the normal body habitus and the absence of secondary sexual characteristics. The psychosexual orientation of the child is distinctly feminine. Statural growth has so far proceeded at a satisfactory rate, and skeletal maturity has progressed normally. The urinary 17-KS excretion is 2.3 mg. per 24 hours. The gonadotropin excretion is 384 mouse units per 24 hours, but despite the menopausal level the patient experiences no hot flashes.

(Right)

FIGURE V—26. Sexual infantilism due to agenesis of the follicular elements of the ovary in a girl of 15 years. Note the short stature, "sphinx neck" and absence of breast development.

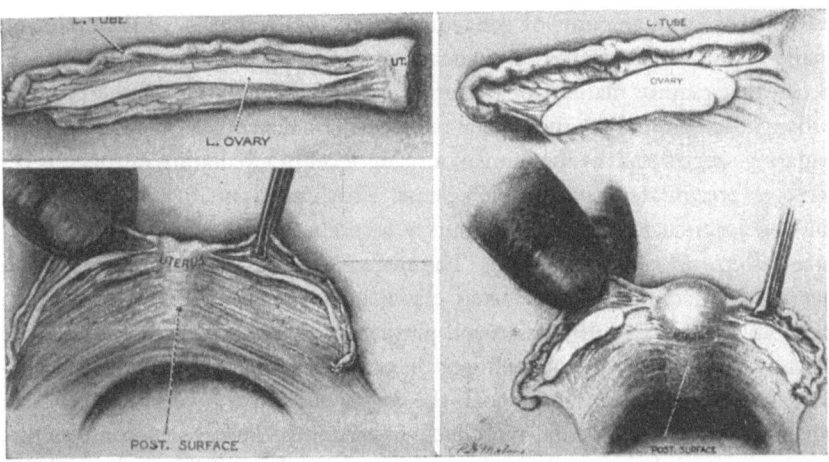

FIGURE V—27. Gross appearance of the uterus and adnexa in a patient with agenesis of the follicular elements of the ovaries (left) compared with those of a normal newborn child (right) drawn to the same scale. From L. Wilkins and W. Fleischmann, *J. Clin. Endocrinol.* 4:357, 1944.

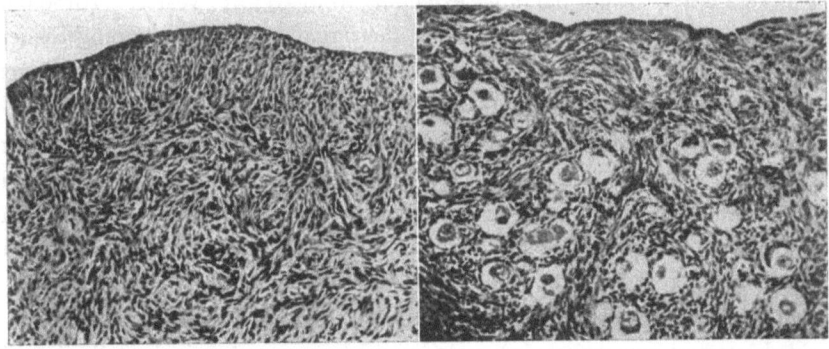

FIGURE V—28. Microscopic appearance of the "ovarian streak" in a patient with agenesis of the follicular elements of the ovary (left) compared with that of the ovary of a normal newborn infant (right). Note the complete absence of germinal epithelium and of Graafian follicles in the defective ovary. From L. Wilkins and W. Fleischmann, *J. Clin. Endocrinol.* 4:357, 1944.

discharge of large amounts of gonadotropins at critical phases of the cycle and smaller maintenance quantities of gonadotropins in the interim phases. In those species that require mating for ovulation, nervous stimulation of the pituitary is thought to bring about the sudden release of gonadotropins; in spontaneously ovulating species such as the human, a rising level of circulating estrogen is believed to precipitate gonadotropin release. Rhythmicity in function, therefore, must be acquired by the female pituitary before a mature gonado-hypophyseal relationship can come into being. The majority of the transitory disorders in menstrual function which characterize adolescence seem ascribable to delay in the establishment of full ovarian and pituitary reciprocity, particularly as these affect ovulation and the functioning of the corpus luteum. Acquired only as viviparity became an evolutionary goal, the corpus luteum is a comparatively late comer among the endocrine reproductive structures. Perhaps in consequence, luteal function is less securely established than follicular function and constitutes the weakest link in the reproductive chain. This is borne out by the fact that luteal function is the last to be acquired in sexual maturation and the first to fail as the menopause approaches. It is seen in the gradual manner in which a given female regains menstrual rhythmicity after a low ebb of sexual activity, as after lactation or after a period of strain or sickness.

In twentieth-century American girls the menarche ordinarily occurs about the age of 13.5 years, the normal range extending from 10 to 17 years.[17a] Although there are authentic instances of normal menstrual function beginning earlier than 10 or later than 17 years, it seems wise to subject individuals who depart from this range to careful study.

Types of Amenorrhea. Amenorrhea should be regarded not as a disease but as a symptom. In this age group it is clinically helpful to distinguish between those patients who have never menstruated (delayed menarche) and those in whom there is a cessation of menses previously present (postmenarcheal amenorrhea).

Delayed menarche. Patients with delayed menarche, in turn, can be subdivided into two categories: (a) cases in which amenorrhea is the reflection of a complete absence of sexual development (i.e., cases of *sexual infantilism*, see above) and (b) cases in which sexual development appears to be normal in all respects except for the occurrence of menstruation.

Congenital defects of the genital tract. In such cases the hypothalamic–pituitary–ovarian mechanism which initiates sexual development has been activated but there is no apparent uterine response to the presence of the sex hormones. Occasionally amenorrhea of this type results from destruction of the

THE OVARIES [349]

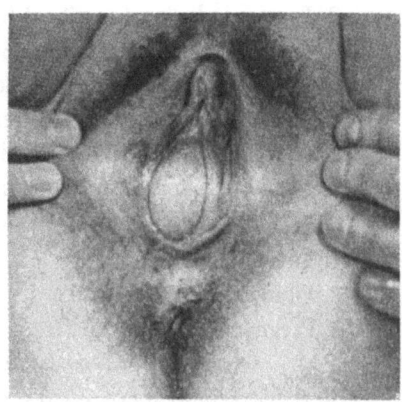

FIGURE V—29. Imperforate hymen in a patient of 27 years, showing the bulging due to retained menstrual accumulation of many years. From E. Novak, *Textbook of Gynecology*, Baltimore, Williams & Wilkins, 1944.

endometrium by a disease such as tuberculosis; in the majority of cases, congenital malformations of the genital tract are responsible. The development and fusion of the Müllerian ducts may be interfered with to such a degree that the uterus is either non-existent or grossly malformed. In less serious cases, the upper genital tract is normal but the egress of menstrual blood is prevented by an obstruction in the lower genital tract, most commonly an imperforate hymen (see Figure 29).[18a] Such cases constitute gynecologic rather than endocrine problems. However, their existence predicates the need for careful examination of the internal and external genitalia of all amenorrheic patients.

Postmenarcheal amenorrhea. In view of the extreme irregularity which often characterizes the immediately postmenarcheal cycles, a diagnosis of postmenarcheal amenorrhea in adolescents is probably unwarranted unless there is an interval of 12 months or more between flows during the first two years, or an interval of six months once the mature pattern of the menses is established.

Postmenarcheal amenorrhea may arise from lesions directly impairing some link in the hypothalamic–pituitary–ovarian mechanism which sustains sexual function or from a variety of disorders whose mode of interference with this mechanism is less clear. Thus, cases of postmenarcheal amenorrhea may be classified as follows:

A. Hypothalamic amenorrhea
   1. Destructive lesions (Froehlich's syndrome)
   2. Functional disturbances (emotional disorders)

B. Pituitary amenorrhea
   1. Destructive lesions

2. Factors inducing functional hypopituitarism
      (a) Thyroid: hyper- and hypothyroidism
      (b) Pancreas: diabetes mellitus
      (c) Adrenal cortex: insufficiency and hyperfunctioning lesions
      (d) Chronic infections and debilitating diseases
      (e) Nutritional disturbances: obesity and undernutrition
   c. Ovarian amenorrhea
   1. Menopause præcox
   2. Fibrocystic disease
   3. Pregnancy

Hypothalamic Amenorrhea

Destructive lesions (Froehlich's syndrome). Froehlich's syndrome, commonly due to a suprasellar cyst, has already been discussed. If the disorder has its onset in childhood, the result is sexual infantilism; if in adolescence, postmenarcheal amenorrhea.

Functional disturbances (emotional disorders) have been given a tentative place under the heading of hypothalamic amenorrhea. Such minor stresses as attending school away from home for the first time or entering upon nurses' training may precipitate transient amenorrhea. Amenorrhea is sometimes an early symptom of more severe psychiatric disturbances such as dementia præcox. Urinary gonadotropin assays are generally normal in such patients.* However, estrogen production is subnormal or nil as can be demonstrated by atropic vaginal smears, a negative "medical" dilatation and curettage or urinary assays for estrogenic hormone (see pages 313, 315, 316). Since it is necessary to supplement FSH with a small quantity of LH to induce estrogen production, it has been suggested that the fundamental defect in such patients is nervous inhibition of LH release.[18 c]

Pituitary Amenorrhea

Destructive lesions. Generalized pituitary deficiency due to destruction of the gland by tumor, infection or infarction is an occasional cause of postmenarcheal amenorrhea in adolescence. Gonadotropins are absent from the urine in such cases. The associated hormonal manifestations are as described for hypopituitary patients in Chapter VII, page 461.

Factors inducing functional hypopituitarism. The miscellaneous disorders which induce functional hypopituitarism and secondary infantilism if their onset is preadolescent induce oligomenorrhea or amenorrhea if their onset is post-

---

* This apparent normality is probably a methodological artefact due to the inability of presently available methods to detect subtle abnormalities in the FSH/LH ratio.

menarcheal. Arrhenoblastoma, a masculinizing ovarian tumor which often has amenorrhea as its first symptom, has intentionally been omitted from consideration because activation of this tumor only rarely[18 b] occurs during the adolescent period or earlier.

Ovarian Amenorrhea

Menopause præcox. This is an exceedingly rare syndrome. For reasons which are totally obscure, the ovary becomes unresponsive to gonadotropic stimulation at some time prior to the normal menopause. Estrogen production ceases, the uterus shrinks, the vaginal mucosa becomes pale and dry (see Figure 31) and the titer of urinary gonadotropins rises to supernormal levels. Demonstrable breast atrophy may or may not occur, depending on the length of time during which the breasts were subjected to normal estrogenic stimulation. If estrogen stimulation is continued for two years or longer, gross atrophy is generally not apparent (see Figure 30). Osteoporosis and senile changes in the skin may presently become demonstrable and constitute a compelling indication for substitution therapy. Curiously, hot flashes are rarely, if ever, experienced by patients with the syndrome.

Fibrocystic disease.[18 d, e] This syndrome, variously known as the Stein-Leventhal syndrome, the "large, pale ovary syndrome," and "cirrhosis of the ovaries" is likewise a rare cause of amenorrhea and oligomenorrhea. The disturbance is thought to be due to a mechanical impediment to ovulation. The ovaries are good-sized and contain follicles, but the capsule is so tough and fibrous that it prevents the follicles from rupturing or even from attaining optimal growth (see Figure 32). Although ovulation is thus inhibited, estrogen production is not entirely suppressed. Atrophy of the sex organs is therefore not observed and the excretion of urinary gonadotropins is normal. Hirsutism without signs of masculinization is sometimes seen.

Pregnancy. It should not be forgotten that pregnancy is an occasional cause of amenorrhea in adolescence. The finding of a soft bluish cervix and an enlarged uterus by pelvic examination should suggest the diagnosis. If necessary, confirmation can be obtained by appropriate tests for the presence of chorionic gonadotropin in the urine.

DIAGNOSIS OF AMENORRHEA. Recognition of the cause of an amenorrhea may in certain instances be possible from the findings of a simple routine examination. In other instances establishment of the diagnosis may require the performance of elaborate and costly laboratory tests. Painstaking scrutiny of each patient is requisite if one is to reduce the number of cases demanding protracted investigation.

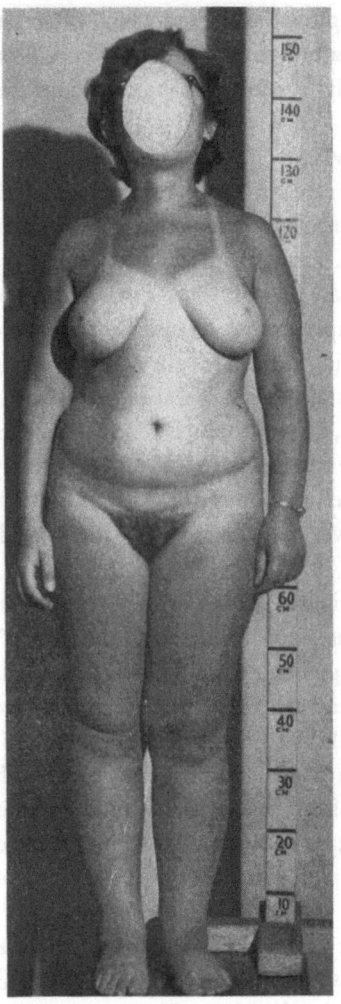

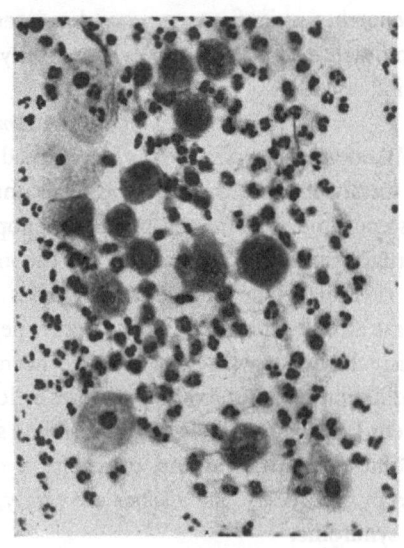

(Right)

FIGURE V—31. Vaginal smear of the patient in Figure 30. The gross appearance of the vagina was suggestive of estrogen deficiency in that the mucosa was pale and dry. The smear confirms the impression of vaginal atrophy. Only breast cells and leukocytes are visible; no cornified epithelial cells are present. Note the resemblance of this smear to that of the prepuberal child shown in Figure 7.

(Left)

FIGURE V—30. Appearance of a girl of 22 years who began to menstruate at the age of 12 and who had a spontaneous menopause at the age of 17. No hot flashes have been experienced by the patient, although the level of urinary gonadotropin excretion is extremely high (192 mouse units per 24 hours). The uterus has shrunk to infantile proportions and the vaginal epithelium has become atrophic (see Figure 31), but the breasts have not regressed. Beginning demineralization of the long bones was demonstrable roentgenographically at the time that this photograph was taken.

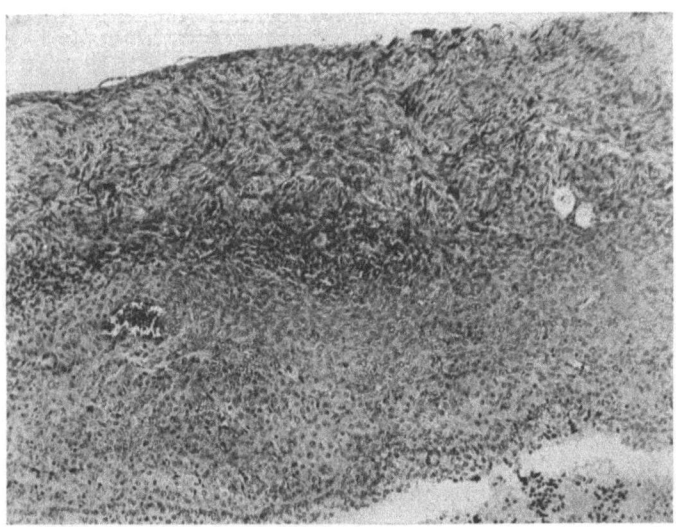

FIGURE V—32. Microscopic appearance of the ovary in fibrocystic disease. Note the extreme fibrosis of the cortex, the trapping of the primordial follicles and the paralutein changes in the theca interna of the follicle at the bottom of the section.

The first essential is an accurate history with emphasis on: (a) the family history as regards endocrine disorders, such as unusually early or late puberty, familial hirsutism and so forth, (b) the character and duration of any illness preceding the amenorrhea, (c) a precise description of the patient's menstrual history—a calendar should be constructed by the physician showing the dates of all periods whose onset can be accurately recalled, the duration and extent of flow, and any mid-cycle or menstrual symptoms (see Figure 33) and (d) the habits of the patient as regards rest, diet and recreation. An attempt should be made to assess the maturity of the patient's emotional adjustment.

A complete physical examination is made with particular attention to the presence of systemic disease, the type of body build, and the presence of the secondary sexual characteristics. The optic fundi are examined, and the visual fields outlined by confrontation. The external genitalia are systematically inspected, and the uterine proportions determined by recto-abdominal examination. If made gently, with care to assure an empty bladder, recto-abdominal examination is surprisingly informative. Vaginal examination may often be foregone unless the preliminary findings suggest the presence of genital abnormalities.

If systematically carried out, even this limited scrutiny will enable certain conditions associated with amenorrhea to be recognized at a glance or diagnosed

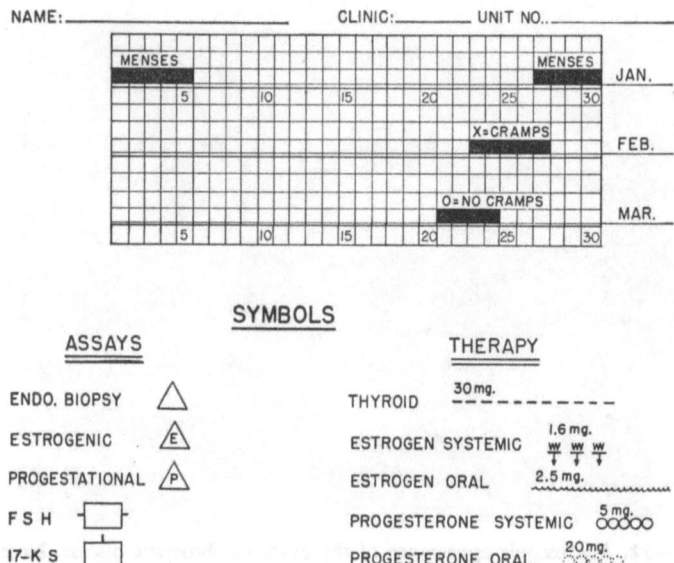

FIGURE V—33. Sample menstrual chart of the type employed at the Massachusetts General Hospital, showing a convenient method for recording menstrual bleeding, endocrine studies and hormone therapy.

after a minimum of investigation: adrenal insufficiency and hyperfunctioning lesions, hyper- or hypothyroidism, diabetes mellitus, chronic infections and debilitating diseases, nutritional disturbances (such as obesity and undernutrition), developmental anomalies of the genitalia and pregnancy.

If the cause of the amenorrhea remains obscure after this preliminary evaluation, it must be sought by means of procedures which test separately each link in the uterine–ovarian–pituitary–hypothalamic chain upon whose integrity normal menstrual function depends. In actual practice, the most important point to determine initially is whether the amenorrhea is ascribable to pituitary or to ovarian failure. This can be ascertained by assaying the urine quantitatively for the presence of the gonadotropic hormones. If the pituitary is at fault, gonadotropins are absent from the urine; if the ovary has failed gonadotropins are present, generally in amounts greatly in excess of normal. For the finer distinctions between the various types of pituitary and ovarian insufficiency, the specific sections to follow should be consulted.

The occurrence of amenorrhea despite normal amounts of gonadotropins in the urine suggests that the hypothalamus may be at fault or that one is dealing with the Stein-Leventhal syndrome. In such instances it is helpful to ascertain whether any estrogen at all is being produced. A variety of methods are available for this purpose (see the section on diagnostic methods), of which one of the simplest is "medical" dilatation and curettage. If the amenorrhea is hypothalamic in origin, bleeding will not follow the administration of progesterone, since estrogen production is entirely in abeyance; if the Stein-Leventhal syndrome is present, withdrawal of progesterone will be followed by bleeding. In rare instances, amenorrhea occurring in the presence of normal gonadotropic function is due to congenital absence of the endometrium or to destruction of the endometrium by a disease such as tuberculosis. The functional capacity of the endometrium itself can be readily tested by providing an adequate stimulus. If estrogen is given, a potentially normal endometrium, no matter how atrophic, will respond with growth and, on withdrawal of the medication, with bleeding. A satisfactory method of carrying out this test is to give 1 mg. of diethylstilbestrol daily for 21 days. The absence of withdrawal bleeding during the next two weeks constitutes strong presumptive evidence for endometrial inadequacy.

TREATMENT OF AMENORRHEA. Rational therapy of the amenorrheas is dependent upon precise diagnosis. In amenorrhea due to serious congenital anomalies of the uterus, it is manifestly impossible to induce menstrual periods with cyclic hormone therapy. If such a patient shows normal feminine secondary sexual development, there is nothing to be gained by hormonal treatment. False amenorrhea due to an imperforate hymen is readily relieved by incision and drainage from below. Hypothalamic amenorrhea due to transient stress is ordinarily self-limited; its duration can often be shortened by judicious reassurance. Prolonged amenorrhea resulting from severe emotional disturbances may, on the other hand, require psychotherapy. Patients with menopause præcox should be given the benefit of cyclic replacement therapy with estrogen, as described for the treatment of ovarian infantilism. If there are good reasons for suspecting the presence of the fibrocystic disease of the ovaries, recourse should be had to laparotomy. Wedge resection of the ovarian capsules will permit ovulation to occur with the establishment of normal menstrual cycles. Amenorrhea associated with the various conditions listed under the heading of "miscellaneous" requires no treatment other than that directed at the primary disorder.

Types of Menorrhagia.[19a] Bleeding which lasts more than seven days, which is sufficient to lower the hemoglobin content of the blood, or which produces dizziness, palpitation, or weakness is arbitrarily considered to be pathologic. The causes of menorrhagia can be classified in many different ways. A classification which is convenient in this age group is the following:

A. Specific endocrinopathies
  1. Ovarian
     (a) Metropathia hemorrhagica
     (b) Granulosa cell tumor
     (c) Fibrocystic disease
  2. Thyroid
     (a) Hypothyroidism
B. Constitutional diseases
  1. Blood diseases
     (a) Associated with thrombocytopenia
        1. Thrombocytopenic purpura
        2. Leukemias
        3. Aplastic anemia
     (b) Unassociated with thrombocytopenia
        1. Pseudo-hemophilia
     2. Liver disease
C. Local pelvic pathology
  1. Carcinoma of the cervix
  2. Sarcoma botryoides
  3. Complications of pregnancy

Specific Endocrinopathies

Ovarian menorrhagia. Functional uterine bleeding, or *metropathia hemorrhagica*,[19 b, c] is a commoner cause of menorrhagia than all the other entities put together. It is characterized clinically by periods of menorrhagia, in which bleeding continues without cramps for weeks or months, alternating with periods of amenorrhea in an otherwise healthy person. In such cases curettage may reveal the endometrium to be either proliferative or atrophic. It is not cast off as during normal menstruation; the bleeding that occurs is oozing from the superficially degenerated endometrial surface. The ovaries lack corpora lutea; usually at least one contains a large follicular cyst filled with fluid of high estrogen content. Hyperestrinism is not present, even in patients whose endometrium is hyperplastic. The condition appears to be due to a decreased or a normal amount of estrogen acting for too long a time, with an absence of progesterone (see Figure 34). The essential defect would seem to be a delay in the establishment of the mature reciprocal pituitary-ovarian relationship. Either ovulation has not occurred, owing to failure of LH to attain a sufficiently high level, or corpus luteum function is not adequately sustained, owing to inadequate levels of luteotropin. Presently available methods of study do not permit a choice be-

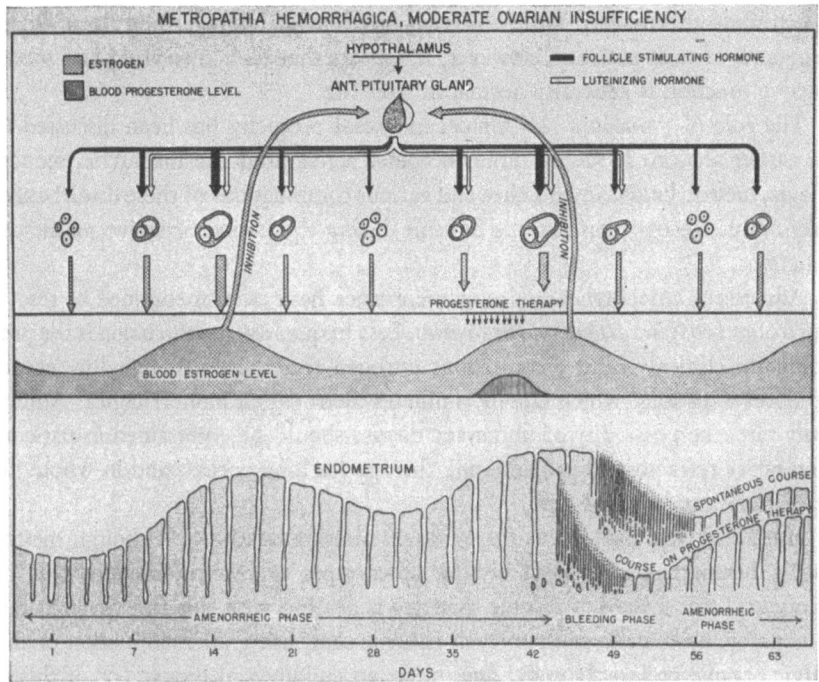

FIGURE V—34. Simplified diagram showing the relations of the hypothalamus, anterior pituitary gland, ovaries and endometrium in an adolescent girl with moderate ovarian insufficiency resulting in metropathia hemorrhagica. Compare Figure 6.

In the above diagram the anterior pituitary, under hypothalamic stimulation, is shown effecting periodic discharge of moderate amounts of follicle-stimulating hormone and small amounts of luteinizing hormone into the circulation. These hormones stimulate the follicles of the ovaries to develop partially and to produce moderate amounts of estrogenic hormone. Luteinizing hormone, however, is never secreted in quantities sufficient to bring about ovulation. Hence, a corpus luteum is never formed and progesterone is never secreted.

In response to the oscillating level of estrogenic hormone the endometrium grows and regresses without bleeding during the first cycle, shown in the left-hand portion of the diagram. Further growth occurs during the second cycle, represented in the right-hand portion of the diagram. The extent of this growth is such that it cannot be sustained when the hormone level declines toward the close of the cycle. Superficial desquamation and bleeding therefore occur, briefly terminating the amenorrheic phase of the disorder. Since ovarian lack is only moderate, estrogen production soon increases again to the point where the hormone level can initiate endometrial growth and thus check bleeding.

If the disorder is temporarily deflected from its spontaneous course by means of progesterone therapy late in the second cycle, additional growth and differentiation of the endometrium occur. When progesterone is withdrawn, the functional layers of the endometrium are desquamated completely.

tween these alternatives. Little objective data is available regarding the ultimate prognosis of such patients. However, it appears that their menstrual and reproductive function is generally normal in later life.

The role of *granulosa cell tumors* in sexual precocity has been discussed in an earlier section. If such a tumor becomes active after the menarche, menorrhagia, metrorrhagia, amenorrhea and various combinations of these disturbances may occur. Recognition may be difficult during the period of active menstrual function.

Adolescent amenorrhea and oligomenorrhea have been mentioned as resulting from *fibrocystic disease of the ovaries*. Less frequently, menorrhagia is the predominant clinical feature; continuous estrogen secretion, although low grade, produces a disorder which closely simulates metropathia hemorrhagica. Admittedly rare, the possibility of fibrocystic disease should be entertained in patients who prove refractory to progesterone therapy for long periods and in whom no other cause can be made out.

DIFFERENTIAL DIAGNOSIS OF OVARIAN MENORRHAGIA. Although metropathia hemorrhagica exceeds all the other types of ovarian menorrhagia in frequency, it is unsafe to assume that one is dealing with this functional endocrinopathy. Systematic study of each patient, comprising an examination of the pelvic organs, preferably under anesthesia, an endometrial biopsy (or, if this is not obtainable, a vaginal smear for estrogen effect) and a determination of the basal metabolic rate should be carried out. Attention should be given to the number of blood platelets, the bleeding and clotting times, clot retraction and capillary fragility. Although in certain instances additional procedures may be required, these studies should enable one to decide into which of the three general categories the problem falls.

Hypothyroid menorrhagia. Little additional comment is required concerning hypothyroidism. Menorrhagia may be associated with mild degrees of thyroid deficiency, and in obscure cases not responding to other forms of treatment, a trial of therapy with 0.1 gm. of desiccated thyroid daily is warranted.

Constitutional Diseases

Blood disorders.[19 d, e] Of the constitutional diseases which have menorrhagia as a symptom, the most important are blood diseases. The diagnostic survey presented on page 356 ordinarily suffices to detect blood dyscrasias such as pseudo-hemophilia, aplastic anemia and leukemia. However, it is not commonly appreciated that idiopathic thrombocytopenic purpura often remains latent for considerable periods. The menorrhagia may appear to respond to progesterone therapy, closely simulating metropathia hemorrhagica. However, in the course of time the bleeding becomes more troublesome and the clinical and laboratory indications of thrombocytopenic purpura become unmistakable. Therefore, patients who are thought to have metropathia hemorrhagica but who do not improve on progesterone therapy should be given the benefit of repeated hematologic evaluation.

Liver disease. When liver disease is severe, menorrhagia occasionally develops in association with a disordered intermediary estrogen metabolism. Sometimes prothrombin time is prolonged. The diagnosis is generally obvious.

Local Pelvic Pathology

Carcinoma of the cervix[19 f] *and sarcoma botryoides.* Finally, there are rare instances in which local pelvic pathology is responsible for menorrhagia in childhood and youth. In early stages both carcinomas and sarcomas of the lower genital tract may have bleeding as their sole manifestation. The prognosis for such tumors is poor, since in most cases they are discovered too late for effective therapy.

Complications of pregnancy may be responsible for bleeding in adolescence, as in later life.

TREATMENT OF MENORRHAGIA.[19 g, h] Inasmuch as metropathia hemorrhagica is ordinarily self-limited, treatment should be conservative. The tragedy of hysterectomy should be avoided at all costs. If a patient is in critical condition from blood loss when first seen, she should be supported by transfusions, and bleeding, if rapid, should be arrested by curettage, which usually affords temporary relief even in cases of thrombocytopenic purpura. The emergency surmounted, the therapeutic goal becomes the induction of periodic endometrial desquamation in as physiologic a manner as possible until the pituitary acquires rhythmicity with respect to gonadotropic function.*

If estrogen secretion is reasonably adequate, as demonstrated by a proliferative endometrium or a well-cornified vaginal smear, all that is required is that progesterone be administered periodically. If progesterone is given intramuscularly† in a dose of 5 mg. daily for five days, menstruation will follow about two days later. The procedure should be repeated at intervals of four to six weeks to prevent excessive proliferation of the endometrium. Many patients will begin to menstruate normally after several courses of such treatment. One can gauge when to terminate therapy by watching for an "escape phenomenon" (see Figure 35).

* If the Smiths' thesis[19 i] is correct (i.e., that the breakdown products of a secretory endometrium act as a stimulus to pituitary secretion, whereas those of a proliferative endometrium do not) periodic transformation to the secretory form may actually accelerate pituitary maturation.

† Secretory changes can be induced in the endometrium by administration of the oral progestin, pregneninolone (see page 300) in large doses. However, the absorption of this compound is so variable that we prefer to administer progesterone by the intramuscular route.

By this is meant a failure to flow within two to four days after withdrawal of progesterone; the reason for the failure to bleed is the occurrence of ovulation and the consequent development of an endogenous source of progesterone, the corpus luteum.

If the level of estrogen secretion is very low, as indicated by an atrophic endometrium or a poorly cornified vaginal smear, bleeding may be more difficult to control. Cyclic progesterone therapy may prove unsatisfactory and even curettage may arrest the bleeding only momentarily. However, such cases often respond well to combined estrogen and progesterone treatment. If the patient is not in critical condition when first seen, bleeding can be arrested within two to five days by giving estrogen in adequate amounts. Diethylstilbestrol in daily dosage of 6 mg. is generally effective; if bleeding has not dwindled by the third day or ceased by the fifth day of treatment, the dosage should be increased by 2 to 6 mg. The effective dose of estrogen, whatever this proves to be, should be continued for three weeks (see Figure 36). At the end of this time stilbestrol should be omitted in order to prevent undue proliferation of the endometrium; withdrawal bleeding ordinarily begins within one to five days after stilbestrol has been withdrawn. Bleeding following estrogen withdrawal may be alarmingly profuse, in which case it may be necessary to re-institute stilbestrol therapy as early as the third day of bleeding. However, if possible, one should permit a five-day withdrawal period before beginning a new 20-day course of stilbestrol. The dosage to be employed in subsequent courses must be determined experimentally for each patient; in successive months, one should reduce the quantity of estrogen as rapidly as possible. Once control of the bleeding has been gained by repeated courses of stilbestrol, progesterone should be administered in a daily dosage of 5 mg. concurrently with estrogen during the last five days of each 20-day course of treatment, when both hormones should be withdrawn simultaneously. Favorable response to this regimen will justify a shift to therapy with cyclic progesterone alone; this, in turn, is continued until an "escape phenomenon" occurs.

Continuous recording of the basal body temperature curve and periodic determination of urinary pregnandiol excretion are helpful in following the course of patients with metropathia. During cycles in which ovulation and corpus luteum production occur, the form of the basal temperature curve changes from the erratic anovulatory to the mature ovulatory pattern. Pregnandiol, initially absent from urine specimens collected late in the cycle, becomes demonstrable.

Even patients who appear to respond dramatically to progesterone therapy have frequent relapses, so that one should indicate at the outset that repeated courses of treatment over a period of years may be necessary.

Bleeding due to idiopathic thrombocytopenic purpura can generally be arrested temporarily by means of curettage, and normal menstrual function restored by splenectomy.

Dysmenorrhea. Disagreeable symptoms of one kind or another are experienced by a large percentage of girls and women at the time of the menses. The symptoms include lassitude, irritability, mild depression, urinary frequency, gastrointestinal disturbances, headache and moderate pelvic discomfort. In a small percentage of women, the pelvic discomfort attains the proportions of severe pain and may prove temporarily incapacitating. Such pain is termed dysmenorrhea.

When dysmenorrhea occurs in the absence of demonstrable pelvic pathology it is designated as "primary"; when associated with organic gynecologic disease, as "secondary." The various pelvic disorders with which secondary dysmenorrhea is sometimes associated (cervical stricture, chronic salpingitis, endometriosis, myomata uteri and, occasionally, uterine retroflexion) are extremely uncommon in adolescence. However, examination of the pelvic organs should not be omitted; it will confirm the diagnosis and reassure the patient.

ETIOLOGY. Little is known regarding the cause of primary dysmenorrhea. However, it appears that the development of cramps is in some way related to the occurrence of ovulation. Bleeding from a proliferative endometrium, developed during a presumably anovulatory cycle, is almost invariably painless. Whether the dysmenorrhea is attributable to a direct action of the luteal hormone on the myometrium or to the breakdown of a secretory endometrium is not clear. However, the fact that normally all demonstrable progesterone is eliminated about two days before the appearance of the menses suggests that cramps result from some action of progesterone rather than to its presence in the system.

CLINICAL MANIFESTATIONS. The clinical evolution of dysmenorrhea in adolescence lends circumstantial support to the concept that ovulation is a *sine qua non* of primary dysmenorrhea. After a year or so of painless periods, the adolescent often begins suddenly to experience cramps. Presumably, the first periods are anovulatory and dysmenorrhea signalizes the beginning of mature ovarian function and corpus luteum formation.

The pain threshold of many patients with dysmenorrhea appears to be abnormally low. Fear and anxiety intensify the pelvic discomfort, and reassurance often affords considerable relief.

The pain of dysmenorrhea is characteristically sharp and cramping, being referred to the mid-line in the lower abdomen; sometimes it is described as a dragging ache in the lower abdomen, radiating to the back and thighs. The time at which the pain begins varies considerably; it may start a few hours before the

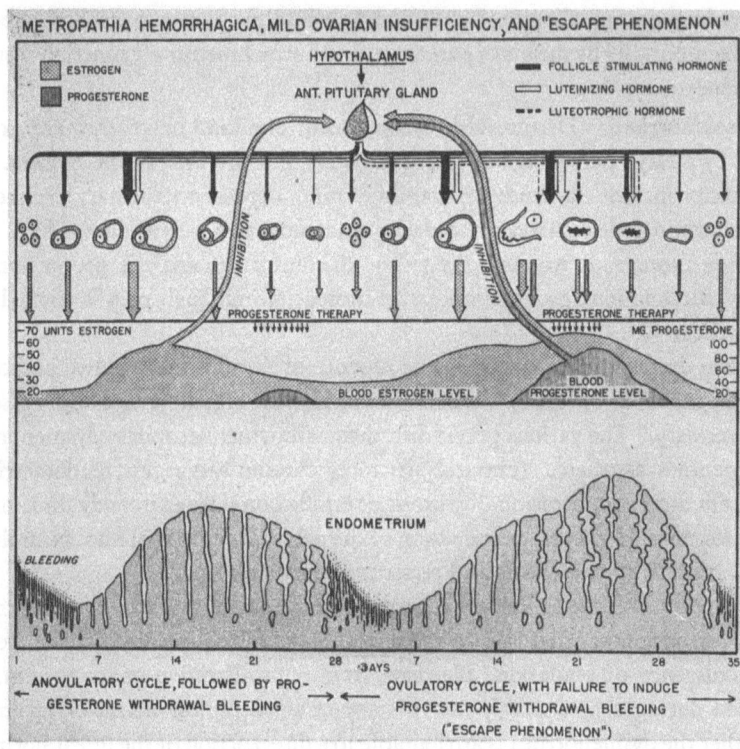

FIGURE V—35. Simplified diagram showing the treatment of metropathia hemorrhagica due to mild ovarian insufficiency and illustrating the "escape phenomenon." For a detailed description of the relations of the hypothalamus, anterior pituitary gland, ovaries and endometrium in this disorder, see Figure 34.

In the above diagram, the patient's response to two courses of progesterone therapy is depicted. The cycle represented in the left-hand portion of the diagram is anovulatory in character, and spontaneous differentiation of the endometrium therefore does not occur. Partial differentiation, however, may be induced by administration of progesterone late in the cycle, and when the hormone is withdrawn extensive endometrial desquamation and bleeding take place.

The cycle shown in the right-hand portion of the diagram is ovulatory, and spontaneous differentiation of the endometrium therefore occurs. In consequence, when additional progesterone is administered and withdrawn late in the cycle, bleeding does not immediately follow; the endometrium continues to be sustained by progesterone secreted by the corpus luteum. The term "escape phenomenon" is employed to denote failure to induce progesterone-withdrawal bleeding under these circumstances.

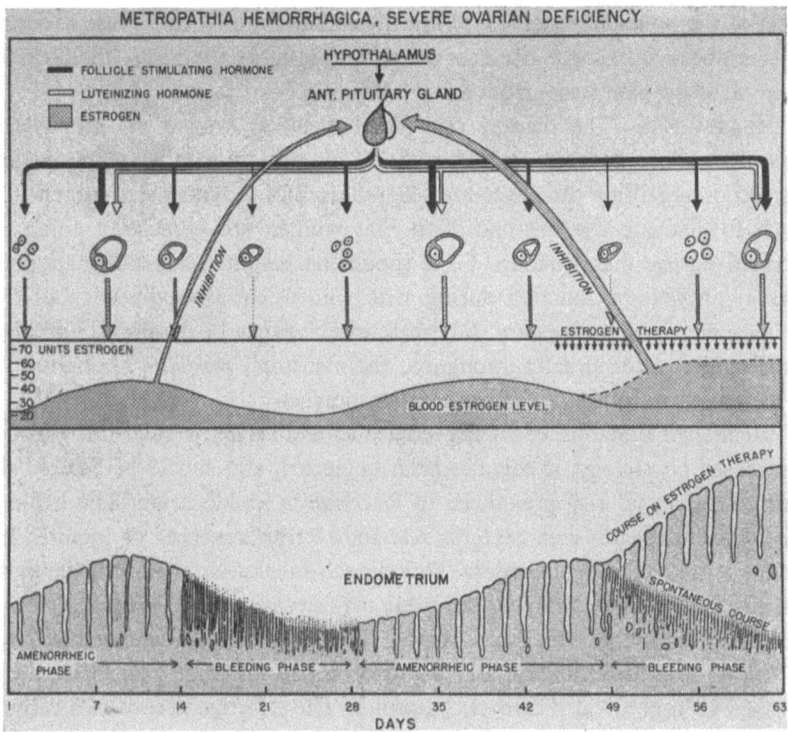

FIGURE V—36. Simplified diagram showing the relations of the hypothalamus, anterior pituitary and endometrium in an adolescent girl with severe ovarian insufficiency resulting in metropathia hemorrhagica. For a representation of these relations in the normal sexually mature female, see Figure 6.

In this figure the anterior pituitary, under hypothalamic stimulation, is shown effecting the periodic discharge of moderate amounts of follicle-stimulating hormone and traces of luteinizing hormone into the circulation. These hormones stimulate the ovarian follicles to develop slightly and to produce small amounts of estrogenic hormone. Owing to deficient secretion of luteinizing hormone, ovulation and corpus luteum formation never occur.

In response to the oscillating level of estrogenic hormone the endometrium alternately grows and regresses. Because ovarian insufficiency is severe, estrogen production increases sluggishly and endometrial growth is slow. Bleeding therefore continues unchecked for prolonged periods. If estrogen therapy is given, as shown in the right-hand portion of the diagram, endometrial growth is stimulated and bleeding promptly arrested.

onset of the flow and continue during menstruation, or it may cease as soon as bleeding begins. In some instances the patient suffers only during the flow. The duration of the pain varies from a few hours to several days.

TREATMENT. The therapy of dysmenorrhea is first of all prophylactic. Primitive taboos concerning menstruation are still influential in our society. Instruction regarding the physiologic significance of the menstrual cycle will do much to dissipate the misconception that women are necessarily ailing and accursed during menstruation. Girls should be taught that menstruation is a normal physiologic function during which no essential modification of their ordinary activities is necessary. Moderate exercise may be continued and warm baths should be taken daily throughout the menstrual period; a hot bath is one of the most comforting measures in dysmenorrhea.

Patients with established dysmenorrhea should be given elementary instruction in sex physiology, if this has been neglected, and should be assured that their pain is in no way prejudicial to marriage or childbearing. The habits of the patient as regards diet, exercise, rest and recreation should be inquired into carefully and rectified if necessary. Periodic self-medication with mild analgesics will provide adequate relief to the great majority of patients during attacks of pain. A prescription which has proved helpful in mild dysmenorrhea is the following: acetylsalicylic acid 300 mg., phenacetin 180 mg., propadrine hydrochloride 40 mg., divided into two capsules. The effective dose is two capsules every two hours for four or five doses.[20a] Narcotics are, in general, contraindicated.

Patients who fail to respond to simple measures can be given an occasional respite from dysmenorrhea by therapy designed to inhibit ovulation. If estrogen is given daily for 25 days, starting on the first day of menstruation, ovulation is prevented, and painless withdrawal bleeding follows.[20b] A variety of estrogenic preparations may be employed for this purpose; diethylstilbestrol in a daily dose of 1 mg. is cheap and satisfactory. Inasmuch as the ovarian-pituitary relationship is insecurely established in adolescence, it seems advisable to withhold estrogen therapy except to enable the patient to attend important school or social functions; in such cases, therapy must be begun four weeks in advance of the anticipated menstruation (see above). In exceptionally severe and protracted cases, presacral neurectomy may deserve consideration.

PROGNOSIS. The prognosis in any given case is uncertain. The dysmenorrhea may disappear with increasing maturity. Marriage, and especially childbirth, often result in elimination of the pain.

HERMAPHRODITISM

Sexual reversal resulting from a demonstrable excess in the titer of circulating heterosexual hormone must be distinguished from congenital intersexuality, or hermaphroditism, unassociated with the presence of excessive heterosexual hormone. In the female, the principal causes of reversal of the first type are: (a) adrenocortical hyperplasia (which may begin either in prenatal or postnatal life), (b) adrenocortical tumors, (c) ovarian arrhenoblastomas, (d) adrenal cell rest tumors and (e) intensive androgenic therapy. Intersexuality of the second type is considered by most authorities to be genetic in origin. However, the theory that temporary hormonal imbalances during pregnancy may be responsible for certain types of pseudo-hermaphroditism, at least, has gained impressive experimental support in recent years.

Classification.[21 a-c] Hermaphroditism is of two types: true and pseudo, or false. True hermaphroditism implies the presence of both male and female gonads; pseudo-hermaphroditism the presence of gonads of only one sex but the possession of genitalia and, at times, secondary sex characters belonging to the opposite sex.

True hermaphroditism can conveniently be subdivided into three categories:
1. Bilateral: testis and ovary on each side, separate or united (ovotestis).
2. Unilateral: testis and ovary, either separate or united, on one side with either testis or ovary on the other.
3. Lateral or alternating: testis on one side, ovary on the other.

The classification of pseudo-hermaphroditism rests upon two essentials, the true sex of the gonads and the character of the other genitalia. One can classify any pseudo-hermaphrodite satisfactorily by the use of two adjectives. The first (masculine or feminine) indicates the nature of the sex gland. The second (external, internal or complete) indicates whether it is the sex of the internal or the external or of both groups of genitalia that differs from that of the gonad.

Thus, a feminine *external* pseudo-hermaphrodite is an individual who possesses ovaries, testes and uterus but whose external genitalia resemble those of the male. The clitoris is hypertrophied, often to penile proportions; the vagina may be absent or may empty into a persistent urogenital sinus. A feminine *internal* pseudo-hermaphrodite possesses ovaries and completely feminine external genitalia. However, vestigial male remnants such as a Gärtner's duct, prostate or vas deferens replace the uterus and tubes. A feminine *complete* pseudo-hermaphrodite is feminine only in the possession of ovaries. The tubes and uterus are hypoplastic or absent and the external genitalia masculine in type. The ovaries may occupy the labia majora, causing it to resemble a scrotum.

True hermaphroditism is extremely rare. Only 40 cases, adequately authenticated by microscopic examination of the gonads, have been reported. The predominant abnormality was the presence of ovotestes, either unilateral or bilateral. Only seven true ovaries and six true testes were found; the remainder (except for four gonads of undetermined type) were ovotestes.

Pseudo-hermaphroditism is far more common. It occurs about once in 1,000 persons. Approximately 75 per cent of patients with pseudo-hermaphroditism are actually males. Ninety per cent of all cases are of the external or the complete types; only 10 per cent are internal in type. However, since the internal type is not clinically recognizable unless there are symptoms leading to operation, its true incidence may be somewhat higher.

DIAGNOSIS. So great is the variation seen in the clinical features that no standard description of any of these types can be given. Because of this variability, many pseudo-hermaphrodites are reared as members of the opposite sex. If, during adolescence, the true sex becomes clearly manifest owing to the appearance of the secondary sexual characteristics, the consequences for the patient may be disastrous. Early diagnosis, therefore, is important from both psychological and sociological points of view. The genitalia of newborn children should be examined with care, and infants who exhibit any sexual variation at birth should be observed and studied until a definite opinion as to their sex can be reached. Certain local abnormalities are suggestive of intersexuality. In the female hypertrophy of the clitoris should arouse suspicion; likewise, the presence of solid bodies in inguinal hernias in young females, particularly in the absence of the menses, should lead to vaginal examination. Urethroscopy occasionally discloses that what was thought to be a normal urethra is actually a persistent urogenital sinus into which a hypoplastic vagina opens. While hormone assays are helpful in distinguishing hormonal from congenital intersexuality, they are of little assistance in determining the true sex in pseudo-hermaphroditism of genetic origin. In a large percentage of cases, only exploratory laparotomy and biopsy of the gonads will establish the diagnosis.

TREATMENT. Cases of hermaphroditism are best managed as individual problems by experienced persons. Most authorities agree that treatment should be designed to help the patient live comfortably in the sexual status which is psychologically most congenial to him. Removal of rudimentary organs of the opposite sex, plastic correction of the external genitalia, and, at times, appropriate hormone therapy may be of great benefit. While the high incidence of dysgerminoma in malformed gonads should be borne in mind, castration should not be carried out routinely.

REFERENCES

1 (a) MOORE, C. R. Sex endocrines in development and prepuberal life. *J. Clin. Endocrinol.* 4:135, 1944.
  (b) PINCUS, G. and THIMANN, K. V. *The Hormones: Physiology, Chemistry and Applications.* New York, Academic Press, 1948.
  (c) HISAW, F. L. Development of the Graafian follicle and ovulation. *Physiol. Rev.* 27:95, 1947.
  (d) ASTWOOD, E. B. Regulation of corpus luteum function by hypophyseal luteotrophin. *Endocrinology* 28:309, 1941.
  (e) AMERICAN MEDICAL ASSOCIATION. *Glandular Physiology and Therapy.* Chicago, A. M. A., 1942.
  (f) ALLEN, E. *Sex and Internal Secretions.* Baltimore, Williams & Wilkins, 1939.
  (g) BURROWS, H. *Biological Actions of the Sex Hormones.* Cambridge Univ. Press, 1945.

2 (a) SMITH, C. A. *The Physiology of the Newborn Infant.* Springfield, Ill., C .C. Thomas, 1945.
  (b) GREULICH, W. W., DAY, H. G., LACHMAN, S. E., WOLFE, J. B. and SHUTTLEWORTH, F. K. A handbook of methods for the study of adolescent children. *Monographs of the Society for Research in Child Development.* Vol. III, No. 2, 1938.
  (c) SHUTTLEWORTH, F. K. The adolescent period; a graphic and pictorial atlas. *Monographs of the Society for Research in Child Development.* Vol. III, No. 3, 1938.
  (d) FRANK, L. K., GREULICH, W. W., BAER, J. L., SEVRINGHAUS, E. L., SHORR, E., WEBSTER, B., BRUCH, H., SCHLUTZ, F. W., GIBSON, S., MOHR, G. and THOM, D. A. Symposium on adolescence. *J. Pediat.* 19:289, 1941.
  (e) STUART, H. C. Physical growth during adolescence. *Am. J. Dis. Child.* 74:495, 1947.
  (f) ASHLEY-MONTAGU, M. F. Adolescent sterility. *Quart. Rev. Biol.* 14:13, 1939.
  (g) REYNOLDS, E. L. and WINES, J. V. Individual differences in physical changes associated with adolescence in girls. *Am. J. Dis. Child.* 75:329, 1948.
  (h) PRYOR, H. B. Certain physical and physiologic aspects of adolescent development in girls. *J. Pediat.* 8:52, 1936.
  (i) NATHANSON, I. T., TOWNE, L. E. and AUB, J. C. Normal excretion of sex hormones in childhood. *Endocrinology* 28:851, 1941.
  (j) CATCHPOLE, H. R. and GREULICH, W. W. Excretion of gonadotrophic hormone by prepuberal and adolescent girls. *Am. J. Physiol.* 129:331, 1940.

3 (a) BARTELMEZ, G. W. Histological studies on the menstruating mucous membrane of the human uterus. *Contrib. Embryol.* 24:143, 1933.
  (b) MARKEE, J. E. Menstruation in intraocular endometrial transplants in the rhesus monkey. *Contrib. Embryol.* 177:219, 1940.
  (c) REYNOLDS, S. R. M. The physiologic basis of menstruation: a summary of current concepts. *J. A. M. A.* 135:552, 1947.

4 (a) REIFENSTEIN, E. C., JR. Endocrinology: a synopsis of normal and pathologic physiology, diagnostic procedures and therapy. *M. Clin. North America* 28:1232, 1944.
  (b) CASTILLO, E. B., DEL, ARGONZ, J. and GALLI MAINI, C. Cytological cycle of the urinary sediment and its parallelism with the vaginal cycle. *J. Clin. Endocrinol.* 8:76, 1948.
  (c) SHORR, E. Evaluation of clinical applications of vaginal smear method. *J. Mt. Sinai Hosp.* 12:667, 1945.
  (d) CAMPBELL, R. E., LENDRUM, F. C. and SEVRINGHAUS, E. L. Endometrial histology and pathology as revealed by the biopsy method. *Surg. Gynec. & Obst.* 63:724, 1936.
  (e) VENNING, E. H. Gravimetric method for the determination of sodium pregnandiol glucuronidate (excretion product of progesterone). *J. Biol. Chem.* 119:473, 1937.
  (f) SOMMERVILLE, I. F., MARRIAN, G. F. and KELLAR, R. J. Rapid determination of urinary pregnandiol; method suitable for routine clinical use. *Lancet* 2:89, 1948.

(g) TOMPKINS, P. The use of basal temperature graphs in determining the date of ovulation. *J. A. M. A.* 124:698, 1944.

(h) KLINEFELTER, H. F., ALBRIGHT, F., and GRISWOLD, G. C. Experience with a quantitative test for normal or decreased amounts of follicle-stimulating hormone in the urine in endocrinological diagnosis. *J. Clin. Endocrinol.* 3:529, 1943.

5 (a) SECKEL, H. P. G. Precocious sexual development in children. *M. Clin. North America* 30:183, 1946.

(b) GESCHICHTER, C. *Diseases of the Breast.* Philadelphia, J. P. Lippincott, 1945.

(c) REUBEN, M. S. and MANNING, G. R. Precocious puberty. *Arch. Pediat.* 39:769, 1922 and *ibid* 40:27, 1923.

(d) WILKINS, I. Abnormalities and variations of sexual development during childhood and adolescence. In *Advances in Pediatrics.* Vol. III. Edited by S. Z. Levine, *et al.* New York, Interscience Publishers, 1948.

6 (a) DOTT, N. M. Surgical aspects of the hypothalamus. In *The Hypothalamus: Morphological, Functional, Clinical and Surgical Aspects.* By W. E. Clark, *et al.* Edinburgh, Oliver & Boyd, 1938.

(b) FORD, F. R. and GUILD, H. Precocious puberty following measles encephalomyelitis and epidemic encephalitis with a discussion of the relation of intracranial tumors and inflammatory processes to the syndrome of macrogenitosomia praecox. *Bull. Johns Hopkins Hosp.* 60:192, 1937.

(c) SCHLESINGER, B. Hydrocephalus with precocious puberty following post-basic meningitis. *Proc. Roy. Soc. Med.* 28:149, 1934.

7   NOVAK, E. The constitutional type of female precocious puberty with a report of nine cases. *Am. J. Obst. & Gynec.* 47:20, 1944.

8 (a) ALBRIGHT, F., BUTLER, A. M., HAMPTON, A. O. and SMITH, P. Syndrome characterized by osteitis fibrosa disseminata, areas of pigmentation and endocrine dysfunction, with precocious puberty in females; report of five cases. *New Eng. J. Med.* 216:727, 1937.

(b) ALBRIGHT, F., SCOVILLE, W. B. and SULKOWITCH, H. W. Syndrome characterized by osteitis fibrosa disseminata, areas of pigmentation and gonadal dysfunction; further observations including report of 2 more cases. *Endocrinology* 22:411, 1938.

(c) LICHTENSTEIN, L. and JAFFE, H. L. Fibrous dysplasia of bone; a condition affecting one, several or many bones, the graver cases of which may present abnormal pigmentation of skin, premature sexual development, hyperthyroidism or still other extraskeletal abnormalities. *Arch. Path.* 33:777, 1942.

(d) FALCONER, M. A., COPE, C. L. and ROBB-SMITH, A. H. T. Fibrous dysplasia of bone with endocrine disorders and cutaneous pigmentation (Albright's disease). *Quart. J. Med.* 11:121, 1942.

9 (a) BLAND, P. B. and GOLDSTEIN, L. Granulosa cell and Brenner tumors of the ovary. *Surg. Gynec. & Obst.* 61:250, 1935.

(b) ZEMKE, E. E. and HERRELL, W. E. Bilateral granulosa cell tumors; successful removal from a child fourteen weeks of age. *Am. J. Obst. & Gynec.* 41:704, 1941.

(c) GEIST, S. H. and SPIELMAN, F. Endocrine tumors of the ovary. *J. Clin. Endocrinol.* 3:281, 1943.

(d) KIMMEL, G. C. Sexual precocity and accelerated growth in a child with a follicular cyst of the ovary. *J. Pediat.* 30:686, 1947.

(e) HARRIS, R. H. Carcinomatous ovarian teratoma with premature puberty and precocious somatic development. *Surg. Gynec. & Obst.* 24:604, 1917 and *ibid* 41:191, 1925.

(f) CRAVEN, J. D. Precocious menstruation. *Am. J. Dis. Child.* 43:936, 1932.

10 KEPLER, E. J., WALTERS, W. and DIXON, R. K. Menstruation in a child aged nineteen months as the result of a tumor of the left adrenal cortex: successful surgical treatment. *Proc. Staff Meet., Mayo Clin.* 13:362, 1938.

11   LINCOLN, E. M., STONE, S. and HOFFMAN, O. R. The treatment of miliary tuberculosis with promizole. *Bull. Johns Hopkins Hosp.* 82:56, 1948.

12   WILKINS, L. and FLEISCHMANN, W. Sexual infantilism in females: causes, diagnosis and treatment. *J. Clin. Endocrinol.* 4:306, 1944.

13 (a) BRUCH, H. Froehlich syndrome; report of the original case. *Am. J. Dis. Child.* 58:1282, 1939.
   (b) GJORUP, E. Hypophyseal nanism resulting from craniopharyngioma. *Acta pædiat.* 27:508, 1940.

14 (a) REILLY, W. A. and LISSER, H. Laurence-Moon-Biedl syndrome. *Endocrinology* 16:337, 1932.
   (b) WARKANY, J., FRAUENBERGER, C. S. and MITCHELL, A. G. Heredofamilial deviations; the Laurence-Moon-Biedl syndrome. *Am. J. Dis. Child.* 53:455, 1937.
   (c) ROTH, A. A. Familial eunuchoidism; the Laurence-Moon-Biedl syndrome. *J. Urol.* 57:427, 1947.

15 (a) WOHL, M. G. and LARSON, E. Diagnosis and treatment of pituitary gland disorders. *M. Clin. North America* 26:1657, 1942.
   (b) ALPERS, B. J. Diagnosis and treatment of pituitary tumors. *M. Clin. North America* 26:1679, 1942.
   (c) WHITE, P. Diabetes in childhood. In *Treatment of Diabetes Mellitus*. By E. P. Joslin, et al. Philadelphia, Lea & Febiger, 1946.

16 (a) TURNER, H. H. A syndrome of infantilism, congenital webbed neck and cubitus valgus. *Endocrinology* 23:566, 1938.
   (b) ALBRIGHT, F., SMITH, P. H. and FRASER, R. A. Syndrome characterized by primary ovarian insufficiency and decreased stature; report of 11 cases with a digression on hormonal control of axillary and pubic hair. *Am. J. M. Sc.* 204:625, 1942.
   (c) VARNEY, R. F., KENYON, A. T. and KOCH, F. C. An association of short stature, retarded sexual development and high urinary gonadotropin titers in women; ovarian dwarfism. *J. Clin. Endocrinol.* 2:137, 1942.
   (d) SCHNEIDER, R. W. and MC CULLAGH, E. P. Infantilism, congenital webbed neck and cubitus valgus (Turner's syndrome). *Cleveland Clin. Quart.* 10:112, 1943.
   (e) WILKINS, L. and FLEISCHMANN, W. Ovarian agenesis: pathology, associated clinical symptoms and the bearing on theories of sex differentiation. *J. Clin. Endocrinol.* 4:357, 1944.
   (f) CASTILLO, E. B., DEL, LA BALZE, F. A., DE and ARGONZ, J. Syndrome of rudimentary ovaries with estrogenic insufficiency and an increase in gonadotropins. *J. Clin. Endocrinol.* 7:385, 1947.

17 (a) ENGLE, E. T. and SHELESNYAK, M. C. First menstruation and subsequent menstrual cycles of pubertal girls. *Human Biol.* 6:431, 1934.
   (b) SHORR, E. Endocrine problems in adolescence. *J. Pediat.* 19:327, 1941.
   (c) HAMBLEN, E. C. *Endocrinology of Woman.* Springfield, Ill., C. C. Thomas, 1945.

18 (a) TOMPKINS, P. The treatment of imperforate hymen with hematocolpos: a review of 113 cases in the literature and a report of 5 additional cases. *J. A. M. A.* 113:913, 1939.
   (b) FLANNERY, W. E. Arrhenoblastoma before puberty. *Am. J. Obst. & Gynec.* 60:923, 1950.
   (c) REIFENSTEIN, E. C., JR. Psychogenic or "hypothalamic" amenorrhea. *M. Clin. North America* 30:1103, 1946.
   (d) STEIN, I. F. and LEVENTHAL, M. L. Amenorrhea associated with bilateral polycystic ovaries. *Am. J. Obst. & Gynec.* 29:181, 1935.
   (e) INGERSOLL, F. M. and MC DERMOTT, W. V. Bilateral polycystic ovaries: Stein-Leventhal syndrome. *Am. J. Obst. & Gynec.* 60:117, 1950.

19 (a) FLUHMANN, C. F. Menometrorrhagia during adolescence. *J. A. M. A.* 135:557, 1947.
(b) ALBRIGHT, F. Metropathia hemorrhagica. *J. Maine M. A.* 29:235, 1938.
(c) TE LINDE, R. W. Endometrial pathology of functional bleeding. In *Menstruation and Its Disorders.* By E. Engle. Springfield, Ill., C. C. Thomas, 1950.
(d) KAHN, M. E. Abnormal uterine bleeding in blood dyscrasias. *J. A. M. A.* 99:1563, 1932.
(e) GOLDBURGH, H. L. and GOULEY, B. A. Postpubertal menorrhagia and its possible relations to thrombocytopenic purpura hemorrhagica. *Am. J. M. Sc.* 200:449, 1940.
(f) POLLACK, R. S. and TAYLOR, H. C. Carcinoma of the cervix during the first two decades of life. *Am. J. Obst. & Gynec.* 53:135, 1947.
(g) CUYLER, W. K., HAMBLEN, E. C. and DAVIS, C. D. Diethylstilbestrol for hemostasis in functional uterine hemorrhage. *J. Clin. Endocrinol.* 2:438, 1942.
(h) RUBENSTEIN, B. B. Treatment of menstrual disorders in adolescent girls. *J. Clin. Encrinol.* 3:163, 1943.
(i) SMITH, G. V. On menstruation. *J. Clin. Endocrinol.* 5:190, 1945.

20 (a) AINLAY, G. W. Palliative treatment of dysmenorrhea with acetylsalicylic acid, phenacetin and propadrine hydrochloride. *Am. J. Obst. & Gynec.* 39:82, 1940.
(b) STURGIS, S. and ALBRIGHT, F. The mechanism of estrin therapy in the relief of dysmenorrhea. *Endrocrinology* 26:68, 1940.

21 (a) CREEVY, C. D. Pseudohermaphroditism; report of 5 cases. *Internat. S. Digest* 16:195, 1933.
(b) WEED, J. C., SEGALOFF, A., WIENER, W. B. and DOUGLAS, J. W. True hermaphroditism; endocrine studies in a case of ovotestis. *J. Clin. Endocrinol.* 7:741, 1947.
(c) YOUNG, H. H. *Genital Abnormalities, Hermaphroditism and Related Adrenal Diseases.* Baltimore, Williams & Wilkins, 1937.

THE TESTES

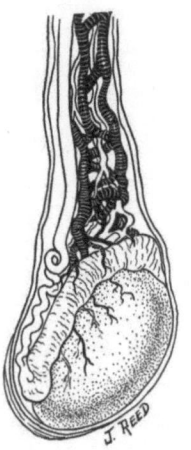

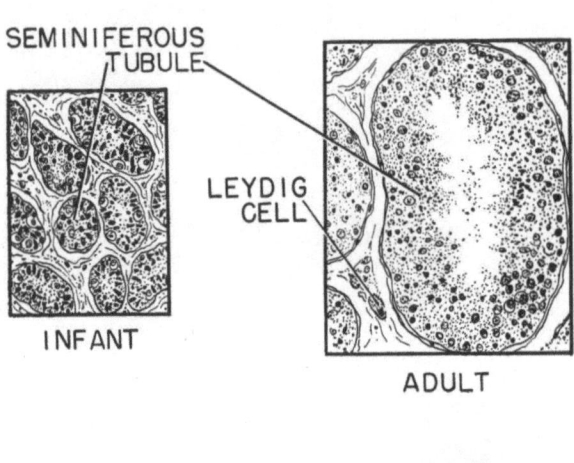

— RELATIVE SIZE OF INFANT AND ADULT TESTES —

CHAPTER VI

THE TESTES

BASIC CONSIDERATIONS

The testes have the primary purpose of inducing maleness and the capacity for reproduction. Testicular hormones also exert a widespread influence upon body economy.

The male gonad is made up of two chief components. One is represented by the interstitial cells of Leydig, which secrete androgens (masculinizing hormones). The other is the testicular tubule, which produces sperm and which may in addition secrete a second type of hormone currently called "inhibin."* Embryologically both of these components arise near the mesonephros in the genital ridge. Since the adrenal cortices arise from adjacent structures, it is not surprising that cells which are histologically indistinguishable from adrenocortical cells are occasionally found in the body of the testes. This nearly common ancestry may account for some of the similarities of chemical structure and physiologic action which hormones produced by testicular interstitial cells show to those produced by certain adrenocortical cells. Normal testicular development and activity is dependent upon specific anterior pituitary gonad-stimulating hormones.

CHEMISTRY OF TESTICULAR HORMONES

The precise nature of the human testicular androgen is not known. However, a potent androgen, testosterone, has been isolated from the testes of bulls.[2] This steroid hormone has a structure reminiscent of adrenocortical hormones (see Chapter III, page 136). The human testicular androgen, like synthetic testosterone, is metabolized and excreted in the urine as neutral 17-ketosteroids. For

* Little is known about this testicular hormone. It appears to be a water-soluble, lipid-insoluble substance present in desiccated bull testes tissue.[1] A further description of its chemical nature must await further studies.

this and other reasons it is generally assumed to be chemically similar to, if not identical with, testosterone.

PHYSIOLOGIC ACTIONS OF TESTICULAR ANDROGENS

General Metabolic Actions. Testosterone prompts *nitrogen anabolism*, as can be demonstrated easily by metabolic balance studies (see Figure 1).[3] It is not known whether this is accomplished by inhibiting protoplasmic catabolism or by stimulating protoplasmic anabolism. The growth-promoting effect is not limited to sex organs but involves the muscles, skeleton and certain other structures.

This protein anabolic action of testosterone can, under certain circumstances, be accompanied by changes in *sugar and fat metabolism*. These are illustrated by studies made on normal fasting men and by observation of a child suffering from progeria. In the former it was noted that testosterone caused not only a decrease in urine nitrogen excretion (see Figure 2), but also a lowering of fasting blood sugar levels (see Figure 3) and an increase in urinary ketone output (see Figure 4). The decreased nitrogen excretion signified that testosterone had acted to inhibit the breakdown of the body's protein stores. Since the body maintains blood glucose levels under conditions of prolonged fasting by protein catabolism (gluconeogenesis from protein), it is not surprising that the blood sugar concentrations tended to fall; and since the organism must derive its energy from either protein, carbohydrate or fat, a reduction in the first two of these components necessarily leads to a compensatory increase in the third component of the metabolic mixture. In other words, the increased ketonuria shown in Figure 4 probably reflects increased mobilization of body fat rather than decreased utilization of ketone bodies or lowered renal threshold for ketone excretion (for related comments see Chapter III, page 150, and Chapter IX, page 543).

These data are interpreted to mean that when testosterone is given under conditions of negative caloric balance, it may accelerate the rate at which body fat stores are depleted. Studies on a progeric child indicate that testosterone tends to prompt a similar phenomenon when given to individuals who are receiving a diet just sufficient to maintain nitrogen and caloric equilibrium. It is seen in Figure 5 that testosterone therapy induced a positive nitrogen balance. This means that a portion of the dietary protein was diverted from the production of energy to the construction of new body protoplasm and was thus equivalent to the subtraction of a portion of the caloric intake. There apparently resulted a caloric deficit which was met by an equicaloric consumption of body depot fat.

Similar changes have been described in experimental animals whose metabolic

The Testes

mixture has been modified by the pituitary growth (protein anabolic) hormone.[4] For related comments, see Chapter VII, page 452.

Testosterone has additional effects upon *electrolyte and water metabolism,* causing more positive balances with respect to sodium, chloride and potassium (Figure 1).[3] Retention of sodium and chloride is accompanied by retention of water, presumably in the extracellular compartment. This action is reminiscent of that described for the adrenocortical Na-K hormone. While the latter prompts diuresis of potassium, testosterone tends to cause retention of potassium. This action of testosterone is probably closely related to the nitrogen anabolic effect described above.* Testosterone can prompt a retention of potassium in relation to nitrogen which is greater than that expected on the basis of normal intracellular composition. In a number of metabolic experiments this has been observed to result in a transient state of marked hypokalemia (see Figure 1†).[6] This hypokalemia is not accompanied by clinical symptoms or electrocardiographic changes.**

Just as potassium is needed for protoplasmic anabolism, so too are such other intracellular electrolytes as phosphorus and magnesium. It is therefore not surprising to learn that testosterone causes phosphorus retention. Phosphorus retention is apt to be in excess of that needed for protoplasmic growth,†† the excess phosphorus being deposited in bones as calcium phosphate.[3]

Actions on Various Body Structures. Androgens effect changes in the musculature, skeleton, kidneys, larynx, skin and hair, as well as the genitalia. In the normal male all of such changes, except those related to the hair and skin, are largely referable to the testicular male hormone. Changes in the skin and hair also are produced by the adrenocortical 17-KS-Gens (see page 156). The actions which bring about these changes may be considered separately as follows.

* Potassium is an important constituent of protoplasm as evidenced by the fact that there are about 100 mEq. in each kg. of fat-free, extracellular water-free, true-muscle tissue. Re-expressed in terms of intracellular water (which comprises about 70 per cent of true-muscle tissue) there are approximately 50 gm. of nitrogen and 143 mEq. of potassium per liter.[5] It is therefore to be expected that about 2.8 mEq. of potassium will be stored with each gram of nitrogen retained.

† Calculations indicate that during the first 80 days of testosterone therapy one patient gained a quantity of nitrogen corresponding to that contained in 3.4 kg. of true muscle. During the same interval he gained potassium in a quantity equal to that present in 6.6 kg. of average normal true muscle. Despite this apparent plethora of potassium, his serum potassium concentration fell temporarily from a normal value of 4.7 to the very abnormally low value of 0.7 mEq. per liter.

** These findings are in marked contrast to those seen in persons who develop intracellular potassium deficiency with or without hypokalemia. Individuals of the latter type are apt to show somatic and cardiac muscle weakness and other evidences of disturbed cellular metabolism (see effects of Na-K hormone excess, Chapter III, page 139).

†† Normally there is 1 gm. of phosphorus for each 15 gm. of nitrogen in true muscle.[5]

Continued on page 381

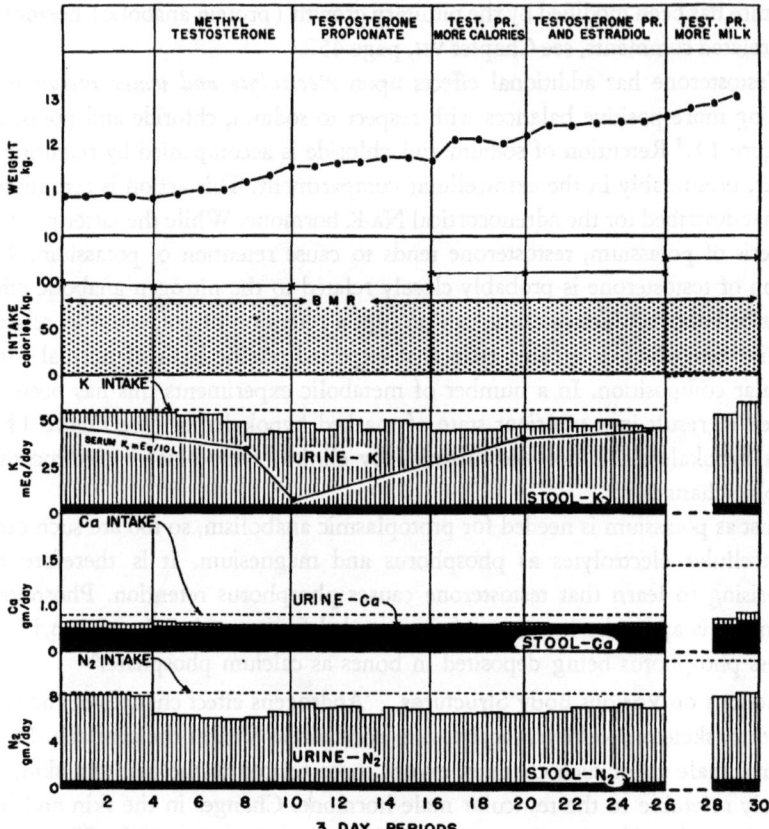

FIGURE VI—1. Production of positive nitrogen balance, positive potassium balance and transitory hypokalemia by testosterone treatment. The regimen is indicated by the first section; in the second section solid circles connected by solid lines indicate changes in body weight. In the third section crosses connected by lines give the caloric intake. The next lower line indicates the basal energy metabolism or output. The following sections of the figure give the daily intake (horizontal broken line), urinary output (vertical lines) and fecal output (solid black area) of, respectively, potassium, calcium and nitrogen. Scales corresponding to each of the foregoing measurements are presented along the left ordinate. When the line indicating the total fecal plus urinary output of a substance reached the line representing the intake of that substance, the patient was in equilibrium with respect to that substance; when the line giving the fecal plus urinary output was lower than the intake (as in periods 4 to 25) the patient was storing the substance at a rate equal to the width of the space between the upper intake line and the lower line defined by urinary plus fecal output.

Also presented in the figure are measurements of serum potassium (solid line connected with solid circles running through the portion of the chart indicated urinary potassium)

FIGURE 1 (continued)

expressed as mEq. per 10 liters according to the scale given for potassium intake and output along the ordinate. Note that testosterone caused an increase in body weight and more positive potassium, calcium and nitrogen balances. It also caused a marked fall in serum potassium concentration from a control level of 4.7 to the low point of 0.7 mEq. per liter. This fall in serum potassium was transient despite continued administration of testosterone. During the period when the serum potassium fell, the patient stored in his body twice the amount of potassium needed for the formation of new muscle as calculated from the nitrogen balance. The fact that the serum potassium fell despite this apparent excess retention of potassium over nitrogen suggests that testosterone may have given body cells an extraordinary avidity for potassium. In other words, the fall in serum potassium was due to migration of potassium from serum to cells rather than from serum to urine as is the case in hypokalemia secondary to desoxycorticosterone intoxication. From N. B. Talbot, A. M. Butler, E. L. Pratt, E. A. MacLachlan and J. Tannheimer, *Am. J. Dis. Child.* 69:267, 1945.

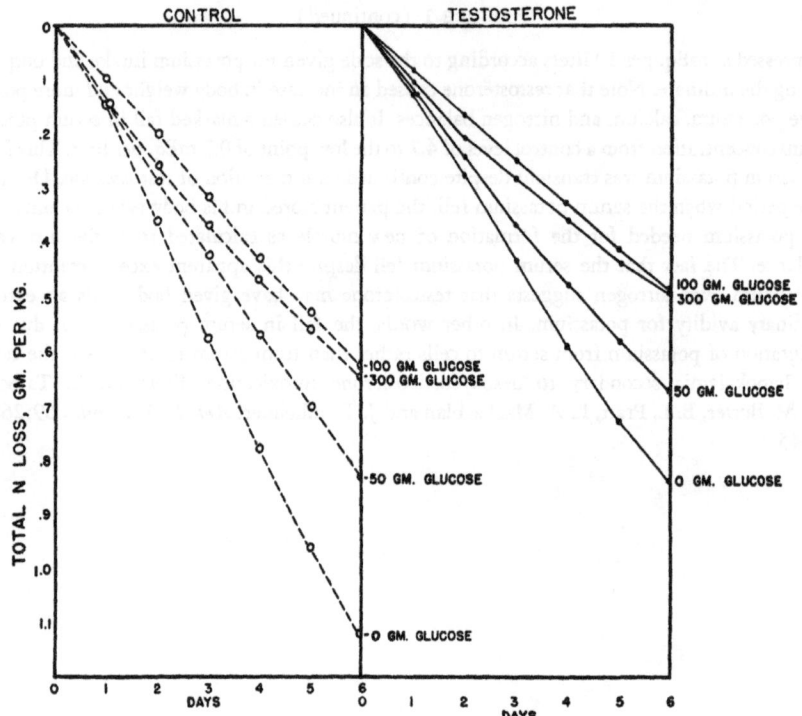

FIGURE VI—2. Effect of 25 mg. of testosterone propionate daily on total urinary nitrogen excretion by subjects receiving various inadequate diets. The left-hand portion of the figure represents control periods; the right-hand portion, periods of testosterone treatment. The periods were of six days' duration as shown along the abscissa. Cumulative nitrogen losses are indicated by the curves coursing downward from left to right. The respective dietary intakes of the individuals studied are indicated by the lower right-hand ends of these curves. Comparison of the 0 gm. glucose (total fasting) curve of the testosterone experiments with the 50 gm. glucose curve of the control experiments shows that testosterone treatment caused as great a reduction in nitrogen output as did the daily administration of 50 gm. of glucose to an otherwise fasting subject.

The above figure and those on the opposite page are from A. M. Butler, N. B. Talbot, E. A. MacLachlan, J. E. Appleton and M. A. Linton, *J. Clin. Endocrinol.* 5:327, 1945.

The Testes

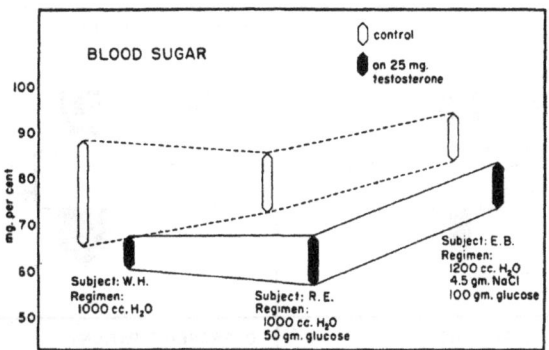

FIGURE VI—3. Effect of testosterone on fasting blood sugar concentrations during periods of inadequate dietary intake. The subjects are the same as those of Figure 2. The length of the double-headed arrows indicates the range of the fasting blood sugar concentrations during the third to sixth days following institution of the regimens indicated along the bottom of the chart. A scale in milligrams of glucose per 100 cc. of whole blood is given along the left-hand ordinate. Note that the subjects had lower blood sugar values when they were receiving testosterone than they did during control periods.

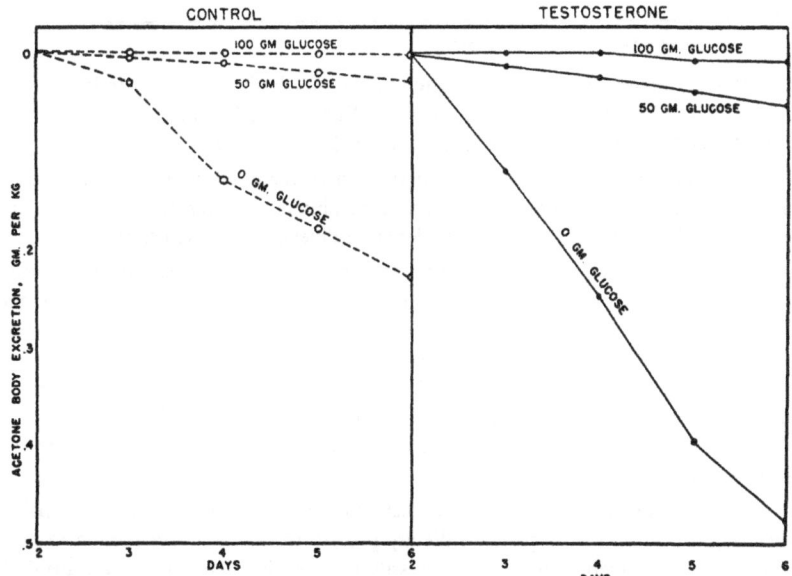

FIGURE VI—4. Effect of testosterone on the urinary acetone-body output of subjects receiving various inadequate diets. The subjects and the experiments of this figure are the same as those of Figures 2 and 3. It can be seen that the urinary acetone-body excretion of the fasting subject (0 gm. of glucose) was doubled when he was treated with testosterone.

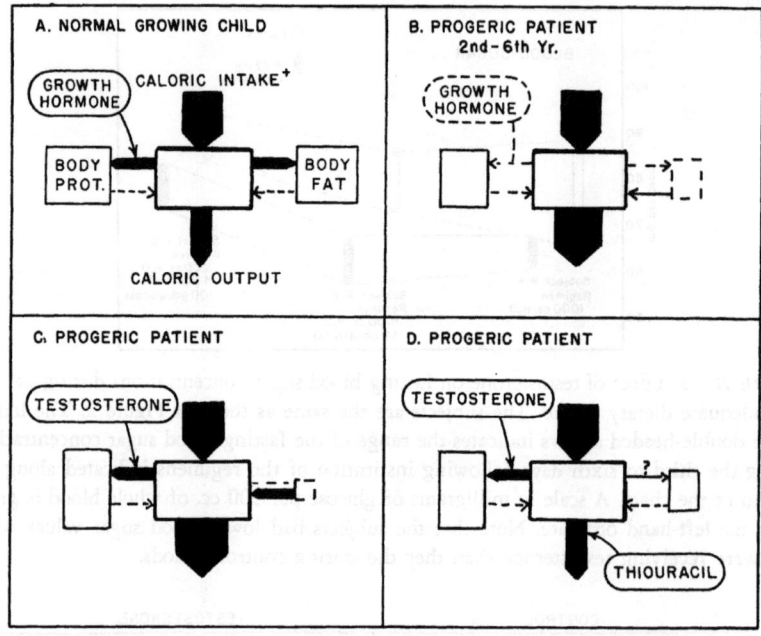

FIGURE VI—5. Diagrammatic representation of the metabolic effects of administered testosterone on a child with progeria. From N. B. Talbot, A. M. Butler, E. L. Pratt, E. A. MacLachlan and J. Tannheimer, *Am. J. Dis. Child.* 69:267, 1945.

SECTION A portrays the conditions which pertain in normally growing children. Here the caloric intake exceeds the caloric output and a surplus is left over for the accumulation of body fat and for protein anabolism under the influence of growth hormones.

SECTION B describes the probable status of a progeric child prior to testosterone treatment as determined by metabolic balance studies. Here the caloric balance was negative (intake slightly less than output). This deficit was met by the combustion of body fat stores. Because of the caloric deficit or some other metabolic disturbance (growth hormone deficiency?; see Chapter VII, Figure 3) his nitrogen balance was in equilibrium rather than positive as in normal growing children. However, this meant that he was able to use his dietary protein exclusively for energy and that he was able to this extent to spare his very limited fat stores.

SECTION C shows that administration of testosterone produced a positive nitrogen balance by diverting a portion of the patient's dietary protein from energy production to protoplasmic synthesis or anabolism. This of necessity reduced the dietary protein available for energy production. The resultant extension of the caloric deficit led to an increase in body fat combustion (i.e., it augmented the rate at which body calory stores were depleted).

Thus it appears that the induction of protoplasmic growth at the expense of body fat stores in a severely depleted subject is physiologically unsound. Ordinarily it is preferable to promote nitrogen anabolism by increasing the caloric intake as discussed in Chapter VII.

Musculature. As a result of their nitrogen anabolic action androgens prompt an appreciable increase in musculature. This is grossly evident in the weight and appearance of bulls as compared to oxen and in the appearance of normal men as compared to boys and eunuchs. It also may be seen in humans to whom testosterone has been given (see Figure 6). There is a limit to the degree of muscular hypertrophy which may be induced by male hormone, but the nature of the limiting factor is not known. In these connections it is noteworthy that preadolescent boys, girls and women in whom androgens are absent can develop and maintain quite a good musculature. It follows that muscular development is not wholly dependent on male hormone.

Skeleton. Since the growth of protein matrix constitutes a fundamental step in skeletal development, the skeletal-growth-promoting action of androgens (see Figure 7) is thought to be related to their protein anabolic effect. This action, like that on the musculature, is potentially limited. One of the limiting factors is epiphyseal closure, which precludes further longitudinal bone growth.

Androgens tend to accelerate epiphyseal calcification and epiphyseal closure (see Figure 8). In patients of both sexes the skeleton is sensitive in this regard during infancy and early childhood, and it may become more sensitive as the individual approaches the adolescent age. Experience with children given testosterone therapy indicates that there may be a lag of 6 to 12 months between the time that the skeleton is first exposed to the male hormone and the time when accelerated maturation becomes evident in skeletal roentgenograms.[7] As will be pointed out below, this phenomenon has an important bearing on the use of testosterone as a growth-promoting agent in dwarfed children (see page 440).

Finally, androgens cause elongation of the face and development of the lower jaw of boys during adolescence (see Chapter III, Figure 51).

Kidneys. Testosterone has been used experimentally as a therapeutic agent in cases of nephrosis and chronic nephritis, since it is known to restore the kidneys of castrated rats to normal size, and even to induce hypertrophy, chiefly by causing overdevelopment of the convoluted tubules.[8] However, in the case of humans, such treatment has not proved of much value.

Larynx. Differences in the pitch and quality of individual men's voices are due to genetic differences in laryngeal structure rather than to differences in the concentration of androgens in the circulation. But in each case the change resulting from laryngeal enlargement at puberty is due to male hormone.

Skin. Androgens as well as certain non-androgenic adrenocortical hormones cause the skin to become coarser in texture and the sebaceous glands to develop secretory activity. Acne may result, especially during the period of sebaceous

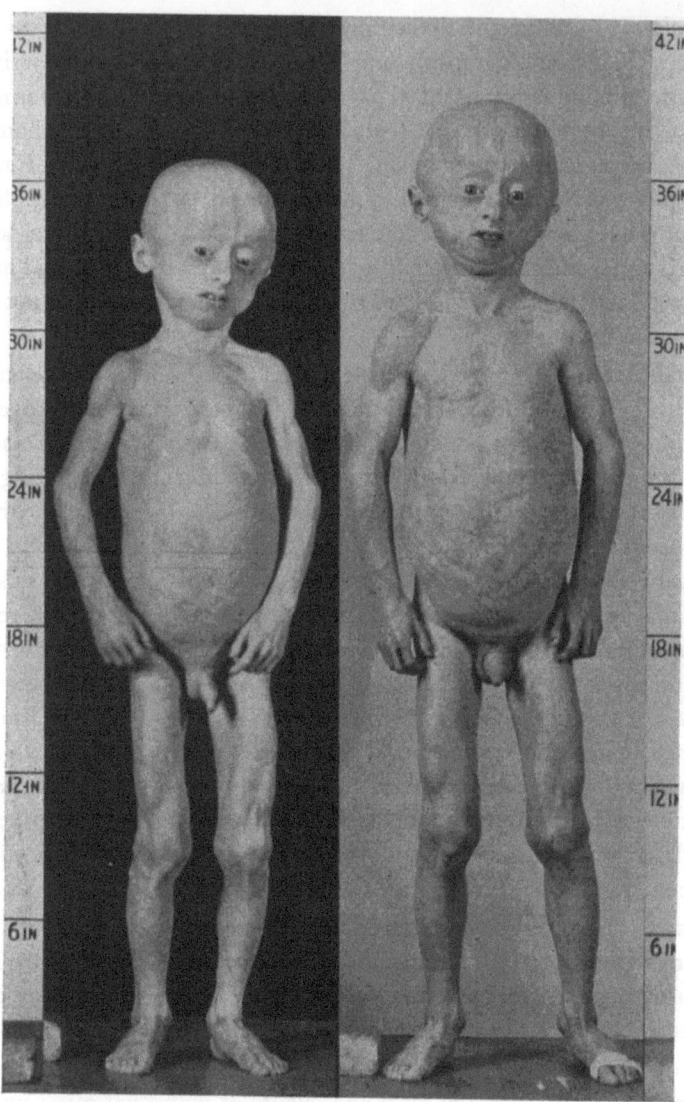

FIGURE VI—6. Effect of testosterone on the muscular development of a six-year-old boy with progeria. From N. B. Talbot, A. M. Butler, E. L. Pratt, E. A. MacLachlan and J. Tannheimer, *Am. J. Dis. Child.* 69:267, 1945

LEFT: The patient's appearance before testosterone therapy.

RIGHT: His appearance after approximately six months of testosterone therapy. Note the increase in musculature, particularly about the shoulder girdles and arms, and in the thighs.

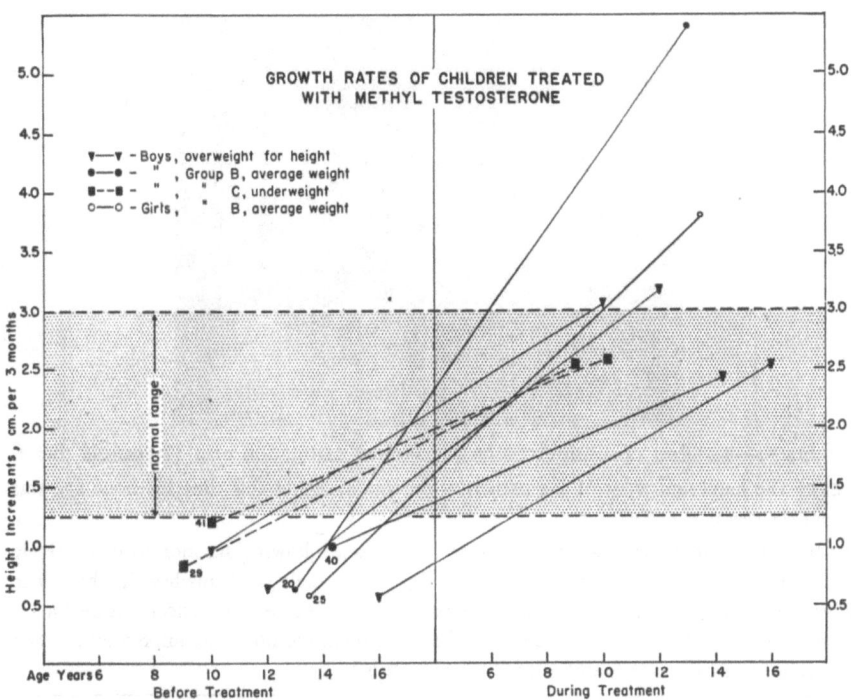

FIGURE VI—7. Effect of oral methyl testosterone therapy on the growth rates of eight dwarfed children, six of whom appeared to be well nourished, and two of whom were thin. Rates of growth were observed over a period of at least six months before treatment was begun and for approximately three months afterward. The shaded area represents approximately the normal range of growth increments. The positions of the symbols of weight status indicate roughly the time at which treatment was started (abscissa). The figures beside the symbols are case numbers. Growth increments are expressed as centimeter per three months (ordinate). It can be seen that in every instance testosterone caused at least a doubling of the growth rate. From N. B. Talbot, E. H. Sobel, B. S. Burke, E. Lindemann and S. B. Kaufman, *New Eng. J. Med.* 236:783, 1947.

gland development. Androgens may also cause dilatation of the capillaries,[9] so that the skin becomes flushed.

Body hair. Androgens ordinarily prompt growth of pubic, axillary and facial hair and cause recession of the hairline over the temples. There are, however, marked differences in the manner in which the hair follicles of various persons respond to this hormone. Thus the American Indian is apt to be beardless because his facial hair follicles are insensitive to androgens, and one occasionally finds patients with axillary alopecia which cannot be eliminated by parenteral

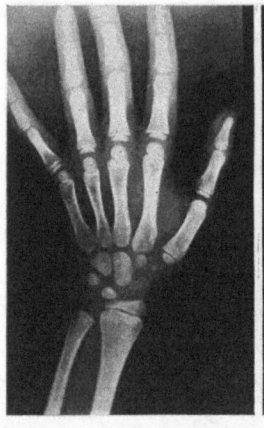 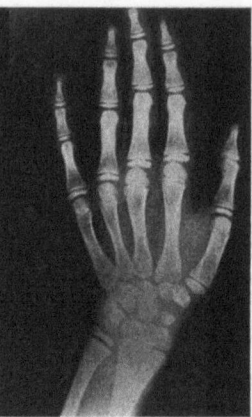

FIGURE VI—8. Effect of testosterone on the skeletal maturation of a 12-year-old dwarf.
LEFT: The hand and wrist of the patient at the age of 12; at this time his bone age was about six years.
RIGHT: The patient's skeletal maturation at 12½ years, following six months of relatively heavy methyl testosterone therapy (50 mg. by mouth daily). Meanwhile his bone age advanced six years. This is to be considered an extreme degree of advancement secondary to testosterone action, but lesser degrees of advancement are noted commonly even when the dose of testosterone is quite small (5 mg. daily).

---

or local administration of testosterone. Contrariwise, the hair follicles over the arms, legs and trunk of certain individuals are unusually sensitive to androgenic action. Such persons show diffuse hirsutism. However, hirsutism by itself should not be considered necessarily indicative of masculinity, for considerable hirsutism may be noted in children and in women who show no clitoral hypertrophy, deepening of the voice or other real evidence of masculinization.

Central nervous system. It is difficult to appraise with accuracy the effect of androgens upon the emotional and intellectual status of children. Objective studies of the intelligence of children with spontaneous sexual precocity indicate that sex hormone has no important effect upon the intelligence quotient.[10] On the other hand, it awakens reproductive instincts and may provoke more aggressive, energetic behavior (see legend to Figure 20).

Secondary sexual characteristics. In boys with normal adrenal cortices, development of the penis, scrotum, prostate and seminal vesicles is very largely, if not entirely, dependent upon testicular androgen action. This means that the anatomic status of these organs ordinarily can be used as a reasonably reliable index of testicular androgen production during childhood and adolescence.

CENTRAL NERVOUS SYSTEM–PITUITARY–GONAD RELATIONS

Observations on children suffering from precocious puberty due apparently to a variety of non-specific central nervous system lesions (see Table 3) strongly suggest that neurologic centers in the hypothalamic region of the brain influence pituitary gonadotropic hormone production. These centers are probably responsible for the initiation of adolescence in the normal child (see Figure 9). The contrary clinical picture of hypogonadism secondary to failure of the central nervous system to activate the pituitary gonadotropic mechanism is thought to occur from time to time, as in patients with the Laurence-Moon-Biedl syndrome. In other words, it appears that just as the gonads will fail to develop unless stimulated by pituitary gonadotropic hormones, the pituitary will fail to develop gonadotropic activity unless activated by appropriate neurologic stimuli.

Anterior Pituitary–Testicular Relations. As described in detail with respect to the ovaries in Chapter V, normal gonadal activity is dependent upon anterior pituitary–gonadotropic hormone stimulation. In the female, when at least a trace of luteinizing hormone (LH) is present, the FSH stimulates the Graafian follicles to develop and secrete estrogens. In the male FSH induces spermatic tubule development and spermatogenesis, while LH stimulates the testicular interstitial cells to develop and secrete androgens. Hence, in dealing with the male, LH is more aptly labeled "interstitial-cell-stimulating hormone," or ICSH.

Parenthetically it may be mentioned that a hormone with an ICSH-like action is also extractable from human urine during pregnancy. Since this is derived from the placental chorion, it is called "chorionic gonadotropin." Because of its similarity of action to pituitary ICSH, it also has been called the "anterior-pituitary-like" hormone. Chorionic gonadotropin is sometimes used in therapy as a substitute for ICSH.

In the male there are reciprocal relations between pituitary activity and gonadotropic hormone production on the one hand and gonadal activity and hormone production on the other. These relations may be divided into two sets. One deals with pituitary FSH and the spermatic tubules; the other deals with interstitial cells and pituitary ICSH. These relations are discussed briefly below. It is to be noted that certain of them obtain only in individuals who have reached adolescent age.

FSH–spermatic tubule relations. Little if any FSH is secreted by the anterior pituitary during the preadolescent period, when the tubules are immature and quiescent. During adolescence the pituitary secretes increased quantities of FSH,

TABLE VI—1. Urinary gonadotropins in normal boys. From E. P. McCullagh, *Recent Progress in Hormone Research*, II, edited by G. Pincus, New York, Academic Press, 1948.

Age, yr.	FSH M.U.*/24 hr.	Age, yr.	FSH M.U./24 hr.
2½	<2	13	26-53
9	6-13	13	26-53
9	6-13	13	26-53
10	<6	13	26-53
	6-13	13	13-26
10	<6	13	26-53
	6-13	13	105-212
10	6-13	14	13-26
10	6-13	14	26-53
10½	>3	14	26-53
			13-26
11	>6	14	13-26
12	26-53	14	26-53
		14	13-26
12	26-53	15	26-53

* Mouse units.

as evidenced by rising urinary excretion values (see Table 1),* and the tubules develop simultaneously (see Figure 10 and Figure 11, right). The last step in the maturation process is spermatogenesis.

Once a boy reaches adolescent age, disturbances of the testicular tubules are apt to prompt marked compensatory alterations in pituitary FSH production. If the individual is castrated or suffers selective damage to the spermatic tubules of the testes, there usually follows a striking increase in urinary gonadotropin excretion to levels of more than 100 mouse units per 24 hours (see Figure 31).

In human adult eunuchoids testosterone prompts a decrease in urinary gonadotropin output only when given in amounts which are considerably larger than those needed to induce a normal degree of masculinization.[11] On the other hand, testosterone in moderate doses can cause a marked decrease in the sperm count of normal adult men.[11]

These observations are difficult to interpret concisely. Presumably FSH production is primarily related to testicular tubule activity. It has been suggested

* Urinary FSH is probably composed of a mixture of gonadotropic hormones with predominantly FSH-like activity. The term "urinary FSH" will be used here interchangeably with true FSH. This is undoubtedly an oversimplification, representing a sacrifice of some degree of accuracy in an attempt to attain clarity. Incidentally, note that these results are expressed on a simple per individual, per 24-hour basis. It would be interesting to know whether assays performed so as to give reliable values expressed on a per square meter of body surface, per 24-hour basis would show similar age differences.

Continued on page 391

The Testes

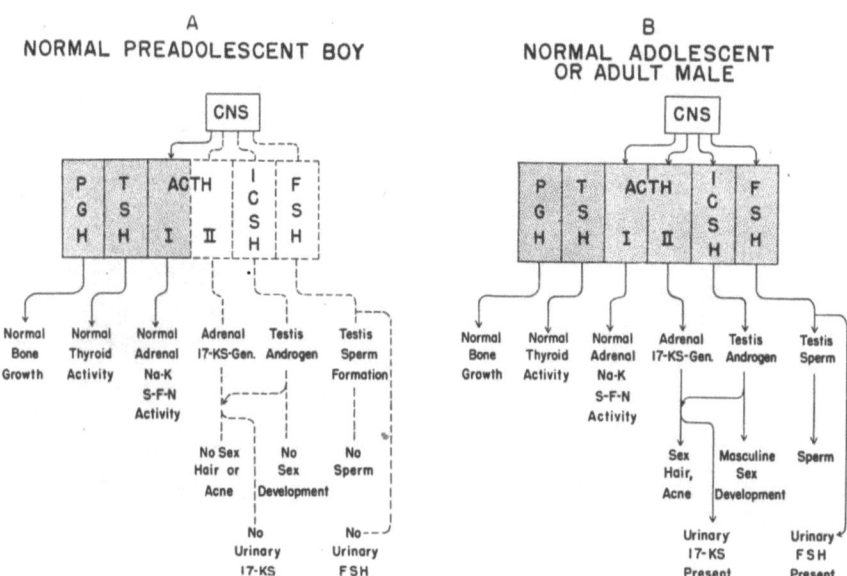

FIGURE VI—9. Diagrammatic representation of differences between preadolescent and adolescent or adult males. In these diagrams the uppermost area labeled CNS stands for the central nervous system; the next lower area represents the anterior pituitary, which is divided into several compartments with individual alphabetic labels; PGH stands for pituitary growth hormone; TSH for thyroid-stimulating hormone; ACTH for adrenocorticotropic hormones; ICSH for interstitial-cell-stimulating hormone; FSH for follicle-stimulating hormone; 17-KS-Gens for adrenocortical urinary 17-ketosteroid precursors; 17-KS for urinary 17-ketosteroids. Note that ACTH is indicated as two distinct hormones (I and II), having separate effects upon adrenocortical activity. The thesis that the human pituitary produces two types of ACTH is based upon indirect evidence (see Chapter III) and should be considered presumptive rather than proved. The arrows coming from these various pituitary areas are thought to exert the effects indicated in the lower section of the diagram. The shaded areas surrounded by solid lines indicate active production of the pituitary hormone or hormones. The white areas and interrupted lines are intended to suggest inactivity.

In the normal preadolescent boy ACTH II and the two gonadotropins ICSH and FSH are inactive, presumably because CNS stimulus is lacking. In consequence, there is little or no adrenocortical 17-KS, testicular androgen or testicular sperm production. In the normal adolescent male the CNS stimulates the pituitary to produce ACTH II and the two gonadotropins just mentioned, with resultant adrenocortical 17-KS, testicular androgen and testicular sperm production. The expected effects of these adrenocortical and testicular hormones on sexual development are indicated. So too is the fact that unlike the normal adolescent and adult male, the normal preadolescent boy has little, if any, 17-KS or gonadotropin (FSH) in his urine.

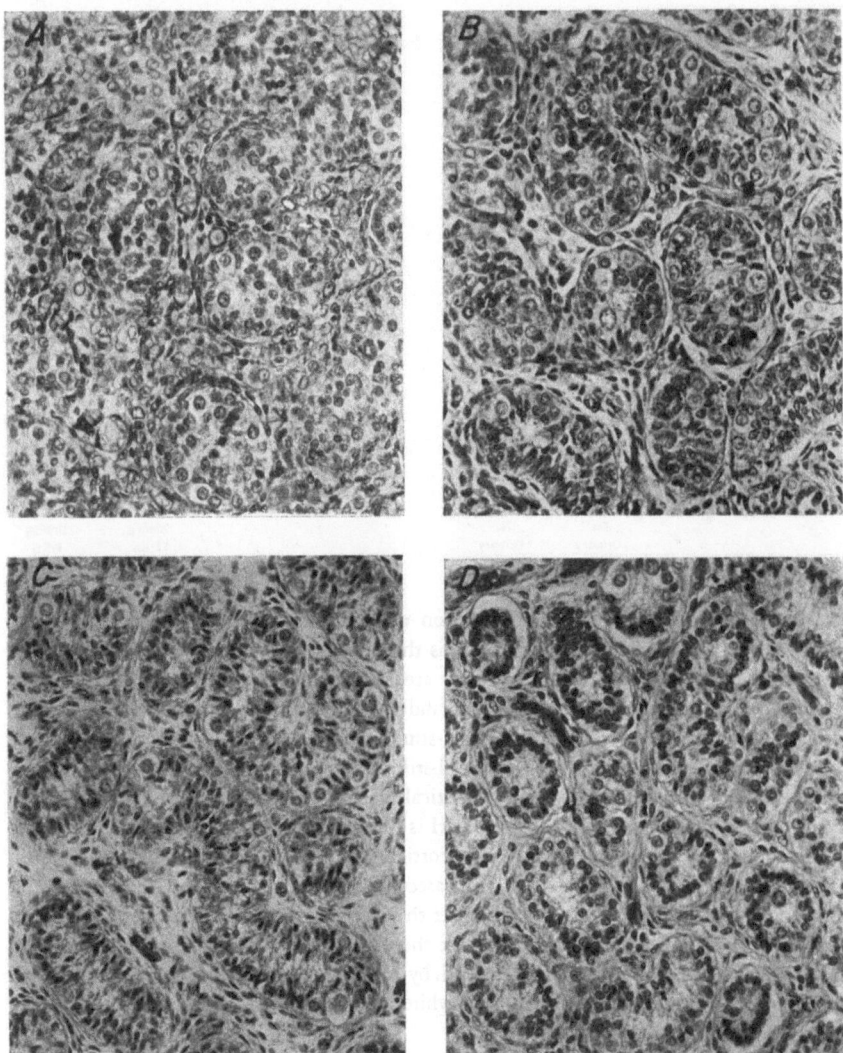

FIGURE VI—10. Testicular biopsies. Magnification x 225.

SECTION A: The fetal testis—seven months' gestation. The tubules are composed of solid masses of cells, including a few large primordial spermatogonia and many small undifferentiated cells. The interstitial tissue is largely cellular and includes some large cells. The interstitial blood vessels are prominent.

SECTION B: The neonatal testis—two days old. The tubules have small, indistinct lumina and include a few prominent spermatogonia and many undifferentiated cells arranged at random. The interstitial tissue is still rather cellular and well vascularized.

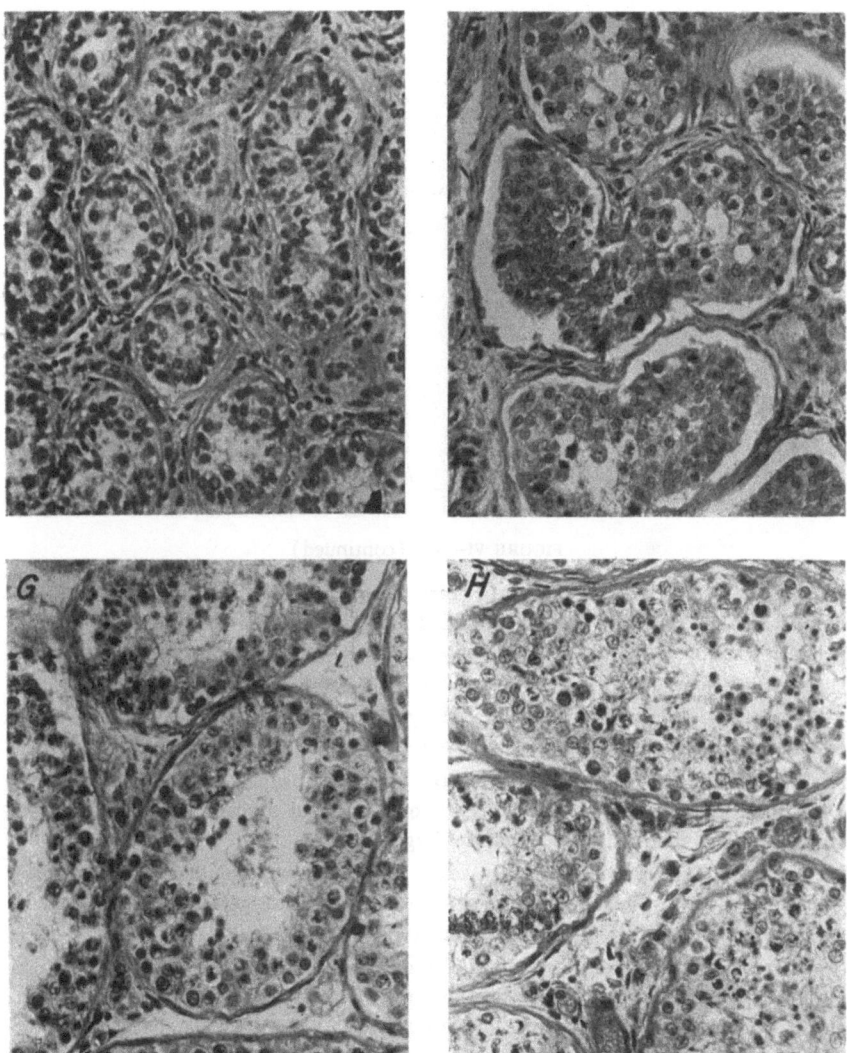

SECTION C: The testis in infancy—one year. The tubules show scant growth, but some of the undifferentiated cells are now oriented in one or two rows about the periphery of each tubule. The spermatogonia remain large with clear cytoplasm. The interstitial tissue is loose, with inconspicuous cells and relatively few capillaries.

SECTION D: The testis in childhood—five years. The tubules have well-defined lumina, about which undifferentiated cells are arranged in a single peripheral layer. The spermatogonia have scant cytoplasm and are less prominent than before. The interstitial tissue is more compact.

Figure 10 continued on page 390

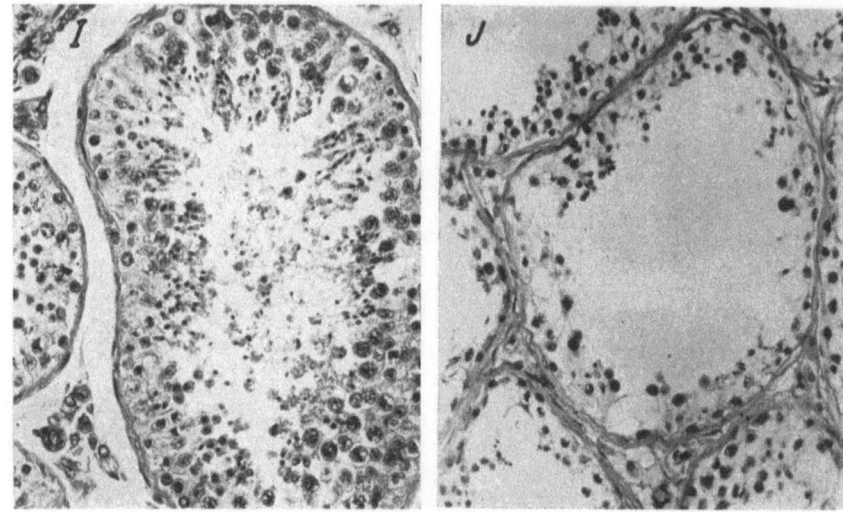

FIGURE VI—10 (continued)

SECTION E: The prepubertal testis—10 years. The tubules are beginning to enlarge. The undifferentiated cells now form several indistinct layers. The spermatogonia are still inactive. The interstitial tissue appears more cellular.

SECTION F: The pubertal testis—13 years. The tubules have enlarged considerably. The undifferentiated cells are in many layers. Many of the spermatogonia are in various stages of mitosis. The interstitial tissue is relatively compressed.

SECTION G: The adolescent testis—15 years. Tubular growth continues. The spermatogonia form many layers, and many are in some phase of mitosis. Mature spermatozoa are present. The interstitial tissue includes large cells.

SECTION H: The adolescent testis—16 years. Tubular growth continues. The spermatogonia form many layers, and many are in some phase of mitosis. Mature spermatozoa are present. The interstitial tissue includes large cells.

SECTION I: The mature testis—32 years. The tubules are of maximal size. There are proportionately fewer spermatogonia than before. Many mature spermatozoa adjoin the lumen. The interstitial tissue is loose and less cellular.

SECTION J: The senescent testis—93 years. The tubules are thin, hollow shells; they include a few spermatozoa, spermatogonia and undifferentiated cells. The interstitial tissue is compressed and fibrotic.

We are indebted to Dr. S. Farber for these photographs and the descriptive comments which accompany them.

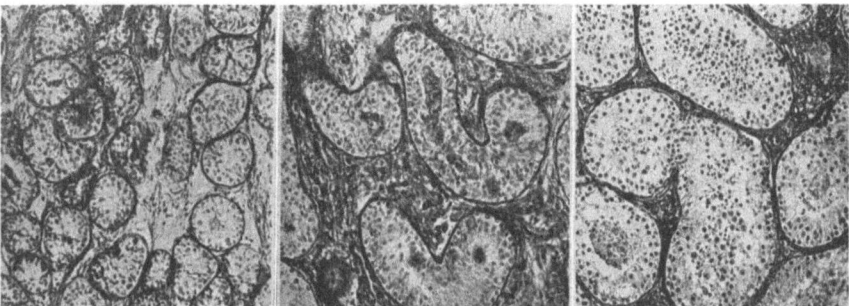

FIGURE VI—11. Testicular biopsies from a patient with hypogonadotropic eunuchoidism before and after gonadotropic hormone. Magnification x 140. From C. G. Heller and W. O. Nelson, in *Recent Progress in Hormone Research*. 3:229, New York, Academic Press, 1948.

LEFT: The patient's appearance before treatment. Note that the seminiferous tubules are of preadolescent appearance and that no Leydig cells are visible in the interstitial tissues.

MIDDLE: Effect of chorionic gonadotropin therapy on the testes. Note that the seminiferous tubules have increased greatly in size but that spermatogenesis has not been stimulated. Note also that the interstitial tissue has increased and now contains Leydig cells.

RIGHT: Appearance of the testes following treatment with chorionic gonadotropin and purified FSH. Note that spermatogenesis has been stimulated.

---

that the tubules secrete a hormone into the blood stream which inhibits FSH production.[11, 12] A possible explanation for the finding that heavy doses of testosterone can inhibit FSH production is suggested by the fact that testosterone is partly metabolized into substances having estrogenic activity.[13] As described in Chapter v, estrogens specifically inhibit production of FSH by the pituitary.

ICSH—Leydig cell relations. Examination of microscopic sections of the testes of normal preadolescent boys indicates that interstitial cells of the Leydig type are absent (see Figure 10, Sections A to F). The testes of older individuals with hypopituitarism and clinical signs of hypogonadism present a similar microscopic appearance (see Figure 11, left). When such persons are treated with the ICSH-like substance known as chorionic gonadotropin, interstitial cell development (see Figure 11, middle) and masculinization occur simultaneously. Chorionic gonadotropin fails to induce masculinization when administered to castrates. Hence it is concluded that this type of gonadotropic hormone, like ICSH, specifically causes the interstitial cells to develop and secrete androgens. FSH is inactive in this respect. In other words, testicular interstitial cell activity is dependent upon ICSH stimulation just as spermatic tubule development depends upon FSH.

With regard to natural, reciprocal relations between testicular androgen and pituitary ICSH production, the following additional information is available. Atrophy of the interstitial cells of adult animals can be induced by giving heavy doses of testosterone.[11] This indicates that androgens inhibit pituitary ICSH production. Although the converse—namely that ICSH production increases after castration—is difficult to certify, it is generally assumed to occur.

Effect of androgens on adrenocorticotropic hormone production. Methyl testosterone in heavy doses can cause a lowering in the urinary 17-KS output of patients with adrenocortical virilism secondary to bilateral adrenocortical hyperplasia.[14]* Testosterone therapy also can result in a lowering of the urinary 11-17-OCS excretion of certain patients with Cushing's syndrome.[15] As discussed in Chapter III, adrenocortical 17-KS-Gens and 11-17-OCS production usually is controlled by pituitary adrenocorticotropins. Hence it is presumed that when testosterone suppresses urinary 17-KS and 11-17-OCS excretion, it does so by inhibiting adrenocorticotropic hormone secretion.

TIMING OF EVENTS DURING NORMAL ADOLESCENCE

This is outlined by Figures 12 and 13 and by Table 2. Related information also is provided by Table 1 and Figure 10 of this chapter and by Figure 13 of Chapter III. Factors responsible for initiating these changes have been considered in the foregoing sections of the present chapter.

Boys differ considerably in the chronologic ages at which these sex maturation changes take place (see Figure 14). Most boys commence to mature between their twelfth and sixteenth years (average, about 14 years). A few otherwise normal boys start to mature several years earlier or later than the ages just stated. In such extreme individuals the family history may be one of similarly early or late adolescence.

Simple adolescent gynecomastia (see Figure 15) is encountered during the middle or late portion of pubescence (Figure 12, Phases 3 and 4) in a large number of normal boys.[16] In this condition, one or both mammary glands undergo hypertrophy for a transient period of one to three years. Usually adolescent gynecomastia subsides spontaneously within two years. When it fails so to do, the patient may be found to have spermatic tubule or other disease (see below under Klinefelter's syndrome).

Another factor to be considered in dealing with physiologically normal ado-

* Methyl testosterone, unlike free testosterone and testosterone propionate, is not metabolized to a urinary 17-KS.

The Testes

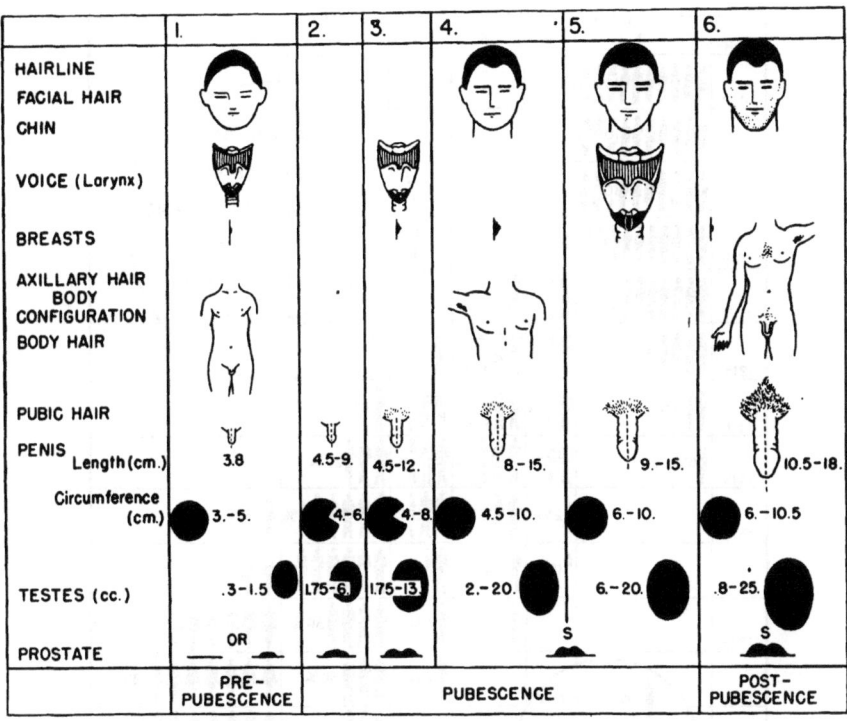

FIGURE VI—12. Diagrammatic representation of the major changes noted during male pubescence. The numbers at the top of the diagram represent maturity classes. The remainder of the diagram is self-explanatory (see also Table 2). From W. A. Schonfeld, *Am. J. Dis. Child.* 65:535, 1943.

lescent boys is pseudo-eunuchoidism. This is characterized by failure of certain end organs, such as the larynx and facial hair follicles, to respond to circulating androgens in an average normal manner. Though these individuals may have a high-pitched, puerile voice or be beardless, they are thoroughly masculine and quite capable of reproduction.

METHODS OF APPRAISING TESTICULAR STATUS

Different tests are used for determining whether the testes are (a) producing androgens, (b) capable of producing androgens or (c) capable of producing sperm.

Appraisal of Testicular Androgen Production. The simplest way to determine androgenic status is by clinical examination of the penis, scrotum and

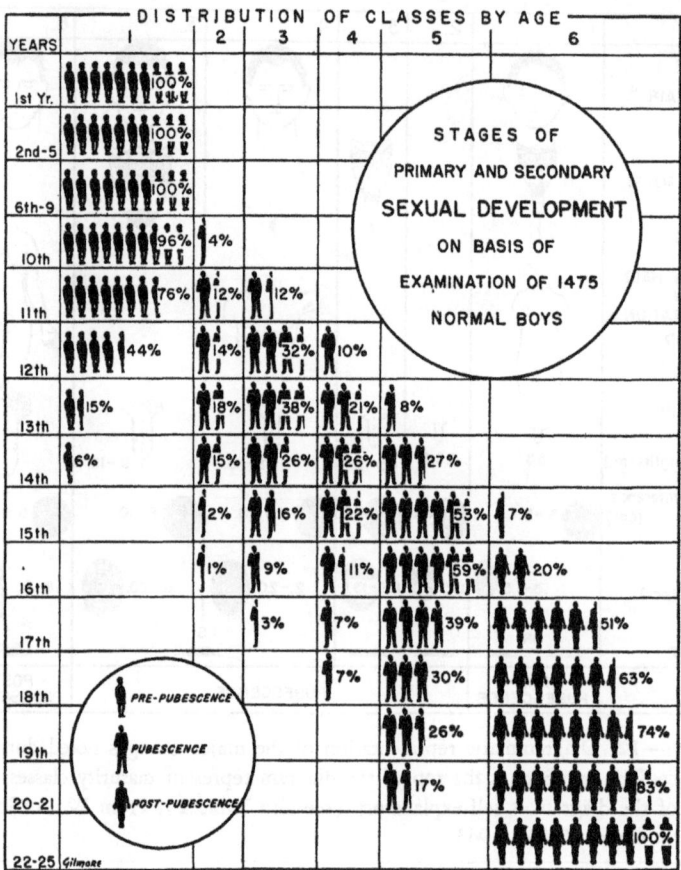

FIGURE VI—13. Diagrammatic representation of the distribution of boys of various ages among the six classes of masculine development indicated in Figure 12. Note that it is exceedingly uncommon for boys under 11 years of age to show evidences of pubescence. Contrariwise, it is exceptional for boys to fail to show at least early evidences of pubescence by the fifteenth year. A few boys are well developed by their twelfth or thirteenth year. From W. A. Schonfeld, *Am. J. Dis. Child.* 65:535, 1943.

prostate. The information thus gained can be compared with the normal standard data of Figure 12. In the absence of androgens, these structures are of puerile size. Adolescent or adult development of these structures signifies androgen activity.

Though masculine development indicates that androgens are present, it does not mean that the androgens are necessarily of testicular origin; in patients with adrenocortical virilism, they are of adrenocortical origin.

TABLE VI—2. The order of appearance of some external changes associated with sexual maturation in boys. Adapted from W. W. Greulich *et al.*, *Monographs of the Society for Research in Child Development*, VII, serial no. 33, 1942.

1. Accelerated growth of the testes, usually followed by that of the penis and scrotum, begins.
2. A conspicuous growth of long downy hair appears on the pubes.
3. Appearance of coarse, long, rather straight pigmented hairs at, and lateral to, the base of the penis follows. These hairs are soon replaced by pubic hairs which are almost completely differentiated.
4. A marked increase in the amount of axillary perspiration with some coarsening of the skin texture is noted.
5. Down on the upper lip, especially at the corners, becomes slightly longer, coarser, and darker.
6. Long, coarse down appears on the extensor surface of the proximal third of the forearm and on the lateral and dorso-lateral surfaces of the distal fourth of the arm.
7. Growth of rather coarse, slightly or moderately pigmented hair on the distal half of the legs and on the distal third of the thighs begins.
8. Long down appears on the side of the face, in front of the ears.
9. Appearance of circumanal hair follows.
10. The pubic region becomes covered with a moderate-to-dense growth of definitive pubic hair. (The hair-covered area now has a concave or approximately horizontal superior border; it does not yet extend laterally onto the adjacent medial surface of the thighs.)
11. Short, fine, pigmented hairs appear in each axilla. (The axillary perspiration has now acquired its characteristic odor.)
12. The voice has deepened perceptibly.
13. Subareolar masses, when present, have usually attained their maximum size.
14. Pubic hair has spread laterally to, or onto, the adjacent medial surface of the thighs and terminal hairs are present along the linea alba. The penis and testes have attained almost their full adult dimensions.
15. A few terminal hairs appear on the sides of the chin and the upper portion of the cheeks just in front of the ears, and the hair on the upper lip becomes coarser and darker.
16. A few terminal hairs appear around the periphery of the areolæ and over the sternum.
17. Formation of the adult type of hairline begins on the forehead (calvities frontalis adolescentium).
18. Almost, or quite, the full amount of terminal hair proper to the young adult is now present on the forearms, arms, legs and thighs.

In interpreting the sequence listed above, it should be remembered that it describes merely the order in which the various developmental features first manifest themselves. Once they have appeared, the further development of each proceeds at the rate proper to itself. The differentiation of those characters that appear early is well under way before some of the later changes are initiated.

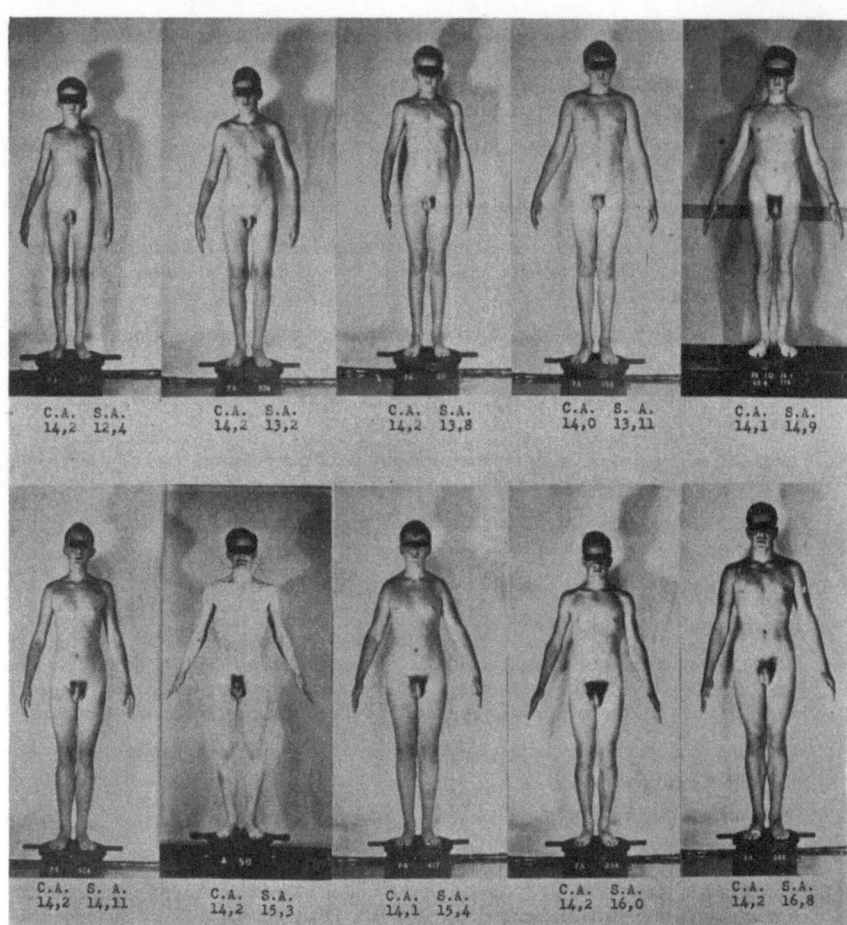

FIGURE VI—14. Photographic illustrations of the fact that there may be wide differences in the physiologic age (sexual maturity status) of boys of the same chronologic age. All the boys shown above were between 14 years, 1 month, and 14 years, 2 months, in chronologic age (CA). Their physiologic age was approximately reflected in their skeletal age (SA), which is indicated at the base of each photograph. From W. W. Greulich, et al., *Somatic and Endocrine Studies of Puberal and Adolescent Boys.* Washington, Society for Research in Child Development (*Monographs* VII:33:3), 1942.

Because the interstitial cells occupy only a small portion of total testicular mass, testicular size *per se* does not always correlate well with testicular androgen production; interstitial cells can undergo considerable development and become quite active functionally without there being an appreciable change in testicular size or consistency (see Table 3). Such interstitial cell development can, how-

THE TESTES   [397]

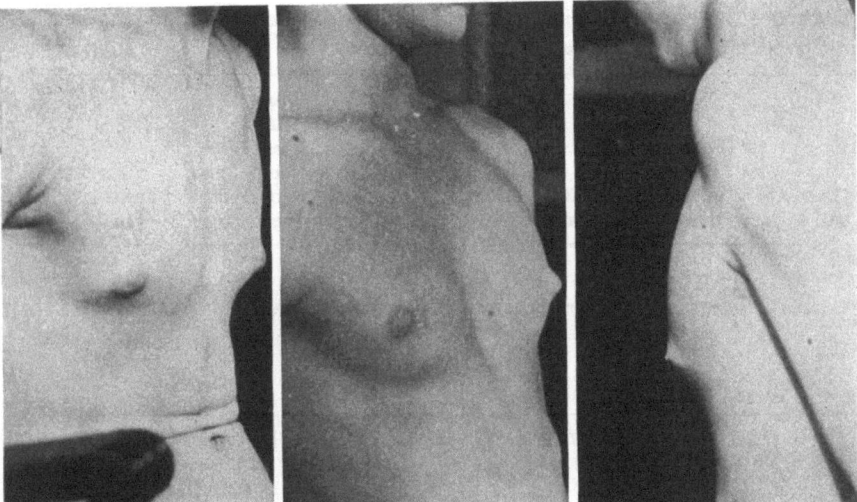

FIGURE VI—15. Adolescent gynecomastia in three healthy pubescent boys. From W. W. Greulich, et al., *Somatic and Endocrine Studies of Puberal and Adolescent Boys.* Washington, Society for Research in Child Development (*Monographs* VII:33:3), 1942.

ever, be detected by microscopic examination of a small testicular biopsy (see Figure 25).

Some additional information concerning testicular androgen production is provided by the excretion values of urinary 17-KS, which are transformation products of adrenocortical and testicular steroid hormones. However, the value of this index of testicular activity is considerably limited by the fact that adrenocortical hormones ordinarily comprise the chief source of these urinary steroids (see Chapter III). Thus the presence even of a normal amount of 17-KS in the urine of a male does not necessarily indicate testicular androgen production (see Tables 7-9). The urinary 17-KS output gives somewhat more reliable information concerning testicular activity when, as in patients with primary hypoadrenocorticism and in boys who have not passed the adrenarche (Chapter III), the adrenal cortices are not contributing to the urinary 17-KS excretion. Rather surprisingly, in young boys with isosexual precocity* due to premature activation of the interstitial cells, the 17-KS output ($\pm$ 0.3 to 3 mg. per day) is usually only slightly elevated above normal limits for age (see Table 3 and Chapter III, Table 6). Such observations suggest that either only a very few milligrams of

* In isosexual precocity the genital structures develop in a normal manner for a person of that sex; by contrast, in heterosexual precocity the development of the sexual characteristics corresponds to that of the opposite sex.   *Continued on page 402*

TABLE VI—3. Representative findings for boys with complete (A) and incomplete (B) true precocious puberty (Table 5, Type 1).

Case no.	Age, yr.	Probable duration	Ht. age	Wt. age	Bone age	Voice	Acne	Muscular development	Penis enlarged	Testis size	Sex hair
A. COMPLETE TRUE PRECOCIOUS PUBERTY
1	10/12	5/12	10/12	9/12				+	+	2×1.5 cm. (6-7 gm.)	+
2	2 9/12	1	3½	6	7	Low	0	+	+	+?	+
3	5		10						+	Adult	+
4	6½	3+			14	Bass	+	+	+	Adult	+ also beard
5	7	4	10½	14	18	Bass		+	+	Adult	+
6	7 8/12	6	9½	10½	11	Bass	0	+	+	Adult	+
7	8	1	11½		9-10	Baritone		+	+	Pecan	+
8	9	¼	8				0?	0?	Slight +	2 cm. long	0?
B. INCOMPLETE TRUE PRECOCIOUS PUBERTY
9	1½	1	2½	3 8/12	2½	Deep	0	+	+	Not enlarged	+
10	1½	½	3½	4½	4	Deep	+	+	+	Slightly enlarged?	+

TABLE VI—3 (continued)

17-KS, mg/ 24 hr.	FSH, M. U./ 24 hr.	Testicular histology		CNS lesion	Source
		Leydig cells	Spermato- genesis		
A. COMPLETE TRUE PRECOCIOUS PUBERTY					
		+	+	Died at 4 yr. with tuberous sclerosis	K. Krabbe, *Encéphale* 281, 1922
1.0	<3	Probably present	Active spermato- cytogenesis	None evident	See Figure 17
23-5.0	17	No hyper- plasia	+	None evident	A. M. Hain, *J. Clin. Endocrinol.* 7:171, 1947
6.0	18			None evident	A. M. Hain, *ibid.* 7:171, 1947
		Adult	+	Ganglio- neuroma	G. Horrax and P. Bailey, *Arch. Neurol. and Psychiat.* 19:394, 1928
1.2	>4 <16 at 9 yr.	Adult	+	None evident	See Figure 20
±40 I. V. an- drogens			+	Glioma	L. M. Weinberger *et. al.*, *Arch. Int. Med.* 67:762, 1941
		Adult ±	Early +	Pinealoma, teratoma	G. Horrax and P. Bailey, *loc. cit.*
B. INCOMPLETE TRUE PRECOCIOUS PUBERTY					
0.1-0.2	<3	Clumps of cells	0	None evident	See Figure 24
0.3		Clumps of cells	0	None evident	

TABLE VI—4. Pseudo-precocious puberty in boys due to testicular interstitial cell tumor (primary hyperleydigism).

Case no.	Age, yr.	Probable age at onset	Ht., cm.	Wt., kg.	Bone age	Penis length, cm.	Sexual hair* P	A	F	Voice change	Size tumor cm.	Urine hormone studies
1	3½	2½	108	21.7	6-7	6	+	0	0	++	2.8×2.5	A-Z neg. 17-KS 64 mg. per 24 hr.
2	5	4	130	27		10	+	0	0	+	1†	Friedman test neg.
3	6	4	130	27	Enlarged		+	0	0		5	Friedman test neg.
4	6⁹⁄₁₂	5½	136	33	Advanced	9.5	+	+	+	++	2.5×1.5	Friedman test neg.
5	9	6	153		Adult		+	+	+		5×4×3.5	
6	9½	5½	143	44.4		9	+	+	+		12×10	
7	11						+		+		10×7	
8	Adult											17-KS 980-1040 mg./24 hr.

* P=Pubic; A=Axillary; F=Facial
† Right testis twice the size of left

TABLE VI—4 (continued)

Effect of removal	Other comments	Source
Pubic hair disappeared; no more excretions; more gentle behavior; testis larger; remaining 17-KS dropped to +10 mg. per 24 hr.		P. Sandblom, *Acta Endocrinol.* 1:107, 1948
Pubic hair disappeared; penis shrank to 8 cm.	Precocious development of tubules; all stages in formation of spermatozoa, but no spermatozoa	C. A. Stewart et al., *Am. J. Cancer* 26:144, 1936
No regression	Slight enlargement of both breasts	L. F. Huffman, *J. Urol.* 45:692, 1941
Hair on upper lip disappeared; voice unchanged; more gentle attitude; remaining testis larger	Heavy musculature	A. A. Werner et al., *J. Clin. Endocrinol.* 2:527, 1942
No regression	Much hair on chest; "powerfully built"; shaves regularly	R. P. Rowlands et al., *Guy's Hospital Rep.* 79:401, 1929
Beard disappeared; remaining testis larger	Very muscular and strong	E. Sacchi, *Riv. Sper. di Freniat.* 21:149, 1895
No regression	Very muscular; severe acne	A. E. Somerford, *Brit. J. Urol.* 13:13, 1941
		E. H. Venning, *Rev. Canad. de Biol.* 1:571, 1942

testicular androgen are needed to cause a marked degree of masculine development or that only a small portion of the androgenic steroid produced by the testes is excreted in the urine as a 17-KS. The former possibility is in keeping with the known weight potency ratio of crystalline testosterone.

In patients with testicular interstitial cell carcinomas, the urinary output of 17-KS may be grossly elevated above normal levels (see Table 4). Presumably in this condition there is marked overproduction of testosterone-like material.

Appraisal of Testicular Capacity to Produce Androgens. The need for making this type of appraisal arises when boys of late adolescent age fail to show signs of masculinization. The question then arises, is the hypogonadism due to primary testicular disease or to failure on the part of the pituitary to secrete gonadotropic hormone (ICSH)?

Figure 16 describes one relatively easy way to find out where the difficulty lies. It is based upon the fact that chorionic gonadotropin acts like ICSH to stimulate androgen production if the testicular interstitial cells are functionally intact. The dose of chorionic gonadotropin is 1,000 I.U. given intramuscularly from three to five times weekly for 6 to 10 weeks. This treatment stimulates normal testes to secrete androgenic hormone, which in turn causes a distinct degree of penile and scrotal development. Chorionic gonadotropin has no effect on eunuchoid patients. Therefore, a positive response to this hormone constitutes excellent evidence that the testicular interstitial cells are intact.

Appraisal of Testicular Tubular Status. Because the testicular tubules do not produce any hormone with clinically discernible effects, it is difficult to appraise tubular status by ordinary clinical examination. Testicular size may be of some approximate diagnostic value because the difference in size of adult as compared with the puerile testis is due in the main to development of the tubules.

As has been mentioned earlier, a much more reliable index of the condition of the testicular tubules is provided by the urinary gonadotropin (FSH) assay. An abnormally high value (i.e., > 100 M.U. per 24 hours) is strong evidence in favor of a presumptive diagnosis of tubular disease. On the other hand, for unknown reasons, certain patients with markedly deranged testicular tubules are found to have essentially normal or low urinary FSH values.

There are two other methods for determining the condition of the tubules. One is the sperm count, a procedure which ordinarily cannot be used in pediatric patients and with relation to which there are no pediatric normal standards. The other is the testicular biopsy. This may reveal a variety of changes including simple immaturity due to lack of FSH (see Figure 11), degeneration without hyalinization, or marked hyalinization (see Figure 35). A variety of intermediate

The Testes

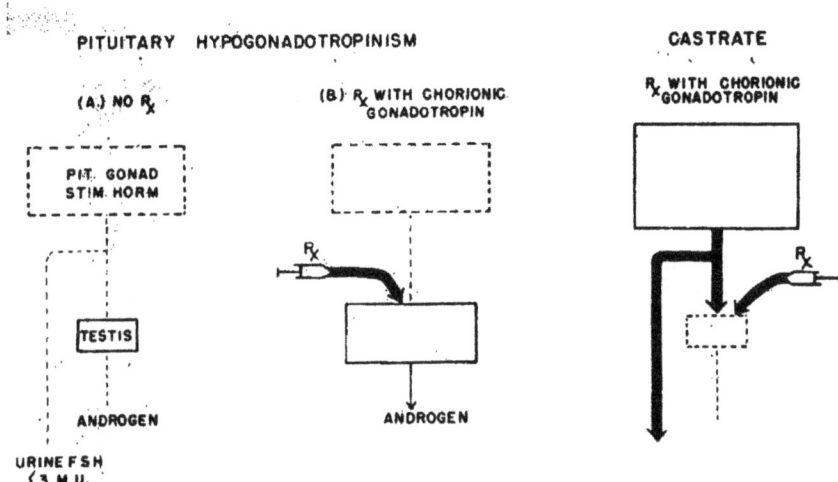

FIGURE VI—16. Diagrammatic representation of the chorionic gonadotropin test. Sections A and B are concerned with secondary testicular–primary pituitary hypogonadotropic hypogonadism. In Section A no pituitary gonad-stimulating hormones are being produced. As a result the urine contains no gonadotropic hormone (FSH). For lack of gonadotropic stimulus, the testes remain quiescent and fail to produce either androgens or sperm. In Section B administration of chorionic gonadotropin acts like pituitary interstitial-cell-stimulating hormone on the testes. The androgens thus produced cause masculine development which is easily recognized clinically.

By contrast, the right-hand diagram shows that in a eunuchoid individual the pituitary is apt to produce increased amounts of gonadotropic hormone with a resultant increase in urinary FSH excretion. But because the testes are absent or defective there is no spermatogenesis or production of androgens. Consequently, chorionic gonadotropin, like endogenous pituitary gonadotropin, is unable to stimulate male hormone production. It, therefore, produces no increase in masculine development when administered to the eunuchoid patient. In summary, masculinization following chorionic gonadotropin therapy indicates that testicular interstitial cells are present and capable of normal function. Failure to respond to gonadotropin indicates primary testicular disease.

---

changes may also be noted in individual patients.

In summary, two chief methods for appraising the condition of the testicular tubules are available: (a) the urinary gonadotropin (FSH) measurement and (b) the testicular biopsy. In older patients the sperm count can also be used. An abnormally elevated FSH value is strongly suggestive of testicular tubule failure. A normal or low value does not rule this condition out. When positive information is wanted, testicular biopsy should be performed.

Continued on page 408

TABLE VI—5. Salient characteristics of various types of isosexual precocity in males.

Type	Alternate name	Cause	Testis size	Signs of masculinization	Spermatogenesis	Urine gonadotropin	Urine 17-KS	Stature	Other information
I. True Precocious Puberty									
A. Hypothalamic									
1. Complete type		CNS lesion or disturbance	Adult	+	+	+	Slightly +	+	Table 4
2. Incomplete type		CNS lesion or disturbance	Slightly +	+	0	0	Slightly +	+	Table 4
II. Pseudo-precocious puberty									
A. Primary testicular	Testicular precocity	Interstitial (Leydig) cell tumor	Usually unilateral tumor	+	0	0	++	+	Table 6
B. Adrenal	Adrenocortical virilism	Adrenocortical hyperplasia or tumor	±N	+	0	0	++	+	Chapter III
C. Medicational									
1. Chorionic gonadotropin		Chorionic gonadotropin therapy	Slightly +	+	0	0	Slightly +	+	
2. Androgens		Testosterone therapy	N	+	0	0	+		

The various symbols have the following meanings: + indicates precocious occurrence or abnormally increased for patient of this age, but within normal adult limits; ++ signifies an increase in output which exceeds normal adult limits; N equals normal for age; 0 equals absent; − equals subnormal.

TABLE VI—6. Salient characteristics of various types of sexual infantilism in males.

Type	Alternate names	Cause	Testis size	Masculinization	Spermatogenesis	Urinary gonadotropin	Urinary 17-KS	Response to CGT* therapy	Stature	Other information
I. Hypothalamic	Froehlich's or Laurence-Moon-Biedl syndrome	Craniopharyngioma; genetic CNS defect	Puerile Puerile	0 or − 0 or −	0 or − 0 ? −	0 or − 0 ? −	− −	Yes Yes ?	− −	See Chapters v and vii
II. Pituitary										
A. Primary type										
1. Generalized	Panhypopituitarism	Pituitary lesion	Puerile	0 or −	0 or −	0 or −	−	Yes	−	Chapter vii, Table 4
2. Specific gonadotropin deficiency	Pituitary infantilism Pituitary eunuchoidism	Pituitary; CNS lesion?	Puerile	0 or −	0	0	Slightly −	Yes	N	Table 7
B. Secondary type, functional										
1. Primary hypothyroid	Athyrosis	Primary hypothyroidism	Puerile	0 or −	0 or −	0 or −	−	Yes	−	See Chapters i, v, and vii
2. Primary caloric undernutrition	Anorexia nervosa	Caloric malnutrition	Puerile	0 or −	0 or −	0 or −	−	Yes	−	
III. Testicular										
A. Generalized	Panhypogonadism, eunuchoidism	Anorchia or destructive lesion of testis	Absent or small	0	0	++	±N	No	N	Table 8
B. Tubules damaged; Leydig cells normal	Sometimes gynecomastia, Klinefelter's syndrome	Destructive lesion of tubules	Small	N or −	0	++	±N		N	Table 9

*CGT = Chorionic gonadotropin.

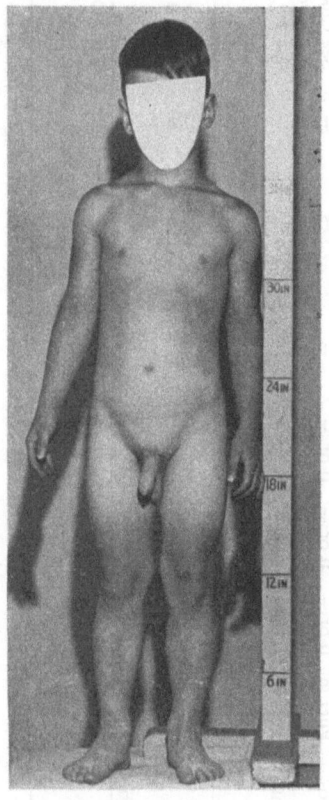

(Left)
FIGURE VI—17. Complete true precocious puberty in a boy of 2%2 years (see Table 3, Case 2).

(Right—opposite page)
FIGURE VI—18. Testicular biopsy from the patient in Figure 17, on which the diagnosis of true precocious puberty was made. Note that the tubules are large and have lumina. Sertoli cells have developed fully and spermatocytogenesis is moderately active, but there are no spermatoids or sperm. The interstitial tissue contains a few fusiform cells, but no fully developed Leydig cells are visible. We are indebted to Dr. R. C. Sniffen for this description.

CASE HISTORY

This patient was born following a normal pregnancy. His weight at birth was 3.4 kg. His early growth and development seemed to proceed normally until, at about 10 months of age, he was noted to have a sparse growth of dark pubic hair. Upon routine examination at one year by his family pediatrician, he was noted to weigh 16 kg. and to have the body of a child of three or four. When he was about 2½ years his mother noted that he had frequent erections and, for the first time, ejaculations of several cc. of seminal fluid. For the salient physical measurements and laboratory findings see Table 3, Case 2.

Generally speaking the child was tall and muscular for his age. His voice was loud and deep but not completely bass. A fine growth of hair appeared over his upper lip; there were sparse growths of pubic and leg hair but none of axillary hair. The hair line at the temples had not recessed. The scrotum was well developed, but the testes were only slightly enlarged. The remainder of the physical examination was not remarkable. Detailed neurologic examination yielded normal results. Intellectual development appeared to be normal for chronologic age. X-ray survey of the skeleton revealed no abnormalities other than acceleration in skeletal development.

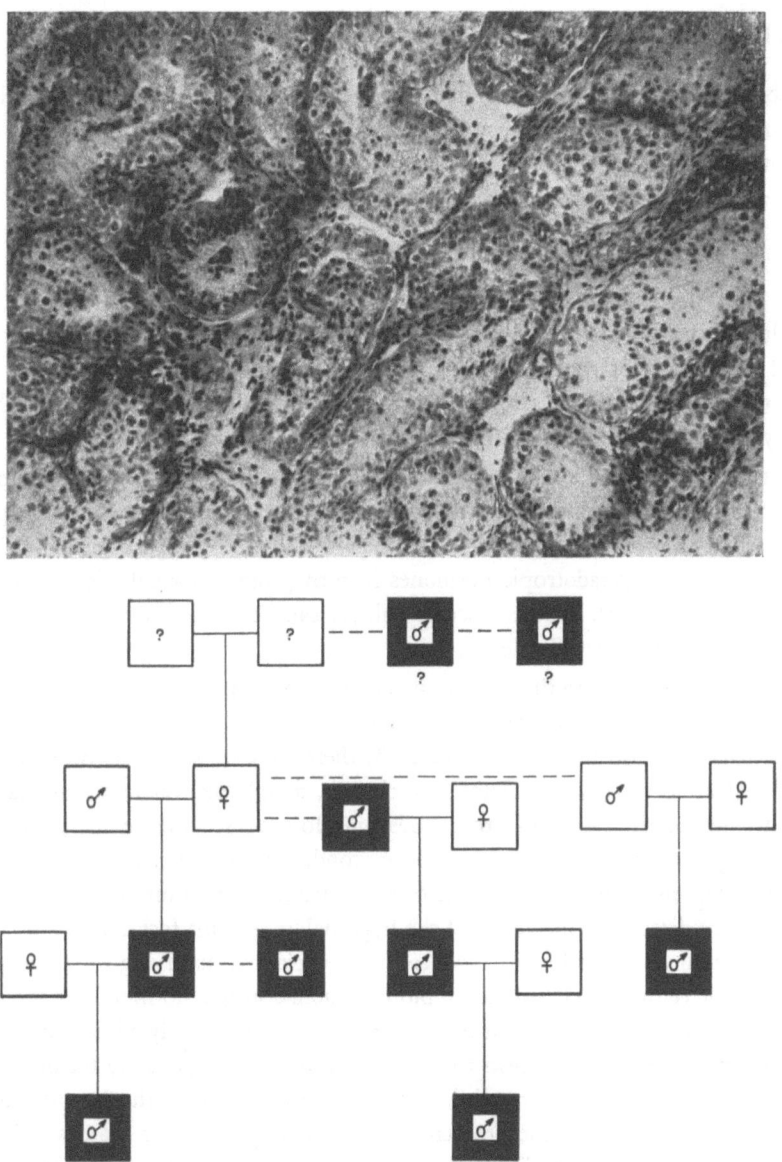

PRESENT PATIENT

FIGURE VI—19. The family tree of the patient with true precocious puberty in Figure 17. Almost without exception the individuals indicated by black blocks had penile and pubic hair growth by the time they had reached the age of four years and bass voices and enough facial hair to shave by the the time they were 10 or 12. Aside from these evidences of physiologic precocious puberty, they were healthy individuals.

CLINICAL CONSIDERATIONS

Tables 5 and 6 set forth in summary form the salient features of the conditions to be considered in the following pages. These summaries conform in arrangement to Figures 11 and 24 of Chapter v. The reader is referred to these figures for a schematic presentation of causal relationships.

ISOSEXUAL PRECOCITY IN MALES

It is not possible to draw a definite and sharp dividing line between physiologic and pathologic early adolescence. Generally speaking, it is unusual for boys to show signs of masculinization before the eleventh year. In boys younger than 10 years such signs may be definitely indicative of pathology.

True Precocious Puberty. This condition originates in the hypothalamus, which activates the pituitary to normal adolescent gonadotropic hormone production at an abnormally early age (see Figure 9 and Chapter v, Figure 11, Condition c). The gonadotropic hormones in turn prompt normal adolescent testicular development. True precocious puberty can be divided into complete and incomplete forms (see Table 3).

Complete form. In this condition adolescence occurs in an essentially physiologic manner at an abnormally early age.

ETIOLOGY. As indicated by Table 3, there may be an authentic lesion in the central nervous system. Tuberous sclerosis, ganglioneuroma and glioma are mentioned in the table; in other cases pinealomas (see Figure 22), internal hydrocephalus, malformations and other conditions have been noted.[17] These diverse lesions appear to have but one characteristic in common, namely, involvement directly or indirectly of the hypothalamus. This fact makes it appear nearly certain that the lesions produce the precocity by modifying the activity of neurologic centers which influence pituitary gonadotropic hormone production.

As illustrated by the patient of Figures 17 to 19, very early adolescence may be a family trait. This suggests that genetic factors are responsible for precocity in certain otherwise healthy children. It also suggests that the hypothalamic changes responsible for the precocity may be functional rather than organic in nature. From the fact that FSH can be demonstrated in the urine of patients with true idiopathic precocity (Table 3, Cases 3 and 4) it seems highly probable that the condition is caused by precocious activation of pituitary gonadotropic hormone production rather than by a hypothetical hypersensitivity of the testicular interstitial cells and spermatic tubules to small amounts of gonadotropic hormone.

CLINICAL MANIFESTATIONS. Many of these are indicated in Table 3, Section A and in the legends of Figures 17 to 23. The condition may start at any time during infancy or childhood. The changes observed correspond approximately to those seen during ordinary adolescence (see Figures 12 and 13; Table 2). Usually the first change to be noted is penile, testicular and scrotal development. Shortly thereafter pubic hair appears and the voice becomes somewhat hoarser or deeper. Accelerated growth in height is commonly evident within a year. In association with this there is an increase in musculature and in body weight. Subsequently, the individual gradually assumes all the physical characteristics of a normal man.

The urinary 17-KS output is found to be increased above the average normal for age and to correspond approximately to the normal for children of equal physiologic age (see Chapter III, Figure 13). It is not markedly increased as in most children with adrenocortical virilism. The urinary FSH output is also elevated to adolescent levels (see Table 1). Testicular biopsy reveals adult-type Leydig cell development and spermatogenesis (Figure 21, left).

DIAGNOSIS. In a boy with isosexual precocity the diagnosis is suggested by the occurrence of testicular development which grossly corresponds to the normal for a pubescent or adult male. The presence of three or more mouse units of FSH per 24-hour urine specimen indicates a hypothalamic–pituitary gonadotropic hormone origin for the disturbance. Demonstration of adult testicular interstitial cell and tubular development in a biopsy specimen indicates that true precocious puberty exists.

Signs of intracranial disease are apt either to be grossly evident or entirely lacking. In patients with evident neurologic disease the signs seen vary so widely according to the nature and extent of the brain lesion as to preclude systematic description. There may be clear signs of intracranial hypertension with extra-ocular disturbances, eyeground and visual field changes and separation of the cranial sutures on the one hand and mental deficiency without localizing neurologic signs on the other. In the case of patients without evident neurologic disease, it usually is not possible to demonstrate a central nervous system lesion even by pneumoencephalography.

TREATMENT. In patients with a manifest neurologic condition, an attempt should be made to locate and, if possible, to eradicate the underlying process. Unfortunately, except for the rare patient with an operable or radio-sensitive tumor (such as a pinealoma), the chances of success are very slim. In the case of patients who lack such a lesion, there appears to be little to be gained by attempts at neurosurgical therapy. Radiation of the pituitary–hypothalamic area has not proved beneficial in the absence of a known lesion and is not recom-

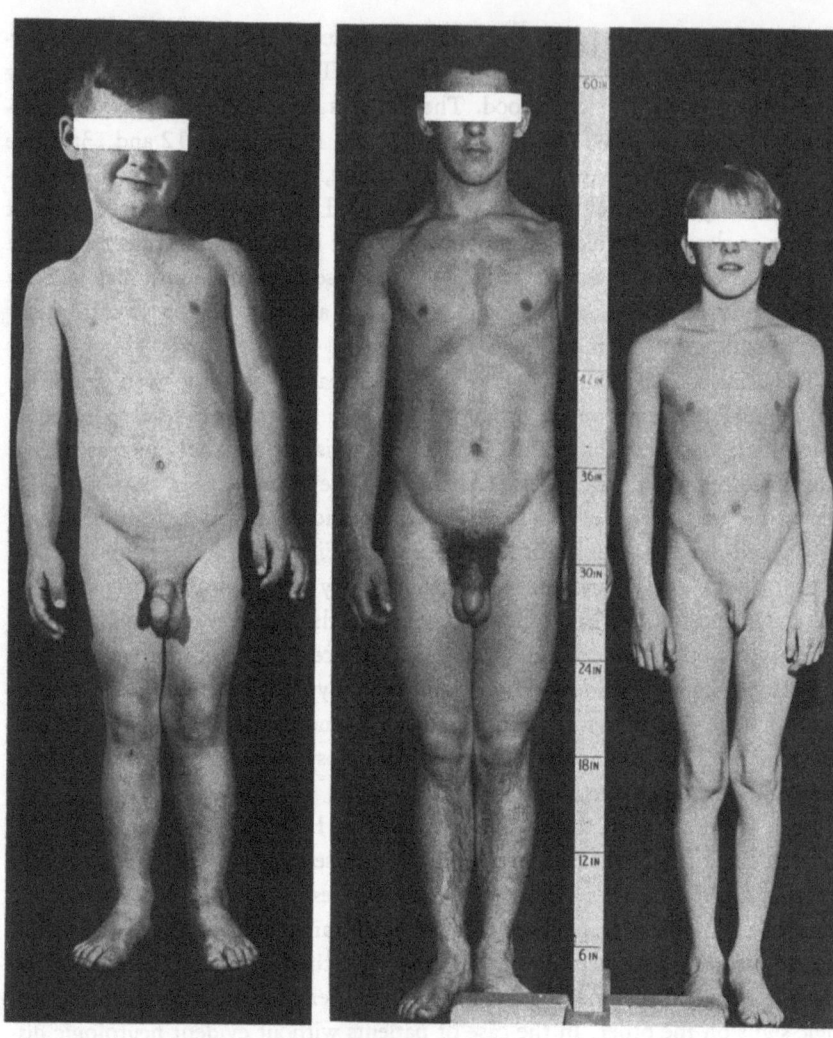

FIGURE VI—20. Complete true precocious puberty (see also Table 3, Case 6).
LEFT: Appearance of the patient at five years of age.
RIGHT: His appearance at 13 years of age. For comparative purposes a normal boy of 13 also is shown.

CASE HISTORY

The parents of this boy first noticed that his penis and testicles were unusually large when he was 1½ years of age. At about three years of age his voice began to deepen, and some pubic and axillary hair growth appeared. Between the ages of three and five, there were questionable episodes of polyuria and polydipsia. At five years he was found to be tall,

CASE HISTORY (continued)

well developed and sexually precocious. His voice was deep, and small growths of pubic and axillary hair had appeared. His penis and testes were of advanced adolescent size.

Of the various measurements and studies made, the following are of the greatest interest. Up to the present time his height age has been approximately two years and his weight age approximately three years in advance of his chronologic age. His bone age, on the other hand, has been markedly accelerated: at seven years of actual age, his bone age was 11; at 10 years of actual age, his bone age was 13; at 12 years of actual age, his bone age was $16^{3}/_{12}$ years.

Testicular biopsy at the age of seven showed spermatogenesis and adolescent development of Leydig cells (see Figure 21). His daily urinary 17-KS output was between 0.8 and 1.2 mg. at eight years, 2.2 and 5.6 mg. at nine years, 1.6 mg. at 10 years and 3.2 mg. at 14 years. At 13 years his urinary 11-17-OCS output was .05 mg. per 24 hours. At nine years there were more than 4 but less than 16 mouse units of gonadotropin (FSH) per 24-hour urine specimen. At no time has it been possible to demonstrate neurologic abnormalities. Electroencephalograms gave essentially normal findings. Pneumoencephalograms done at five and six years of age, respectively, revealed only questionable dilatation of the third cerebral ventricle. The possibility of diabetes insipidus was ruled out by finding the urine specific gravity to be as high as 1.030 on numerous occasions.

The patient has always been in the best of health. His intellectual status has been normal (IQ 109). In an effort to control his condition by hormonal means, he was given 1 mg. of stilbestrol daily for a period of three months when he was 9 years of age. This treatment failed to result in any major changes in his behavior, although it was reported that he showed an increased tendency to fall asleep earlier at night and was perhaps less energetic during the day. On the other hand, it did prompt both early mammary gland development and testicular changes (Figure 21). In other words, it appeared that continuous stilbestrol therapy probably would result in a considerable degree of feminization and might in addition cause permanent damage to presumably normal testes. This seemed an excessively high price to pay for temporary suppression of precocious masculinization. Administration of stilbestrol was therefore discontinued.

The patient's only real difficulty was in the social sphere. He seemed to get more than the usual pleasure out of fights with other boys. He also ran away from home several times. Once he was picked up by police while watching the windows of a near-by nurses' dormitory. On another occasion, when he was 13 years old, school authorities found contraceptives in his pockets. The problems arising out of these various episodes were managed successfully by Dr. E. Lindemann of the Massachusetts General Hospital psychiatric service, who assumed that this boy's behavior expressed in a straight-forward manner the discrepancy which existed between his judgment on the one hand and the kinds of activity made possible by his precocious somatic development on the other. Specific efforts were made to provide him with opportunities for strenuous physical activity in the form of boxing and other sports. In addition, the school authorities were persuaded that it was not possible for him to sit still in school for prolonged periods and that he should be given opportunities to move around and expend energy in various useful and constructive ways. With the aid of these measures his difficulty gradually disappeared.

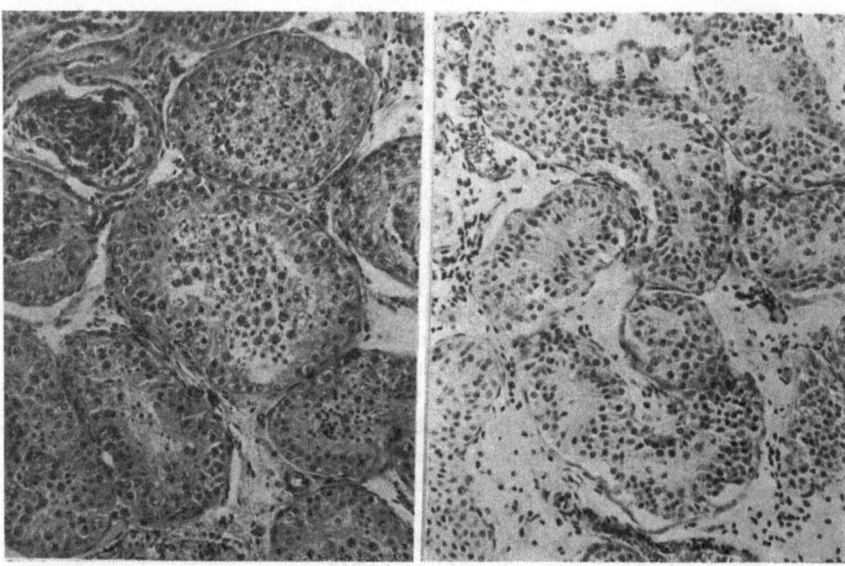

FIGURE VI—21. Testicular biopsies from the patient of Figure 20 with complete true precocious puberty before and after the administration of stilbestrol. We are indebted to Dr. R. C. Sniffen for these descriptive comments.

LEFT: Biopsy obtained before treatment. Note that the tubules are large, and that active spermatogenesis has occurred. A few small groups of large interstitial cells are present.

RIGHT: Biopsy obtained after a month of treatment with 1 mg. of stilbestrol daily. Note the marked involution of the testes. Only a few of the tubules now have lumina. Spermatids and sperm have disappeared. The tubular cells are desquamating. The interstitial tissue is loose and infiltrated by lymphocytes and plasma cells. No morphologically distinct Leydig cells are visible.

mended. Neither is estrogenic treatment advised. While it may act to suppress pituitary gonadotropic hormone production and hence to suppress masculinization, it also tends to cause degenerative changes in the spermatic tubules (see Figure 21, right).

Practically speaking, the most important therapeutic contribution usually can be made in the socio-psychologic sphere. These children have the vigor, energy and drive characteristic of normal male adolescence, but retain the intelligence characteristic of their actual age.[10] As a consequence, they are likely in a quite innocent manner to become "peeping Toms" or to show other manner of socially unacceptable attention to the opposite sex. Moreover, they are apt to have so much pent-up physical energy that they find it exceedingly difficult to remain quiet at school for the usually required periods. These tendencies lead to much distress unless the true and incidentally transient nature of these boys' problems are carefully explained to parents, police and school authorities. If, however, such children can be provided with safe and acceptable outlets for physical energy through sport activities, special assignments in school and so forth they may pass through without serious mishap the difficult period during which their emotions and intelligence are catching up with their somatic development.

PROGNOSIS. The outlook for boys with true precocity who do not have an evident neurologic lesion is about as follows: although they are exceptionally tall during early childhood, they are apt because of precocious fusion of long bone epiphyses to stop growing before they have attained full adult stature. Consequently, as adults they tend to be stocky and to have relatively short extremities. They remain permanently masculinized in the normal adult sense. Like certain adults who become bald and appear older than their years at a relatively early age, some of these precocious children may look 30 or 40 years old when they are no more than 15 or 16 years old. We remember vividly our feeling of incredulousness in talking to and examining one such 16-year-old boy who had matured spontaneously in early childhood. It didn't seem possible that this apparently middle-aged man was in fact only of adolescent age. Though his appearance belied his true age, his reactions and behavior were in keeping with it.

It is most unusual for patients who fail to show neurologic disturbances at the onset of the precocity to develop such disturbances in subsequent years. Patients with obvious neurologic signs have a poor prognosis, for they are apt to succumb to their neurologic ailment within a few years.

Incomplete form. Figure 24 and Section B of Table 3 present information concerning boys who, like the patients just described, showed gross signs of precocious masculine development. However, they differed from the foregoing patients in certain respects. The testes, instead of being precociously enlarged in proportion to the external genitalia, were of normal size for age. Biopsy examination of testis tissue showed the interstitial cells to be precociously developed in pseudo-hyperplastic clumps. However, the tubules were of relatively immature size and appearance. There was no sign of spermatogenesis (see Figure 25).

All these findings can be explained by assuming that these patients were producing ICSH, but not FSH.* ICSH causes adult Leydig cell development and androgen production, but not spermatic tubule development. Leydig cell development is not productive of an appreciable increase in testicular size. Hence, the finding that the testes of these patients were of approximately normal size for

* Urine assays showed that there were less than 3 mouse units of gonadotropin per 24-hr. urine sample.

Continued on page 418

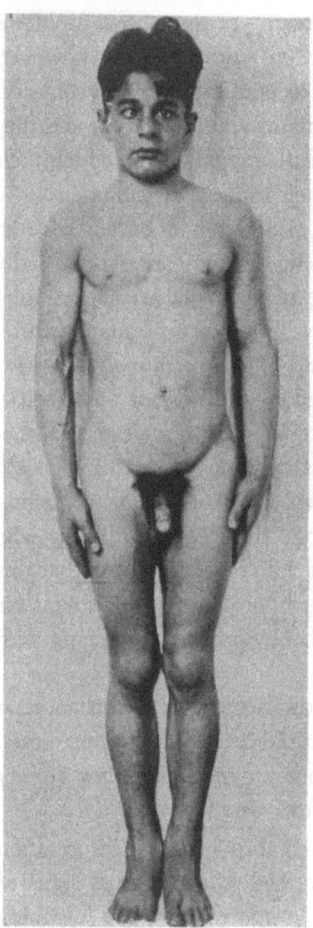

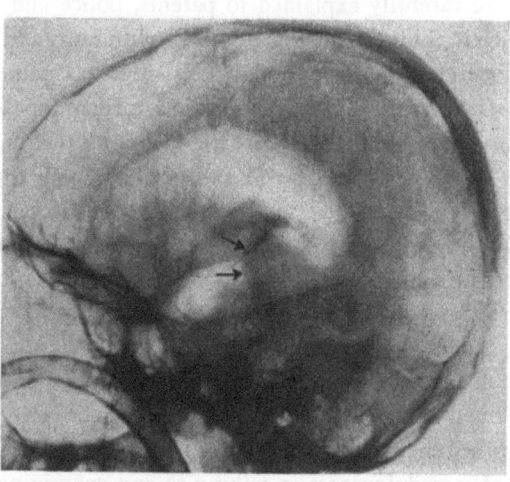

(Right)
FIGURE VI—23. Ventriculogram of the patient in Figure 22. The arrows point to the shadow of a tumor (pinealoma) bulging into the posterior end of the dilated third ventricle.

Figures 22 and 23 are from G. Horrax, *Arch. Neurol. and Psychiat.* 35:215, 1936.

(Left)
FIGURE VI—22. Complete true precocious puberty due to a central nervous system lesion in a boy of 10 years.

CASE HISTORY

The patient commenced to grow rapidly in height, to gain weight and to develop musculature at nine years of age. At about the same time his genitalia rapidly approached adult proportions, and his voice became bass. For three weeks before admission to the hospital he complained of headaches and for 10 days double vision had been noted. On physical examination he weighed 35 kg. and was 144 cm. tall. His development corresponded to that of a boy 16 years old. His blood pressure was 114/76. The right pupil did not react to light and accommodation as well as the left. External rotation of the right eye was poor. The outlines of the optic disks on both sides were obliterated, and the retinal vessels were markedly enlarged and tortuous. Ventriculo-encephalograms showed dilated ventricles and a large mass bulging into the posterior portion of the third ventricle.

CASE HISTORY (continued)

A decompression operation, followed by roentgen treatment, resulted in temporary improvement. The boy's parents were reluctant to have a radical operation performed until the simpler procedure had been tried.

A personal communication from Dr. Horrax states that one year later a large pinealoma was removed. It is noteworthy that the patient's precocity was not specifically due to the pinealoma, but to a lesion of the central nervous system which caused disturbances in hypothalamic nuclei. In these connections, it is also interesting to note that pinealomas rarely cause precocity in females. It is therefore suggested that the pineal gland may be so located within the central nervous system that it is much more apt to impinge upon nervous pathways affecting ICSH production than upon those affecting FSH production. Hence a lesion activating ICSH production would not prompt sexual precocity in the female, although it would in the male.

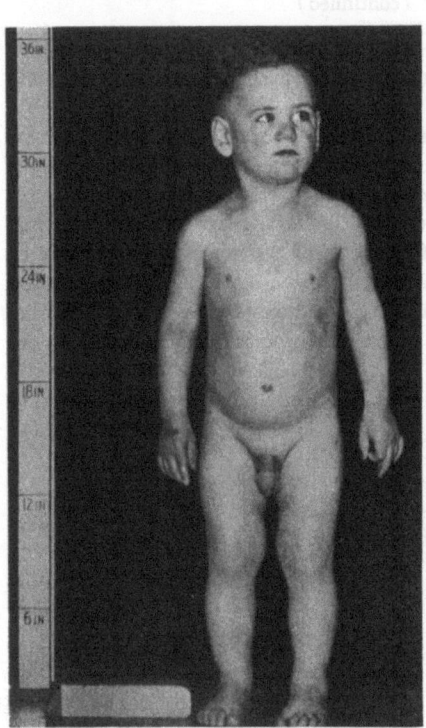
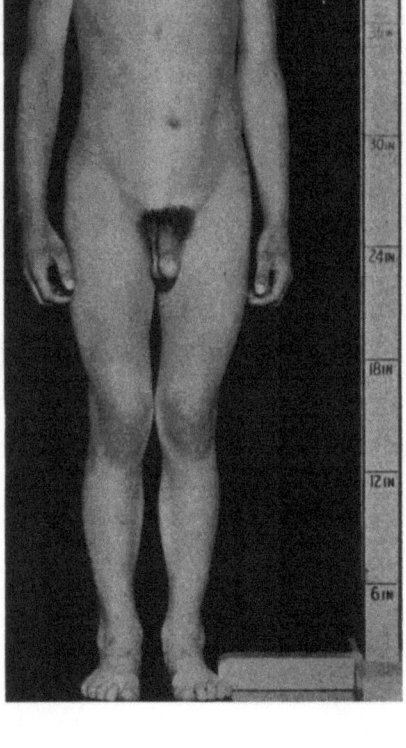

FIGURE VI—24. Incomplete true precocious puberty (see Table 3, Case 9).
LEFT: The patient's appearance at 1½ years.
RIGHT: His appearance at 5½ years.

CASE HISTORY

Precocious penile development was noted when the patient was six months of age. Pubic hair appeared at one year. At 1½ years his voice was somewhat deep. Aside from these abnormalities his history was not remarkable. At 1½ years he was very vigorous and strong, with heavily developed musculature. His measurements indicated that he was above average in weight (13.5 kg.) and in height (95 cm.). His penis was 5.5 cm. in length, but his testes were of normal size for his age. Pubic hair had begun to appear but no axillary hair or acne. The only abnormality revealed by roentgenograms of the skeleton, including the skull, was that his bone age corresponded to that of a boy of 2½ years. A lumbar puncture

The Testes

CASE HISTORY (continued)

yielded normal spinal fluid. Pneumoencephalograms and intravenous pyelograms yielded normal results. His urinary 17-KS output was between 0.1 and 0.2 mg. per 24 hours. His urinary gonadotropin (FSH) was less than 3 mouse units per 24 hours. The adrenal glands were explored by Dr. O. Cope through a wide transverse abdominal incision; both glands were found to be of normal size and texture. An adrenal biopsy revealed nothing abnormal. A testicular biopsy performed by Dr. F. Simmons and interpreted by Dr. R. C. Sniffen (see Figure 25) revealed large blocks of interstitial cells of Leydig type and showed an increase in the size of the tubular lumina but no spermatogenesis. On the basis of the foregoing it appeared that the patient's precocity was of central origin.

After consultation with Drs. J. Mixter and G. W. Holmes, it was decided to give the pineal region a total of 800 roentgens. This therapy failed to exert any beneficial influence upon the course of the disease. At five years of age, the patient measured 108 cm. in height and weighed 23 kg. His bone age was 8 years and his 17-KS output ranged between 0.6 and 1.6 mg. per 24 hours. At 5½ years of age he measured 137 cm. in height and weighed 32 kg. By this time his voice was quite deep and his muscles very powerful. He had a little facial acne, and the hair line over his temples had begun to recede. He still had no axillary hair growth, and his testes were still essentially normal in size. His urinary gonadotropin output was negative for 6.5 mouse units per 24 hours. At seven years of age he measured 144 cm. in height and weighed 38.5 kg. At this time his testes were of early adolescent size.

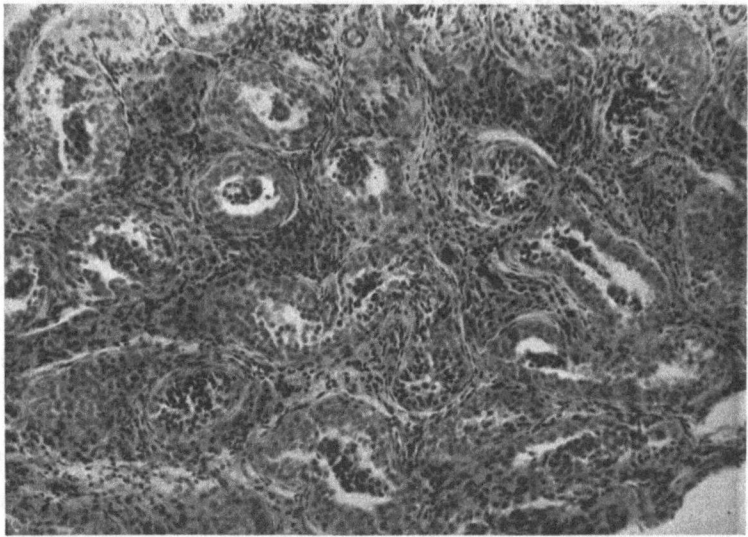

FIGURE VI—25. Testicular biopsy from the patient in Figure 24. Note the pseudo-hyperplastic masses of interstitial cells lying between the relatively undeveloped and inactive testicular tubules. Magnification x 70.

age. Hence, also, the pseudo-hyperplastic appearance of the Leydig cells shown in the testicular biopsies. The 30- to 60-fold increase in testicular volume which occurs during adolescence is due largely to spermatic tubule growth. As a result of this growth, the Leydig cells of the normal adult testis are thinly distributed. In adults with hyalinized testicular tubules the Leydig cells appear pseudo-hyperplastic and clumped as in the patients under consideration here (see Figure 35).

Boys with this condition are particularly to be distinguished from those with pseudo-isosexual precocity of adrenocortical origin, since the two types of patient may be of nearly identical external appearance (compare the patient of Figure 24, this chapter, with the patient of Figure 43, Chapter III). In children of preadolescent age with adrenocortical virilism, however, the urinary 17-KS output is apt to be higher and testicular biopsy usually reveals neither Leydig cell development nor spermatogenesis.

It is probable that patients with the incomplete form of isosexual precocity ultimately develop all the characteristics of the complete, true form.

Pseudo-Precocious Puberty. Children with this condition (Chapter V, Figure 11, Conditions E, G and H) present much the same external appearance as children with true precocious puberty. The difference is to be found in the origin of the precocity. In pseudo-precocious puberty, male hormone production is occurring unnaturally as a result of a primary disturbance in the testes, in the pituitary adrenocorticotropin–adrenal cortex system, or as a consequence of treatment with chorionic gonadotropin or androgenic hormone. Because the hypothalamic–pituitary gonadotropin mechanism is not activated as in the case of patients with true precocious puberty, there is no spermatogenesis and capacity to procreate is not established.

Primary testicular precocity due to an interstitial (Leydig) cell tumor. This is a rare condition, characterized by precocious masculine development in association with testicular tumor (see Table 4 and Chapter V, Figure 11, Condition E). The clinical picture is illustrated by the patient of Figure 26, which resembles that of patients with other types of masculine precocity. They tend to be tall and heavily muscled for their age and to show pubic and axillary hair growth, accelerated skeletal development and so forth. In the few instances of this condition where the urinary 17-KS output has been measured, a high value has been found. Urinary gonadotropic hormone measurements have given negative results.

Testicular interstitial cell tumors are of firm-to-hard consistency. They do not transilluminate well. While they may be expected to vary in size and configuration, they tend to cause a relatively even enlargement of the involved gonad.

The diagnosis rests upon biopsy examination (see Figure 27), in which hyperplasia of Leydig cells (see Figure 25) and hyperplasia of adrenocortical rest cells (Chapter III, Figure 52) are to be distinguished from Leydig cell cancer.

Treatment for Leydig cell cancer is surgical excision. If this is done before metastases have occurred,* the prognosis is good. Hirsutism and other signs of precocious masculinization will recede (see Figure 26, right). The urinary 17-KS output also may be expected to drop toward or to normal levels and to remain there unless remnants or metastases of the tumor remain. In this connection it is somewhat surprising to note that the 17-KS output of the patient of Figure 26 failed to fall to normal levels following surgical removal of his presumably unilateral Leydig cell tumor. Preoperative 17-KS values ranged between 50 and 60 mg. per day; postoperatively for a period of one year the values ranged between about 10 and 20 mg. per day. Despite the persistent elevation in urinary 17-KS output to normal adult levels, he lost almost all evidences of precocious masculine development including pubic hair growth. No clear explanation for this paradox is available, though the possibility of a coexistent adrenocortical derangement is suggested by the fact that one of this patient's adrenal glands was thought upon histologic examination to be "malformed" and to show evidences of "circulatory disturbances."

Adrenocortical virilism. This condition is considered in Chapter III. It is mentioned here to call attention to its importance in the differential diagnosis of isosexual precocity in the male.

Medicational precocity. When chorionic gonadotropin first became available, some rather extreme degrees of pseudo-precocious puberty were produced with its aid.[18] No difficulty should be encountered in determining whether such medication has been given.

This condition is of particular interest because of the fact that biopsies of the testes of patients who have received heavy chorionic gonadotropin therapy (see Figure 11, middle) are reminiscent of those obtained in the case of children with spontaneous incomplete precocity (see Figure 25).

Following withdrawal of chorionic gonadotropin treatment, children of prepubescent age tend to show marked regression in the signs of precocious masculinization. Boys of pubescent age may, however, continue to undergo normal adolescent development.

With one exception the foregoing comments hold also for boys rendered sexually precocious by androgenic hormone (testosterone) therapy. The exception lies in the fact that testosterone constitutes "substitution" therapy at a lower

---

* Leydig cell tumors can metastasize to the liver and thence to other organs.

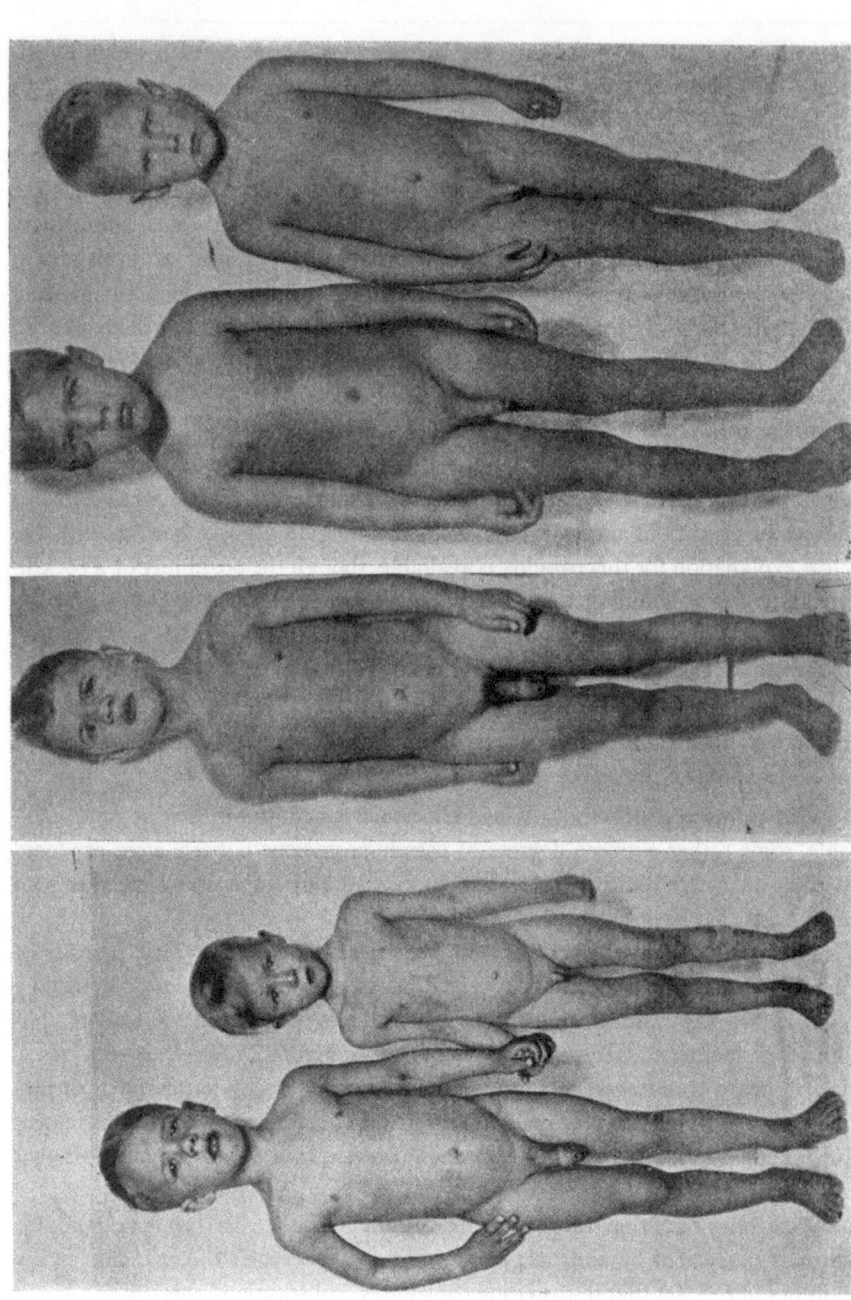

FIGURE VI—26. Sexual precocity due to a testicular interstitial cell tumor. From P. Sandblom, *Acta endocrinologica* 1:107, 1948.
LEFT: The patient at 2³⁰/₁₂ years, with a normal boy of the same age for comparison.
MIDDLE: The patient at 3½ years.
RIGHT: The patient one year postoperatively, at 4½ years, with a normal boy of the same age for comparison.

CASE HISTORY

The patient developed normally until 2²/₁₂ years, when he began to gain in weight and height at an abnormally accelerated rate. In five months he gained 4 kg, and during the following three months he gained another 4 kg. His facial expression became coarse and his skin seborrheic. Coincidentally, his voice began to deepen. At 2⁸/₁₂ years it was noted that his external genitals were enlarged, and he became frequently sensitized to erections. At 2¹⁰/₁₂ years pubic hair began to grow. He became ill-tempered, difficult to manage, and lost interest in playing with other children. At 2¹¹/₁₂ years on physical examination he measured 108 cm. and weighed 21.7 kg. His face showed some acne. His voice was breaking and tended to be bass. His musculature was unduly developed and was remarkably firm. His penis measured 6 cm. in length; the left testis was the size of a small plum; the right testis, about half as large. There was some pubic but no axillary hair. X-ray studies failed to reveal any abnormalities other than an advance in bone age to about 6½ years. His urinary 17-KS output was 23 mg. per 24 hours. His IQ was 111.

A consultant suspected an adrenal tumor. When an exploratory operation was performed, the right adrenal appeared to be entirely normal. Since the left adrenal was of firmer texture and had an indurated area the size of a pea, it was removed. Recovery was uneventful. Microscopic examination of the gland showed the capillaries of the cortex to be widened and parenchyma to be reduced. In some areas the blood had escaped among the cells of the reticular zone. The pathologic diagnosis was adrenal malformation with circulatory disturbances.

During the five postoperative months the patient grew 10 cm. in height and gained 4½ kg. in weight. Sexual tendencies became more marked, as evidenced by daily erections and sexual advances to adult women. His temper also became worse. His urinary 17-KS output increased to 64 mg. per 24 hours. On the other hand, no gonadotropic hormones could be found in the urine. The right testis remained approximately the same, but the left testis grew somewhat firmer in consistency. It was then suspected that a tumor was present. When the left testis was removed, a round tumor the size of a plum was found in the center of the gland. It was separated from the remainder of the organ by a connective tissue capsule. Adjacent testicular tissue was of normal appearance and showed no signs of spermatogenesis. The microscopic appearance of the tumor is shown in Figure 27.

Postoperatively the patient's urinary 17-KS output dropped to between 10 and 20 mg. per 24 hours, at which general level it remained for the ensuing year. His rapid growth ceased immediately. His mind returned to the childish state, and he lost his tendency to erections and his interest in the opposite sex. After a few months his voice became lighter in quality and he commenced to play with other children. His facial skin became smooth and soft. His pubic hair disappeared, but his penis remained approximately 7 cm. in length. The remaining testis was thought to have become slightly larger.

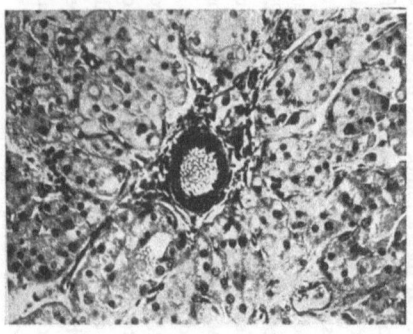 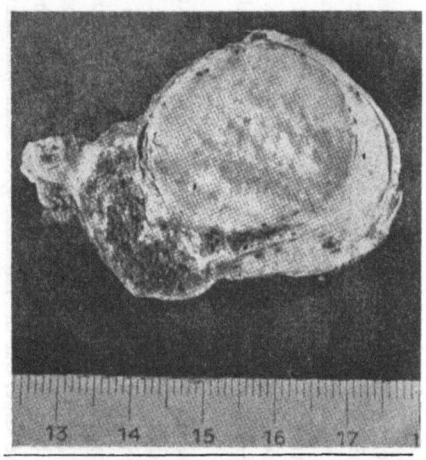

FIGURE VI—27. Cross section of the testicular tumor from the patient in Figure 26. LEFT: Magnification x 260.

level (see Chapter V, Figure 11, Condition H) than is the case with chorionic gonadotropin therapy (see Figure 16, this chapter). Under the former circumstance the testes are being precociously stimulated to activity; in the latter, they remain quiescent.

SEXUAL INFANTILISM–HYPOGONADISM WITH FAILURE OF SEXUAL DEVELOPMENT OR ASPERMATOGENESIS

The line of demarcation with respect to chronologic age between physiologic and pathologic retardation of adolescence in boys is not sharp. The great majority of healthy boys show some definite evidence of testicular androgen production (such as penile development) by the time they are 16 or 17 years old. A few boys do not start to mature until an even later age. Approximately speaking, therefore, failure to show signs of testicular maturation and androgen production by the age of 17 years suggests that something may be wrong. The potential existence of a disturbance in gonad function may, of course, be suspected and diagnosed in boys of younger age, especially when signs of primary panhypopituitarism or anorchia are grossly evident.

In broad terms there are three possible causes for failure of sexual development. These are indicated diagrammatically in Figure 24 of Chapter V and in outline form in Table 6.

Hypothalamic Infantilism. In this condition (Chapter V, Figure 24, Condition C), there is failure of sexual development because of a disorder in the hypothalamic centers which control gonadotropin production by the pituitary. As a result of this disorder there is no adolescent increase in the production of gonadotropins and hence no testicular male hormone production or spermatogenesis.

Sexual infantilism of hypothalamic origin bears a close clinical resemblance to that seen in children and adolescents with generalized pituitary deficiency. When due to a craniopharyngioma, there are apt to be signs of an expanding lesion in the suprasellar region, in addition to evidences of generalized pituitary insufficiency. For further information concerning the diagnosis and management of this disease, see Chapter VII, page 462, and below under pituitary infantilism, primary type. When due to a genetic defect of the type represented in patients with the Laurence-Moon-Biedl syndrome, mental deficiency, retinitis pigmentosa, obesity and other deformities are evident. For further comments on this condition, see Chapter V, page 341, and Chapter VII, page 472.

Pituitary Infantilism, Primary Type. This condition is due to a lesion in the anterior pituitary body (Chapter V, Figure 24, Condition D). As a result of the primary disturbance there is failure in the production of gonadotropins and hence failure of gonadal development as outlined in the preceding section. Since such a lesion can injure both the hypothalamus and the pituitary, a few patients probably suffer simultaneously from "hypothalamic" and "pituitary" infantilism.

As described diagrammatically in Figure 28, pituitary deficiency can be either generalized (Section A) or fractional (Section B).

Generalized pituitary deficiency (panhypopituitarism). The manifestations of this condition are multiple, owing to the fact that in addition to gonadotropic hormone deficiencies, there are deficiencies in pituitary growth hormone (with stunted growth in children), lack of thyroid-stimulating hormone (with evidences of secondary hypothyroidism) and lack of adrenocorticotropins (with evidences of secondary hypoadrenocorticism). For a general consideration of hypopituitarism, see Chapter VII. For a description of the secondary hypothyroid and secondary hypoadrenocortical aspects of the disease, see Chapters I and III. The present section will be concerned chiefly with the hypogonadal portion of the picture.

CLINICAL MANIFESTATIONS. The clinical picture presented by children with this condition is illustrated by the patient of Figure 30 with its accompanying legend.

The gonadal status of such patients is somewhat variable. In the preadolescent period the genital structures correspond to the normal for age, but sexual maturation fails to take place during adolescence. However, in contrast to patients with primary testicular infantilism there may be minimal evidence of testicular development and activity. That is, the testes may develop to a size larger than

Continued on page 428

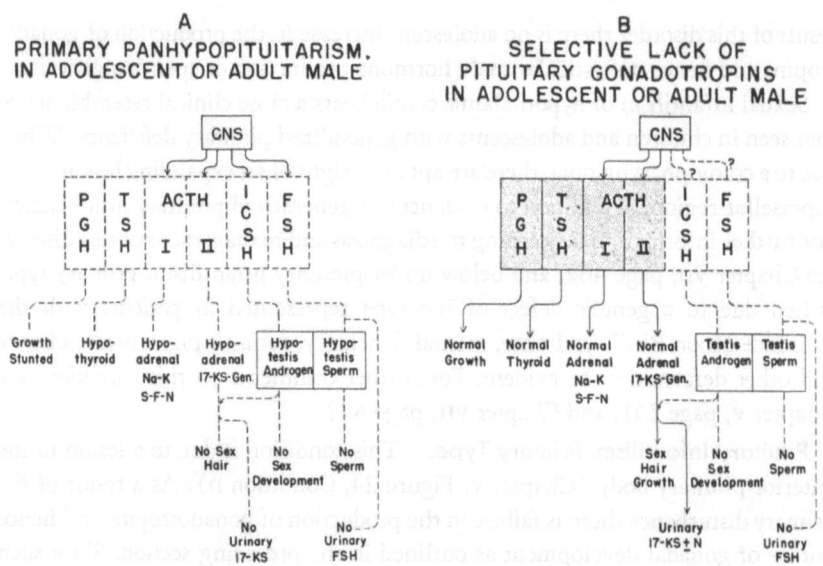

FIGURE VI—28. Diagrammatic representation of the characteristics of panhypogonadism secondary to primary hypopituitarism. The design of this diagram corresponds to that of Figure 9.

SECTION A describes the status of a patient with complete hypopituitarism. Note that there is a lack of thyroid-stimulating, adrenocorticotropic and gonadotropic hormones (ICSH and FSH). As a consequence of these pituitary hormone deficiencies, the patient's growth is stunted and he has secondary hypothyroidism, secondary hypoadrenocorticism and secondary hypogonadism. Because the adrenal cortices produce no 17-ketosteroid precursors (17-KS-Gens) and the testes produce no androgens, masculine sexual development does not take place. There is no sex hair growth, no spermatogenesis, very low 17-KS output and no excretion of urinary gonadotropin (FSH) (see also Figure 16).

SECTION B describes the status of patients whose pituitary function is normal except for gonadotropic production. As shown by the interrupted lines running from the central nervous system (CNS) to the pituitary interstitial-cell-stimulating hormone (ICSH) and follicle-stimulating hormones (FSH), it is possible that hypopituitarism of this type is secondary to failure on the part of the hypothalamus to stimulate pituitary ICSH and FSH production. Because of the gonadotropic hormone lack, the testes remain immature, as in preadolescent children (see Figure 9). On this account there is no masculine sexual development, spermatogenesis or excretion of urinary gonadotropin (FSH). On the other hand, because adolescent-type adrenocorticotropic hormone (ACTH II) production does occur, the adrenal cortices produce 17-KS-Gens, which in turn prompt sex hair growth and give rise to nearly normal urinary 17-KS excretion values.

The Testes

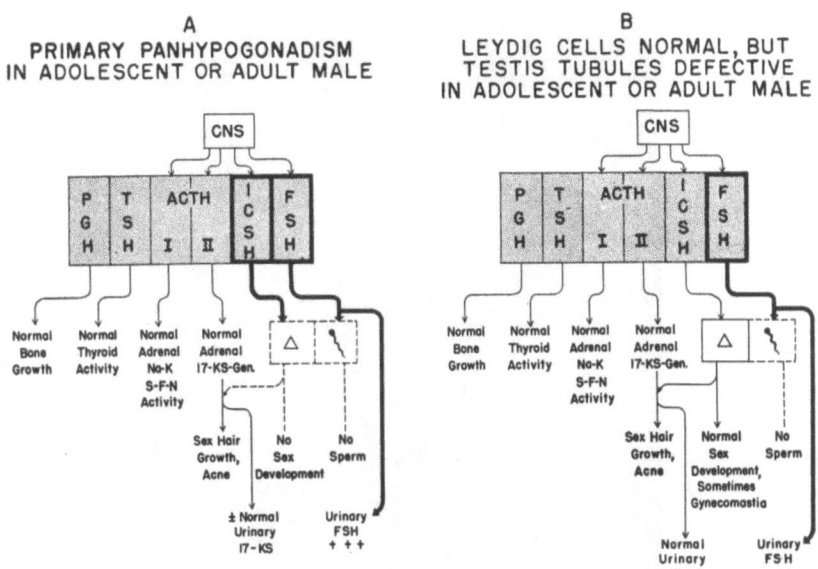

FIGURE VI—29. Diagrammatic representation of primary panhypogonadism. The design of this figure corresponds to that of Figure 9.

SECTION A describes the changes which occur in eunuchoid patients. It is seen that there is a compensatory increase in pituitary interstitial-cell-stimulating hormone (ICSH) and follicle-stimulating hormone (FSH) production. The increase in ICSH must still be considered a probable rather than a proven phenomenon. The FSH increase is demonstrable by urinary gonadotropin (FSH) assay. Because the testes are absent, these gonadotropic hormones have no effect and there is no masculine sexual development. Spermatogenesis does not occur, but there may be some sex hair growth and acne secondary to normal adrenocortical 17-ketosteroid precursor (17-KS-Gens) production. The remainder of this diagram indicates normal relations and activities.

SECTION B describes the conditions presumed to exist in males with normal Leydig cells but defective spermatic tubules. In this diagram note that FSH, but not ICSH, production is increased. Note also that the Leydig cells produce androgens which contribute (a) to sex hair growth, acne and urinary 17-KS excretion and (b) to normal masculine sexual development. Sometimes these patients have gynecomastia. For further comment, see text, page 437.

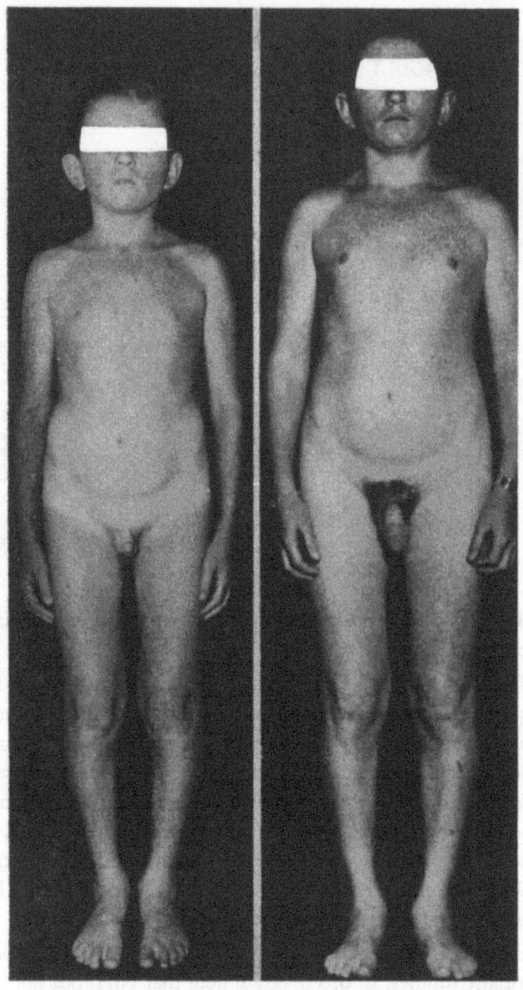

FIGURE VI—30. Apparent generalized idiopathic pituitary insufficiency with sexual infantilism in a male aged 23.
LEFT: Appearance of the patient before treatment.
RIGHT: His appearance after a year of testosterone therapy.

CASE HISTORY

The patient had always been undersized for his age. He was born after a seven months' pregnancy which was terminated because of nephritis in the mother. At birth he weighed approximately 1.2 kg. There were no neonatal difficulties of note. At one year of age his appearance was more like that of a normal month-old baby. After that time he grew at the rate of approximately 2.5 cm. per year. During childhood he was always lean, never

CASE HISTORY (continued)

obese. One testicle descended when he was six years old and the other when he was about eight. He has never had any spontaneous development of masculine sexual characteristics. Thus, he has shown chronic retardation of the somatic growth and maturation. On the other hand, his intellectual development has been satisfactory. A review of the family and past history failed to reveal any additional information of note.

On physical examination at 23 years of age the patient was found to be 143.5 cm. tall and to weigh 35.8 kg. His muscular development was rather poor. The subcutaneous fat appeared to vary from adequate to somewhat excessive. There was no evidence of axillary hair, pubic hair or penile growth. Other findings were not remarkable. Laboratory studies revealed that urine was normal, hemoglobin 12 gm. per cent, the NPN 34 mg. per cent, serum cholesterol 250 mg. per cent. Serum electrolyte values were within normal limits. The serum protein-bound iodine was 3.2 micrograms per cent, a slightly subnormal value suggestive of mild hypothyroidism. The urinary 17-KS output was 0.6 mg. per 24 hours, a very low reading. The urinary gonadotropin (FSH) assay was negative for 6.5 mouse units per 24 hours. The BMR was −24 per cent. X-rays of the skull failed to indicate any abnormalities except that the frontal sinuses were undeveloped and the ethmoid and sphenoid were somewhat small. The bone age as determined from roentgenograms of the hand and wrist was approximately 14 years. The patient was treated with thyroid in doses up to 60 mg. per day without marked benefit. Administration of testosterone (in the form of pellets and oral methyl testosterone) induced masculinization, as shown in the right-hand photograph.

that characteristic of childhood, but smaller than that seen in normal adolescents and adults. In addition, there may be minimal evidence of penile development and of pubic hair growth. When such signs of development are seen, they indicate that failure in the production of gonadotropins is relative rather than absolute.

DIAGNOSIS. Laboratory studies and clinical tests are usually needed to certify this diagnosis. From the specific point of view of anterior pituitary–gonadal status, the urinary FSH test is helpful. In patients with marked hypopituitarism, assays reveal that there are less than 3 mouse units in a 24-hour urine specimen. In less extreme cases there may be 3, but less than 6, mouse units present. The urinary 17-KS output is very low (< 1 mg. per day) in panhypopituitary patients. Testicular biopsy reveals simple retardation in development (see Figure 11, Section A). In contrast to patients with primary testicular infantilism, these patients undergo masculinization when subjected to the chorionic gonadotropin test (page 402).

TREATMENT AND PROGNOSIS. In this condition therapy and recovery depend in part upon the nature of the primary pituitary disturbance and in part upon the age of the patient. If there is an authentic destructive lesion of the anterior pituitary, the prognosis for spontaneous remission of the hypopituitary state is poor. In such patients chronic substitution therapy, starting at about 14 years, is usually needed to bring about and maintain masculinization. If objective evidence of a lesion in the region of the pituitary is lacking, there is a greater possibility that the hypopituitarism is functional in nature, resulting from a potentially correctible defect such as hypothyroidism, malnutrition, chronic infection (see below under pituitary infantilism). Occasional individuals with apparent primary, idiopathic panhypopituitarism undergo a spontaneous remission between 20 and 25 years of age for no known reason.

Assuming hypopituitarism to be due to intrinsic pituitary disease, there are two possible types of treatment. One consists in the administration of a hormone such as chorionic gonadotropin. This is equivalent to providing a substitute for ICSH. At present, because of limitations in supply, it is not possible to provide FSH substitution therapy. This method of treatment is physiologically sound and has the potential advantage of prompting normal adult testicular activity, including spermatogenesis. From the practical standpoint, however, it is difficult to carry out, for this type of hormone must be given intramuscularly three or four times weekly. In the case of chorionic gonadotropin an effective dose is 500 I.U. Furthermore, unless the hormone given is of human origin (as is chorionic gonadotropin), it is apt as a foreign protein to induce the formation of antibodies. These can inactivate the administered hormone. For such reasons gonadotropic substitution therapy is ordinarily used only over short periods of time for diagnostic or special therapeutic purposes.

Testosterone administration comprises a more convenient method of inducing masculine development. The indications and dosages are with one possible exception essentially as outlined below for primary testicular hypogonadism (page 436). This exception pertains to patients of adolescent age with apparent hypopituitarism of unknown origin. Because some of these patients are potentially capable of spontaneous adolescence, it appears desirable to treat them intermittently rather than continuously until no reasonable possibility of spontaneous recovery remains. Therefore, from about age 15 methyl testosterone in daily oral doses of 10 to 20 mg. may be given for periods of two or three months and then omitted for alternate periods of equal or longer duration. If natural pituitary and gonadal activity has become established, the patient will not show signs of regression in masculine development. If natural activity has not become established, such signs may appear within three to six months.

In the treatment of dwarfed panhypopituitary patients, especially, testosterone dosage should be considered with relation to stature and skeletal development. Such relations are discussed in another section (page 440).

Specific, selective or fractional gonadotropin deficiency (Figure 28, Section B; Table 7). There are occasional patients who resemble those with panhypopituitarism in that (a) they show no masculine development, (b) their urinary gonadotropic output is subnormal and (c) their response to the chorionic gonadotropic hormone test (see page 402) is positive, but who differ in that they fail to present gross evidence of deficiency in pituitary growth hormone (dwarfism), adrenocorticotropic hormone (very low urinary 17-KS, etc.) or thyrotropic hormone (dwarfism, etc.).

ETIOLOGY. The cause of fractional hypopituitarism is difficult to define. Congenital pituitary defects, nutritional disturbances, derangements in thyroid and adrenal function and chronic disorders such as diabetes mellitus and renal disease, as well as various acute illnesses, have been mentioned as possible causes.[19] Occasionally the condition may represent an early phase of panhypopituitarism due to a destructive lesion of the hypophysis.

TREATMENT. Therapy for this type of hypogonadism is the same as for hypogonadism secondary to generalized anterior pituitary deficiency. Again, it is to be remembered that most boys of adolescent age with apparent sexual retardation are physiologically slow maturers, in some cases in accordance with familial pattern.* On this account, it usually is best to give intermittent treat-

* Opposite genetic tendencies with resultant early adolescence are also seen occasionally (see Figure 19).

TABLE VI—7. Male eunuchoidism due to selective lack of pituitary gonadotropins with normal testes as evidenced by positive response to chorionic gonadotropin therapy (hypogonadotropic hypogonadism).* Data from R. W. Fraser et al., J. Clin. Endocrinol. 1:234, 1941.

Case no.	Age, yr.	Ht., cm.	Ht. age	Wt., kg.	Bone age	Penis size	Testis size	Sexual hair † P	A	F	Urinary 17-KS output Mg. per 24 hr.	After CGT** therapy
1	21	184	Adult	65.6	Retarded	Infantile	Infantile	S	N	–	4.8	Rise in 17-KS output
2	24	172	Adult	63.5	Retarded	—	Small	S	–	–	3.5	Rise in 17-KS output
3	28	171	Adult	55.5	Retarded	Infantile	Infantile	S	N	–	4.2	Clinical response
4	29	186	Adult	74.5	Retarded	Small	Small	S	N	S	6.4	Indefinite
5	34	167	Adult	68.2	—	Infantile	Infantile	S	N	–	3.9	Rise in 17-KS output
6	35	174	Adult	74.2	Retarded	—	Olive stone	N	N	–	3.0	Slight rise in 17-KS output

* Like the patients of Table 8, these subjects were of essentially normal stature and showed sparse pubic and axillary hair growth but little or no penile growth. They differed from these patients in their tendency to have no urinary gonadotropins, to respond to chorionic gonadotropin therapy and to have lower urinary 17-KS values. These findings indicate that the eunuchoidism in the present cases was due to a deficiency of pituitary gonadotropins. The fact that the urinary 17-KS output was not very low plus the fact that the patients were of normal stature indicates that they were not suffering from a marked degree of pituitary growth and adrenocorticotropic hormone deficiency as is the case in patients with full-blown panhypopituitarism (Chapter VII, Table 4). On the other hand, the fact that their urinary 17-KS values were somewhat lower than normal suggests that in association with the gonadotropin lack there also was a mild degree of adrenocorticotropic hormone deficiency.
† P = Pubic; A = Axillary; F = Facial; S = Sparse; N = None.
** CGF = Chorionic gonadotropin.

ment, preferably with chorionic gonadotropin (see page 428) until the likelihood of a spontaneous cure has dwindled to very small proportions (i.e., until the patient is 18 or 20 years old). Thereafter, one may be obliged to prescribe chronic maintenance therapy with one of the testosterone compounds.

Pituitary Infantilism, Functional Type, Secondary to Athyrosis and Nutritional Deficiencies. Sexual infantilism of this type (see Chapter V, Figure 24, Condition E) is mentioned here for differential diagnostic purposes. Primary athyrosis and caloric undernutrition may lead to functional hypopituitarism with consequent failure to produce gonadotropic hormones. Sexual infantilism results as it does in patients with hypothalamic and pituitary infantilism. For other information concerning the diagnosis and management of these conditions, see under physiologic hypopituitarism, Chapter VII, page 472.

The Testes

Testicular Infantilism. In this condition (Chapter v, Figure 24, Condition F), although the hypothalamus and the anterior pituitary function adequately, sexual development fails to proceed normally because of a primary defect in the testes. As shown diagrammatically in Figure 29, the testes may be totally destroyed or absent (panhypogonadism, Section A) or the testicular tubules may be damaged while the interstitial cells remain intact (selective hypogonadism, Section B).

Panhypogonadism (Figure 29, Section A). This term signifies that both the tubules and the interstitial cells are destroyed or absent as a consequence of testicular agenesis (congenital anorchia), castration, trauma, torsion of the spermatic cord, hemorrhage, tumor, idiopathic fibrosis, faulty surgery or other lesion. Acquired testicular disease may involve only one gonad; in constitutional testicular disease both gonads are apt to be involved. It is only when both testes are damaged that generalized symptoms and signs of hypogonadism become evident.

CLINICAL MANIFESTATIONS. The clinical picture presented by children with panhypogonadism is illustrated by the patient of Figure 31. His growth and maturation up to adolescent age were essentially normal. He had no complaints and behaved exactly like a normal boy. Had he been allowed to progress to adult age without treatment, his physical characteristics probably would have corresponded to those of an adult eunuch.

In adult eunuchs there is failure of penile, scrotal and prostate development, the voice is of puerile pitch, the musculature is poorly developed and fusion of the skeletal epiphyses is delayed (see Table 8). On the other hand, though there may be no normal adolescent growth spurt, growth in height continues at an approximately normal rate through adolescence, so that normal adult stature is usually attained at an approximately normal age. Though the delay in skeletal maturation and epiphyseal fusion mentioned above presumably offers a continued opportunity for growth, only a few eunuchoid individuals actually do grow to an exceptionally tall stature. Because of the delay in epiphyseal closure there is, however, a tendency for eunuchs and eunuchoids to have relatively long extremities.[20]

Such patients eventually develop a sparse growth of pubic and axillary hair. Present evidence indicates that this is caused by the normal adrenocortical 17-KS-Gens. As shown in Table 8, the urinary 17-KS output usually is within normal limits. On the other hand, urinary FSH values tend to be abnormally high. Precise information concerning the earliest age at which one may expect to find elevated urinary FSH values in boys with primary hypogonadism is not known. Limited experience suggests that gonadotropins appear in the urine of these patients at about the same age that they would appear if the testes were

Continued on page 436

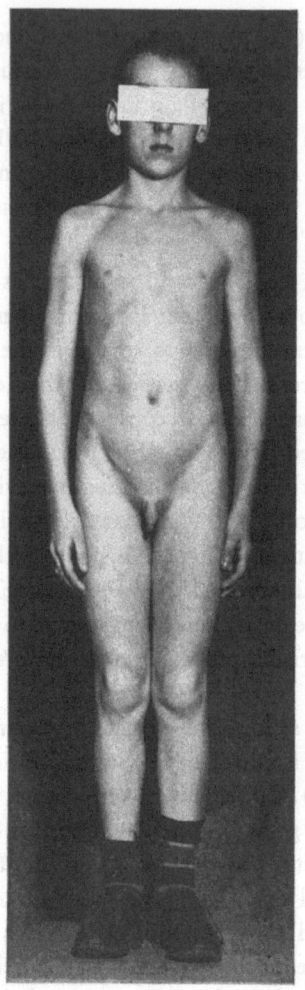
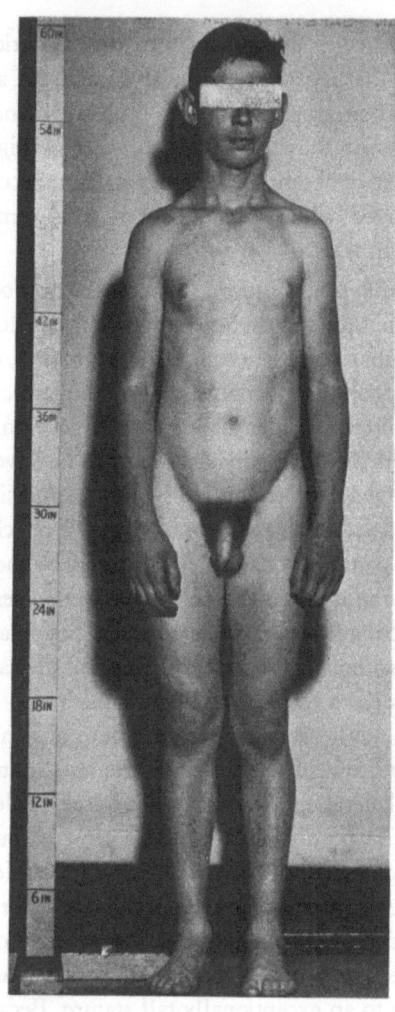

(Left)
FIGURE VI—31. Idiopathic testicular atrophy in a boy of 12 years.
(Right)
FIGURE VI—32. Idiopathic gynecomastia in a boy of 18 years with normal spermatogenesis.

CASE HISTORY (FIGURE 31)

When the patient was one month of age, it was noted that his testes were very small and undescended. At an orchiopexy, performed when he was 12 years of age, his right testicle was found to be markedly atrophic. When first seen in this clinic at the age of 12½ years, he was a lean, healthy-looking boy in no distress. He measured 143 cm. in height and weighed 35 kg. These measurements placed him in the lower 10 percentile group with respect to height and weight. His body proportions were approximately normal. He showed no evidence of secondary sexual development, and both testes were exceedingly small.

Otherwise, the findings of the physical examination were not remarkable. Roentgenograms of his hand and wrist revealed that his bone age corresponded with his actual age of 12 years. The urinary 17-KS output was 3.3 mg. per 24 hours, and the urinary gonadotropin (FSH) output 190 mouse units per 24 hours. On the basis of these findings a diagnosis of testicular atrophy was made.

In order to avoid interference with spontaneous maturation, no therapy was given until the patient was 15 years of age. At that time the urinary 17-KS and gonadotropin output values were found to be exactly as previously reported. Now, however, his bone age corresponded to the average for normal boys of 13½ years. On physical examination he showed a small growth of pubic hair but no evidences of penile development; neither testicle could be found. Since there appeared to be little likelihood of spontaneous sexual development, he was started on 20 mg. of methyl testosterone by mouth daily. Within three months there was a definite increase in penile size and in pubic hair growth.

After six months of therapy, the scrotum was found to be well developed, and axillary hair growth had begun. However, the testicles could not be found. After two years of therapy the patient became quite thoroughly masculinized, as evidenced by adult development of his penis, scrotum and pubic and axillary hair. In addition, his voice had deepened and he had commenced to shave. Though testosterone had thus induced masculinization, it failed to cause the urinary gonadotropin output to fall to normal levels (see text). At 17 years he measured 166 cm. in height and weighed 53 kg. These measurements, like those above, placed him at the 10 percentile level with respect to height and weight.

The patient's emotional adjustment to his difficulty has been quite good. He participates actively in athletics, but he exercises great care to hide himself when taking a shower in the company of others and makes every effort to see that no one knows about the absence of his testicles. He does not seem disturbed with the thought that maintenance of his masculine development probably will depend to a considerable extent upon continuous testosterone therapy.

CASE HISTORY (FIGURE 32)

The patient was first seen at the age of 12 years because of stunted growth. His history indicated that he had suffered severe nutritional privation between the ages of one and three years. Extensive studies failed to reveal any organic disease. Because it was thought that he might be a pituitary dwarf, he was treated intermittently with methyl testosterone between the ages of 12 and 14 years. The dose administered ranged between 10 and 30 mg. per day. This treatment caused an increase in growth rate and masculine development. After three courses of testosterone it was found that he was growing spontaneously at a normal rate. Accordingly, testosterone treatment was discontinued. Between the patient's fourteenth and sixteenth years no abnormalities were noted. However, when he was about 16 years of age, he began to develop bilateral gynecomastia. This has persisted up to the present. At the age of 20 he now measures 138 cm. in height and weighs 48 kg. As shown by the above photograph, he is alert and healthy in appearance. Aside from the gynecomastia, no abnormalities have been found on physical examination. His urinary gonadotropin (FSH) output is between 13 and 52 mouse units per 24 hours. His 17-KS is between 12 and 13 mg. per 24 hours and his urinary 11-17-OCS is 0.1 mg. per 24 hours. A recent testicular biopsy revealed many Leydig cells and moderately well-advanced spermatogenesis. His sperm count is normal (82 million sperms per cc.).

TABLE VI—8. Male eunuchoidism of primary testicular origin with positive urinary gonadotropin assays and failure to respond to chorionic gonadotropin therapy (hypergonadotropic hypogonadism).*

Case no.	Age, yr.	Ht., cm.	Wt., kg.	Bone age	Penis size	Testis size	Sexual hair† P	A	F	Urinary gonadotropin	Urinary 17-KS mg/24 hr.	Response to CGT** therapy	Source
1	12	143	35	12	Puerile	None	N	N	N	190 M. U.	3.3	—	Case 471,276 MGH
2	19	158	51.3	Adult	3.8 cm.	None	S	S	N	High	5.8	None	C. G. Heller et al., J. Clin. Endocrinol. 3:573, 1943.
3	20	171	—	Adult	Small	Fibrous remnant	S	—	N	30 M. U. per 100 cc.	2.4	—	R. W. Fraser et al., J. Clin. Endocrinol. 1:234, 1941.
4	21	180	100	Adult	3.8 cm.	None	S	S	N	High	11.8	None	C. G. Heller et al., loc. cit.
5	24	176	58.5	Adult	Infantile	None	S	S	N	High	14.4	None	Ibid.
6	24	174	72.0	Adult	Infantile	None	S	S	N	High	10.2	None	Ibid.
7	25	186	41.7	Adult	Infantile	None	S	—	N	Positive	8.4	None	R. W. Fraser et al., loc. cit.
8	29	179	60.8	Adult	Small	1 cm.	S	S	N	Positive	—	—	C. S. Byron et al., J. Clin. Endocrinol. 1:359, 1941.
9	31	186	90.0	Adult	6.0 cm.	1 cm.	S	S	S	25 R. U. per L.	—	—	S. A. Vest et al., J. Urol. 40:154, 1938.
10	35	172	85.5	Adult	3.8 cm.	Atrophic	S	S	N	High	8.4	None	C. G. Heller et al., loc. cit.
11	57	149	56.5	12	2.5 cm.	Atrophic	S	S	N	High	7.4	None	Ibid.

Iliac crests open: Case 4 Bone age, Case 5 Bone age, Case 6 Bone age, Case 11 Bone age. Retarded: Cases 3, 7, 8, 10.

* Note that these patients, though of normal adult stature, had small penises and small or absent testes. These findings plus the fact that the urinary gonadotropin output was high and the response to chorionic gonadotropin therapy negative indicate that the testes were severely damaged or absent. The urinary 17-KS were therefore probably derived from adrenocortical 17-KS-Gens. The fact that the 17-KS output values were essentially within normal limits indicates that there was no adrenocorticotropin deficiency. The adrenocortical 17-KS-Gens presumably caused the growth of pubic and axillary hair. Note, however, that they failed to prompt penile development.

† P = Pubic; A = Axillary; F = Facial; S = Sparse; N = None.   **CGT = Chorionic gonadotropin.

TABLE VI—9. Clinical manifestations of patients with a testicular tubule defect, normal Leydig cells and gynecomastia. Data from H. F. Klinefelter et al., *J. Clin. Endocrinol.* 2:615, 1942. See also C. G. Heller and W. O. Nelson, *J. Clin. Endocrinol.* 5:1, 1945.

Case no.	Age, yr.	Onset of puberty, yr.	Gynecomastia noted, yr.	Ht., cm.	Bone age	Testis size	Masculine development	Urinary FSH M.U./24 hr.	Urinary 17-KS mg/24 hr.	Comments
1	17	13	13	181.1	Normal	Very small	Normal	235	7.2	Mumps at age 2 without orchitis
2	18	14	14	170.7	Normal	Extremely small	Normal	640	*	No mumps; congenital syphilis
3	22	14	17	175.4	Normal	Extremely small	Normal	150	7.2	Mumps without orchitis
4	24	14	18	182.2	Normal	Very small	Normal	—	4.8	Obese; right hemianopsia
5	28	14	18	177.0	Delayed	Very small	Subnormal	—	4.6	Feebleminded
6	30	13	14	183.5	Normal	2 cm.	Normal	200	13.1	Narcolepsy; renal stones
7	33	13	16	182.2	—	Small	Normal	270	9.6	Mumps without orchitis
8	35	14	16	177.5	Normal	Very small	Normal	330	10.3	Mumps without orchitis; obese
9	38	12	18	171.6	—	Extremely small	Normal	—	9.2	Cystic disease of lung

* The pretreatment assays of 1.2 and 2.4 mg. averaging 1.8 mg. per 24 hours are thought to be due to faulty technique and are not included. Later assays, after four to six weeks without treatment, ranged from 4.3 to 9.0 mg., with an average of 5.7 mg. per 24 hours.

normal (see Table 1). However, we have observed one anorchic boy who excreted at least 6 mouse units of urinary gonadotropin (FSH) per 24 hours at the age of 6. Once gonadotropin appears in the urine, it is apt to rise to abnormally high levels if the gonads are defective.

Chorionic gonadotropin therapy does not induce masculinization in this type of patient. Exploration either fails to reveal the presence of any testicular tissue or discloses only fibrotic remnants.

TREATMENT. Therapy for panhypogonadism consists in the administration of testosterone starting at about 14 years of age. This will bring about and, if continued, will maintain adult masculine development. It will not, of course, impart the ability to procreate. While the drug can be given intramuscularly in oil as testosterone propionate (5 to 25 mg. three times a week) or as pellets of testosterone implanted subcutaneously (five to ten 75 mg. pellets are effective for a period of about three months),[21] the simplest form of therapy appears to be methyl testosterone by mouth.* Unless there is a particular reason for hurry, 10 mg. of methyl testosterone taken daily are sufficient to bring about gradual masculinization. Provided the epiphyses are widely open, this dose usually will induce a spurt in growth and some acceleration in skeletal maturation. Larger doses (i.e., 30 or more mg. daily) will prompt more rapid sex and skeletal development but will not induce a correspondingly rapid rate of growth in stature. Growth in stature ceases when skeletal maturation is completed, as evidenced by epiphyseal closure. Thus, for the younger patient who has yet to attain adult stature, use of the smaller dose appears preferable.† For the older patient who already has grown as tall as he wishes and who is anxious to become masculinized promptly, larger doses are in order. Definite changes, including penile size, may be looked for within 3 to 6 months on the smaller doses and within about 6 to 10 weeks on the larger doses.

PROGNOSIS. With respect to masculinization the prognosis is good as long as treatment is continued. If therapy is withdrawn, there is apt to be considerable regression in masculinity. Early in therapy this is evidenced by recession of pubic hair and shrinkage in the penis, scrotum and prostate. After prolonged therapy

---

* Roughly speaking, in terms of daily dosage testosterone propionate given intramuscularly is from two to four times as potent as an equal weight of methyl testosterone given orally. Testosterone taken as linguets which are allowed to dissolve slowly after being placed under the tongue exerts more of an effect than the same dose swallowed into the stomach. Maximum nitrogen anabolic action is attained with daily doses ranging between 10 and 25 mg. of testosterone propionate given intramuscularly and 25 and 90 mg. of methyl testosterone given orally. The maximum nitrogen-retaining effect of testosterone may "wear out" gradually after several months.

† The use of testosterone as a growth-promoting agent is considered separately at the end of this chapter (see page 440).

THE TESTES						[437]

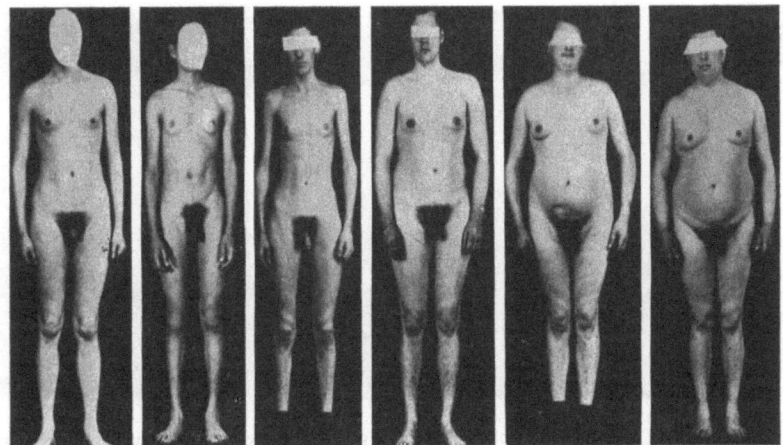

FIGURE VI—33. Appearance of six patients with normal Leydig cells but defective spermatic tubules and increased urinary gonadotropin (FSH) output and gynecomastia. From H. F. Klinefelter, E. C. Reifenstein and F. Albright, *J. Clin. Endocrinol.* 2:615, 1942.

these structures, as well as the bass voice and beard, may remain fairly well developed although volume of ejaculate and potentia coeundi may diminish.

Testicular tubule deficiency (aspermatogenesis) with normal interstitial cell function and sometimes with gynecomastia (Figure 33). This condition differs from the foregoing in that though patients become masculinized, they remain sterile. Some also have gynecomastia (the Klinefelter syndrome).[12] Except when gynecomastia is present, patients with this disease are apt to be considered normal until they marry and it is discovered that they are sterile. The following comments will therefore be restricted largely to gynecomastia in association with a lesion of the testicular tubules.

ETIOLOGY. The cause of such lesions is not known. There is no evidence, clinically or histologically, that they result from inflammatory disease. Neither is there any clear suggestion that the condition is usually due to a prior episode of mumps or other viral disease. Spermatic duct obstruction does not play a role. While cryptorchidism after the onset of adolescence sometimes seriously interferes with spermatogenesis, it does not ordinarily result in gynecomastia.

The cause of the gynecomastia is also unknown. One theory postulates that it is due to a disturbance in androgen metabolism secondary to a lack of "inhibin" (see page 373),[12] another that it is due to excess pituitary mammotropic hormone.

CLINICAL MANIFESTATIONS. In testicular tubule deficiency the clinical picture (see Table 9) includes (a) normal or nearly normal development of

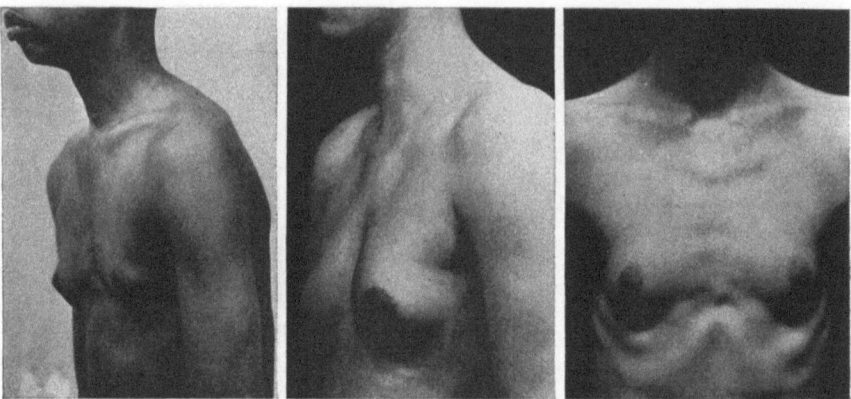

FIGURE VI—34. Close-up views of the chests of three of the six patients of Figure 33. From H. F. Klinefelter, E. C. Reifenstein and F. Albright, *J. Clin. Endocrinol.* 2:615, 1942.

the masculine secondary sexual characteristics (Figure 33), (b) gynecomastia (Figure 34), (c) abnormally small testes, (d) abnormally elevated urinary FSH output, (e) normal to moderately low urinary 17-KS excretion and (f) hyalinization of the seminiferous tubules (see Figure 35).

Puberty starts in a normal manner when the individual is between 12 and 14 years of age. The gynecomastia, which always is bilateral, becomes evident from one to six years later—usually attaining maximum development within six years of the onset of puberty. In about 25 per cent of the cases observed it is present in mild degree; in the remainder the development of the breasts is that of adolescent girls. The areolæ are enlarged but are not remarkably pigmented. There is no mammary secretion. The breasts are not tender unless hit or manipulated. Masculine underdevelopment of moderate degree has been noted in some cases; most patients are normally masculinized.

The testes are normally descended, of normal consistency and normally sensitive to pressure. However, they are small in size, measuring about 1.5 by 1.0 by 0.5 cm. (0.75 cc.) in comparison with those of a normal adult, which vary from 5 by 3 by 2 cm. to about 5 by 3 by 3 cm. (30 to 45 cc.).

As in castrate and eunuchoid patients the urinary output of FSH is abnormally elevated. This deviation is presumably demonstrable only in patients who have reached adolescent age. The reason why the urinary 17-KS output of some of these individuals is slightly to moderately below average normal is not known.

The structural defects in the testes are readily demonstrable in testicular biopsy specimens. The tubules of individual patients are involved to a variable

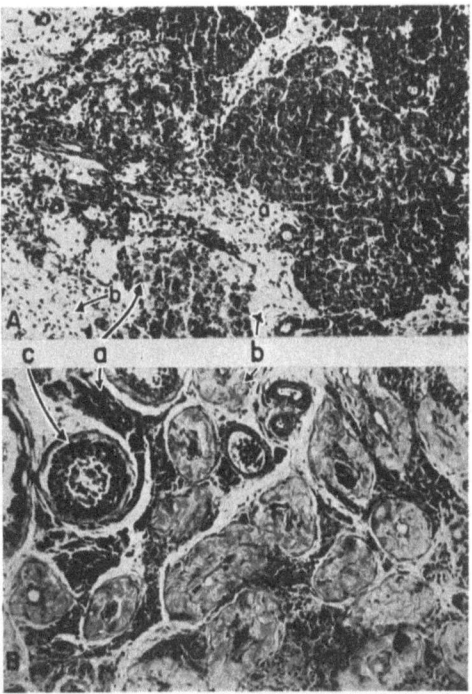

FIGURE VI—35. Testicular biopsy from a patient with Klinefelter's syndrome: (a) Leydig cells, (b) completely hyalinized tubules, (c) partially hyalinized tubule. Note that the Leydig cells in Section A almost suggest adenoma formation. From H. F. Klinefelter, E. C. Reifenstein and F. Albright, *J. Clin. Endocrinol.* 2:615, 1942.

extent, some showing partial and some showing complete hyalinization (see Figure 35). Normal spermatogenesis is never present. The hyaline tissue stains pink with eosin and like collagen with phosphotungstic acid and aniline blue. Frequently fine granules of unknown nature are present in the hyaline tissue. The interstitial cells are numerous and give a false impression of hyperplasia. This pseudo-hyperplastic appearance is explained by the fact that the total volume of the testes of such a patient is only 1/30 to 1/60 of that of a normal adult. Consequently, the interstitial cells appear to be 30 to 60 times more numerous than is usually the case. A similar concentration of interstitial cells is evident in the testes of boys with incomplete true precocious puberty (see Figure 25).

Breast tissue biopsy shows some ductal hyperplasia with marked proliferation of periductal connective tissue. These changes are thought to be radically different from those produced by the administration of estrogenic hormone. Estrogens cause more ductal hyperplasia and less periductal connective tissue.

DIAGNOSIS AND DIFFERENTIAL DIAGNOSIS. The occurrence of gynecomastia, small testes and abnormally elevated urinary FSH excretion in a normally masculinized patient is strongly suggestive of defective testicular tubules. The diagnosis is confirmed by microscopic examination of testicular tissue.

Defective spermatogenesis plus increased urinary FSH excretion may occur in the absence of gynecomastia. However, as mentioned before, it is not likely that this type of disturbance will be recognized during childhood or adolescence.

Conversely, gynecomastia may occur in the absence of testicular tubule disease. In fact, physiologic, adolescent gynecomastia is found in conspicuous form in about 50 per cent of normal boys (see Figure 15). It is usually most evident at a time when masculine development is well under way. As a rule, physiologic gynecomastia recedes within a period of two or three years to the point where it no longer is detectable by palpation, and by the twentieth year of life to a vestigial stage.[16]

Persistent gynecomastia is seen occasionally in patients who have no demonstrable testicular defects (see Figure 33). In addition, it may occur as a manifestation of testicular interstitial cell tumors and chorionepitheliomas.[22] In the latter condition the breasts may secrete, the areolæ are enlarged and pigmented and the urine contains excessive amounts of estrogen and chorionic gonadotropin.* Other rare causes of gynecomastia are adrenocortical cancer and hyperplasia, estrogen therapy (see legend of Figure 20), desoxycorticosterone acetate treatment, cirrhosis of the liver, pituitary tumors, thyrotoxicosis and atrophy of the testis following radiation.[22]

TREATMENT. No satisfactory method of treatment for the testicular defect has been found. Moreover, there is no dependable hormonal therapy for the gynecomastia. Estrogen administration aggravates this condition, and progesterone usually fails to ameliorate it. However, as methyl testosterone in oral doses of 20 to 40 mg. per day sometimes causes a reduction in gynecomastia within three to six months, it should therefore be tried before surgery is resorted to. Cosmetically satisfactory effects may be accomplished by surgical mastectomy via an incision at the margin of the nipple areola.

CLINICAL USE OF TESTOSTERONE AS A GROWTH-PROMOTING AGENT

As outlined in an earlier section of this chapter, under certain circumstances testosterone administration accelerates skeletal growth (see Figure 7). Testosterone also causes an acceleration in the rate of skeletal maturation (see Figure 8). But neither testosterone nor any other growth-promoting factor is capable of inducing much linear growth once skeletal maturation has progressed to the point where closure or fusion of the skeletal epiphyses has occurred.† Since

---

* This substance is measurable by the Aschheim-Zondek test.

† Testosterone also may fail to prompt growth in patients with chondrodystrophy or the like.

ultimate stature is the product of two variables—(a) rate of growth and (b) duration of growth—it is important to consider the relative effects of testosterone upon them. This has been done in a controlled study on a group of nutritionally stunted children between six and ten years of age.[7 b] The results obtained may be summarized as follows:

Testosterone invariably caused an increase in growth rate from subnormal to normal or slightly supranormal levels. This effect was as great in children given 5 mg. of methyl testosterone by mouth daily as in those given 10, 20 or 30 mg. per day. The effect was evident within three months of starting treatment.

Testosterone also caused an acceleration in the rate of skeletal maturation as judged by study of roentgenograms of the hand and wrists with relation to Todd's normal standards. This effect was about as noticeable in those subjects who were given daily doses of 5 mg. as in those receiving larger doses. This tendency to acceleration in skeletal maturation became roentgenologically evident in some patients during the period of therapy; in others it became noticeable only at the end of a 6-to-12-month follow-up period. Available evidence fails to indicate any subsequent compensatory lag in skeletal maturation.

When average changes in rate of growth in height (expressed in terms of years of height age*) were related to average changes in rate of skeletal maturation,† it was found that in two-thirds of the cases testosterone had brought about a relatively greater increase in the rate of skeletal maturation than in the rate of growth in height.

When this phenomenon occurs spontaneously, as in congenital adrenocortical virilism (Chapter III, Figure 46), growth tends to be unusually rapid during the early phase of childhood, but to be checked by precocious epiphyseal closure before a normal adult stature has been attained. It appears that the same sort of thing happens in children treated with testosterone. This means that although testosterone treatment causes a temporary growth spurt, it may do so at the expense of a decrease in ultimate stature.

Comments on the Use of Testosterone as a Protein Anabolic Agent in Debilitated Patients. Evidence presented in an earlier section of this chapter indicates (a) that testosterone causes protoplasmic anabolism even under conditions of negative caloric balance and debility and (b) that this protoplasmic anabolism may be at the expense of an equicaloric drain on body fat stores.

Survival of the organism may depend upon its ability to obtain enough fuel to meet its energy needs. Since the debilitated patient has usually lost most of

* The height age of a child is equal to the average chronologic age of normal children of the same height and sex.

† Taking into account the delayed effects of testosterone upon skeletal maturation rate.

his depot fat, he lacks adequate reserves of fuel to meet his energy needs. To hasten the rate at which these are expended by giving testosterone under conditions of inadequate caloric intake would appear unphysiologic and contrary to the best interests of the organism. Moreover, there is no clear evidence that testosterone treatment hastens wound-healing or causes new protoplasm to be laid down in areas of greatest need.

As discussed in Chapter VII (page 478), providing depleted subjects with an adequate caloric intake plus a reasonable protein, mineral and vitamin intake commonly leads not only to replenishment of the body's calory stores, but also to a satisfactory rate of protoplasmic anabolism and wound-healing. This physiologic means of fostering recovery is considered the therapeutic method of choice. Certainly it should be tried before resorting to testosterone.

COMMENTS ON CRYPTORCHIDISM

Cryptorchidism is usually not due to an endocrine disturbance. Although persistence of cryptorchidism into adult life results in failure of spermatogenesis, it does not interfere with testicular androgen production. When this condition has resulted in spermatic tubule degeneration, there is apt to be a compensatory increase in FSH production, as in the case of the patients of Tables 8 and 9 (see also Figure 31).

Cryptorchidism is of two chief types: (a) true cryptorchidism, or ectopic testis, and (b) pseudo-cryptorchidism.

True Cryptorchidism. In this condition normal descent of one or both testes is impeded by some mechanical lesion. The gonad may escape from the inguinal canal and become bound by adhesions in an adjacent ectopic position. Alternatively, it may be retained within the inguinal canal or abdominal cavity because of fibrous bands, short spermatic cord or other defect. Such testes fail to descend when the perineum is warmed and cannot be pushed into the scrotum by gentle digital pressure. Only rarely can they be made to descend by chorionic gonadotropin or testosterone therapy.

Cryptorchid patients often have an associated inguinal hernia which may be either microscopic or macroscopic in size. When hernia repair *per se* is indicated in a cryptorchid boy, the need for herniorrhaphy should determine the time for orchiopexy.

In the case of boys who do not have a gross hernia, therapy varies according to the clinical findings. If the undescended testis or testes can be located, but cannot be moved into normal position by manual pressure, there is little to be gained by giving hormonal therapy. Such individuals should be subjected to surgical orchiopexy before they attain adolescent status (i.e., 10 or 12 years of age). If the undescended testis cannot be found upon physical examination after application of heat to the perineum (see below under pseudo-cryptorchidism), chorionic gonadotropin may be used for differential diagnostic purposes when the patient reaches the age of 9, 10 or 11. In the case of bilateral cryptorchidism its administration will indicate whether or not the patient is suffering from anorchia (see Figure 16); in that of unilateral cryptorchidism, whether the testis is capable of natural descent.

If chorionic gonadotropin treatment fails to cause descent of the gonad, but indicates that testicular tissue is present, surgical exploration becomes indicated. Patients who show no response to the standard therapeutic test with chorionic gonadotropin are investigated as outlined above under testicular sexual infantilism.

Following orchiopexy, the prognosis is good with respect to male hormone production. On the other hand, it must be guarded with respect to spermatogenesis. Unfortunately we have no clear evidence that this guarded prognosis can be improved appreciably by early operation.

Pseudo-Cryptorchidism. By contrast pseudo-cryptorchidism is characterized by the fact that the testes are intermittently withdrawn from the scrotum into the inguinal canal by the cremasteric muscles. When these muscles are caused to relax by application of a hot water bottle to the perineum for a period of 5 to 10 minutes or by placing the patient in a hot bath for a similar period of time, the testes descend spontaneously to, or almost to, their normal scrotal position. In such cases when the patient reaches adolescence, male hormone acts to keep the testes permanently within the scrotum. This same reaction can be produced at an earlier age by chorionic gonadotropin or testosterone therapy. Descent of the testes under the influence of such therapy merely indicates that these organs would have descended spontaneously in a similar manner at a later date. Pseudo-cryptorchidism therefore requires no treatment.

REFERENCES

General References

ALLEN, E., DANFORTH, C. H. and DOISY, E. A. *Sex and Internal Secretions.* Baltimore, Williams & Wilkins, 1939.

BURROWS, H. *Biologic Actions of Sex Hormones.* 2d ed. New York, Cambridge Univ. Press, 1949.

Specific References

1 (a) MARTINS, T. and ROCHA, A. Influence de la castration, des greffes et des implantations des gonades sur le lobe antérieur de l'hypophyse. *Compt. rend. Soc. de biol.* 105:793, 1930.

(b) MC CULLAGH, D. R. and WALSH, E. L. Experimental hypertrophy and atrophy of the prostate gland. *Endocrinology* 19:466, 1935.

2   DORFMAN, R. I. Biochemistry of androgens. In *The Hormones: Physiology, Chemistry and Applications*. Vol. I. Edited by G. Pincus and K. V. Thimann. New York, Academic Press, 1948.

3 (a) KENYON, A. T., SANDIFORD, I., BRYAN, A. H., KNOWLTON, K. and KOCH, F. C. The effect of testosterone propionate on nitrogen, electrolyte, water and energy metabolism in eunuchoidism. *Endocrinology* 23:135, 1938.

(b) KENYON, A. T., KNOWLTON, K., SANDIFORD, I., KOCH, F. C. and LOTWIN, G. A comparative study of the metabolic effects of testosterone propionate in normal men and women and in eunuchoidism. *Endocrinology* 26:26, 1940.

(c) ALBRIGHT, F., PARSON, W. and BLOOMBERG, E. Cushing's syndrome interpreted as hyperadrenocorticism leading to hypergluconeogenesis: results of treatment with testosterone propionate. *J. Clin. Endocrinol.* 1:375, 1941.

4   SAMUELS, L. T. The relation of anterior pituitary hormones to nutrition. In *Recent Progress in Hormone Research*. Vol. I. Edited by G. Pincus. New York, Academic Press, 1947.

5 (a) TALBOT, N. B., BUTLER, A. M. and MAC LACHLAN, E. A. The effect of testosterone and allied compounds on the mineral, nitrogen and carbohydrate metabolism of a girl with Addison's disease. *J. Clin. Invest.* 22:583, 1943.

(b) REIFENSTEIN, E. C., JR., ALBRIGHT, F. and WELLS, S. L. The accumulation, interpretation and presentation of data pertaining to metabolic balances, notably those of calcium, phosphorus and nitrogen. *J. Clin. Endocrinol.* 5:367, 1945. Correction *ibid* 6:232, 1946.

6   BUTLER, A. M., TALBOT, N. B. and MAC LACHLAN, E. A. Effect of testosterone on concentration of potassium in serum. *Proc. Soc. Exper. Biol. & Med.* 51:378, 1942.

7 (a) HOWARD, J. E., WILKINS, L. and FLEISCHMANN, W. The metabolic and growth effects of various androgens in sexually immature dwarfs. *Tr. A. Am. Physicians* 57:212, 1942.

(b) SOBEL, E. H., RAYMOND, C. S., QUINN, K. V. and TALBOT, N. B. Relative effects of methyl testosterone upon the rate of growth and the rate of skeletal maturation of stunted children. (To be published.)

8 (a) SELYE, H. The effect of testosterone on the kidney. *J. Urol.* 42:637, 1939.

(b) SELYE, H. Effect of hypophysectomy on morphological appearance of kidney and on renotropic action of steroid hormones. *J. Urol.* 46:110, 1941.

(c) KLOPP, C., YOUNG, N. F. and TAYLOR, H. C., JR. The effects of testosterone and of testosterone propionate on renal functions in man. *J. Clin. Invest.* 24:189, 1945.

(d) KOCHAKIAN, C. D. The role of hydrolytic enzymes in some of the metabolic activities of steroid hormones. In *Recent Progress in Hormone Research*. Vol. I. Edited by G. Pincus. New York, Academic Press, 1947.

9   HAMILTON, J. B. The role of testicular secretions as indicated by the effects of castration in man and by studies of pathological conditions and the short lifespan associated with maleness. In *Recent Progress in Hormone Research*. Vol. III. Edited by G. Pincus. New York, Academic Press, 1948.

10   GESELL, A., THOMS, H., HARTMAN, F. B. and THOMPSON, H. Mental and physical growth in pubertas præcox; report of fifteen years' study of a case. *Arch. Neurol. & Psychiat.* 41:755, 1939.

11 (a) MC CULLAGH, E. P. Sex hormone deficiencies; some clinical considerations. In *Recent Progress in Hormone Research*. Vol. II. Edited by G. Pincus. New York, Academic Press, 1948.

(b) HECKEL, N. J. Production of oligospermia in a man by the use of testosterone propionate. *Proc. Soc. Exper. Biol. & Med.* 40:658, 1939.

12 (a) KLINEFELTER, H. F., JR., REIFENSTEIN, E. C., JR. and ALBRIGHT, F. Syndrome characterized by gynecomastia, aspermatogenesis without A-leydigism, and increased excretion of follicle-stimulating hormone. *J. Clin. Endocrinol.* 2:615, 1942.

(b) HELLER, C. G. and NELSON, W. O. Hyalinization of the seminiferous tubules associated with normal or failing Leydig cell function; discussion of relationship to eunuchoidism, gynecomastia, elevated gonadotropins, depressed 17-ketosteroids and estrogens. *J. Clin. Endocrinol.* 5:1, 1945.

13   DORFMAN, R. I. and HAMILTON, J. B. Urinary excretion of estrogenic substances after the administration of testosterone propionate. *Endocrinology* 25:33, 1939.

14 (a) REIFENSTEIN, E. C., JR., FORBES, A. P., ALBRIGHT, F., DONALDSON, E. C. and CARROLL, E. Effect of methyl testosterone on urinary 17-ketosteroids of adrenal origin. *J. Clin. Invest.* 24:416, 1945.

(b) GARDNER, L. I., SNIFFEN, R. C., ZYGMUNTOWICZ, A. S. and TALBOT, N. B. Follow-up studies in a boy with mixed adrenal cortical disease. *Pediatrics* 5:808, 1950.

15 (a) TALBOT, N. B., ALBRIGHT, F., SALTZMAN, A. H., ZYGMUNTOWICZ, A. S. and WIXON, R. The excretion of 11-oxycorticosteroid-like substances by normal and abnormal subjects. *J. Clin. Endocrinol.* 7:331, 1947.

16   GREULICH, W. W., DORFMAN, R. I., CATCHPOLE, H. R., SOLOMON, C. I. and CULOTTA, C. S. Somatic and endocrine studies of puberal and adolescent boys. In *Monographs of the Society for Research in Child Development.* Vol. VII. Serial no. 33, 1942.

17 (a) WEINBERGER, L. M. and GRANT, F. C. Precocious puberty and tumors of the hypothalamus; report of a case and review of literature, with pathophysiologic explanation of precocious sexual syndrome. *Arch. Int. Med.* 67:762, 1941.

(b) RUSSELL, W. O. and SACHS, E. Pinealoma; a clinico-pathologic study of 7 cases with a review of the literature. *Arch. Path.* 35:869, 1943.

18   THOMPSON, W. O. and HECKEL, N. J. Precocious sexual development from an anterior pituitary-like principle. *J. A. M. A.* 110:1813, 1938.

19 (a) FRASER, R. W., FORBES, A. P., ALBRIGHT, F., SULKOWITCH, H. W. and REIFENSTEIN, E. C., JR. Colorimetric assay of 17-ketosteroids in urine; a survey of the use of this test in endocrine investigation, diagnosis and therapy. *J. Clin. Endocrinol.* 1:234, 1941.

(b) NELSON, W. O. and HELLER, C. G. The testis in human hypogonadism. In *Recent Progress in Hormone Research.* Vol. III. Edited by G. Pincus. New York, Academic Press, 1948.

20   TALBOT, N. B. and SOBEL, E. H. Endocrine and other factors determining the growth of children. In *Advances in Pediatrics.* Vol. II. Edited by S. Z. Levine, *et al.* New York, Interscience Publishers, 1947.

21 (a) REIFENSTEIN, E. C., JR. The protein-anabolic activity of steroid compounds in man. *Transactions of the First Conference on Bone and Wound Healing; Supplement A.* New York City, Josiah Macy, Jr. Foundation, 1942.

(b) HOWARD, J. E. and JEWETT, H. J. Clinical studies with male hormone; therapeutic use of pellets of testosterone propionate. *J. Clin. Endocrinol.* 2:107, 1942.

22 (a) HUFFMAN, L. F. Interstitial cell tumor of the testicle; report of a case. *J. Urol.* 45:692, 1941.

(b) GILBERT, J. B. Studies in malignant testis tumors: syndrome of choriogenic gynecomastia; report of 6 cases and review of 129. *J. Urol.* 44:345, 1940.

(c) SIMPSON, S. L. and JOLL, C. A. Feminization in a male adult with carcinoma of the adrenal cortex. *Endocrinology* 22:595, 1938.

(d) GLASS, S. J., EDMONDSON, H. A. and SOLL, S. N. Sex hormone changes associated with liver disease. *Endocrinology* 27:749, 1940.
(e) DAVIDOFF, L. M. Studies in acromegaly; the anamnesis and symptomatology of 100 cases. *Endocrinology* 10:461, 1926.
(f) MOEHLIG, R. C. Pituitary tumor associated with gynecomastia. *Endocrinology* 13:529, 1929.
(g) STARR, R. Gynecomastia during hyperthyroidism; report of two cases. *J. A. M. A.* 104: 1988, 1935.

23 MAC COLLUM, D. W. Clinical study of spermatogenesis of undescended testicles. *Arch. Surg.* 31:290, 1935.

THE ANTERIOR PITUITARY

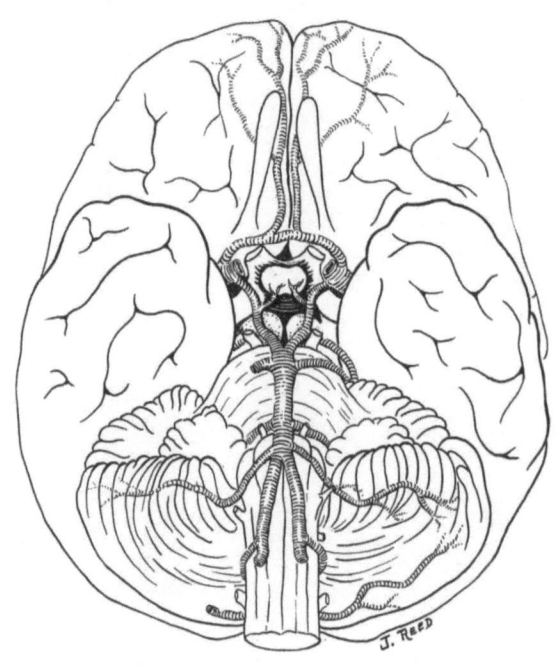

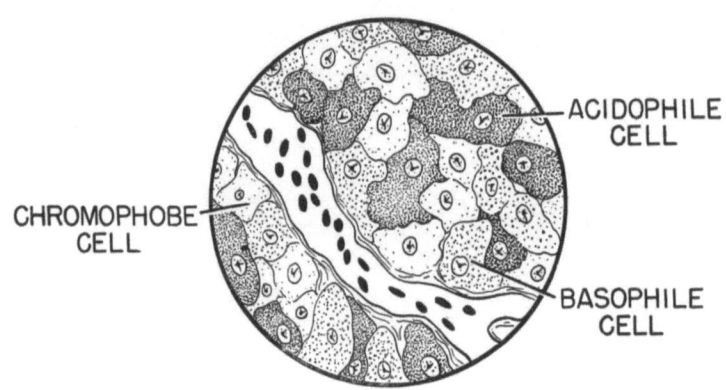

CHAPTER VII

THE ANTERIOR PITUITARY

BASIC CONSIDERATIONS

The pituitary gland is a small structure lodged in the hollow of the sella turcica of the sphenoid bone. In the adult it weighs about half a gram. It is composed of two distinctly different parts—the glandular anterior portion (adenohypophysis) and the posterior neural portion (neurohypophysis) (see Chapter VIII). Lying between these is a less-well-understood area called the pars intermedia.

The adenohypophysis arises from a long upward evagination (Rathke's pouch) of the ectoderm of the stomodeum just in front of the buccopharyngeal membrane. Normally the attachment of the epithelial portion of the pituitary to the buccal epithelium becomes attenuated and is finally broken during the prenatal period of development. Occasionally, however, islands of Rathke's pouch cells may be left resting in the pharyngeal wall or enclosed in the sphenoid bone. It is these cells which sometimes give rise to a craniopharyngioma.

The anterior pituitary contains cells of three types: acidophilic (or eosinophilic), basophilic and chromophobic. This terminology is not entirely accurate, for modern histologists do not always employ both acid and basic dyes in the differential staining of pituitary tissue. Nevertheless, it is so firmly established by long usage that it has not yet been supplanted by a more accurately descriptive one.

The two chromophilic types of adenohypophyseal cell are thought to be responsible for the production of anterior pituitary hormones; the chromophobic cells are generally considered to be endocrinologically inactive. This thesis has stemmed largely from observations on patients with eosinophilic, basophilic and chromophobic adenomas. The eosinophilic adenoma is apt to be seen in association with gigantism or acromegaly. The basophilic adenoma may be associated with evidences of Cushing's syndrome. The chromophobic adenoma characteristically fails to give rise to somatic changes suggestive of excess anterior pituitary hormone production. On the contrary, it is more likely to be accompanied by signs of hypopituitarism. These are presumed to be due to mechanical compression and hence destruction of endocrinologically active adenohypophyseal cells by the chromophobe tumor.

Table 1 indicates the names of the major types of anterior pituitary hormone and their chief actions.[1 a-c] It also indicates that most of these hormones have been considered in previous chapters of this book in connection with the target glands which fall under the control of the respective specific pituitary tropic hormones. Though only the pituitary growth hormone (PGH) is considered in detail in the present chapter, certain over-all comments concerning anterior pituitary function may be in order.

As shown in Table 1, the anterior pituitary occupies a crucial position in body economy. It elaborates hormones which profoundly influence either directly or indirectly by way of other endocrine glands almost every organ in the body. In general, the rate of growth of a structure or the activity of a gland which is under pituitary control waxes and wanes in proportion to the intensity of the pituitary stimulus. The pituitary itself, however, is also the target of various neural and humoral stimuli which inhibit or augment the activity of the adenohypophysis. Thus, the anterior pituitary is not necessarily to be considered the master organ. Rather it appears that supreme control resides in the hypothalamus of the central nervous system. It is the latter organ which determines the general level of specific pituitary activities. For example, during preadolescence the central nervous system directs the pituitary to remain quiescent with regard to gonadotropic hormone production. When adolescent age is reached, the central nervous system causes the pituitary to prompt sexual development by the production of appropriate gonadotropic hormones and of a presumably specific adrenocorticotropic hormone (see Chapter VI, Figure 9).

Once pituitary activity has been "turned on" in these regards, there develops an interrelation between pituitary-tropic-hormone production on the one hand and target-gland-hormone production on the other. If the secretory activity of the target gland is insufficient to maintain a satisfactory concentration of target gland hormone in the circulation, there is a compensatory increase in pituitary-tropic-hormone production. This is clearly illustrated in patients with gonadal failure (see Chapter V, Figure 25; Chapter VI, Figure 29). Contrariwise, when the rate of production of hormone by a target gland becomes excessive, there is a compensatory decrease in pituitary-tropic-hormone production (Chapter III, Figure 38). As a consequence of this check-and-balance mechanism, the respective concentrations of the various hormones under pituitary-tropic-hormone control are normally maintained within optimal limits. This means that the

TABLE VII—1. Types of adenohypophyseal hormones. Data from H. B. Van Dyke, *The Physiology and Pharmacology of the Pituitary Body*, Chicago, The University of Chicago Press, 1936-1939.

Name of hormone	Abbreviations	Action	Where considered
1. Thyroid-stimulating	TSH	Thyroid gland development; thyroid hormone production and secretion	Chapter I
2. Gonadotropins			
(a) Follicle-stimulating	FSH	Development of ovarian follicles; testicular spermatogenesis	Chapter V Chapter VI
(b) Luteinizing or interstitial-cell-stimulating	LH ICSH	Ovarian corpus luteum formation; testicular interstitial (Leydig) cell development; male hormone production and secretion	Chapter V Chapter VI
(c) Luteotropic		Production of progesterone by corpus luteum	Chapter V
3. Mammotropic		Mammary gland development	Chapter V
4. Adrenocorticotropins (Specific subtypes postulated, but not proved)	ACTH	Adrenocortical development; adrenocortical hormone production and secretion	Chapter III
5. Pituitary growth or somatotropic (also glycotropic?) (also renotropic?)	PGH	Body protoplasmic including skeletal growth; hyperglycemic anti-insulin action; renal function action	Present chapter

pituitary in conjunction with the hypothalamus on the one side and subsidiary target glands on the other constitutes a major bodily homeostatic mechanism.

THE PITUITARY GROWTH HORMONE (PGH)[1c]

Chemical Nature. Like other anterior pituitary hormones, PGH is a protein substance. It has now been isolated from alkaline extracts of animal pituitary tissue in crystalline, electrophoretically and isoelectrically homogenous form. Though its molecular weight (about 45,000) and physicochemical characteristics are approximately known, its exact structure has not been determined. Like many other proteins, it is destroyed by trypsin and pepsin digestion. Hence the hormone is ineffective when given by mouth. It is, however, biologically active when administered parenterally.

Physiologic Actions. In contrast with the other anterior pituitary hormones, PGH acts directly upon certain body structures rather than indirectly via subsidiary endocrine glands. Its actions may be considered under several subheadings.

Action on somatic structures and related metabolic phenomena. PGH is a protoplasmic anabolic hormone. This action is revealed by symmetrical growth of the skeleton (which has a protoplasmic framework), muscles and splanchnic organs, including the liver and thymus.[1c] It can lead to remarkable degrees of gigantism (see Figure 14) in individuals with open epiphyses and to acromegaly in mature individuals whose skeletal epiphyses have closed.

The growth-promoting effects of PGH also are reflected in metabolic measurements. There is a more positive nitrogen balance and a lowering in blood amino acid concentration. Rats treated with PGH also show a marked increase in serum inorganic phosphorus concentration* and in serum alkaline phosphatase activity. Contrary changes are observed when PGH activity is eliminated by hypophysectomy.

In the opposite sense, it is noted that young hypophysectomized animals show a marked reduction in somatic growth rate. This reduction is not eliminated by correcting the hypothyroidism and hypoadrenocorticism which occur as a result of the hypopituitarism.[2] However, it is overcome by the administration of pituitary extracts which contain the growth hormone in highly purified form.[1c]

Effects of PGH upon body composition. As mentioned above, PGH in some wise diverts dietary protein from catabolic, or energy-producing, to anabolic, or tissue-building, channels of metabolism. This results in striking differences in body composition. These can be demonstrated under a variety of experimental circumstances. Thus, it has been shown (a) that under conditions of inadequate caloric intake (negative caloric balance) hypophysectomized animals catabolize more of their body protein and less of their body fat than do intact controls,[3] (b) that under conditions of forced high caloric feeding (positive caloric balance) hypophysectomized animals anabolize less new protein, but more body fat, than intact controls and (c) that administration of PGH causes normal and hypophysectomized rats to gain more protein and less fat than do comparable controls (see Figure 1).[1c, 3]

These data indicate that even under conditions of positive caloric balance the body's synthesis of proteins is considerably limited in the absence of such an anabolic hormone as PGH (see also under protein anabolic action of testosterone, Chapter VI, page 374). Moreover, under conditions of negative caloric balance, lack of protein anabolic hormone is apt to result in increased protoplasmic catabolism.

Lack of influence of PGH upon certain structures and phenomena.[1, 2] PGH does not induce development of the thyroid, adrenal cortices, gonads or of male

---

* Adult acromegalic human patients show a similar tendency to hyperphosphatemia.[1d]

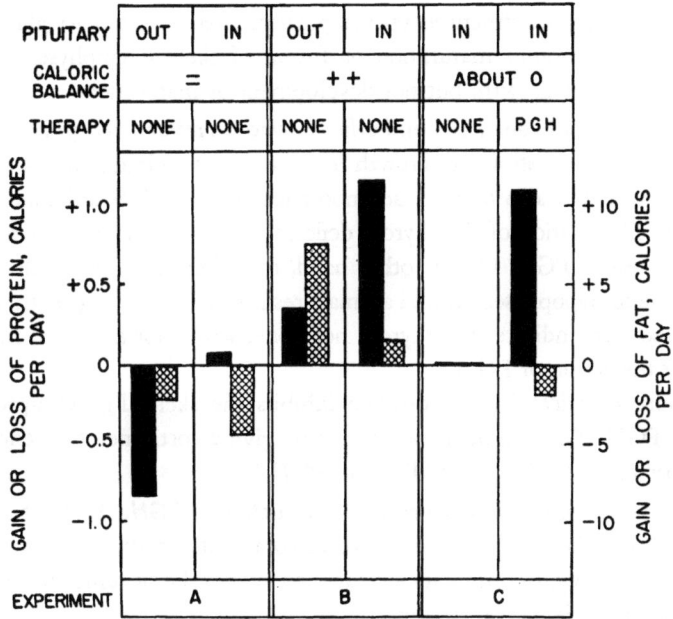

FIGURE VII—1. Effects of hypophysectomy and of pituitary (growth hormone) extract treatment upon body composition of rats. The top segment of the figure indicates whether the animals were intact or hypophysectomized. The second section indicates approximately whether the caloric balance was negative, positive or zero. Therapy is indicated in the third section. The bars indicate respective gains and losses of protein (black bar) and fat (cross-hatched bar) expressed in terms of caloric equivalent per rat per day, assuming 4 calories per gram of protein and 9 calories per gram of fat.

In Experiment A, under conditions of negative caloric balance, hypophysectomized animals lost much more protein but less fat and incidentally fewer total calories than pair-fed controls.

In Experiment B, under conditions of strongly positive caloric balance, hypophysectomized rats gained much less protein and much more fat than pair-fed intact controls.

In Experiment C, the administration of a preparation containing pituitary growth hormone caused a very considerable increase in protein storage. In these animals, which were approximately in caloric equilibrium, this gain in protein was at the expense of an approximately equicaloric loss of body fat.

The data of the above experiments are from the following sources:

Experiment A: M. Lee and G. B. Ayres: *Endocrinology*, 20:489, 1936.

Experiment B: L. T. Samuels, *Recent Progress in Hormone Research*, vol. I, New York, Academic Press, 1947.

Experiment C: F. G. Young, *Biochem. J.* 39:515, 1945.

or female accessory sex structures (penis, prostate, uterus, mammary gland, etc.). Neither does it prompt maturation or fusion of skeletal epiphyses. In other words, it promotes growth, but not development or maturation.

Interrelations between PGH and other hormones influencing growth. PGH can, as stated above, stimulate growth in hypophysectomized animals who lack not only PGH, but also thyroid, adrenocortical and, in older animals, gonadal hormones. Elimination of the thyroid deficiency in such animals increases their responsiveness to PGH. On the other hand, the administration of thyroid hormone alone to hypophysectomized animals results in very little growth acceleration. These facts indicate that thyroid hormone, while not a growth hormone, facilitates the action of PGH.[2]

The adrenocortical S-F-N hormone inhibits the skeletal-growth-promoting action of PGH. This can be demonstrated by giving cortisone or adrenocorticotropic hormone (ACTH) in addition to PGH.[4]

Factors which may influence rate of production of PGH. Lack of information makes it difficult to offer unequivocal comments on this important aspect of PGH physiology. Certain data appear, however, to be of sufficient interest to deserve at least brief consideration.

It appears that estrogenic hormone inhibits PGH production by the pituitary. This is suggested by the fact that estrogen treatment results in a marked decrease in the rate of growth of experimental animals.[5] The same phenomenon has also been noted in adolescent girls given estrogen therapy. Estrogen does not, however, prevent administered PGH from inducing accelerated somatic growth.[5] In other words, it inhibits the production, but not the action of PGH. An exception to this statement occurs when estrogen acts to cause closure of skeletal epiphyses.

Thyroid hormone also may exert some influence upon the rate of production of PGH. It is well known that primary athyrosis results in a marked slowing of growth. It also is known that athyrotic individuals can be made to grow if given PGH (see above) or testosterone (unpublished observations). In other words, it seems that the failure of athyrotic individuals to grow may be due not only to the fact that thyroid lack renders end organs less susceptible to the growth-promoting effects of PGH, but also to a diminution in the rate of production of PGH.

When thyroid-deficient individuals are rendered euthyroid by appropriate thyroid hormone substitution therapy, there follows a transient period of very rapid growth (see Chapter I). It is not known whether this is due to a release of pent-up end organ urge to grow or to a transient overproduction of PGH. Medicational thyrotoxicosis fails to result in growth acceleration. Hence, it is presumed that thyroid in excess does not favor overproduction of PGH.

Heredity, possibly acting via the hypothalamus, may play some role in determining PGH production rates. Unfortunately, objective information concerning this question is totally lacking.

Nutrition, especially caloric balance, is known to bear a systematic relation to the nitrogen balance of the growing child.[2] This is illustrated by the data of Figure 2. Here it can be seen that under conditions of constant nitrogen intake, there was a distinct tendency for the nitrogen balance to become more positive as the caloric balance was rendered more positive by the addition of non-protein calories to the diet. Under conditions of constant caloric intake, doubling the nitrogen intake had no more than a transient ($\pm$ 18-day adjustment period) influence upon the nitrogen balance. In other experiments it was found that reducing the protein intake under conditions of constant caloric intake also caused only a transient change in nitrogen balance, provided the protein intake was kept above minimum adequate levels. Whether the changes in nitrogen balance should be attributed directly to the differences in caloric balance or to changes in PGH production, as suggested in the theoretic diagrams of Figure 3, remains to be determined by direct measurements of PGH activity.

Possible influence of PGH on carbohydrate metabolism and pancreatic islet function. Extracts rich in PGH contain a substance which tends to raise blood glucose concentration.[6] It is not entirely clear whether this is actually an action of PGH or whether the glycotropism is due to another pituitary hormone with physicochemical properties so similar to those of PGH that the two cannot readily be separated. For comments on possible modes of action of this pituitary principle, see Chapter IX.

METHODS OF APPRAISING ANTERIOR PITUITARY STATUS

To indicate here in detail all the various procedures which may be used to appraise anterior pituitary status would be to repeat much of the information presented elsewhere in this volume. Figure 4 and Table 2 illustrate this fact in a summary manner. They also call attention to the fact that but few direct methods for measuring the rates of production of the various anterior pituitary hormones are available as yet. Consequently, pituitary status must to a large extent be appraised indirectly by studying the condition of the thyroid, adrenal cortices and gonads.

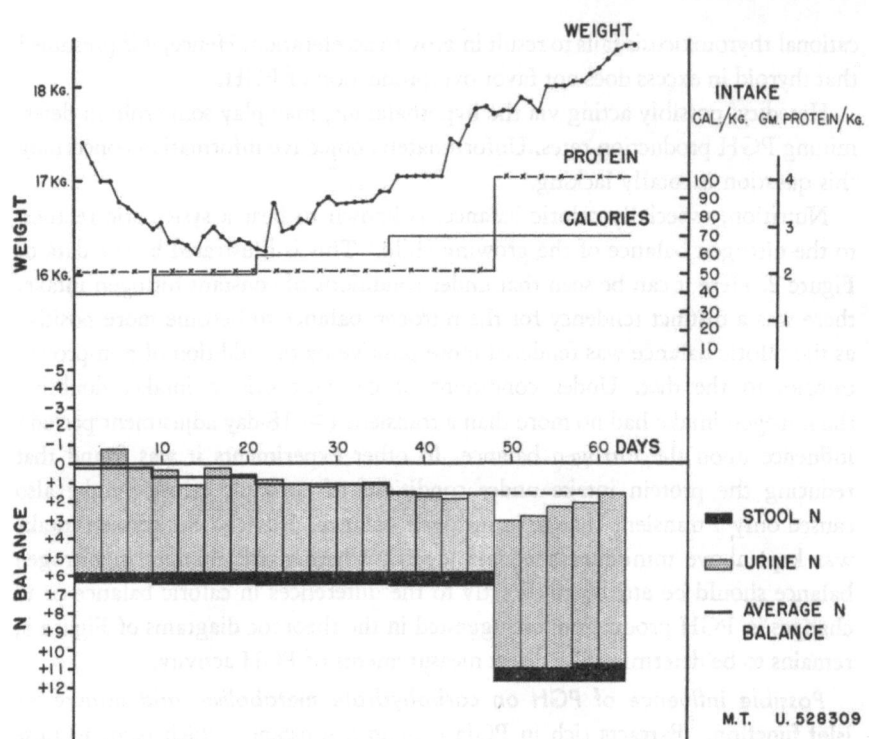

FIGURE VII—2. Relations between caloric intake, protein intake and nitrogen balance in a growing child. During the first 48 days of study the protein intake was constant at about 2 gm. per kg. per day; during the remaining period of approximately 15 days it was 4 gm. per kg. per day. During the first 36 days the caloric intake was increased stepwise from 40 to 70 calories per kg. per day. Nitrogen intake is indicated by the distance between the horizontal line intersecting the left-hand scale at zero and the bottom of the blackened area. Balance is indicated by the difference between intake and stool plus urinary nitrogen output. The average output for each interval of constant caloric intake is indicated by the solid black horizontal lines which intersect the upper portion of the shaded areas representing urinary nitrogen output. Observe that increases in caloric balance were accompanied by stepwise increases in nitrogen balance. When, during the last 15 days of study, the protein intake was doubled, there was a transient increase in nitrogen balance. However, by the last three days of this regimen, nitrogen balance was exactly the same as that observed before the increase in protein intake.

In addition to endocrine evidences of a pituitary lesion there are occasionally local manifestations of an expanding lesion in the region of the sella turcica. The commonest cause of such manifestations is the craniopharyngioma.[7] Because the local symptoms and signs of this lesion are fairly representative of those seen

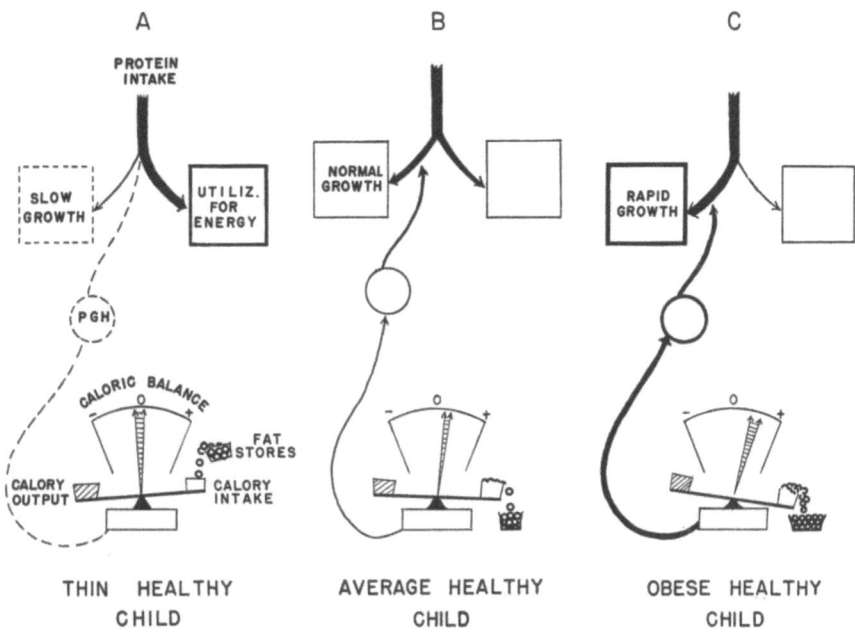

FIGURE VII—3. Diagrammatic representation of possible relations between caloric balance and pituitary growth hormone (PGH) production and protoplasmic growth rate.

SECTION A: The solid arrow at the top of the diagram indicates that protein intake can be used for either protein anabolic or energy purposes. The scale at the bottom of the diagram shows that when the caloric intake is less than the caloric output the negative balance thus produced results in an obligatory expenditure of body fat. It is suggested that under these circumstances PGH production is relatively small but sufficient to prevent the large nitrogen losses indicated in the extreme left section of Figure 1.

SECTION B: Here it is suggested that under conditions of average normal caloric intake and average normal positive caloric balance: (a) surplus calories are stored as body fat and (b) the pituitary tends to produce more growth hormone. This hormone in turn causes a larger proportion of the dietary protein to be utilized for growth purposes and correspondingly less to be used for energy production.

SECTION C: These considerations are extended here to suggest that, under conditions of strongly positive caloric balance, there is an increased stimulus to pituitary growth hormone production with resultant rapid protoplasmic growth.

---

in patients with true pituitary tumors, they are outlined in some detail below. In addition it is noteworthy that they comprise one of the commonest causes of authentic organic primary hypopituitarism.

As with pituitary adenomas, at first the commonest neurologic symptoms of

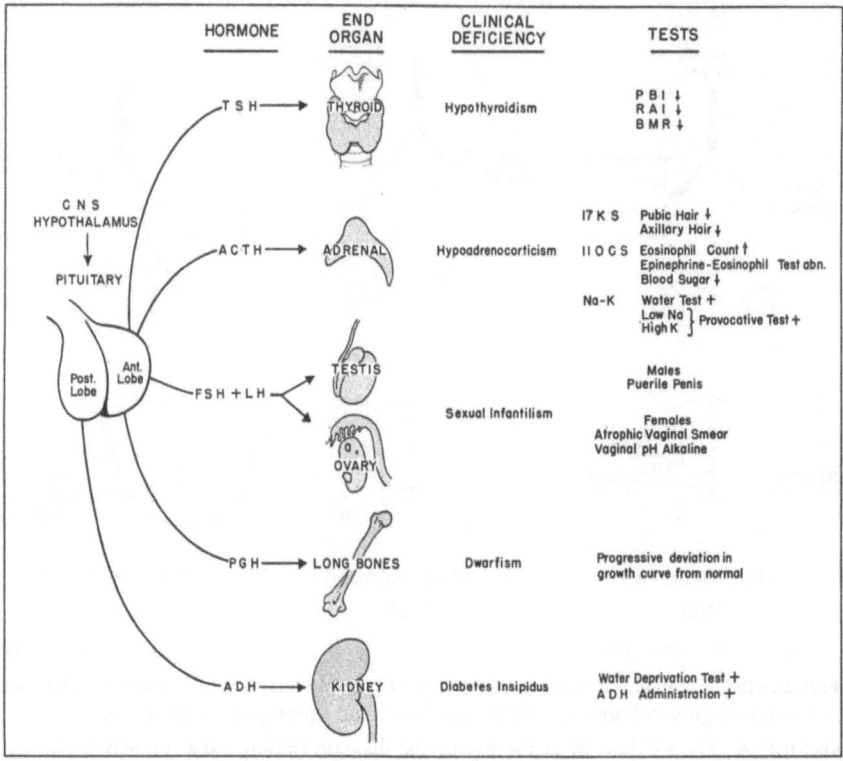

FIGURE VII—4. Diagrammatic indication of types of change noted in patients with generalized pituitary insufficiency.

craniopharyngioma are headache and vomiting. These are followed by progressive loss of vision and blindness due to pressure on the optic chiasm. When the craniopharyngioma is suprasellar, the chiasm is pushed downward and forward, so that defects of the lower quadrant visual field appear early and bitemporal hemianopsia later. When the tumor is of asymmetrical shape, right or left homonymous hemianopsia may result from one-sided optic tract damage. Less commonly, craniopharyngiomas are intrasellar or subchiasmal and expand anteriorly. Then they may press upward on the chiasm and produce various bizarre visual field defects. At times no visual field defects can be demonstrated. At others, compression of optic pathways may lead to primary optic atrophy.

When large craniopharyngioma cysts develop, they may invaginate the floor of the third cerebral ventricle, either filling its anterior portion or blocking one of the interventricular foramina. These may result in acute hydrocephalus with

TABLE VII—2. Methods of appraising anterior pituitary status, exclusive of general physical examination and of local examinations for pituitary tumor or central nervous system lesion.

Aspect of anterior pituitary function	Question of Too much	Question of Too little	Possible clinical condition	Types of diagnostic procedure used	See also
TSH	+		Thyrotoxicosis	Serum protein-bound iodine, BMR, RaI uptake Response to KI therapy	Chapter I
		+	Hypothyroidism	Serum protein-bound iodine, alkaline phosphatase, cholesterol Response to thyroid therapy	
ACTH	+		Adrenocortical virilism Precocious adrenarche	Urinary 17-KS	
	+		Cushing's syndrome	Urinary 11-17-OCS, eosinophil count	Chapter III, Table 3
		+	Hypoadrenocorticism (Hypoglycemia)	Epinephrine-eosinophil test, ACTH-eosinophil test, urinary 17-KS, CHO tests, etc.	
Gonadotropins	+		Sexual precocity Castrate	Urinary gonadotropins (FSH); gonad biopsies	
		+	Sexual infantilism	Urinary gonadotropins (FSH); in males chorionic gonadotropin test	Chapters V and VI
PGH	+		Too tall	Growth rate measurements; rule out masculine sexual precocity	Below in this chapter
		+	Too short	Growth rate measurements; rule out epiphyseal fusion, chondrodystrophy, renal disease, hypothyroidism, etc.	

signs of intracranial hypertension. In addition, or instead, irritation or destruction of various parts of the hypothalamus may lead to hyperthermia, hypersomnia, increased appetite with tendency to excessive body weight gain, diabetes insipidus or to autonomic epilepsy characterized by a mixture of sympathetic and parasympathetic reactions. If the cyst ruptures, irritating material liberated into the ventricles or subarachnoid space causes a severe aseptic ventriculitis or meningitis.

Roentgenograms of the skull aid in the diagnosis of this condition. Calcification within or above the sella turcica (see Figure 5) is observed in the majority of cases. Evidence of increased intracranial pressure (separation of sutures, convolutional atrophy, erosion of clinoid processes) and of enlargement of the sella turcica also may be seen.

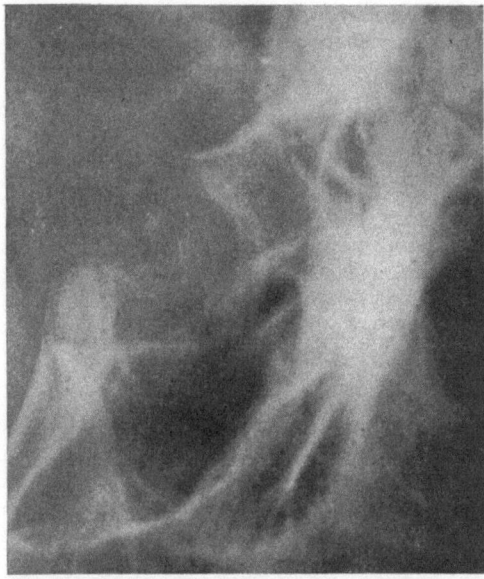
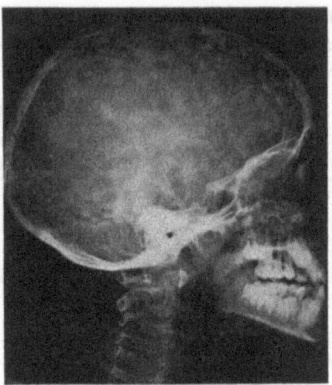

FIGURE VII—5
Craniopharyngioma.

RIGHT: Note the hammered-silver appearance of the cranium, the separation of the sutures and the erosion of the clinoid processes.
LEFT: Observe the three flecks of calcification in the region of the diaphragma sellæ.

CLINICAL CONSIDERATIONS

For reasons outlined above (see page 450), the present considerations will be limited to certain conditions not discussed elsewhere in this book.

Table 3 sets forth in outline form the types of pituitary condition which may be encountered, plus some of the causes and a partial list of corresponding clinical diagnoses. Note that there are two chief types of hypopituitarism and of hyperpituitarism. One, called the pathologic type, is characterized by the fact that the pituitary has failed as a homeostatic organ and is no longer working for the best interests of the organism. The other, called the physiologic type, is characterized by the fact that pituitary activity has been modified or altered in accordance with the needs of the body. Pathologic hypo- and hyperpituitarism can be caused either by intrinsic pituitary defects or by failure of an extrapituitary mechanism to stimulate the pituitary in accordance with physiologic requirements. On the other hand, physiologic hypo- and hyperpituitarism are always functional in nature and are brought about by the normal operations of the body's defense mechanisms.

TABLE VII—3. Outline of pituitary conditions and their causes.

Condition	Causes	Clinical diagnosis
I. Hypopituitarism A. Pathologic type: 1. Primary, organic	Destructive lesion of pituitary such as tumor (craniopharyngioma, hamartoma, dermoid, epidermoid, lipoma, ectopic pinealoma, Hand-Schüller-Christian deposits, eosinophilic granuloma), hemorrhage, infarct, infection	Hypopituitarism, pituitary dwarf, pituitary infantilism, etc.
2. Secondary, functional	Disturbance in neuro-regulatory centers (idiocy, destructive brain lesions)	Hypothalamic sexual infantilism
B. Physiologic type: 1. Secondary, functional	Primary athyrosis Caloric undernutrition	Athyrosis Anorexia nervosa; Nutritional dwarfism
II. Hyperpituitarism A. Pathologic type: 1. Primary, organic	Eosinophilic adenoma Basophilic adenoma	Pituitary gigantism Cushing's syndrome
2. Secondary, functional	Hypothalamic lesion (tumor, cyst, encephalitis, hydrocephalus, pinealoma, etc.)	True sexual precocity
B. Physiologic type: 1. Secondary, functional	Stress Caloric hypernutrition	Alarm reaction Physiologic accelerated adolescence of obesity

PATHOLOGIC HYPOPITUITARISM

Primary Organic Hypopituitarism (Simmonds' Disease).[8 a] The literature contains numerous reports of cases of presumed true, organic hypopituitarism. Relatively few of them, however, are sufficiently well documented to be considered reasonably authentic. This is an inevitable consequence of the fact that suitable procedures for appraising pituitary function in all its aspects have not been generally available.

CLINICAL MANIFESTATIONS. Patients with primary hypopituitarism fall into two chief groups. In one there are gross symptoms and signs of an expanding lesion in the region of the sella turcica; in the second, such signs and symptoms are either totally lacking or so subtle as to escape attention unless a careful search is made for them. In the former group the local manifestations of an intracranial lesion may so predominate the total clinical picture that evidences of pituitary dysfunction command only secondary attention. In the latter group, however, the manifestations of pituitary hypofunction are paramount. These two forms of this disease will be considered separately in the following paragraphs.

Hypopituitarism with signs of an expanding lesion in the region of the sella turcica (Froehlich's syndrome).[8,b] The neurologic manifestations presented by patients with an expanding lesion in the region of the sella turcica have been outlined in an earlier section (see page 456). Children with this disease tend to be considerably short for their chronologic age and to be overweight for their height (see Table 4; Figures 6 and 7). When, however, intracranial disease results in anorexia or vomiting, the patient may be cachectic rather than normally nourished or obese. In patients of advanced adolescent or older age, genital development and pubic and axillary hair growth are either totally lacking or appreciably below par. Roentgenograms reveal retardation in skeletal maturation (see Figure 8). Various special tests of endocrine function reveal changes similar to those outlined in the following section for patients with idiopathic hypopituitarism. Occasional patients may have signs of posterior pituitary insufficiency.

When signs of an expanding intracranial lesion are evident, the problem presented is largely in the neurosurgical realm. This aspect of the problem should be referred to a competent neurosurgeon. The associated endocrine problems of greatest immediate importance are apt to be with relation to the pre-, intra- and postoperative management of diabetes insipidus and of secondary hypoadrenocorticism. For a discussion of the diagnosis and management of diabetes insipidus, the reader is referred to Chapter VIII; for information concerning the diagnosis and treatment of hypoadrenocorticism secondary to primary pituitary failure, he is referred to page 469 of the following section and to Chapter III.

Hypopituitarism without signs of a lesion in the region of the sella turcica (idiopathic, primary hypopituitarism). Hypopituitary patients who lack obvious local signs of intracranial lesion usually come to the physician with retarded physical growth and development as their chief complaints. In many instances the time of onset cannot be dated accurately. Rather in such a case, the parents are apt to say that their child appeared to be normal as an infant and that retardation was not apparent until he was two or more years old. Later, he seemed to lag behind schedule in sexual development. Rarely are there complaints of mental retardation or sluggishness, of easy fatigability, constipation, sensitivity to cold weather, dizziness or faintness before breakfast (due to hypoglycemia), of gastrointestinal disturbances, renal disturbances or other such functional difficulties. This is another way of saying that these patients ordinarily lack symptoms grossly suggestive of hypothyroidism, hypoadrenocorticism or diabetes insipidus.

TABLE VII—4. Primary hypopituitarism due to authentic pituitary lesions.

Case no.	Sex	Age at onset	Age, yr.	Ht., cm.	Ht. age	Wt., kg.	Wt. age	Bone age	Sexual development	Comments
1	F	3	5	87.6	2	13.5	2½	—	—	Rathke's pouch cyst removed at 3½ yr.
See H. Cushing, *Brit. M. J.* 2:1, 48, 1927
2	F	6	9	124	7	42	12½	—	—	Bullet entered sella turcica at 6 yr.
See H. Cushing, *The Pituitary Body and Its Disorders*, Philadelphia, Lippincott, 1912; O. Madelung, *Verhandl. d. deutsch. Gesellsch. f. Chir.* 33:16, 1904
3	M	±3	7	104	4	18.2	5			Rathke's pouch cyst removed at 7 yr.
			12	114.6	5½	24.6	7½	6	—	
4	F	9	10¼	120	6½	22.2	7			Chromophobe adenoma removed; adenoma recurred
			15⅓	130.6	8	30.4	9½	8-9	—	
See H. Cushing, *Arch. Int. Med.* 51:487, 1933
5	F	8-9	12	115	5¾	20.9	6¼	Retarded	—	Calcium deposit in enlarged sella
See I. P. Bronstein, N. D. Fabricant, *Am. J. Dis. Child* 60:1140, 1940
6	F	9	14¾	142.5	10½	42.6	12½	13-14	—	Suprasellar cyst curetted at 14⅓ yr.
See E. K. Shelton, et al., *Am. J. Dis. Child* 47:719, 1934
7	F	11	18	129	8½	30	9½	Retarded	Slight	Calcification within enlarged sella; pituitary tumor at autopsy. Minimal breast development; sparse pubic hair
See J. A. Buchanan et al., *Endocrinology* 24:565, 1939
8	M	11	19	143.5	10¾	30.7	9¾	—	Infantile	Craniopharyngioma partially removed at 11 yr.
See R. W. Fraser et al., *J. Clin. Endocrinol.* 1:234, 1941
9	F	12-13	20	135	9	Mod. obesity	—	Retarded *	Slight	Calcification above and to the right of sella turcica on x-ray. Sparse pubic hair
See E. Gjörup, *Acta pædiat.* 27:508, 1940
10	F	18?	26	142.1	10½	34.2	10¾	Retarded *	Infantile	Calcified craniopharyngioma at autopsy
See J. E. Farber et al., *J. Clin. Endocrinol.* 1:688, 1941
11	M	—	46	122	6¾	37.8	12	Retarded *	—	Calcified pituitary cyst; ballooned sella turcica
See S. Buxton et al., *Brit. J. Surg.* 27:18, 1939, 1940

* Epiphyses not fused.

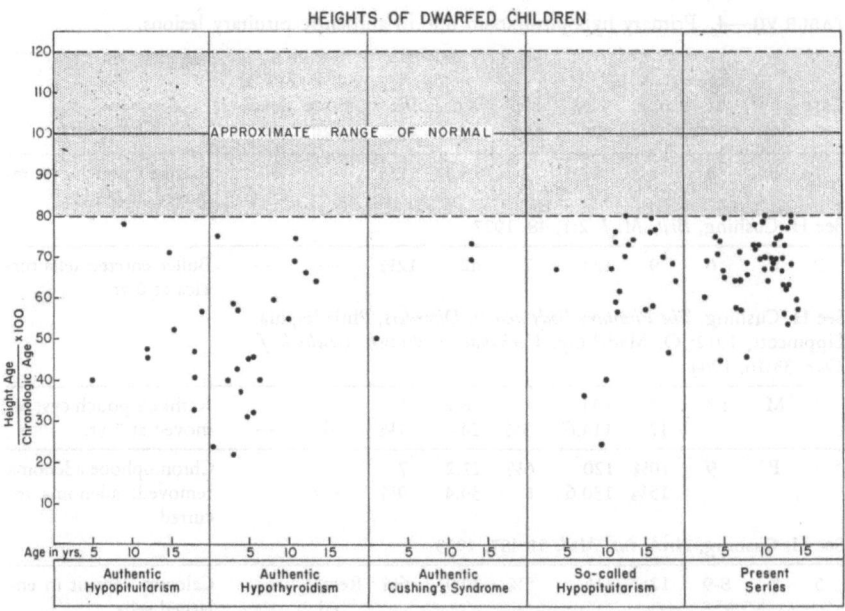

FIGURE VII—6. Heights of dwarfed children. The height age of a child is found by determining the average age of normal children of the same height and sex. Note the consistent tendency to dwarfism in patients with authentic hypopituitarism. Similar degrees of dwarfism may be observed in children with hypothyroidism, Cushing's syndrome, so-called hypopituitarism (i.e., the diagnosis was presumptive) and in children suffering from caloric undernutrition (indicated by the term "present series"). From N. B. Talbot, E. H. Sobel, B. S. Burke, E. Lindemann and S. B. Kaufman, *New Eng. J. Med.* 236:783, 1947.

In fact, they usually seem quite healthy aside from their developmental retardation.

PHYSICAL EXAMINATION. Many of these children have a subtly similar appearance (see Figure 9); like the patients of Table 4, they are markedly and symmetrically short for their age and are usually overweight for their height. Their faces have a full, rather youthful shape. The head is of normal size, the hair of normal texture. Examination of the eyes, including extra-ocular movements, eyegrounds and visual or confrontation fields, reveals no abnormalities. Dentition is sometimes retarded. The tongue is of normal size, the voice of normal juvenile quality. The thyroid may or may not be barely palpable; it is not goitrous. Examination of the lungs, heart, blood pressure and abdomen yields negative results. There is little if any adolescent development of the secondary sex organs; pubic, axillary and leg hair growth is very sparse or absent. The

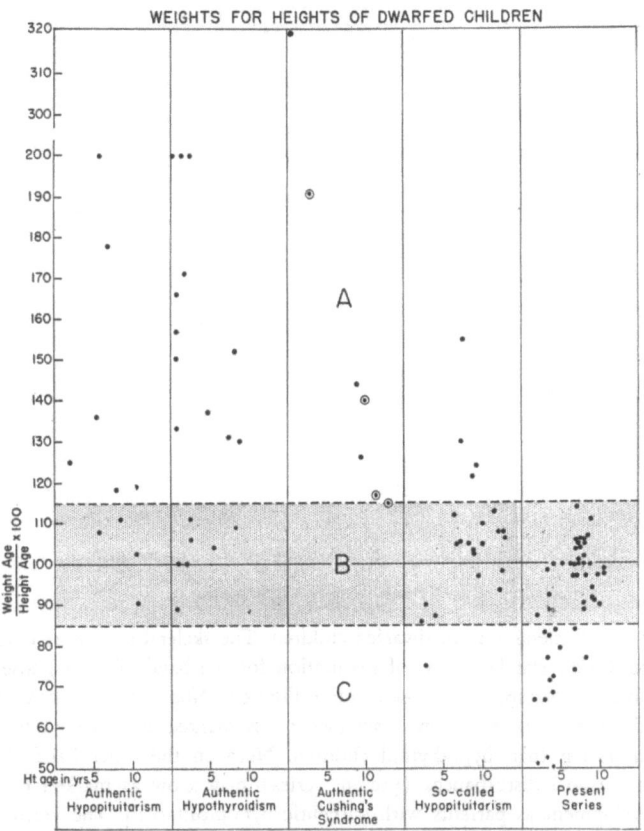

FIGURE VII—7. Weights of various types of dwarfed children. Area A includes patients considered to be overweight for their height; area B includes patients whose weight is within normal limits for height; area C includes patients who are underweight for height. The circled points represent children with Cushing's syndrome who were not dwarfed and so emphasize the fact that there is a tendency to be overweight in this condition. From N. B. Talbot, E. H. Sobel, B. S. Burke, E. Lindemann and S. B. Kaufman, *New Eng. J. Med.* 236:783, 1947.

skin, while warm and moist, is likely to be of a fine, soft, smooth texture, comparable to that seen in infants and young children. It is free from acne, and there is no odor to the axillary sweat as in normal adolescents and adults. On the other hand, it sometimes has a yellowish hue due to hypercarotenemia.

LABORATORY STUDIES. Routine tests of blood, urine and stools give essentially normal results. The serum total protein, non-protein nitrogen, inorganic

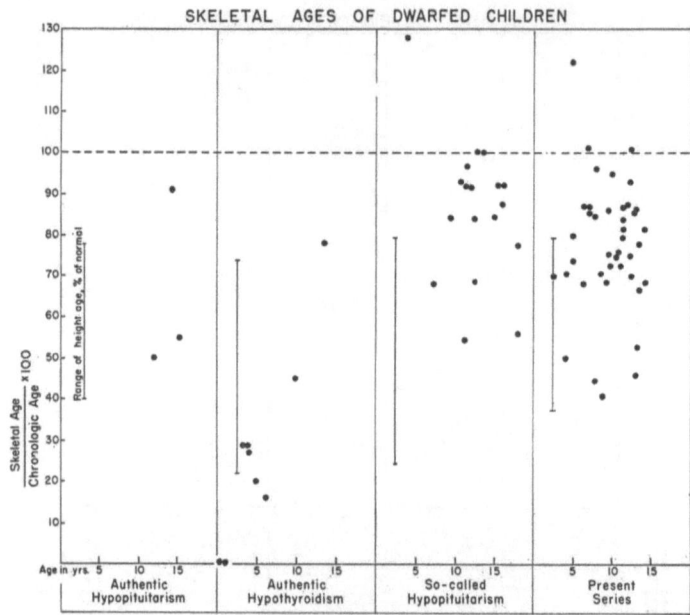

FIGURE VII—8. Skeletal ages of dwarfed children. The skeletal ages were determined by reference to Todd's standard atlas of maturation for the hand. The diagnoses indicated along the abscissa correspond to those given in Figure 6. Note that patients with authentic or so-called hypopituitarism show a somewhat less marked tendency to retardation in skeletal maturation than hypothyroid children. Note on the other hand that patients suffering nutritional disturbances (present series) may show as marked retardation in skeletal development as patients with authentic hypopituitarism. The vertical lines appearing in each section indicate the range in height age (expressed as per cent of average normal) for the patients whose bone ages are represented in that section. From N. B. Tablot, E. H. Sobel, B. S. Burke, E. Lindemann and S. B. Kaufman, *New Eng. J. Med.* 236:783, 1947.

phosphorus, total calcium, sodium, potassium, chloride and bicarbonate concentrations usually are within normal limits. Roentgenograms commonly reveal that skeletal development is retarded (usually by three or more years) with relation to normal for chronologic age. Very occasionally epiphyseal dysgenesis is found (see Chapter I, Figure 3).

Tests to determine endocrine status. The appropriate tests for determining endocrine status in relation to hypopituitarism are summarized in Figure 4 and Table 2. Here it is indicated that no clinical method for appraising *PGH status* other than by body growth measurements is available as yet. Appraisal of such measurements is greatly facilitated by use of a growth chart such as that shown

The Anterior Pituitary

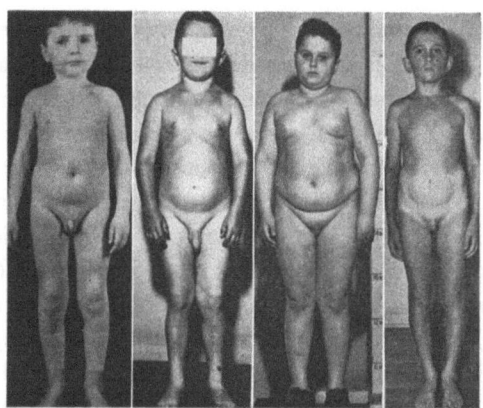

FIGURE VII—9. Idiopathic hypopituitarism in male patients of various ages (left to right: 11, 15, 15 and 24 years). All these individuals were dwarfed and sexually puerile but well-nourished and alert. Compared with adults with panhypopituitarism they appear disconcertingly healthy; they are not juvenile replicas of the pale, lethargic, parchment-skinned adult with Simmond's disease.

---

in Figure 1 of the Appendix. *TSH status* is evaluated indirectly with the aid of such indices of thyroid gland function (Chapter I) as the serum protein-bound iodine measurement, which may be slightly subnormal; serum carotenoids, which may be abnormally elevated; serum cholesterol, which is most commonly within normal limits, but which may be abnormally elevated as in primary athyrosis; and serum alkaline phosphatase activity, which is apt to be within normal limits rather than abnormally low as in most cases of primary athyrosis. In the absence of TSH, radioactive iodine uptake by the thyroid is abnormally low. *ACTH status* is appraised with the aid of certain tests indicated in Table 3 of Chapter III. The epinephrine-eosinophil test gives results indicative of either anterior pituitary or adrenocortical failure. The urinary output of 17-KS and of 11-17-OCS-like substances tends to be abnormally low.* By means of the ACTH test one can determine whether the difficulty lies within the pituitary rather than the adrenal cortices. Application of the insulin tolerance test may yield some additional information. Both adrenocortical S-F-N hormone and pituitary glycotropic hormone lack tend to render patients unusually sensitive to the hypoglycemic effects of a standard dose of insulin.[8c] The insulin tolerance test is listed in Table 3 of Chapter III. *Gonadotropin status* is evaluated both by inspection of the patient for signs of sexual development and by measurements of urinary gonadotropin output (see

---

* These tests, particularly the former, are of less value in patients under 12 years of age than in older patients (Chapter III, Figure 13).

Chapters V and VI). It must be remembered, however, that the latter are sometimes misleading. Dr. Fuller Albright has observed high urinary gonadotropin values in menopausal women with extensive destructive lesions of the anterior pituitary gland. Apparently small remnants of pituitary tissue can secrete considerable amounts of gonadotropin (100 mouse units per day).

DIFFERENTIAL DIAGNOSIS. Table 5 lists the major conditions which, like hypopituitarism, may result in stunted growth. The conditions bearing the closest resemblance to primary idiopathic hypopituitarism are (a) short stature in an otherwise normal individual, (b) physiologic retarded adolescence in a healthy child, (c) short stature in association with ovarian agenesis and (d) functional hypopituitarism secondary to malnutrition, hypothyroidism, hypothalamic or other chronic debilitating disturbances (see below).

TREATMENT. The problem of treating hypopituitary patients can be approached from two points of view: (a) pituitary hormone and (b) pituitary target-gland hormone therapy. The former may be considered direct, the latter indirect substitution therapy. These two methods of treatment are considered briefly in the following paragraphs.

Pituitary hormone therapy. If perfectly accomplished, pituitary hormone therapy would cause a return to normal of thyroid, adrenocortical and gonadal function. In addition it should provide the organism with optimal amounts of PGH. Until very recently it was practically impossible to attain this goal, since no potent pituitary hormone preparations suitable for clinical use could be obtained. At present adrenocorticotropic hormone (ACTH) preparations of well-standardized potency are generally available. Efforts also are being made to produce clinically effective thyrotropic, gonadotropic and pituitary growth preparations; these are available only in small amounts for special study purposes.

A substance with properties like those of the pituitary testicular interstitial-cell-stimulating hormone (ICSH), namely human urinary chorionic gonadotropin, has been on the market for some time. Like pituitary hormones, it must be given parenterally to be effective. This method of administration and its relatively high cost have limited its use to short-term therapeutic test procedures (see Chapter VI, page 428). For long-term maintenance, the tendency has been to give gonadal hormones, which can be taken by mouth (see below and Chapter VI).

Pituitary target-gland hormone therapy. It is usually possible to eliminate the most distressing manifestations of pituitary gland failure by means of appropriate target-gland substitution therapy as considered in the following paragraphs.

Caution should be used in administering *thyroid hormone* to persons having or suspected of having primary hypopituitarism, since in this condition full therapeutic doses can produce hypoadrenocorticism with fatal outcome (see Chapter III, Figure 37). Serious difficulties are not likely to develop if the response to the epinephrine-eosinophil test is normal, but in any case they can be avoided by starting medication at a very low level—namely 6 to 9 mg. of USP thyroid per m^2 per day. This is approximately one-tenth of the estimated maintenance dose required by a patient with primary athyrosis. If the initial dose is well tolerated for a period of two weeks, it may be increased by an equal amount and the patient observed for another two weeks. Similar stepwise increments in dosage can be made up to the point where the patient either is taking a full maintenance dose or has begun to develop such signs of intolerance as weakness, faintness, dizziness, pallor, excess weight loss or nutritional disturbances (see also under hypoadrenocorticism, Chapter III).

Concerning the desirability of using thyroid medication, the following may be said. It is sometimes very difficult to distinguish between patients with primary hypopituitarism and secondary hypothyroidism on the one hand and patients with primary hypothyroidism and secondary hypopituitarism on the other. This diagnostic problem is encountered most often in patients of adolescent and older age; it is not so apt to be found in younger individuals. One of the simplest and surest ways to make a *differential diagnosis* is to give thyroid hormone and observe its effect upon the patient. If the patient is suffering from simple, primary hypothyroidism, definite improvement will become evident within three to six months (see Chapter I). By contrast, if the patient has primary hypopituitarism, he will show only vague and indefinite improvement or develop some of the untoward manifestations mentioned above. In the former instance, continuation of the thyroid medication at full-dose levels is clearly indicated. In the latter instance, it usually appears that thyroid hormone treatment had best be reduced and continued only if it appears to have some beneficial influence.

Patients with primary hypopituitarism usually do not need chronic maintenance treatment with *adrenocortical hormones*. On the other hand, the adrenocortical hormone requirements of hypopituitary patients increase under certain conditions (e.g., severe infection, a major operation such as removal of a craniopharyngioma or thyroid therapy). Since a patient with primary hypopituitarism has a limited ability to produce ACTH and hence to increase adrenocortical secretory activity in accordance with need, he may develop signs of acute hypoadrenocorticism during periods of unusual stress. Such hypoadrenocorticism is recognized and combatted as outlined in Chapter III.

As hypopituitary patients reach middle or late adolescent age, *gonad-hormone substitution therapy* becomes indicated. In boys methyl testosterone by mouth

TABLE VII—5. Causes of short stature.

Condition	Alternate name	Indicated by
A. Genetic (page 475)	Hereditary short stature	Family history and absence of other abnormalities
B. Nutritional insufficiency		
1. Starvation (page 473)	Nutritional dwarf	History and physical examination
2. Steatorrhea (page 86)	Celiac syndrome; pancreatic fibrosis	Fatty stools; absence of duodenal enzymes
3. Diabetes mellitus (page 577)		Glycosuria; glucose intolerance
C. Hypothalamic disturbance		
1. Organic lesion (page 462)	Froehlich's syndrome	Suprasellar calcification; erosion of clinoids; visual field changes
2. Congenital defect (page 472)	Laurence-Moon-Biedl syndrome	Low IQ; obesity; retinitis pigmentosa; polydactylism
3. True precocious puberty (pages 321, 408)		History of early sexual development; closure of skeletal epiphyses
D. Hypopituitarism, anterior (page 462)	Pituitary dwarf	Epinephrine-eosinophil test; signs of sexual infantilism; hypothyroidism, etc.
E. Hypopituitarism, posterior (page 520)	Diabetes insipidus	Polydipsia; polyuria; inability to concentrate urine without becoming dehydrated
F. Hypothyroidism (page 14)	Cretinism; juvenile myxedema	General retardation of somatic and skeletal development; low PBI, hypercarotenemia; low alkaline p-ase, etc.
G. Hyperparathyroidism		
1. Primary (page 122)		Serum Ca +, P −
2. Secondary (page 82)	Vit. D lack rickets	Serum Ca normal or −, P −, alk. p-ase +; x-ray changes
	Renal rickets	Same as above plus signs of renal impairment with NH_4Cl tolerance −, urea clearance −, etc.
H. Hyperadrenocorticism		
1. Excess S-F-N hormone (page 235)	Cushing's syndrome	Buffalo obesity; chronic eosinopenia; urinary 11-17-OCS +
2. Abnormal androgen production (page 234)	Adrenocortical virilism	Urinary 17-KS+ ; 17-KS pattern abnormal; precocious epiphyseal closure

TABLE VII—5 (continued)

Condition	Alternate name	Indicated by
I. Primary skeletal defects		
1. Ovarian agenesis (page 344)	Ovarian dwarfism	High urinary FSH; signs of ovarian estrogen action lacking
2. Pseudo-hypoparathyroidism (page 111)		Serum Ca −, P +, x-ray changes
3. Chondrodystrophies*		X-ray changes
4. Osteogenesis imperfecta*		X-ray changes
J. Miscellaneous		
1. Galactosemia, galactosuria (page 552)		Special urine sugar test
2. Glycogen storage (page 580)	von Gierke's disease	Epinephrine-glucose tolerance test
3. Cardiac, intestinal, hepatic or renal insufficiency*		
4. Chronic infection*		History and physical examination
5. Sex hormone therapy		History of therapy; precocious closure of epiphyses
6. Progeria†		Physical examination as per Chapter VI, Figure 6

*See D. J. McCune. *Clinics* 2:380, 1943.
†See N. B. Talbot, A. M. Butler, E. L. Pratt, E. A. MacLachlan and J. Tannheimer. *Am. J. Dis. Child.* 69:267, 1945.

TABLE VII—6. Causes of tall stature.

Condition	Indicated by	See page
A. Pituitary gigantism	Changes in visual fields, eyegrounds, sella turcica, etc.	481
B. Functional or hereditary tall stature	Family history; and absence of signs of organic disease	492
C. True precocious puberty	Normal sexual development occurring at abnormally early age	321, 408
D. Pseudo-precocious puberty	Accelerated sexual development	
1. Testicular type	Unilateral testicular tumor	418
2. Adrenal type	Pseudo-hermaphroditism or masculinization in girls; masculinization without testicular development in boys	224
3. Ovarian type	Precocious feminine development plus tumor in ovary	330

causes a satisfactory degree of masculine development (see Chapter VI). In girls stilbestrol is ordinarily sufficient to bring about definite evidences of feminization within a few months (see Chapter V).

Comments on the promotion of growth in hypopituitary patients. PGH substitution therapy is not as yet clinically practicable. This is unfortunate, for PGH is the only agent known to be capable of stimulating growth without at the same time accelerating skeletal maturation.

The only other available growth-promoting agent is testosterone. As described in Chapter VI, this hormone not only causes an increase in the growth rate, but also considerable acceleration in skeletal maturation. The latter action may so shorten the patient's growth period that he can never attain even the minimum normal adult stature (see Chapter III, Figure 46). Testosterone is therefore of dubious value as a growth-promoting agent. Moreover, girls become masculinized when treatment is continued for more than a few months. Estrogenic hormone fails to prompt as much of a growth spurt as testosterone, but shares with this androgen the tendency to accelerate skeletal maturation. Thyroid therapy likewise fails to prompt an increase in the growth rate of hypopituitary patients.

PROGNOSIS. It is difficult to predict the outcome in the case of patients treated for primary organic hypopituitarism until they are between 20 and 25 years. If they have shown no signs of spontaneous remission by then, it is probable that they never will. Up to that time, however, there is at least a remote possibility that certain patients will spontaneously grow and mature in a nearly normal manner.[8e] If they do not undergo such a spontaneous remission, the tendency is toward permanent somatic infantilism unless substitution treatment with sex hormones is undertaken. Therapy with these hormones produces a sterile dwarf of mature appearance. The intellect is not grossly impaired.

Secondary Functional Hypopituitarism. This condition is presumed to exist in certain patients who show in addition to signs of pituitary failure gross mental deficiency (as in the Laurence-Moon-Biedl syndrome), cerebral agenesis or other severe type of central nervous system lesion. Obesity, hypogonadism, polydactylism, retinitis pigmentosa, or enlarged parietal foramina and microphthalmos are likely to be present.[9] It is included here mostly for purposes of classification. The clinical manifestations are as described above for patients with primary hypopituitarism without signs of a lesion in the region of the sella turcica.

PHYSIOLOGIC HYPOPITUITARISM

Various extrapituitary factors may lead to a functional decrease in pituitary activity. Two examples of this condition are considered below.

Hypopituitarism Secondary to Primary Athyrosis. This condition is identical with that described under the heading of primary athyrosis in Chapter I. Difficulties in distinguishing it from primary hypopituitarism are encountered most often in patients of adolescent age (see above under treatment with thyroid hormone).

Hypopituitarism Secondary to Undernutrition (Starvation and Anorexia Nervosa). Prolonged periods of inadequate dietary intake can result in signs of decreased pituitary activity.[2, 8a, 10] The intensity of the signs tends to be roughly proportional to the degree of caloric undernutrition. This condition may arise from such widely variable causes as poverty, emotional anorexia, intestinal insufficiency and chronic illness.

CLINICAL MANIFESTATIONS. The signs and symptoms may likewise vary, depending upon the nature of the underlying cause and the degree of deprivation. Surveys of the dietary intake of a representative group of children of the type under consideration reveal that the outstanding nutritional defect may be caloric lack. When this is so, clinical signs of protein, mineral and vitamin deficiency are not present. When the malnutrition is due to famine or chronic intestinal deficiency, multiple nutritional defects are to be expected.

Most commonly children with functional hypopituitarism secondary to undernutrition are abnormally small and moderately thin (Figures 6, 7 and 10). The thinness is evidenced by their lack of subcutaneous tissue as well as by the fact that they tend to be underweight for height (see Figure 7). They are otherwise healthy in appearance, alert and active. Routine clinical study usually fails to reveal significant organic disturbances in any of the body systems (brain, heart, lungs, kidneys, gastrointestinal tract, skeleton, exocrine or endocrine glands) although skeletal and sexual maturation may be retarded (see Figure 8).

In contrast to the foregoing, patients with severe malnutrition show much more marked clinical changes (see Figure 12). The patient is thin, gaunt and listless. He has lost all sense of humor. Constipation is sometimes severe. Body temperature falls to subnormal levels; rectal readings as low as 94°F. have been recorded. The pulse is slowed to about 40 beats per minute. The blood pressure is at low normal levels. The skin is cool, rough and dry. Sexual development is arrested.

LABORATORY TESTS. In patients with dietary deficiencies the epinephrine-eosinophil and insulin tolerance tests usually give normal results (see Chapter III, Table 3).[8] The serum protein-bound (thyroid hormone) iodine concentration either is within normal limits or is slightly subnormal. The urinary 17-KS output values of patients over 13 or 14 years of age are lower than normal for age, but average higher (i.e., $>$ 1 mg. per day) than those seen in patients with

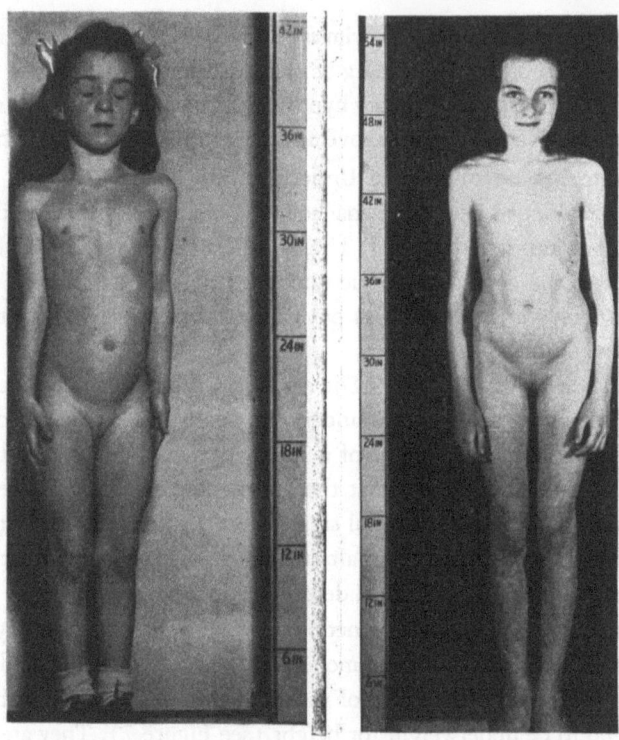

FIGURE VII—10. Functional hypopituitarism secondary to caloric undernutrition with retarded growth and maturation in two physically and mentally healthy girls. Both patients gained, grew and matured satisfactorily following improvement in caloric intake.
LEFT: Actual age 7 years, height age 3½, weight age 2, bone age 6 years.
RIGHT: Actual age 15½ years, height age 12, weight age 10, bone age 13 years. Serum protein-bound iodine 6 μ per cent; 17-KS 3 mg. per 24 hours; urinary gonadotropin (FSH) 6.5 mouse units per 24 hours. Note the paucity of subcutaneous tissue.

primary athyrosis and primary hypopituitarism. In patients of adolescent age the urinary gonadotropic hormone (FSH) output may be more (3 mouse units per day) than zero, but less than normal. In association with these findings there may be minimal clinical evidence of early sexual development (penile and testis growth in the male; vaginal pH and cell changes plus mammary development in the female).

DIAGNOSIS. The diagnosis is a presumptive one and is arrived at by a process of exclusion. It is not tenable in the case of patients who are obviously well-nourished and overweight for height. Neither is it logical in the case of patients who have signs of a destructive lesion in the brain. However, patients with

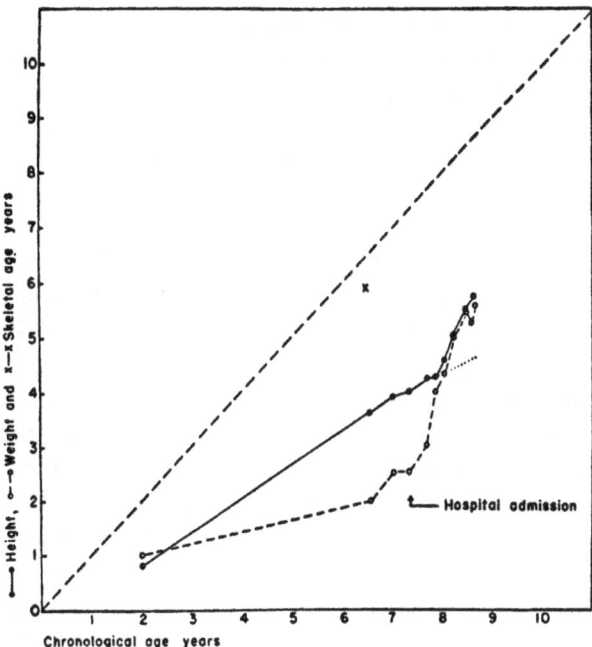

FIGURE VII—11. Growth in height and gain in weight of a child (Figure 10, left) with nutritional dwarfism before and after hospital admission, when dietary intake was increased. Results are expressed as height age (black circles connected by solid line) and weight age (white circles connected by interrupted line) plotted according to the scale of the ordinate against chronologic age (abscissa). One measurement of skeletal age is represented (x). The diagonal dash line indicates where the weight age and skeletal age symbols should fall if the patient were average normal for age and sex. Note that about six months following a marked increase in the rate of weight gain there was a correspondingly marked increase in the rate of height gain. From N. B. Talbot, E. H. Sobel, B. S. Burke, E. Lindemann and S. B. Kaufman, *New Eng. J. Med.* 236:783, 1947.

various organic diseases of the central nervous system sometimes develop a clinical picture which is superficially indistinguishable from that seen in patients with advanced anorexia nervosa. The diagnosis in such cases may depend upon the performance of a lumbar puncture or pneumoencephalogram.

Hereditary small stature[8 d] and hereditary tendencies to normal but relatively retarded adolescence may be very difficult to distinguish from functional hypopituitarism secondary to caloric malnutrition. Valid differentiation can be had only by observing the effects of higher caloric feeding.

Primary hypopituitarism usually can be ruled out by application of the epinephrine-eosinophil and insulin tolerance tests. In mildly to moderately undernourished patients gross signs of thyroid deficiency are totally lacking. The administration of thyroid hormone to such patients produces neither good nor bad effects. In cases of severe depletion reduction of thyroid function of moderate degree may occur as a result of homeostatic adjustments. Such a reduction in thyroid activity is considered normal for the circumstances even though it is accompanied by many of the symptoms and signs of ordinary, primary hypothyroidism. Primary hypothyroidism can be ruled out either by observing the patient's response to an adequate dietary intake or by performing radioactive iodine uptake studies. As discussed in Chapter I, it is considered inadvisable to give thyroid hormone treatment for diagnostic purposes to patients with marked evidences of caloric undernutrition.

Careful studies of patients with apparent caloric malnutrition and presumed functional hypopituitarism reveal that a small percentage are suffering from renal disturbances. These may be so subtle as to escape attention unless urea clearance and other tests of renal tract status are carried out (see Chapter II). One patient was found to have cystinuria. Others have had advanced pyelonephritis, some with calculus formation. In still others conditions involving various body systems have been discovered. On these accounts it is believed that the abnormally small, thin child should be subjected to a thorough medical check-up.

TREATMENT. When hypopituitarism is due simply to caloric lack, it can be assumed that any observed deviations in endocrine gland activity are of a homeostatic rather than of a pathologic nature. The problem therefore is not primarily an endocrine one, but lies in the areas of nutrition, economics, emotions or genetics. When the caloric undernutrition is due to poverty or poor planning, its correction is apt to require social services; when due to emotional disturbances, the aid of a child psychiatrist may be needed. In a small percentage of these patients the latter may be able to eliminate emotional anorexia with relatively little effort. In the remaining cases a great deal of intense psychiatric work may be required to make any progress whatsoever.

Presently available PGH preparations are of no value. The clinical usefulness of the more refined and potent extracts currently being developed remains to be demonstrated.

PROGNOSIS. Even in cases of severe anorexia nervosa, resumption of normal feeding habits is followed by a rapid gain in weight and by rapid disappearance of listlessness, hypothermia, bradycardia and other changes. In due course complete physical and functional normalcy is attained. But if the anorexia persists, the outcome may be fatal.

In cases of mild-to-moderate undernutrition, the outlook is less forbidding. When economic or emotional factors can be found and eliminated, a rapid

The Anterior Pituitary

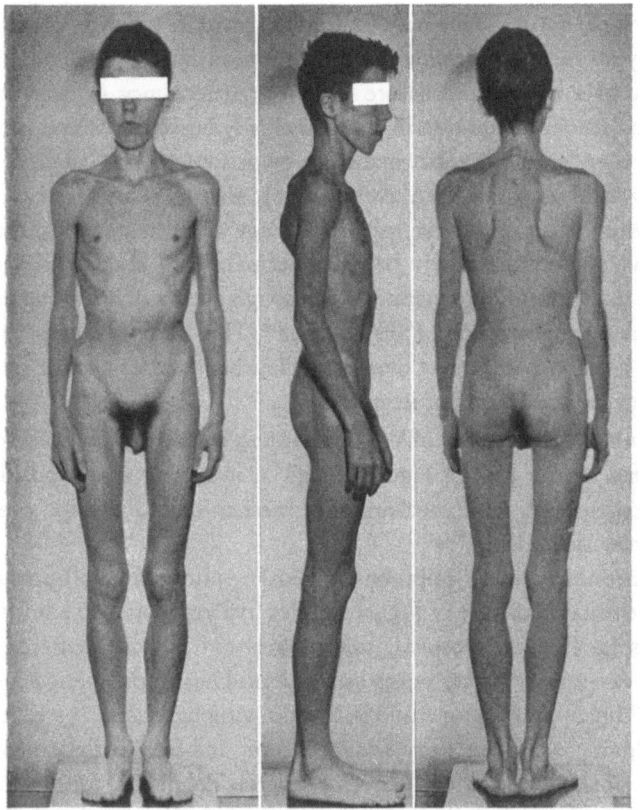

FIGURE VII—12. Anorexia nervosa in a boy of 14 years.

CASE HISTORY

The patient was apparently well until the age of 13, when he became mentally depressed and lost his appetite. During the three months prior to hospitalization he became lethargic and very constipated. Although he had weighed 46 kg. and measured 140 cm. at age 13½, when first seen at our clinic, he weighed 33 kg. and measured 156 cm. On physical examination, he presented the appearance shown in the figure. His temperature was 94° by mouth, pulse 42 and blood pressure 90/70; his respirations were 16. His motions and speech were slow; his skin was cool, dry and of coarse texture. Laboratory studies indicated normal renal function, serum protein, NPN and electrolyte values. An epinephrine-eosinophil test gave normal results. The 17-KS output was 4 mg. per 24 hours. Serum protein-bound iodine (4.3 gamma per cent) and radio-active iodine uptake were normal. The BMR was −46 per cent. All other findings were essentially negative. He was successfully persuaded to eat more while in the hospital. Following this he began to gain weight rapidly and to lose the physical and functional manifestations of extreme undernutrition.

gain in weight occurs. This may be followed within a period of six to twelve months by an increase in growth and maturation rates (see Figure 11). Even if nothing of a therapeutic nature is done, the tendency in mild cases is for growth and sexual maturation to progress slowly but surely. Occasional patients of this type undergo a late but marked growth spurt during adolescence; some eventually attain a taller than average adult stature. The majority, however, stop growing before they have reached average adult height. In most instances sexual development ultimately becomes normal. Very occasionally, girls grow to normal stature but fail to mature, even though eventually showing abnormally high urinary gonadotropin (FSH) output.* This finding suggests either that they were born with imperfect ovaries or that their ovaries became permanently damaged during the period of inanition.

Note on the Acceleration of Wound-healing by Increasing Caloric Balance. As indicated by the data of Figures 1 and 2, it is clear that a positive caloric balance acts through some mechanism or mechanisms to prompt a tendency to protoplasmic anabolism.

This phenomenon has important clinical application as illustrated by the severely debilitated patient of Figure 13. For five years prior to admission to the Massachusetts General Hospital, this ten-year-old boy had suffered from the results of extensive thermal burns on his legs. During this period he was subjected to 25 skin-grafting operations, mostly without success. As time went on, despite a high protein diet, heavy chemotherapy and frequent plasma and whole blood transfusions, he gradually became severely debilitated for lack of calories. Not only did skin grafts fail to take, but donor sites began to slough. When first seen here, a major portion of his back (from which skin for grafting purposes had been taken) was a raw mass of infected granulation tissue. Examination revealed the boy to be reduced almost literally to skin and bones. It was therefore obvious that he had gradually burned up almost all his caloric stores (fat and protein) because of caloric undernutrition and that he had lost all capacity for wound-healing as a result. Accordingly, he was placed on a high caloric regimen.† At first, it was necessary to use tube-feeding. Later he was able to take adequate amounts of food by mouth. Within a few days after the high caloric regimen was started, the wounds commenced to take on a healthier appearance. Within

---

* Dr. Fuller Albright had encountered four such patients.

† The high caloric mixture employed had the following composition per liter: evaporated milk 600 cc.; 40 per cent cream 40 cc.; vegetable puree 35 cc.; two eggs; Karo syrup 70 gm.; brewer's yeast 7 gm.; sodium chloride 3.5 gm. water q.s. ad 1,000 cc. This mixture had a caloric value of about 1,450 calories per liter. Initially the patient was given about 800 calories per m^2 per day. At approximately three-day intervals the intake was increased by 400 calories per m^2 until an intake of about 2,000 calories per m^2 per day was reached.

The Anterior Pituitary [479]

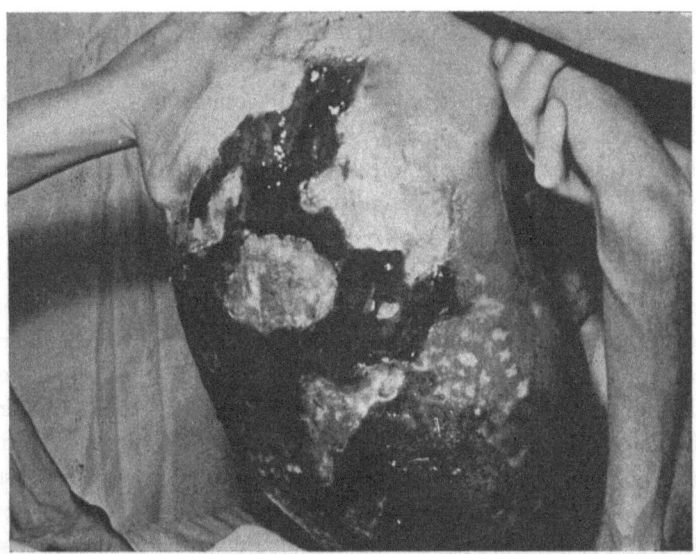

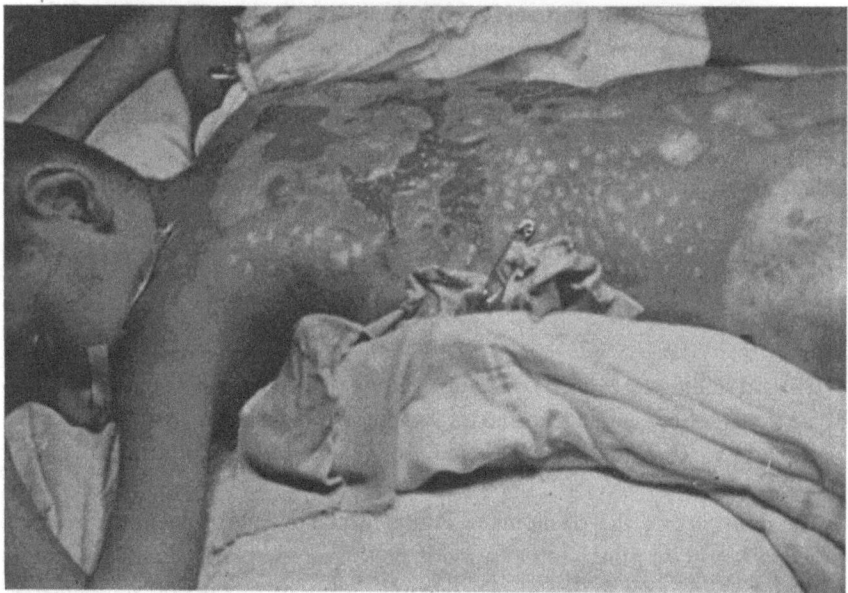

FIGURE VII—13. Effect of improving caloric balance on wound-healing of a boy with thermal burns of long standing. In the upper figure observe the extensive raw wound of the back and the marked thinness of the arms. In the lower figure note the increase in subcutaneous fat and the extensive wound-healing which became evident after about three months of high caloric feeding. For further comments see text. We are indebted to Dr. B. Webster for the opportunity to present these photographs.

three weeks about two-thirds of the old donor sites had begun to heal spontaneously. Subsequently, skin grafts took successfully.

The observations on this patient invite certain comments. First, it is clear that the institution of a dietary regimen which was *known* to provide an adequate caloric intake resulted not only in weight gain but also in rapid wound-healing. An increase in caloric balance accomplished favorable changes which could not be attained by the administration of protein, minerals and vitamins under conditions of inadequate caloric intake. Second, there was no need to supplement the high caloric regimen with administration of exogenous growth hormone. On the contrary, as indicated in Figure 1 of this chapter and Figure 5 of Chapter VI, administration of a nitrogen (protoplasmic) anabolic hormone accelerates body fat catabolism in subjects receiving an inadequate caloric intake. This, in turn, results in more rapid depletion of the patient's fat (caloric) stores. By increasing total energy output, thyroid therapy may do likewise. Complete exhaustion of the body's caloric stores under conditions of negative caloric balance inevitably results in death. It therefore appears unphysiologic and harmful to give growth hormone (PGH or testosterone) or thyroid to a depleted patient whose caloric intake is less than his caloric expenditure. Moreover, it is probably unnecessary to give growth hormone to induce protoplasmic anabolism once the caloric balance has been rendered positive. It thus would appear desirable to withhold growth hormone therapy until it has been found that correction of caloric deficit fails to result in satisfactory wound-healing and protoplasmic growth.

COMMENTS ON THE SELECTIVE OR FRACTIONAL NATURE OF HYPOPITUITARISM IN CERTAIN PATIENTS

Clinical studies suggest that it is unusual for a patient to exhibit signs of failure of all the anterior pituitary hormones (panhypopituitarism). More commonly, while some are lacking, others are being produced in adequate or nearly adequate amounts.

For examples of the phenomena indicated above, the reader is referred to Chapters V and VI, where information is presented concerning individuals who are normal except for failure of gonadotropic hormone production and hence of sexual maturation. Another example is provided by the occasional child in whom moderately advanced adolescent sexual development precedes adolescent adrenocortical activity (see Chapter III, Figure 53). This condition is mentioned to suggest that dissociations in the respective pituitary functions may occur normally. Whether short stature in otherwise healthy children and adolescents some-

The Anterior Pituitary

times is due to a selective lack of pituitary growth hormone is uncertain. It is known only that such children can be made to grow more rapidly when artificially stimulated by an exogenous growth-promoting agent (see Chapter VI, Figure 7). This fact suggests that the spontaneous rates of growth of these children would be greater if their own pituitaries were producing larger amounts of growth hormone.

Somewhat selective changes in the respective production rates of the several anterior pituitary hormones appear to occur as compensatory phenomena under certain circumstances. Figure 38 of Chapter III suggests, for example, that in patients with adrenocortical cancer there may be a marked reduction in adrenocorticotropic hormone production. Similarly, in the patient with gonadal tumor there is apt to be a suppression of gonadotropic hormone production. On the other hand, the castrate produces unusually large amounts of gonadotropins (see Chapters V and VI). Thyrotropic hormone secretion is sometimes inhibited by thyroid therapy (see Chapter I).

Adrenocortical, gonadal and thyroid hormones may act to influence the rate of production of more than a single pituitary-tropic-hormone. For example, estrogens may inhibit not only gonadotropic, but also growth hormone production (see above, page 454). Simultaneously, they may stimulate adrenocorticotropic hormone production.

The foregoing very incomplete list of endocrine interrelations is presented to call attention to the intricate nature of these phenomena. More detailed consideration of them must await the acquisition of additional information.

PATHOLOGIC HYPERPITUITARISM

As discussed above under clinical considerations, pathological hyperpituitarism may be divided into two types, (a) primary organic and (b) secondary functional hyperpituitarism.

Primary Organic Hyperpituitarism. This condition may be seen in patients with eosinophilic or basophilic adenomas of the adenohypophysis. Basophilic adenomas are sometimes found in association with Cushing's syndrome.[11]* For a discussion of this condition, turn to Chapter III. Eosinophilic adenomas cause tall stature in children and gigantism in adolescents. In older persons whose skeletal epiphyses are fused eosinophilic adenomas cause acromegaly.

Pituitary gigantism (eosinophilic adenoma). This is a rare condition, there

---

* When this occurs, some authors use the term "Cushing's disease." At present it is not clear whether an adenoma is ever primary. It seems more probable that adenomas develop as a result of hyperadrenocorticism. They rarely are of sufficient size to produce local signs.

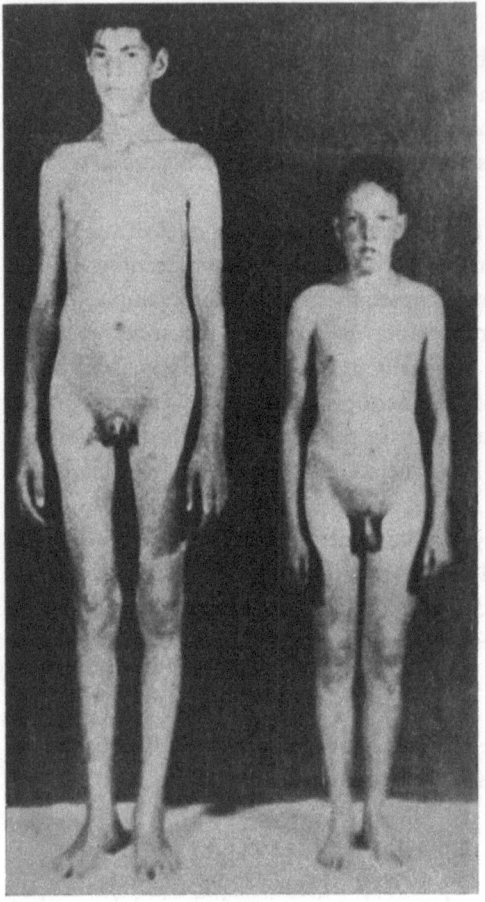

FIGURE VII — 14. A 15-year-old giant and a normal boy of the same age. Note the absence of signs of sexual development. Note the great increase in the stature of the patient relative to the normal control. Note also that this increase is not accompanied by any signs of sexual development. From L. M. Hurxthal, *J. Clin. Endocrinol.* 3:12, 1943.

being only a small number of cases on record in the world literature. Sample data on such patients are presented in Figures 14 and 15 and Table 7.

CLINICAL MANIFESTATIONS. The signs and symptoms of pituitary gigantism are interesting in their simplicity. There is (a) rapid growth of the skeleton and supporting mesenchymal structures, but (b) no acceleration of skeletal maturation and (c) usually no gross evidences of hyperthyroidism, hyperadrenocorticism or hypergonadism (sexual precocity). In fact, sexual development may be retarded. Occasionally there are signs of an expanding lesion in the region of the pituitary (see page 456).

Stated in other words, some patients with primary organic hyperpituitarism appear to be suffering almost exclusively from excess PGH production. Other patients, especially adult acromegalics, may show evidences of excess thyrotropic and adrenocorticotropic hormone in addition to signs of excess growth hormone.

The Anterior Pituitary

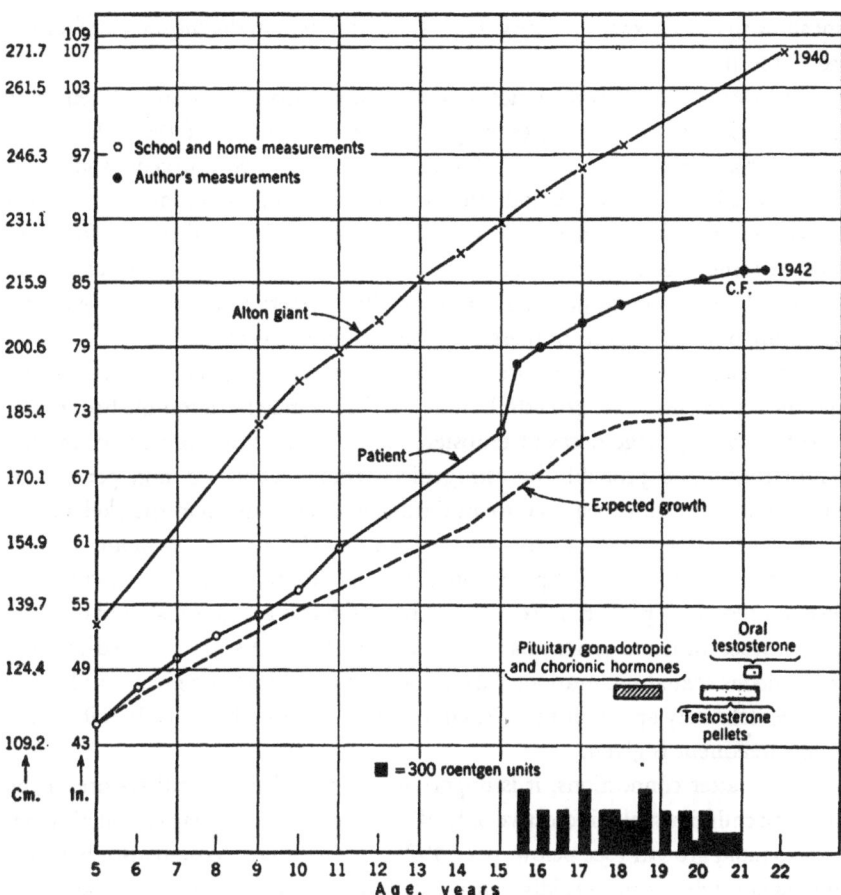

FIGURE VII—15. Gigantism resulting from pituitary adenoma. The growth chart of the Hurxthal giant (labeled "patient"; see also Figure 14) and the Alton giant shows that the Alton giant grew at a rate of about 12 cm. per year from his fifth to his ninth year and about 6 cm. per year from his ninth to his twenty-second year. Hurxthal's giant also attained excessive stature through abnormally rapid growth, but therapeutic closure of the epiphyses by means of androgenic hormone therapy apparently succeeded in limiting the duration of growth. From L. M. Hurxthal, *J. Clin. Endocrinol.* 3:12, 1943, as adapted by N. B. Talbot and E. H. Sobel, *Advances in Pediatrics*, II, New York, Interscience Publishers, 1947.

DIAGNOSIS. In the absence of definite local manifestations of a pituitary adenoma, the diagnosis of eosinophilic adenoma with primary pituitary gigantism can only be considered possible or presumptive. The diagnosis is suggested by a growth curve similar to those of Figure 15 in the case of a patient who does not show signs of sexual precocity. For a list of differential diagnostic possibilities, see Table 6.

TREATMENT. Therapy varies with the clinical manifestations. When there is substantial evidence of an eosinophilic tumor, radiation of the sella turcica may be considered. The advice of a radiologist and neurosurgeon should be sought in this connection. As indicated in Figure 15, radiation cannot be counted on to exert a strikingly beneficial influence upon body growth rate. Moreover, there is some risk of injuring pituitary basophils as well as eosinophils if very heavy radiation is undertaken. Surgery usually is reserved for patients who are becoming blind as a result of pressure upon the optic nerves.

Hormonal therapy may be used to hasten epiphyseal fusion (see Figure 15) and thus to stop skeletal growth. Epiphyseal fusion may be accomplished within a year or two by large doses of testosterone (about 100 mg. per day of methyl testosterone) and probably by estrogenic hormone (about 5 mg. per day of stilbestrol). The time required to attain this end depends upon the skeletal development of the patient at the onset of therapy. Estrogenic hormone may, in addition, act to inhibit PGH production. Gonadal hormone therapy also prompts pseudo-precocious puberty in young patients.* On this account it should be withheld at least until the patient has attained adolescent age and has failed to show spontaneous sexual maturation. Furthermore, it should not be given until it has become definitely apparent that the child will attain a pathologically tall stature unless treatment is given.

In the latter connections, it is important to recognize that tall stature in the growing child is usually indicative only of good health and perhaps a genetic tendency to rapid growth (see below, page 492). It is to be emphasized also that most individuals who grow rapidly during childhood stop growing spontaneously before they have become true giants. This is especially so in the case of children who undergo adolescence at an average normal or earlier than average age. See also below under secondary functional (pathologic) and functional (physiologic) hyperpituitarism.

Secondary Functional Hyperpituitarism. This condition originates in the hypothalamus or adjacent areas of the brain. The resultant clinical picture is well represented by children with true precocious puberty as described in Chapters V and VI. There has been much speculation on the possibility that conditions such as thyrotoxicosis, adrenocortical virilism (with bilateral adrenocortical hyperplasia) and diabetes mellitus of the juvenile type may likewise be due to functional pathologic hyperpituitarism secondary to an extrapituitary disturbance. There is no proof that these hypotheses are correct.

* In males estrogen causes gynecomastia and testicular atrophy (see Chapter VI, Figure 21).

TABLE VII—7. Pituitary gigantism.*

Case no.	Sex	Probable age at onset	Age, yr.	Ht., cm.	Wt., kg.	Bone age	Sexual hair † P	A	F	Genitalia	Comments	Source
1	M	Infancy	11.5	208	112	11	—	—	—	—	Sella turcica enlarged	L. H. Behrens et al., *Endocrinology* 16:120, 1932; C. L. Humberd, *J.A.M.A.* 108:544, 1937
			13.5	222	—	—	M	N	N	Penis, 10 cm.		
			18	251	179	—	—	—	—			
2	M	4-5	15	198	85	13	N	N	N	Small	Sella turcica enlarged	L. M. Hurxthal, *J. Clin. Endocrinol.* 3:12, 1943
			20.5	217	—	—	—	—	—			
3	M	8	15	192	92	—	—	—	—	—	Sella turcica enlarged; visual field defects	H. Cushing, *The Pituitary Body and Its Disorders*, Philadelphia, Lippincott, 1912
4	F	—	18	203	—	—	—	—	—	—	Sella turcica enlarged	W. Hutchinson, *N. York M. J.* 72:89, 1900
5	M	13	18	216	138	—	—	—	—	Backward development	Acromegalic features; pituitary tumor at autopsy	C. L. Dana, *J. Nerv. & Ment. Dis.* n.s. 18:725, 1893; W. Hutchinson, *N. York M. J.* 72:89, 1900
			19	223	146	—	—	—	—			
6	M	—	20	233	138	Retarded **	—	—	—	—	Sella turcica enlarged	W. Robinson, *Brit. M. J.* 1:560, 1921
7	M	—	22-24	230	—	Retarded **	—	—	—	—	Acromegaly; large sella; kyphoscoliosis	J. McFarland, *Tr. & Stud. Coll. Physicians, Philadelphia* 6:148, 1938
8	M	15	36	251	124	Retarded **	S	N	N	Penis small; testes atrophic	Large sella; collapsed pituitary cyst	H. Cushing, *Arch. Int. Med.* 51:487, 1933

* In addition to being tall, patients tend toward retarded sexual and skeletal development. ** Epiphyses not fused.
† P = Pubic; A = Axillary; F = Facial; M = Moderate; S = Scant; N = None.

PHYSIOLOGIC HYPERPITUITARISM

This condition is the counterpart of physiologic hypopituitarism as described earlier in this chapter. A good example of the phenomenon is provided by the "alarm reaction" as described in Chapter III. Here stress temporarily evokes a marked increase in pituitary adrenocorticotropic hormone for the homeostatic purpose of increasing the adrenocortical hormone output in accordance with the body's needs. Other less-well-defined presumptive examples are seen (a) in children who eat too much, become obese and show accelerated growth and development and (b) in children who simply attain an unusually tall stature. These conditions are considered below.

Functional Hyperpituitarism Secondary to Caloric Hypernutrition (Simple Dietary Obesity). It is presumed that just as the tendencies to short stature and retarded adolescence seen in patients with caloric undernutrition may be explained by functional (physiologic) hypopituitarism, the opposite tendencies seen in healthy obese children may be explained by functional (physiologic) hyperpituitarism. Such hyperpituitarism is thought to be the result rather than the cause of the hyperalimentation and adiposity.

The healthy obese child tends to be taller for chronologic age than the average non-obese child.[12] Obese children also tend to undergo adolescence at an earlier than average age, and their skeletal development and urinary 17-KS output may correspond to the average normal for children one or more years older. In other words, the trend in obese children is toward accelerated, normal physical growth and maturation.

ETIOLOGY. The clinical histories of such obese children may yield interesting information. If due care is taken, it is almost always possible to elicit a story of overeating. Sometimes this is told spontaneously; at others, it is vigorously denied. When denied, skillful questioning may be needed to obtain a clear picture of past and present food habits.

The exact sources of excess calories vary somewhat. Most commonly the greatest excesses are accounted for by carbohydrates, especially sweets and starchy foods (potatoes, rice, macaroni, spaghetti, cereals, breads, pastries, candies and the like). High-fat foods (butter, cream, salad oils, etc.) frequently play a role, the tendency being to combine them with starches (butter on bread, cream on cereal and so forth).

The reasons for overeating are legion.[12] In certain instances, eating simply constitutes a major family pleasure. In certain others, there has developed the idea that a good appetite insures good health. This belief often grows in the minds of parents who have suffered the loss of another child through illness or accident. Psychiatric studies reveal that a good many obese children result from an unplanned and unwanted pregnancy. This can culminate in emotional rejection of the child by the parents. In such cases the mother and father may have an unconscious sense of guilt because of their inability to feel affection. In an effort to salve their conscience, parents may give such children excessive physical attention in the form of food. Children who are insecure, worried, overprotected or bored tend spontaneously to eat for the comfort, pleasure and satisfaction which derives from the taste of food and the sensation of a full stomach.

These factors have been mentioned to suggest that it is usually possible to find some reasonably acceptable cause for obesity other than a mysterious "glandular disturbance." To be sure, there are rare patients who develop a morbid appetite because of a hypothalamic lesion involving neurologic centers which control appetite. Likewise, there are rare patients whose obesity is due in part to a reduction in energy output secondary to thyroid hormone deficiency (see Chapter I) and there are the very rare patients who show excess weight gain as a manifestation of Cushing's syndrome (see Chapter III) or chronic hyperinsulinism (see Chapter IX). The incidence of these conditions relative to simple dietary obesity is, however, extremely low.

In these connections it appears to be true that obesity *per se* is always due to an excessively positive caloric balance and that it can be corrected by placing patients on a regimen which renders their caloric balance negative. Apparent exceptions to this statement are almost always explained by abnormal or unusual retentions of water within the body. Such retentions, which may be of several weeks' duration, ordinarily account for any temporary failures to lose weight after the dietary intake has been suitably restricted. It further appears that certain people require fewer calories per square meter per day to maintain caloric equilibrium than do others. This difference means that some people have a lower energy output per square meter per day than other equally normal persons. To some extent these differences in energy output are attributable to differences in physical activity, psychic tension and the like. Whether they are also explainable in part by differences in metabolic status it is difficult to say, but it is interesting to recall that the basal metabolic rates of normal individuals vary as much as plus or minus 15 to 20 per cent from the average for all normal persons. There is little to suggest that thyroid hormone is the chief determinant of this phenomenon in normal individuals. The possibility that other endocrine factors are of importance remains to be investigated.

[488]   CHAPTER VII:

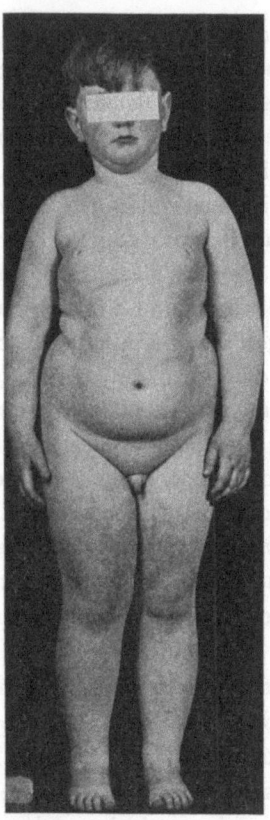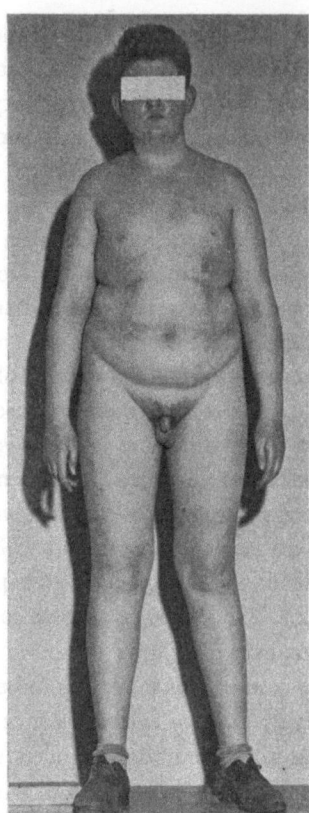

FIGURE VII—16. Physical appearance of two boys of 6 and 18 years suffering from obesity due to overeating. Note that the excess adipose tissue is generally distributed over the trunk and extremities and that it does not involve the face and neck as in patients with Cushing's syndrome (Chapter III, Figure 47). The accumulations of subcutaneous fat are particularly heavy in the regions of the breasts and hips. In these patients the breast adiposity could be distinguished from true gynecomastia by the absence of palpable mammary gland tissue.

CLINICAL MANIFESTATIONS. The configuration of the ordinary obese child is usually similar to those shown in Figure 16. The excess fat is generally distributed over the body, but may accumulate particularly in the region of the breasts and hips. Except in girls of adolescent age, it is rare to find any palpable mammary gland tissue (i.e., gynecomastia).

As mentioned previously, the tendency is toward tall stature, but exceptions to this rule are encountered from time to time. Examination of the head and eyes reveals no evidence of an intracranial lesion. The thyroid is not remarkable.

Except for a tendency to pseudo-hypertension,* the cardiovascular and respiratory systems are normal. The abdomen is usually too thickly padded with fat to permit adequate examination. Pubic and axillary hair growth is either normal for age or precociously developed. The genitalia usually correspond to the normal for age, although a fair degree of variability is to be expected as in other normal children (see Chapter VI, Figures 12 and 13). In males the penis is often so imbedded in fat that it appears to be abnormally small. When the fat at the base is pushed back, the organ is seen to be of normal size.

The skin usually is of normal juvenile or adolescent texture. It is not dry, cold and sand-papery as in patients with hypothyroidism. There may be silvery pink striæ distensæ over the breasts, thighs and lower abdomen, but there are not the purplish, depressed striæ of Cushing's syndrome (see Chapter III, Figure 49). Quite frequently one finds the fingernails of obese children chewed to the quick. This usually is a manifestation of emotional tension. Occasionally other more gross evidences of tension such as nervous tics may be noted.

LABORATORY STUDIES. Roentgenograms and other tests fail to reveal any gross deviations from the normal other than a tendency toward accelerated skeletal maturation. Studies of thyroid status yield essentially normal results. Other measurements designed to give direct or indirect information concerning pituitary status (Table 2 and Figure 4) not only fail to indicate hypopituitarism but sometimes even indicate mild physiologic hyperpituitarism. For example, the urinary 17-KS output of very obese children frequently corresponds to the average for normal children a few years older.

DIFFERENTIAL DIAGNOSIS. Most of the factors involved in differential diagnosis have been implied in the foregoing sections. In tall obese children showing advanced maturation, the diagnosis rests between simple dietary obesity with physiologic hyperpituitarism and true precocious puberty (see Chapters V and VI). In the obese child of normal or short stature who shows advanced skeletal and sexual development, the same differential diagnosis holds. In addition, one may search for such causes of short stature as precocious epiphyseal closure and chondrodystrophy. In the obese child who is of short stature and who shows retardation of skeletal and sexual development or other signs of abnormal development, the possibility of primary organic hypopituitarism, primary hypothyroidism, primary central nervous system disease (such as the Laurence-Moon-Biedl syndrome), ovarian agenesis, Cushing's syndrome or other systemic disease should be considered carefully (see Table 5).

* Obese individuals may appear to have hypertension when blood pressure cuffs of standard breadths are employed. The apparent hypertension usually disappears if a suitably broad cuff is used.

TREATMENT. Patients with dietary obesity often pose a difficult therapeutic problem. In about a third of the cases a cure can be effected by awakening a sense of pride in personal appearance. When the nature of the trouble is explained, simple dietary advice and encouragement are all that is needed. In the other two-thirds, there are problems underlying the tendency to overeat which are so complex as to require expert psychiatric management. Even with such aid, a number of these patients appear totally resistant to treatment.

In most instances there is no need for a rigid dietary regimen. On the contrary, it often is better to tell the patient which foods are of high and which are of low caloric content. He (or his parents) are then urged to use good sense in menu selection. The fact that sizable amounts of lean meat, white fish, leafy vegetables and the like can be eaten for purposes of filling the stomach is mentioned in order to show the patient that it is more a matter of what he eats than how much

TABLE VII—8. Fruits classified by carbohydrate content (A) and average composition of common foods (B). From E. H. Rynearson and C. F. Gastineau, *Obesity*, Springfield, Thomas, 1949.

A. FRUITS CLASSIFIED BY CARBOHYDRATE CONTENT

1. *Fresh or juice-packed*

5 per cent	10 per cent	15 per cent	20 per cent
Rhubarb	Blackberries	Apples	Bananas
	Cantaloupe	Apricots	Grapes
	Cranberries	Blueberries	Plums
	Gooseberries	Cherries	
	Grapefruit	Currants	
	Honeydew melon	Huckleberries	
	Lemons	Pears	
	Limes	Raspberries	
	Oranges		
	Peaches		
	Pineapple		
	Strawberries		
	Watermelon		

2. *Water-packed*

5 per cent	10 per cent	15 per cent	20 per cent
Apricots	Applesauce	Kadota figs	
Blackberries	Cherries, black		
Cherries, red	Fruit for salad		
Cherries, white	Pears		
Loganberries	Pineapple		
Peaches	Plums		
Raspberries	White grapes		
Strawberries			

TABLE VII—8 (continued)

	B. AVERAGE COMPOSITION OF COMMON FOODS Per 100 gm. of food		
	Carbohydrate, gm.	Protein, gm.	Fat, gm.
Vegetables and fruits:			
3 per cent vegetables	3	1	0
6 per cent vegetables	6	1	0
15 per cent vegetables	15	2	0
20 per cent vegetables			
Potato	20	2	0
Shelled beans	20	7	0
Green corn	20	3	1
5 per cent fruits	5	1	0
10 per cent fruits	10	1	0
15 per cent fruits	15	1	0
20 per cent fruits	20	2	0
Cereals and breadstuffs:			
Breakfast cereals, dry	76	11	3
Breakfast cereals, cooked	11	1	—
White bread	52	9	2
Whole wheat bread	48	10	4
Rye bread	52	6	3
Wheat flour	76	11	1
Soda crackers	73	10	11
Dairy products:			
Whole milk	5	3	4
Skimmed milk	5	3	1 *
Cream, light or coffee	4	3	20
Cream, heavy or whipping	4	3	30
Buttermilk	5	3	1 *
Cheese, cheddar type	2	24	32
Cottage cheese, dry	4	20	1
Cottage cheese, creamed	4	20	5
Eggs, each	—	6	6
Meats and fish:			
Meat, cooked, very lean	—	25	5
Meat, cooked	—	25	15
Meat, cooked, very fat	—	25	30
Fish, miscellaneous	—	20	3
Oysters	4	6	1
Liver	4	20	4
Cooked bacon	—	25	50
Fats:			
Butter or oleomargarine	—	—	81
Lard or bacon fat	—	—	100
Olive oil and other oils	—	—	100
Mayonnaise	3	2	78
Peanut butter	21	26	48

* There is a negligible amount of fat in commercially separated milk.

he eats. Table 8 gives lists of the relative caloric values of commonly used foods.

In making dietary recommendations to obese patients, it is helpful to remember that when food has been a major source of satisfaction, restriction of intake creates a need for some sort of substitute pleasure or satisfaction. At times it may appear that the adiposity is of lesser importance than the problems created by attempts to control body weight. This is especially so in mentally deficient children and in children with severe emotional disturbances. Moreover, it is to be remembered that children can "grow into" their weight if weight is held stationary. Gradual weight reduction is preferable to rapid weight loss under most circumstances, and it is much better to undertake a regimen which can be adhered to than to start a rigid regimen and subsequently break it.

Supplementary medication with thyroid, benzadrine and other agents is not recommended. Except when specifically lacking, thyroid hormone is of no value. At times, however, it may appear desirable to rule out all possibility of hypothyroidism by therapeutic trial of this hormone. For a description of this procedure and comments on the interpretation of results obtained, see Chapter I. If a therapeutic trial with thyroid hormone fails to indicate that hypothyroidism has existed, the hormone should be discontinued.

PROGNOSIS. The healthy fat child develops into a normal, though sometimes adipose, adult. If the obesity persists into adult life the patient is more likely to develop hypertension, diabetes mellitus and menstrual disturbances than the person of normal weight.

Functional Hyperpituitarism with Tall Stature. It is unusual for boys to complain that they are too tall, but healthy adolescent girls occasionally complain of unusual height. Not infrequently these patients give a family history of tall stature in close relatives. Complete history, physical examination and laboratory study fail to reveal any pathology. It may be presumed, therefore, that these children have grown rapidly either because the pituitary gland has been producing PGH at an unusually rapid rate or because the end organs have been unusually responsive to growth hormone action.

The problem presented by such individuals usually falls more in the psychiatric than in the medical realm. In some instances it is found that it is really the parents who are concerned about the child's stature. The parents' reaction may date back to childhood experiences of their own and may consist in a desire to spare their offspring the embarrassment which they once felt as a consequence of being taller than their friends. If clarification of such relations fails to solve the problem, other factors may be considered. First, it is possible to make an approximate guess regarding a child's ultimate stature by relating present height, present skeletal age and menarcheal age. Growth in boys ceases when the skeletal

The Anterior Pituitary

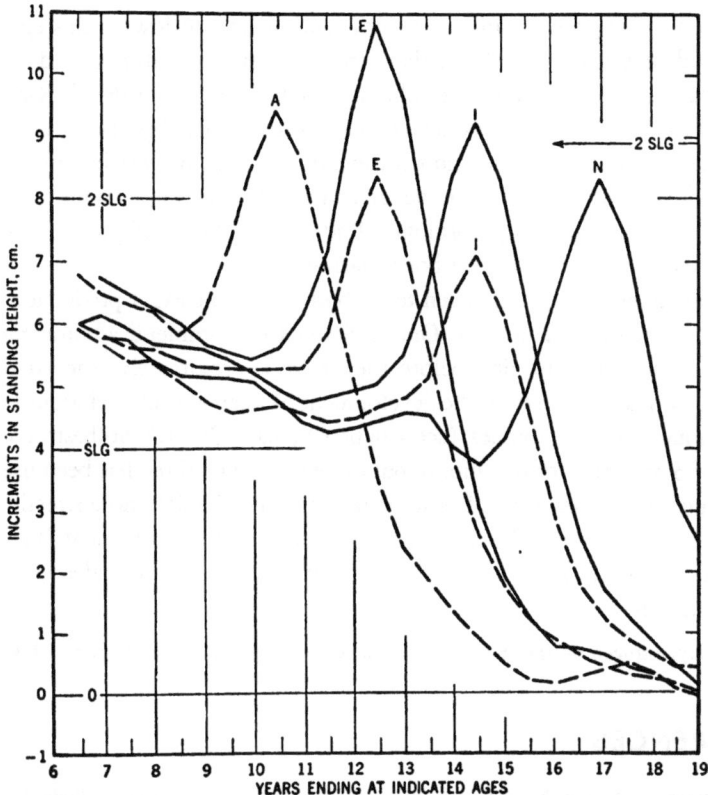

FIGURE VII—17. Average annual increments in standing height of girls (- - -) and boys (—·—) having their maximal growth at the ages of 10½ (A), 12½ (E, E), 14½ (I, I) and 17 (N) years, respectively. The abbreviations SLG and 2SLG represent straight line growth and twice straight line growth of girls 8 to 17 years old (i.e., if growth were plotted as a straight line, average growth would equal SLG and more rapid growth would show values above SLG). In girls maximum growth rates are noted at about the time of the menarche; growth ordinarily ceases five years later. In boys maximum growth ceases about five years after spermatogenesis. From F. K. Shuttleworth, *Sexual Maturation and the Physical Growth of Girls Age Six to Nineteen*, (Washington, Society for Research in Child Development, *Monographs* II: 5, 1937), as adapted by N. B. Talbot and E. H. Sobel, *Advances in Pediatrics* II, New York, Interscience Publishers, 1947.

age reaches about 18 years. In girls a skeletal age of 16 years marks the end of the growth period. Thus if a girl has a skeletal age of 14 years, it is safe to say she should stop growing within approximately two years. Further, as shown in Figure 17, it can be predicted that she should not grow more than about 2.5 cm. during this interval. If she has already passed the menarche, it also can be pointed out that growth rate decelerates continuously following this episode.

Should circumstances indicate that further increase in stature would be highly undesirable, therapy designed to inhibit growth may be considered. X-ray treatment of the pituitary and of skeletal epiphyses is considered potentially too harmful to be recommended. Radiation of the pituitary must be very intense to inhibit the production of growth hormone, and in so doing it is apt also to inhibit the secretion of other pituitary hormones. Radiation of the epiphyses may result in serious damage to the adjacent bone marrow.

As mentioned earlier, estrogen tends both to inhibit PGH production and to accelerate skeletal maturation. One hesitates to recommend administration of estrogenic hormone to girls before they have approximately reached the menarche, for fear of upsetting the development of normal cyclic relations between the pituitary and the ovaries (see Chapter V, page 364).* Stilbestrol in daily doses of 3 to 5 mg. for one month out of every two or three has been used with some success in a few girls of post-menarcheal age. To date no distressing complications have arisen. On the other hand, this form of treatment is still considered potentially hazardous and one to be employed only under exceptional circumstances.

* In boys estrogen treatment may damage the testicular tubules (see Chapter VI, Figure 21).

REFERENCES

1 (a) VAN DYKE, H. B. *The Physiology and Pharmacology of the Pituitary Body.* Univ. Chicago Press. Vol. I, 1936; Vol. II, 1939. (A new edition is in press.)
  (b) LI, C. H. and EVANS, H. M. Chemistry of anterior pituitary hormones. In *The Hormones: Physiology, Chemistry and Applications.* Vol. I. Edited by G. Pincus and K. V. Thimann. New York, Academic Press, 1948.
  (c) LI, C. H. and EVANS, H. M. The biochemistry of pituitary growth hormone. In *Recent Progress in Hormone Research.* Vol. III. Edited by G. Pincus. New York, Academic Press, 1948.
  (d) REIFENSTEIN, E. C., JR., KINSELL, L. W. and ALBRIGHT, F. Observations on the use of the serum phosphorus level as an index of pituitary growth hormone activity; the effect of estrogen therapy in acromegaly. *Endocrinology* 39:71, 1946.

2   TALBOT, N. B. and SOBEL, E. H. Endocrine and other factors determining the growth of children. In *Advances in Pediatrics.* Vol. II. Edited by S. Z. Levine, *et al.* New York, Interscience Publishers, 1947.

3   SAMUELS, L. T. The relation of the anterior pituitary hormones to nutrition. In *Recent Progress in Hormone Research.* Vol. I. Edited by G. Pincus. New York, Academic Press, 1947.

4 (a) WELLS, B. B. and KENDALL, E. C. The influence of corticosterone and c-17-hydroxy-dehydrocorticosterone (compound E) on somatic growth. *Proc. Staff Meet., Mayo Clin.* 15:324, 1940.
  (b) BECKS, H., SIMPSON, M. E., LI, C. H. and EVANS, H. M. Effects of adrenocorticotropic hormone (ACTH) on the osseous system in normal rats. *Endocrinology* 34:305, 1944.

5 GRIFFITHS, M. and YOUNG, F. G. Assay of hypophyseal growth-promoting extracts employing rats treated with diethylstilboestrol. *J. Endocrinol.* 3:96, 1942.

6 WILHELMI, A. E., FISHMAN, J. B. and RUSSELL, J. A. A new preparation of crystalline anterior pituitary growth hormone. *J. Biol. Chem.* 176:735, 1948.

7 (a) BAILEY, P., BUCHANAN, D. N. and BUCY, P. C. *Intracranial Tumors of Infancy and Childhood.* Univ. Chicago Press, 1939.
  (b) INGRAHAM, F. D. and SCOTT, H. W., JR. Craniopharyngiomas in children. *J. Pediat.* 29:95, 1946.
  (c) GORDY, P. D., PEET, M. M. and KAHN, E. A. The surgery of the craniopharyngiomas. *J. Neurosurg.* 6:503, 1949.

8 (a) ESCAMILLA, R. F. and LISSER, H. Simmonds' disease: a clinical study with review of the literature; differentiation from anorexia nervosa by statistical analysis of 595 cases, 101 of which were proved pathologically. *J. Clin. Endocrinol.* 2:65, 1942.
  (b) BRUCH, H. The Froehlich syndrome; report of the original case. *Am. J. Dis. Child.* 58:1282, 1939.
  (c) FRASER, R. W., ALBRIGHT, F. and SMITH, P. H. Carbohydrate metabolism: the value of the glucose tolerance test, the insulin tolerance test and the glucose-insulin tolerance test in the diagnosis of endocrinologic disorders of glucose metabolism. *J. Clin. Endocrinol.* 1:297, 1941.
  (d) WILKINS, L. Genetic and endocrine factors in the growth and development of childhood and adolescence. In *Recent Progress in Hormone Research.* Vol. II. Edited by G. Pincus. New York, Academic Press, 1948.
  (e) BRONSTEIN, I. P. and CASSORLA, E. Pituitary dwarfism: spontaneous correction. *J. Pediat.* 28:618, 1946.

9 (a) WARKANY, J., FRAUENBERGER, G. S. and MITCHELL, A. G. Heredofamilial deviations: the Laurence-Moon-Biedl syndrome. *Am. J. Dis. Child.* 53:455, 1937.
  (b) WARKANY, J. and WEAVER, T. S. Heredofamilial deviations: enlarged parietal foramens combined with obesity, hypogenitalism, microphthalmos and mental retardation. *Am. J. Dis. Child.* 60:1147, 1940.

10 (a) MASON, K. W. and WOLFE, J. M. Physiological activity of hypophysis of rats under various experimental conditions. *Anat. Rec.* 45:232, 1930.
   (b) WERNER, S. C. Failure of gonadotropic function of rat hypophysis during chronic inanition. *Proc. Soc. Exper. Biol. & Med.* 41:101, 1939.
   (c) MULINOS, M. G. and POMERANTZ, L. Pseudo-hypophysectomy; a condition resembling hypophysectomy produced by malnutrition. *J. Nutrition* 19:493, 1940.
   (d) KLINEFELTER, H. F., JR., ALBRIGHT, F. and GRISWOLD, G. C. Experience with quantitative test for normal or decreased amounts of follicle stimulating hormone in urine in endocrinological diagnosis. *J. Clin. Endocrinol.* 3:529, 1943.
   (e) BUTLER, A. M., RUFFIN, J. M., SNIFFEN, M. M. and WICKSON, M. E. Nutritional status of civilians rescued from Japanese prison camps. *New Eng. J. Med.* 233:639, 1945.
   (f) TALBOT, N. B., SOBEL, E. H., BURKE, B. S., LINDEMANN, E. and KAUFMAN, S. B. Dwarfism in healthy children; its possible relation to emotional, nutritional and endocrine disturbances. *New Eng. J. Med.* 236:783, 1947.

11 (a) CUSHING, H. *The Pituitary Body and Its Disorders.* Philadelphia, J. P. Lippincott, 1912.
   (b) CUSHING, H. "Dyspituitarism": twenty years later, with special consideration of the pituitary adenomas. *Arch. Int. Med.* 51:487, 1933.

12 (a) BRUCH, H. Obesity in childhood: I. Physical growth and development of obese children. *Am. J. Dis. Child.* 58:457, 1939; III. Physiologic and psychologic aspects of the food intake of obese children. *Ibid* 59:739, 1940; BRUCH, H. and TOURAINE, G. Obesity in childhood: V. The family frame of obese children. *Psychosom. Med.* 2:141, 1940.
   (b) TALBOT, N. B. Obesity in children. *M. Clin. North America* 29:1217, 1945.
   (c) RYNEARSON, E. H. and GASTINEAU, C. F. *Obesity.* Springfield, Ill., C. C. Thomas, 1949.

THE POSTERIOR PITUITARY

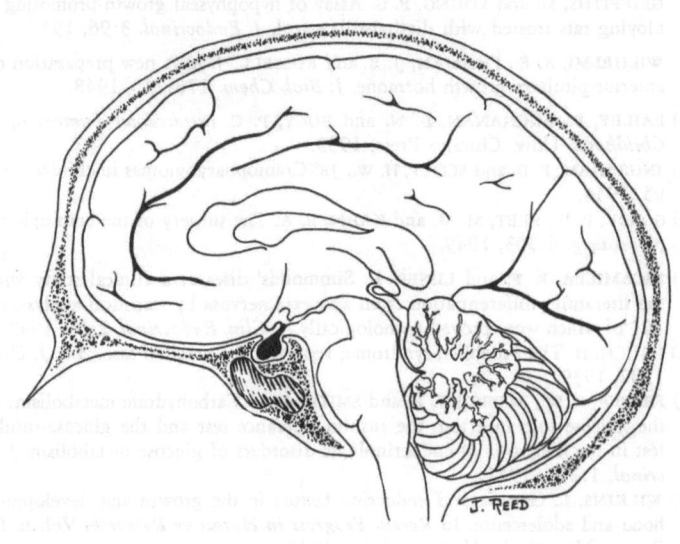

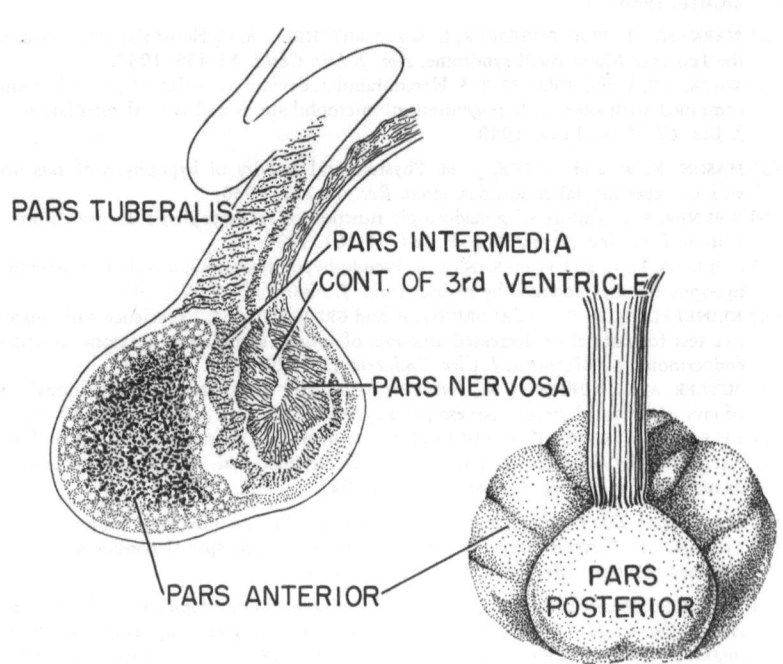

CHAPTER VIII

THE POSTERIOR PITUITARY

BASIC CONSIDERATIONS

DEVELOPMENT AND STRUCTURE OF THE POSTERIOR LOBE

The posterior lobe of the pituitary develops in the embryo as a pouch or infundibulum from neural tissue of the floor of the hypothalamus. In the area of the sella turcica this structure encounters Rathke's pouch, the anterior lobe anlage, which simultaneously pushes up from the roof of the primitive pharynx. The infundibulum invaginates Rathke's pouch from above and behind and thus becomes almost completely invested with anterior lobe tissue. Nevertheless it retains its hypothalamic connections, which become the pituitary stalk. The secretory function of the posterior pituitary depends upon the integrity of this stalk through which pass efferent nerve fibers from the supra-optic and paraventricular nuclei of the hypothalamus. The blood supply of the posterior lobe is derived from branches of the vertebral arteries approaching it from below and behind. By contrast, the anterior lobe receives its blood supply from two arterioles which descend the pituitary stalk carrying blood which has already circulated through parts of the hypothalamus. Thus, while the interior pituitary lacks neural connections with the brain, humeral pathways develop to form intimate links between this organ and the hypothalamus.

Structurally the fully developed posterior lobe consists of a meshwork of loose neuroglial cells, or neurocytes, invested by a thin epithelial layer. The simple microscopic appearance of the tissue gives little suggestion of its complex physiologic activity.

HORMONES OF THE POSTERIOR LOBE

Simple aqueous extracts of fresh posterior lobe tissue contain protein material of large molecular size. This material has biological activity at three different sites. It acts at the kidney to inhibit water diuresis. It causes the muscularis of arterioles to contract, thus effecting an increase in blood pressure. In addition, it acts on the musculature of the pregnant uterus to bring about contraction. Upon hydrolysis, the active material of simple tissue extracts yields two chemically similar polypeptides with molecular weights of approximately 2,000. One of these, oxytocin, causes uterine contraction, but has little or no vasopressor or antidiuretic activity. The other polypeptide, vasopressin, is a potent vasoconstrictor and antidiuretic substance but is essentially free of oxytocic activity. Efforts to fractionate vasopressin into compounds possessing only antidiuretic or vasoconstrictor activity by physicochemical means have not been successful.[1]

Physiologic studies strongly suggest that the posterior pituitary can secrete a specific antidiuretic and a separate, specific oxytocic hormone. Thus intravenous administration of hypertonic saline solution prompts release of maximal quantities of antidiuretic hormone without evidence of simultaneous oxytocin release. If hypertonic saline administration is followed by electrical stimulation of nervous pathways to the posterior pituitary, oxytocin appears in the peripheral blood but without a further increase in antidiuretic hormone concentration.[2] Furthermore, the absence of a rise in blood pressure when conditions favor an increase in endogenous secretion of antidiuretic hormone suggests that the posterior pituitary can release antidiuretic hormone independent of pressor material.

This chapter will be largely concerned with the antidiuretic hormone, which appears to play a fundamental role in the moment-to-moment control of the body's water metabolism. A discussion of the limited pharmacologic applications of the other principles of posterior pituitary extracts will be mentioned in a later section (page 535).

PHYSIOLOGY OF THE ANTIDIURETIC MECHANISM

Antidiuretic hormone determines the relation between water and solutes in urine and thus, indirectly, their relation in all body fluids. The concept of the relation between water and solutes is made difficult by the fact that we ordinarily think of a variable quantity of solute and a fixed quantity of vehicle or solution. The hypothalamic-neurohypophyseal system determines volumes of solution relative to essentially constant quantities of solutes measured in terms of milliosmoles.*

The hypothalamic-neurohypophyseal system is activated to increase antidiuretic hormone production when, as in dehydration, the water component of the

---

* Milliosmole is a unit of measure of total osmotic activity of a mixture of solutes. Abbreviated mosM.

body fluid is proportionately diminished. Hormone released in response to this stimulus acts at the kidney to increase water reabsorption. The water thus "restored" to the body favors a return to normal of the relation of water to solutes in body fluids (see Figure 1).

In the following sections these relations will be considered in more detail. The action of the antidiuretic hormone will be discussed first. Secondary effects of hormonal action will be considered next and factors responsible for changes in the rate of production of antidiuretic hormone last.

Action of the Antidiuretic Hormone on the Kidneys. For convenience in presentation, this subject will be considered under a number of headings below.

Renal mechanisms.[3] Figure 2 shows in simplified, diagrammatic form some of the renal mechanisms which determine urine volume and concentration. The renal glomeruli filter from plasma a volume of solution amounting to about 100,000 cc. per m^2 per day. Except for the fact that it is nearly protein free, this glomerular filtrate is similar in solute composition to plasma. Glomerular filtrate has about 3.2 cc. of water to each milliosmole of total solute. Stated conventionally, the 100,000 cc. of glomerular fluid filtered per m^2 per day contain approximately 31,000 mosM of solute.

As this glomerular filtrate passes down through the upper portion of the kidney tubule, about 85 per cent of the water and 97 per cent of the solutes are reabsorbed into the circulation. This commonly is labeled "obligatory" water reabsorption. So far as is known, antidiuretic hormone plays no direct role in these phenomena. There remains a residue of water (15 per cent of 100,000 cc., or 15,000 cc.) and of solutes (3 per cent of 31,000 mosM, or approximately 1,000 mosM) which now must pass through the lower renal tubule before leaving the kidney as urine. The quantity remains essentially unaltered as the solutes pass through the lower nephron, where presumably certain important processes such as the substitution of ammonium ion for fixed-base radicles takes place. These processes alter the composition but do not appreciably affect the total osmotic activity of the solute residue. Eventually, a variable fraction of the 15,000 cc. of water is reabsorbed. This variable, or "facultative," reabsorption of water in the lower renal tubule is determined largely, though not exclusively, by the action of antidiuretic hormone.

Action of the antidiuretic hormone on the renal mechanisms. Antidiuretic hormone enables the lower renal tubule to reabsorb a large proportion of the 15 liters of water per m^2 per day that are delivered to it from the upper tubule. Maximally effective quantities of hormone permit the lower tubule to reduce the ratio of water to solutes to a minimum of 0.66 cc. per mosM (1.5 mosM per

CHAPTER VIII:

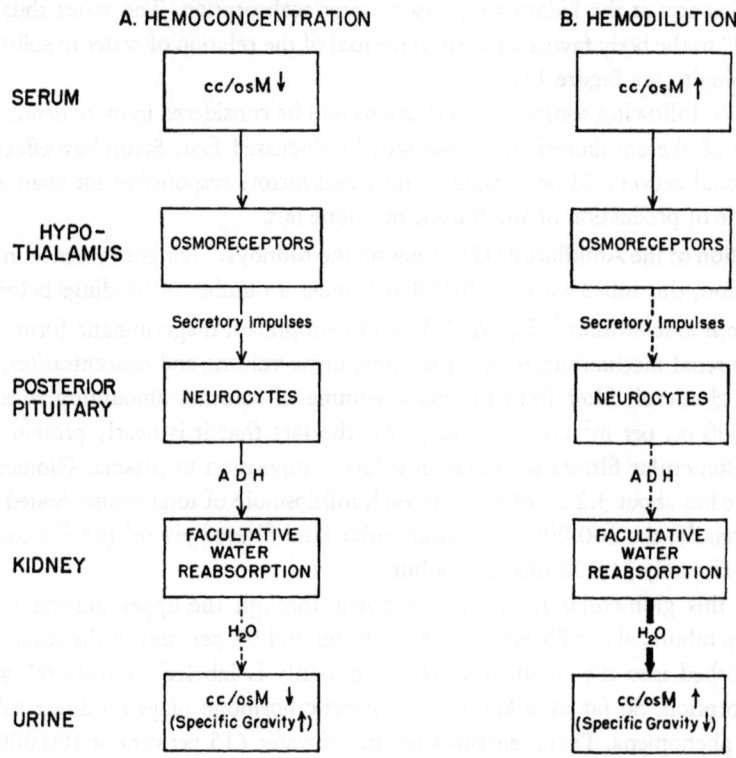

FIGURE VIII—1. Diagrammatic representation of hypothalamic-neurohypophyseal control of water metabolism.

SECTION A: A fall in serum water relative to solutes (dehydration) stimulates "osmoreceptors" of the hypothalamus to send secretory impulses to the neurocytes of the posterior pituitary, and thus increases antidiuretic hormone production. The hormone is carried to the kidney by the blood stream and there acts to increase facultative water reabsorption. A highly concentrated urine is eliminated.

SECTION B: The water content of serum relative to solutes is high (hyperhydration). The hypothalamic osmoreceptors fail to stimulate the posterior pituitary neurocytes under these circumstances. No antidiuretic hormone is released. In the absence of antidiuretic hormone the kidney secretes a dilute urine. As in Section A a change in the ratio of water to solutes in serum results in a corresponding change in the relation of water to solutes in urine.

The Posterior Pituitary

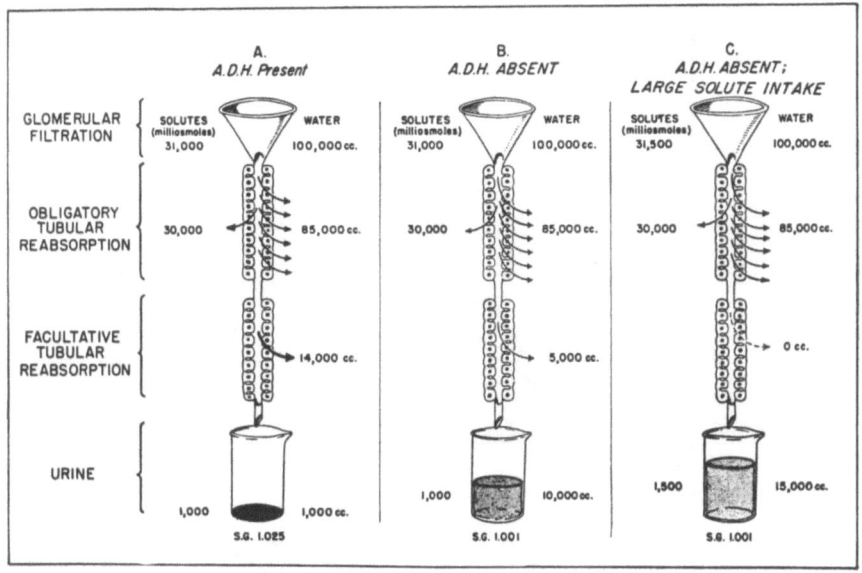

FIGURE VIII—2. Diagrammatic representation of factors regulating facultative water reabsorption (the values shown are per m^2 per 24 hours). Note that in all three instances the functions of the glomerulus and upper tubule are constant. Glomerular fluid containing water and solutes in the amounts indicated passes first into the upper tubule. Here essentially all the solute reabsorption takes place and the greater portion of filtered water is removed simultaneously by obligatory reabsorption.

SECTION A: Moderate quantities of antidiuretic hormone are assumed to be present. Under the influence of the hormone water entering the lower tubule is reabsorbed until a certain osmotic concentration is reached. The osmotic concentration is dependent upon the amount of antidiuretic hormone present, and in this instance it is shown to be 1 mosM per cc. The water and solutes remaining after facultative reabsorption are excreted together as relatively concentrated urine.

SECTION B: It is assumed that water intake is just sufficient to meet urine water needs. Water is reabsorbed in the lower tubule until an osmotic pressure of 0.1 mosM per cc. is reached. This is the highest value normally attainable in the absence of antidiuretic hormone. In the presence of 1,000 mosM, a relatively large volume (10,000 cc.) of dilute urine results. But this urine volume is not necessarily maximal.

SECTION C: The urine volume can be increased to a ceiling value of approximately 15,000 cc. per m^2 per 24 hours by imposing a solute load of 1,500 mosM per m^2 per 24 hours. Under this circumstance facultative reabsorption of water drops to zero.

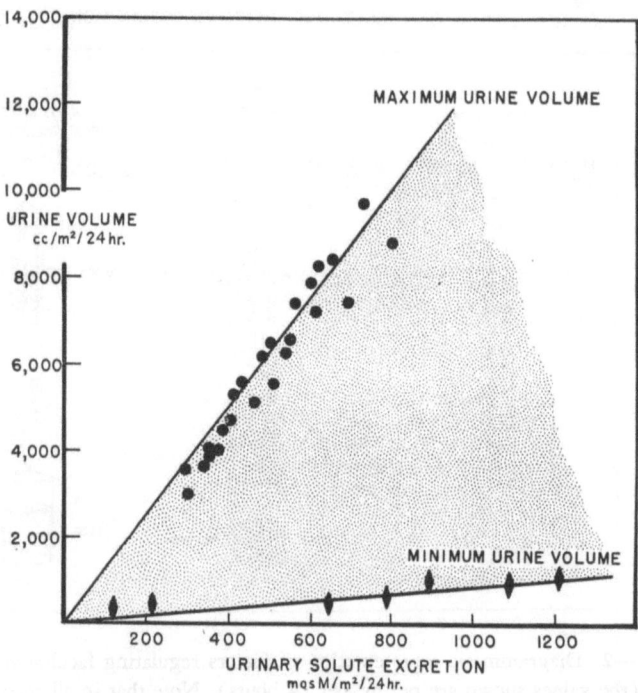

FIGURE VIII—3. Relation of maximum and minimum urine volume to solute load. Urine volume is shown on the ordinate, and urinary solute excretion on the abscissa. The points defining the upper boundary of the stippled area represent observations on hyperhydrated normal individuals excreting maximum volumes of urine. Those defining the lower boundary represent observations on hydropenic individuals excreting minimal urine volumes. The stippled area represents the range of variation in urine volume permitted the normal individual by the posterior pituitary-renal mechanisms. Note that a small solute excretion permits maximum water conservation on a limited water intake. However, when solute excretion is small, only a limited diuretic response to a large intake of water is possible. While the maximum diuretic response to a large water intake is much enhanced when solute excretion is increased, it is also evident that a much larger minimal water intake is necessary to meet the renal water requirement and prevent dehydration. From J. D. Crawford, E. J. Schoen and A. P. Nicosia, *Proc. Soc. Pediat. Research*, May, 1951.

---

cc.).[4a] Under this circumstance a urine solute residual of 1,000 mosM per m^2 per day is excreted in a urine volume of 670 cc.; 14.33 liters of water per m^2 per day are returned to the body (see Figure 2, Section A).

In the absence of antidiuretic hormone the lower renal tubule can reabsorb water from the fluid delivered it only until the water/solute ratio is reduced to approximately 10 cc. per mosM.[4b] Hence, under the conditions of Figure 2, Section B, the elimination of 1,000 mosM of solute describes an obligatory urine volume of 10,000 cc. per m² per day.

Relative to plasma with a normal water/solute ratio of 3.2 cc. per mosM,[4 c] urine excreted in the presence of abundant antidiuretic hormone contains less water than solutes (0.67 cc. per mosM). Neglecting extrarenal water losses and assuming a constant, ordinary intake of water and solutes, passage of urine of this type tends to raise the ratio of water to solutes in plasma. Urine excreted in the absence of hormone contains more water than solutes (10 cc. per mosM). The secretion of this type of urine will tend to lower the ratio of water to solutes in plasma. Changes in the rate of water outflow in relation to solute outflow in urine thus provide a means for regulating the relation of water to solutes in plasma and, indirectly, in all body fluids.*

Relations between antidiuretic hormone, solute load and minimum urine volume. The solutes requiring excretion by the kidney (here termed solute load) and antidiuretic hormone are inseparable determinants of minimal urine volume (see Figure 3). The foregoing discussion has suggested that when the solute load is constant there is an inverse proportionality between urine volume and antidiuretic hormone activity. Solute load, however, is seldom constant. When antidiuretic hormone activity is fixed, variations in solute load cause directly proportional variations in urine volume (see Figure 4). Hence the excretion of a urine of minimal volume is dependent upon maximal antidiuretic hormone influence and minimal solute load.

Urine solute load is determined by dietary intake and by metabolic forces operating within the body. The dietary contribution to urine solute load is least when only carbohydrate and fat are eaten. These nutrients are metabolized almost exclusively to carbon dioxide and water. Because the carbon dioxide is excreted largely by way of the lungs, the solute residue presenting for renal elimination is very small. Endogenous contributions to urine solute load are least when enough carbohydrate is given to prevent ketosis and to minimize protein catabolism.† By such means the total solute load for renal elimination can be reduced to about 200 mosM per m² per day. Under conditions of full antidiuretic hormone activity, this amount of solute can be excreted in a urine volume of only 135 cc. per m² per day (1.5 mosM per cc.).

* Ketosis is prevented and protoplasmic catabolism reduced to minimal values by provision of 60 grams of glucose per m² per day (see Chapter VI, Figures 2 and 4).

† Until recently it has been assumed that osmotic equilibrium is maintained at all times between plasma, other extracellular fluids and intracellular fluids by mechanisms described in Chapter III, Figure 10. There is evidence, however, which suggests that exceptions to this thesis may be encountered. For instance, current studies indicate that liver cell fluid may be distinctly hypertonic as compared with serum.[4 d]

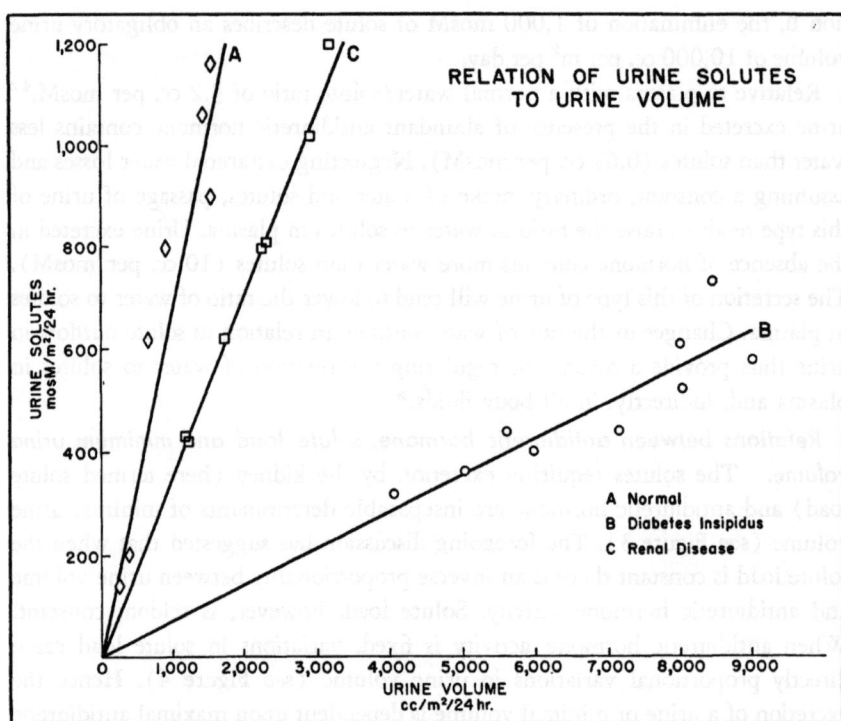

FIGURE VIII—4. Relation of urine solutes to urine volume in patients with diabetes insipidus and renal disease. The urine solute output is shown on the ordinate; the urine volume on the abscissa. The points connected by line A represent observations on normal individuals. Here it can be assumed that antidiuretic influence was approximately constant, since water conservation of moderate degree is a normal characteristic. The points connected by line B represent observations on a patient with diabetes insipidus. Antidiuretic influence may be assumed minimal in this patient. The points which define line C represent observations on a patient with renal disease unable to respond to antidiuretic hormone. Note that when antidiuretic influence is constant, urine volume varies in proportion to the solute load. Furthermore, note that a given solute load may be excreted with a decreasing expenditure of water as antidiuretic hormone influence is increased. From J. D. Crawford, N. B. Talbot, C. U. Lowe and A. M. Butler. Unpublished observations.

Larger solute loads result from feeding diets of high protein and mineral content.* They also occur under conditions of prolonged fasting when endogenous protein catabolism and ketosis occur.[5]

* Minerals and organic solutes, particularly urea, are liberated by protein digestion; both those contained in free form in the diet and those released from organic combination by digestion of dietary protein are largely eliminated by way of the urine.

Relations between antidiuretic hormone, solute load, water load and maximum urine volume. The relation between water and solutes in the urine of patients with antidiuretic hormone insufficiency (simple diabetes insipidus) is not entirely fixed. Under conditions of water restriction, urine water may be reduced to a minimum of about 7 cc. per mosM, while under conditions of large water intake urine water may rise to a maximum of about 15 cc. per mosM. No clear explanation for this phenomenon is available at the present time. It is more of physiologic than of clinical importance. Accordingly, it will be ignored in the following paragraphs and the average values will be given.

Figure 2 shows that urine volumes do not necessarily reach 15,000 cc. per m^2 per day in the absence of antidiuretic hormone. According to Section B of that figure a urine volume of 10,000 cc. per m^2 per day would be expected in an individual excreting 1,000 mosM per m^2 per day (1,000 mosM x 10 cc. per mosM). Reductions of the solute load to 200 mosM per m^2 per day by the means described above would reduce the urine volume to but 2,000 cc. per m^2 per day. Only if such an individual were excreting 1,500 mosM, would the urine volume increase to the maximum of 15,000 cc. per m^2 per day (Section C, Figure 2). Larger solute loads, however, would be intolerable, for even in the absence of antidiuretic hormone the kidney is incapable of excreting urine at a rate exceeding about 15,000 cc. per m^2 per 24 hours.*

The ingestion of water in excess of body capacity for water elimination regularly results in signs of water intoxication, including hemodilution, tissue edema, convulsions and death (see Figure 5).

Even within the limits just described the normal organism has a large reserve capacity for solute elimination. Theoretically, the normal individual abundantly supplied with antidiuretic hormone could excrete, in 15,000 cc. of urine, a total of 15,000 x 1.5 or 23,000 mosM of solute, a value approximately 30 times greater than the average normal requirement (about 700 mosM per m^2 per day). Ordinarily this average load is eliminated in about 1,000 cc. of urine, or approximately 7 per cent of potentially available urine water.

Quantitative and temporal aspects of antidiuretic hormone action. Figure 6 presents observations which suggest that antidiuretic hormone exerts an all-or-none type of action on the kidney tubules. The administration of an antidiuretic

* In the absence of antidiuretic hormone it appears to be impossible, figuratively speaking, to crowd more than 1 mosM of solute into 10 cc. of water in lower tubular fluid. Consequently, no increase in urine concentration results from augmentation of the solute load. The materials which cannot find space in the urine accumulate in the body. Sometimes this leads to hemoconcentration and thirst and hence to excess water intake. Serious disturbances in body economy result whenever maximum renal capacity for either water or solutes is exceeded.

[506]   CHAPTER VIII:

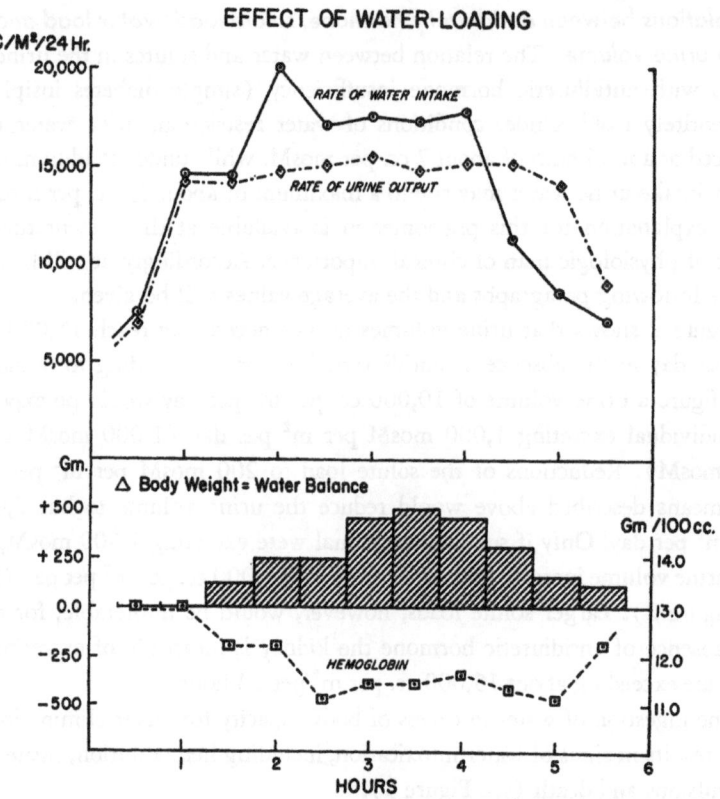

FIGURE VIII—5. Renal limitation of maximal urine volume. The subject of this experiment was a patient with diabetes insipidus. In the upper portion of the figure the rates of water intake and urine output are shown on the ordinate. In the lower portion of the figure the left- and right-hand ordinates give changes in body weight and hemoglobin concentration respectively. The abscissa indicates time in hours. Extra-renal water losses over the experimental period have been assumed negligible and hence change in weight has been used as an index of water balance. Note that renal water excretion kept pace with increasing water intake until a rate of 15,000 cc. per m² per 24 hours was reached. Renal water output then remained essentially constant even though the rate of intake was maintained significantly in excess of output. The failure of the rate of urine output to increase above this plateau value is apparently due to a renal limitation (see text). This experiment was terminated before serious consequences of water retention were observed. In Figure 10 similar data are shown from an experiment in which an animal was forced to develop marked water intoxication. From J. D. Crawford and N. B. Talbot. Unpublished data.

The Posterior Pituitary

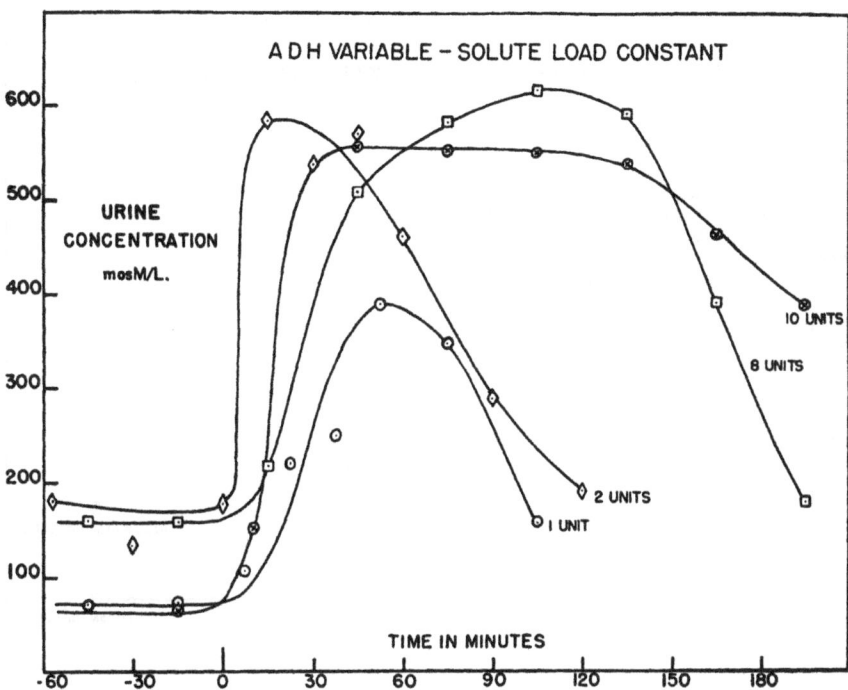

FIGURE VIII—6. Relation of pitressin dosage to duration of antidiuresis. The subject of this experiment was a patient with diabetes insipidus taking a diet with a urine solute residue of approximately 1,000 mosM per m^2 per day. Urine concentration and time in minutes are shown on the ordinate and abscissa respectively. The curves obtained after administration of pitressin in doses of 1, 2, 8 and 10 units are plotted on these coordinates. Note that approximately the same maximum urine concentration was attained in each instance, but that the period of time during which maximally concentrated urine was excreted was roughly proportional to the size of the pitressin dose. From J. D. Crawford. Unpublished data.

---

hormone preparation to an individual with posterior pituitary insufficiency results within a few minutes in a marked decrease in the ratio of water to solutes in urine or, in more familiar terms, a marked increase in urine concentration and decrease in urine volume. If the dose is small, this increase in urine concentration persists for only a short time. If the dose is larger, the degree of urine concentration is approximately the same but of longer duration.

The duration of action of a given dose of antidiuretic hormone seems to bear an inverse relation to the size of the solute load presenting for excretion per unit of time (see Figure 7). In other words, more antidiuretic hormone is needed to

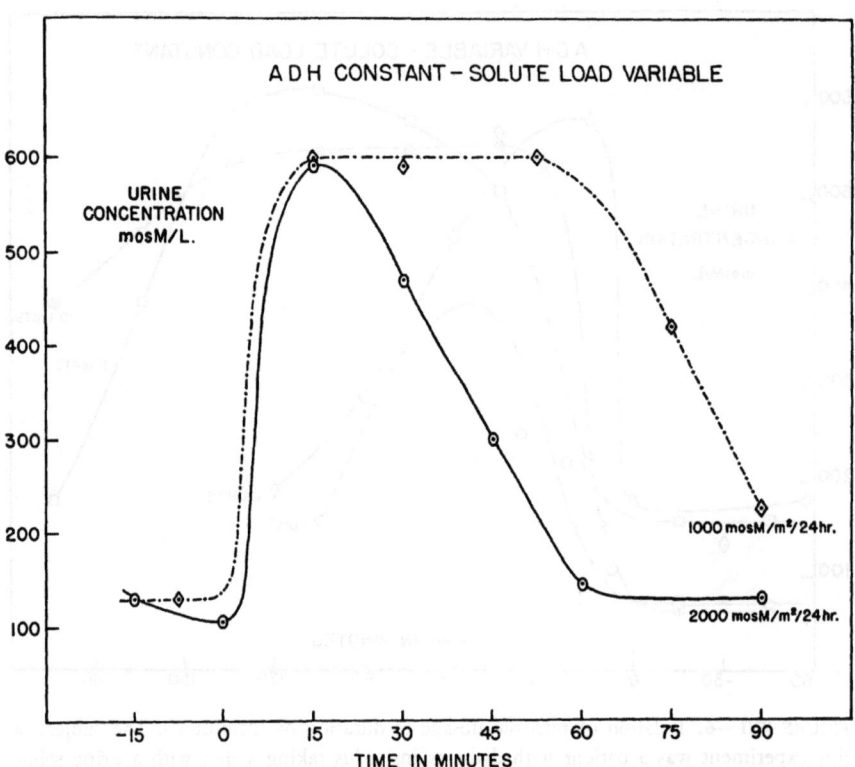

FIGURE VIII—7. Relation of urine solute excretion to duration of pitressin antidiuresis. The subject of this experiment was the same as in Figure 6. The effect of 2 units of pitressin was studied when the patient was on two different diets providing respectively 1,000 and 2,000 mosM per m² per day for renal excretion. Note that in both instances administration of pitressin resulted in approximately equal increases in urine concentration (ordinate). The duration of action (abscissa) was significantly greater when the patient was taking the low solute diet than when he took the diet with a high solute residue. From J. D. Crawford. Unpublished data.

eliminate a maximally concentrated urine containing 2,000 mosM of solute per m² per day than a similarly concentrated urine containing only 1,000 mosM. Such observations suggest that antidiuretic hormone determines renal capacity for osmotic work as regards water reabsorption.[6a] They further suggest that antidiuretic hormone may be produced in proportion to osmotic demands.[6b, c]

Relations between antidiuretic hormone and urine solute composition. In the foregoing sections it has been assumed that antidiuretic hormone does not

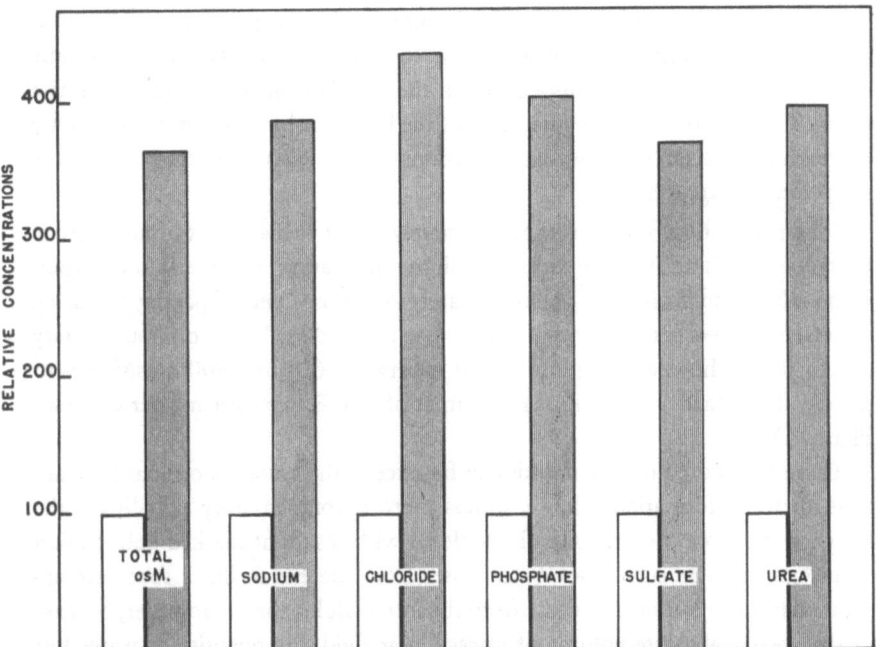

FIGURE VIII—8. Effect of antidiuretic hormone on renal solute excretion. The subject of this experiment was a normal individual. Two urine specimens were collected over consecutive 15-minute periods. The first collection was made at the height of a water diuresis. One unit of pitressin was injected intravenously immediately after termination of the first collection. The urine volume of the first specimen was 158 cc., while that of the second was 40 cc. The two specimens were analyzed for total solutes and for several different individual constituents. The figure shows that the total and the various individual solute concentrations increased about fourfold after pitressin administration; the absolute rate of solute output was essentially unchanged. This is interpreted to mean that pitressin caused an increase in tubular water reabsorption with but little effect upon the reabsorption of solutes. From J. D. Crawford. Unpublished observations.

---

influence renal solute output either quantitatively or qualitatively. This assumption is approximately in keeping with available facts. Although administration of large amounts of commercially prepared posterior pituitary extracts* may result in increased excretion of certain solutes, especially chloride ion,[7 a] smaller, more physiologic doses have insignificant chloruretic effects (see Figure 8).[7 b-d] Moreover, antidiuretic material extracted from the urine of dehydrated but otherwise normal individuals appears to have no chloruretic effect.[7 e, f]

* These extracts are probably relatively impure and may contain physiologically active substances other than antidiuretic hormone.

Secondary Effects of Antidiuretic Hormone. In the prolonged absence of antidiuretic hormone, losses of water due to inefficient facultative renal tubule reabsorption have far-reaching effects on the metabolism of the individual as a whole. Conversely, excessive quantities of the hormone have opposite but equally far-reaching effects. These secondary actions will be discussed separately in the succeeding paragraphs.

Effects of antidiuretic hormone deficiency. The initial effect of antidiuretic hormone lack is an increase in urine volume in relation to urine solute output. If the solute load is minimal (approximately 200 mosM per m^2 per day), a urine volume of 2 liters per m^2 per day results (see page 502). Under ordinary dietary circumstances, however, the solute load is between 600 and 800 mosM per m^2 per day. Such loads result in urine volumes of 6 to 8 liters per m^2 per day (see Figure 4).

These losses of water by the kidney far exceed the amounts ordinarily available for urine formation. Hence, unless there is compensatory polydipsia, the body's water stores become rapidly depleted with resultant marked dehydration (see Figure 9). In such cases water losses from the extracellular space are approximately proportional to those from the intracellular space. However, because of the greater absolute volume of intracellular fluid, the quantity of water lost from the cellular compartment exceeds that lost from extracellular sources.[8] The transfer of water from the intracellular to the extracellular space, where it is available to meet renal water needs, is accomplished by the maintenance of an extracellular osmolar concentration which is slightly greater than that in intracellular fluid (see Figure 9 and Chapter III, Figure 10). In the acute experiment of Figure 9 (this chapter) the dissociation between potassium and nitrogen losses seen in more chronic dehydration is not evident (see Chapter IX, Figure 2).

The dehydration results in hemoconcentration and particularly a rise in serum sodium. The immediate result of these changes is a marked increase in thirst.[8] A large water intake secondary thereto ordinarily prevents the extreme dehydration which occurs when water is withheld. Interestingly, patients with diabetes insipidus also develop anorexia. As described above, moderate anorexia results in a reduction of urine solute output and hence in minimal obligatory urine volume. In patients with long-standing diabetes insipidus this anorexia becomes selective. Foods of high metabolite and mineral residue (particularly protein and salty foods) are specifically avoided. In their stead a diet consisting largely of carbohydrates, which are relatively low in mineral content (potatoes, rice, bread, macaroni, fruits) and fats, is chosen.[9a]

A further change noted under these conditions is a decrease in the rates of extrarenal water loss. Sweating is almost never observed in patients with a deficiency of antidiuretic hormone.[9 b] The water content of the stools is also apt to be diminished.[9 c]

Effects of excessive quantities of antidiuretic hormone.[9 b, 10 a, b] Administration of posterior pituitary extracts to normal individuals in excess of need results in abnormal water retention. At first the volume of extracellular fluid becomes overexpanded. Within a short time, however, osmotic forces cause a portion of the surplus water to move into the intracellular compartment of the body (see Chapter III, Figure 10). Both extracellular and intracellular edema results.*

Extension of these changes to toxic degrees is normally prevented by avoidance of water (i.e., lack of thirst). On the other hand, if this natural protective reaction is by-passed and water ingestion in excess of needs is continued, body metabolism becomes seriously disturbed. Cerebral edema, convulsions and death ensue.

Control of Posterior Pituitary Activity by the Hypothalamus.[11] Transection of the pituitary stalk, interruption of the fiber tracts leading from the supra-optic and paraventricular nuclei of the hypothalamus or destruction of these nuclei themselves all lead to a deficiency in antidiuretic hormone similar to that seen after removal of the posterior pituitary. The secretory activity of the neurocytes in the posterior pituitary thus appears to be under the control of nervous impulses from the hypothalamus. In the absence of stimulation by such impulses, no antidiuretic hormone is released from the gland and the neurocyte content of antidiuretic material rapidly diminishes. When stimulation is absent over long periods, the neurocytes undergo morphologic changes suggestive of degeneration.

Factors Which Stimulate the Neurohypophyseal Mechanism.[12 a] Two factors, namely emotional stress and hemoconcentration, induce antidiuretic hormone secretion. Rage, fear and excitement are examples of the first type of stress that can elicit this response. Physical exercise, epinephrine and a variety of noxious drugs and stimulants have a similar effect.

An increase in serum osmolar concentration (decrease in the ratio of water to solutes in serum) can be produced artificially, as by the intravenous administration of concentrated sucrose solution, or can occur spontaneously as a result of negative water balance. When serum osmolar concentration is elevated, as by the intravenous administration of concentrated sucrose solution, increased antidiuretic hormone action is evidenced by the prompt appearance of concentrated urine. In a previously well-hydrated subject, the increase in urine

---

* Extrarenal water losses may be markedly increased by administration of posterior pituitary extracts. Profuse sweating as well as diarrhea and vomiting may be induced. Since available extracts contain the oxytocic principle as well as certain other substances, it is not clear whether these extrarenal water losses result directly from antidiuretic hormone action.

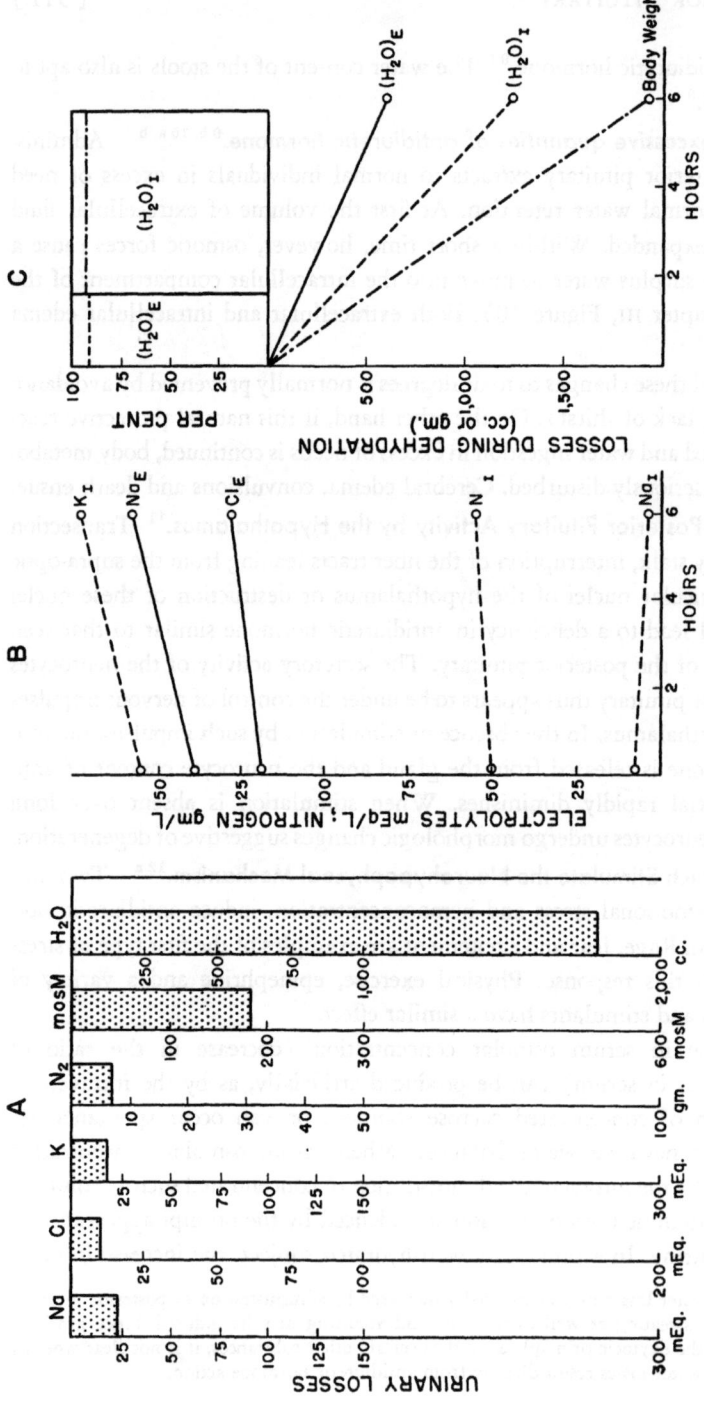

FIGURE VIII—9. Metabolic changes in water deprivation in diabetes insipidus. The subject of this experiment was a patient with diabetes insipidus deprived of food and water for a period of six hours (see also Figure 12).

SECTION A shows the urinary losses of sodium, chloride, potassium, nitrogen, total solutes and water plotted on individual ordinates which indicate the approximate relative distribution of these substances in body fluids. Note that the losses of the various individual solutes are nearly proportional to one another and that they are small in relation to the loss of water.

SECTION B shows the calculated changes in the concentration of these solutes in body fluids. Note that there are approximately proportional increases in intracellular and extracellular fluid solute concentrations with the exception of intracellular sodium, which appeared to be leaving cell fluid.

SECTION C: The calculated losses of intracellular and extracellular water are shown on the lower ordinate. The upper ordinate shows per cent changes in total extra- and intracellular fluid volumes. Note that although the absolute loss of intracellular water is approximately twice that of extracellular water, per cent losses from original volumes are almost equal. From J. D. Crawford, C. U. Lowe and N. B. Talbot. Unpublished observations.

concentration is proportionally far greater than the increase in serum osmolar concentration. In fact, the increased osmolar concentration due to the sucrose is rapidly overcome by the increased renal water economy.

If the hypertonic solution is injected directly into the internal carotid artery of an experimental subject, a marked antidiuresis occurs even if osmolar concentration elsewhere in the body has not been increased. Such observations indicate that there are hypothalamic "osmoreceptors" which are sensitive to small changes in osmolar concentration of the fluid in which they are bathed (see Figure 1). It appears that when the fluid reaching these receptors has an osmolar concentration of less than 310 mosM per liter the hypothalamic cells remain quiescent and little or no antidiuretic hormone is secreted. Contrariwise, when the osmolar concentration of the fluid reaching the cells is increased above this critical value, impulses are sent to the neurocytes of the posterior pituitary, which then discharge antidiuretic hormone into the circulation.

These receptors have not been identified histologically, but certain functional peculiarities of the system have been defined. The receptors respond to a variety of hypertonic solutions infused via the internal carotid artery. Initially, the response appears to be a function of the total osmolar concentration rather than the chemical composition of the solution. Prolonged infusion experiments suggest, however, that chemical composition of the infusate is important. Sodium salts appear to cause continued stimulation proportional to osmolar concentration over relatively long periods. Urea solutions, on the other hand, appear to have a diminishing effect with time. This behavior of the hypothalamic osmoreceptors is reminiscent of the behavior of the kidneys toward urea. The kidneys, it will be remembered, offer urea a position in urine proportional to its osmotic importance when a urea load is at first imposed. Later urea appears to be tucked into the same osmotic space as the major electrolytes sodium and potassium.[12 b]

A further peculiarity of the hypothalamic osmoreceptors is evident in the difference in behavior occasioned by suddenly, as contrasted with slowly, effected changes in serum osmolar concentration. Acute increases regularly result in an increase in antidiuretic hormone production; changes occurring over days or weeks cause a much smaller response than equal changes occurring over a period of minutes or hours.[12 c] In other words, the system may under certain circumstances fail to respond adequately to a serious need for water conservation or, conversely, for water elimination.

Elimination and Inactivation of Antidiuretic Hormone. Material with antidiuretic properties similar to those of posterior pituitary extract is found in the urine of normal individuals. The rate of renal excretion of this antidiuretic material is increased by restriction of water and decreased when water is given in excess of needs. It disappears from the urine entirely when need for conserving water is eliminated by a very large intake. The amount of antidiuretic material in urine bears a relation to the solute content. Urine passed during a given period when the solute load is large contains more of such material than that passed during the same length of time and at the same concentration but under conditions of decreased load. Thus the amount excreted in urine appears to bear a relation to the state of hydration and to the need for "renal osmotic work" (see page 508).[13]

Antidiuretic material is regularly absent from the urine after destruction of the posterior pituitary. When posterior pituitary extracts are administered, an increase in antidiuretic activity is detectable in urine subsequently excreted. However, the activity of material thus recovered is less than that of the injected extract. The ratio of material recovered to material administered diminishes as the dose increases.[13] These observations give additional evidence for the identity of the antidiuretic material in urine with that secreted by the posterior pituitary. They suggest that the disappearance of antidiuretic material from the urine when need for water conservation is eliminated can be explained by postulating prompt cessation of hormone production. On the other hand, the fact that the well-hydrated individual excretes only a fraction of administered hormone suggests that excesses are partially inactivated or destroyed within the body.

Studies of the inactivation of antidiuretic hormone by various tissues suggest that an important role is played by the liver.[14 a, b] Liver tissue as well as cell-free hepatic extracts can rapidly inactivate large quantities of posterior pituitary extract. Initially, the original antidiuretic activity of posterior lobe extracts may be recovered by elution from the liver proteins. With the passage of time, a diminishing fraction of the original activity is recoverable by this means. Such loss of activity can be prevented by heating the liver extract before adding antidiuretic material. Hence, liver proteins appear to have not only a capacity for rapid inactivation of antidiuretic hormone by adsorption, but also a capacity for slow enzymatic destruction of adsorbed material.

The quantitative importance of these processes in the living subject has not been determined. It is of interest, nevertheless, to note that antidiuretic hormone has been found in increased concentrations in the blood and urine of patients with hepatic insufficiency.[7 f] Furthermore, patients with severe liver disease are apt to show a marked delay in diuresis after administration of a water load.[7 f, 14 c, d] Such deficiencies in water excretion have sometimes dramatically responded to administration of crude liver extracts.[14 d, e]

The Role of the Adrenal Cortex in Water Metabolism.[15 a, b] In patients with progressive cerebral lesions the large volumes of urine which are seen characteristically after destruction of the posterior pituitary are no longer observed when there is subsequent destruction of the anterior pituitary gland. Similar changes are noted in experimental animals when first the posterior and then the anterior pituitary or adrenal cortices are removed. If such animals are treated with adrenocortical extract, the water metabolism typical of posterior hypophysectomy reappears. Theoretically, treatment of totally hypophysectomized animals with pituitary adrenocorticotropic hormone should also result in return of symptoms of posterior pituitary hypofunction. In practice, the demonstration of this phenomenon is difficult, owing to contamination of available adrenocorticotropic hormone preparations with antidiuretic material of posterior lobe origin.

The tendency for hypoadrenocorticism, whether primary or secondary to panhypopituitarism, to cause the disappearance of the polyuria of simple posterior pituitary insufficiency may be explained by the following factors. To begin with, it will be remembered that urine volume is the product of two variables, urine solute output and the relation of urine water to urine solutes expressed as the ratio cc. per mosM. Removal of either the adrenals or the anterior pituitary, if the posterior pituitary has already been removed, does not alter to an important extent the average water solute ratio in urine. However, both adrenalectomy and hypophysectomy are apt to lead to a reduction in urine solute excretion. It appears likely that this diminished solute output, referable to a decrease in appetite, is a major factor in the disappearance of polyuria when the individual with diabetes insipidus becomes totally hypophysectomized. Large volumes of urine can be restored by urging a diet which increases solute excretion to normal levels.

The adrenocortical hormones appear to have an additional effect on water metabolism quite apart from their influence on solute excretion. This effect can be illustrated by observations under three sets of circumstances. First, individuals with simple adrenocortical insufficiency are unable rapidly to dilute their urine in response to a sudden water load. In association with this phenomenon it has been found that after water-loading antidiuretic material fails to disappear as promptly from these individuals' blood as from that of normal subjects. However, it is not known whether, under these circumstances, the abnormal persistence of antidiuretic material is the result of excessive production or delayed inactivation. Secondly, stressed individuals with evidence of physiologic hyperadrenocorticism are frequently observed to excrete large volumes of relatively dilute urine even when dehydrated. Such individuals have been found to have large quantities of antidiuretic material in their blood and urine, indicating an abundant endogenous supply. Furthermore, they fail to show more than a limited response to administered hormone. These observations suggest some type of antagonism between the adrenocortical and posterior pituitary hormones at the level of the kidney. Finally, it has been noted that patients with diabetes insipidus complicated by primary adrenocortical failure or hypoadrenocorticism secondary to panhypopituitarism exhibit a sluggish diuretic response to water-loading which is qualitatively similar to that seen in simple hypoadrenocorticism. It is difficult to explain this phenomenon by any of the mechanisms mentioned above. Thus, it can be seen that the interrelations of the posterior pituitary, adrenal cortices and anterior pituitary are complex and not completely understood.

Summary Remarks on Limits of Control of Water Homeostasis by the Posterior Pituitary. In the foregoing sections the mechanisms by which the posterior pituitary mediates antidiuresis have been outlined. It is apparent that the normal function of the system is to maintain within an optimum range the water content of extracellular and, indirectly, of intracellular fluid in relation to the solutes which they contain. The lability and the efficiency of the system is manifest by the normal constancy of body water despite wide variations in the rates of water intake, extrarenal water loss and urinary solute output. As is true with respect to other homeostatic systems, the posterior pituitary–renal system can operate to protect the constancy of body water supplies only within certain readily defined limits.

In the normal individual maximum water economy is a function of proper operation of the antidiuretic mechanism and of the solute load requiring renal excretion. Maximum urine concentration achieved in the presence of abundant supplies of antidiuretic hormone is in the neighborhood of 1,500 mosM per liter. Solutes presenting for renal excretion can be reduced to approximately 200 mosM per m^2 per day. The sum of minimal urine volume (135 cc.) and extrarenal water requirements (500 cc. per m^2 per day) then yields a figure of approximately 635 cc. per m^2 per day for the lowest water intake permitting survival without dehydration.

In the absence of antidiuretic hormone water excretion is limited by low rates of solute output. This is because a volume of not more than 10 cc. of water can accompany each solute milliosmole. Hence, when solute excretion is reduced to 200 mosM per m^2 per day maximum urine volume is limited to approximately 2,000 cc. per m^2 per day. Calculations similar to those used above to define the minimal water intake permitting survival without dehydration show that with a solute load of 200 mosM per m^2 per day the maximal water intake tolerated without overhydration is 2,500 cc. per m^2 per day.

In the absence of antidiuretic hormone proportionally larger volumes of urine can be excreted as the solute output is increased until the ultimate limit of 15,000 cc. per m^2 per day is reduced. This limit is imposed by the participation of 85 per cent of the glomerular filtrate water in obligatory tubular reabsorption. While this maximal volume of urine can contain only 1,500 mosM of solute per m^2 per day when antidiuretic is absent, much larger amounts of solute can be excreted when antidiuretic hormone is available. Efforts to increase urine volume above the maximum defined by the kidney are unavailing and result in serious consequences including water intoxication, circulatory collapse, hematuria and death (see Figure 10).

Within these wide limits the normal posterior pituitary–renal system maintains essential constancy of body water stores. An increase in serum osmolar concentration of as little as 2 per cent activates the posterior pituitary to increased production of antidiuretic hormone. Within as short a period as 10 minutes increased conservation of water is indicated by excretion of a more concentrated urine. Conversely, a decrease in serum osmolar concentration of similar proportions is sufficient to inhibit antidiuretic hormone production. Beginning elimination of the excess water may be shown by a fall in urine concentration within a period of 20 to 30 minutes.[12a]

Symptoms of antidiuretic hormone lack are ordinarily absent if the lesion fails to destroy or cause degeneration of less than approximately 95 per cent of the secretory neurocytes of the posterior pituitary.[11] In experimental animals lesions which destroy a significant portion but less than 95 per cent of the posterior pituitary produce signs of antidiuretic hormone deficiency only if the solute load is markedly increased.[16] These observations suggest that maintenance of normal water homeostasis requires only a small fraction of the maximal potential capacity of the hypothalamic-neurohypophyseal system.

CLINICAL CONSIDERATIONS

Some of the conditions in which polyuria is apt to be the chief complaint are classified in Table 1. Here also are listed certain characteristics of each condition which are helpful in differential diagnosis. Detailed descriptions of these conditions will be found in the ensuing paragraphs.

HYPOFUNCTION OF THE POSTERIOR PITUITARY

Posterior pituitary hypofunction is manifest by the events described earlier in connection with antidiuretic hormone deficiency (see page 510). It may be

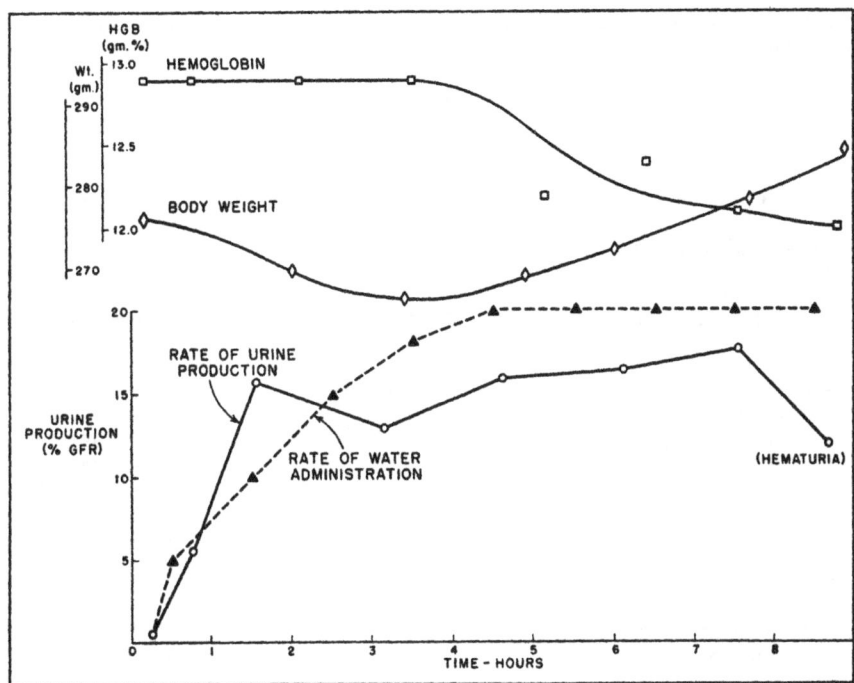

FIGURE VIII—10. Induction of water intoxication. The above experiment, carried out in a normal rat, is comparable to that of Figure 5. It shows in addition nearly the full range in adaptative response of a subject with normal posterior pituitary function. In the early hours of the experiment the rate of urine output kept pace with the increasing rate of water administration, so that there was no dilution of body fluids. Hemoglobin concentration remained constant. The initial weight loss is accounted for by extra-renal losses as well as by renal losses slightly in excess of intake. After approximately two hours the rate of urine production reached the physiologic maximum (approximately 15 per cent of glomerular filtration rate). However, there was an increase in body weight owing to continued administration of water. Simultaneously there was a dilution of body fluids, as indicated by the fall in hemoglobin concentration. These changes were poorly tolerated; the animal eventually showed a fall in urine volume, hematuria and convulsions. Observations of J. D. Crawford and N. B. Talbot as set forth in *Pediatrics* 6:1, 1950.

the result of an organic lesion or of a functional disorder. Organic lesions causing loss of water economy may be located in or adjacent to the posterior lobe itself or may be present in the paraventricular and supra-optic nuclei of the hypothalamus. Lesions located so as to interrupt the nervous pathways traversing the floor of the third ventricle and pituitary stalk likewise result in loss of posterior pituitary activity. Functional reduction in antidiuretic hormone production occurs

TABLE VIII—1. Classification and characteristics of several conditions in which polyuria may be the presenting complaint.

Condition	Urine concentration	Response to Posterior pituitary extract *	Response to Water deprivation †	Blood NPN	Remarks
A. Hypofunction of posterior pituitary					
1. Primary diabetes insipidus	<1.005	N **	0	Low	X-rays may show lesion in area of optic chiasm or sella turcica
2. Functional psychogenic polydipsia	<1.005	N	N	Low	History usually suggests emotional instability. Physical examination may show evidence of inanition but not dehydration
B. Non-neurohypophyseal					
3. Nephrogenic diabetes insipidus	<1.005	0	0	Low	Usually seen in males; often familial; present at birth
4. Pannephritis	1.010	0	0	N or high	Usually there is a clear-cut history of renal disease
5. Adrenocortical alarm reaction	1.015	—	—	N	Relative resistance to antidiuretic hormone

* See page 521. † See page 524. ** N = Normal; — = subnormal; 0 = essentially no response

when the intact neurohypophyseal system lacks the osmotic stimulation which normally operates almost continuously to cause hormone secretion.

Pathologic Posterior Pituitary Hypofunction (Diabetes Insipidus) (Table 1, Condition 1).[4b, 17a] This is a rare disturbance, which may be seen at any age. It occurs somewhat more frequently in boys than in girls. Once it develops it is almost always permanent.

ETIOLOGY. The cause of diabetes insipidus is variable. In childhood the most common neoplastic lesions occurring in or encroaching upon the hypothalamic-neurohypophyseal system are craniopharyngiomas, eosinophilic granulomas, medulloblastomas and "metastatic" pinealomas (see Figure 11). Diabetes insipidus has been seen after severe head trauma, particularly after fracture through the base of the skull. It also may occur as a result of a pyogenic abscess adjacent to the posterior lobe. Not infrequently the cause is obscure, there being no demonstrable organic lesion in the hypothalamic or posterior pituitary areas. Such cases are classified under the somewhat unsatisfactory term "idiopathic" (see Figure 12).

CLINICAL MANIFESTATIONS. Symptoms usually develop suddenly, so that the patient is able to date the beginning of the disorder accurately. The most prominent of these are polyuria and polydipsia. The average urine volume is from 8 to 10 liters per m^2 per day immediately after onset. The water intake necessary to maintain hydration is correspondingly great. Children with this disease have such an urgent thirst that when parents attempt to curb it they find it necessary to watch the child continuously. Hospitalized patients have been known to steal water from neighboring bedside tables, water faucets, toilets, flower vases—in fact, from almost every conceivable source. Water restriction is of no therapeutic value. When used for diagnosis it results in dehydration and may lead to manic behavior.

The constant need for water intake and elimination is accompanied by a disturbance of sleep habits, increasing fatigue and irritability. Loss of appetite is characterized by the specific anorexia described earlier (page 510). Fatigue in itself may act further to decrease dietary intake. Nausea is frequent in the morning, when patients are usually most dehydrated.

Constipation, skin dryness due to lack of sweat formation, diminished skin elasticity and reduced mucous membrane moistness resulting from dehydration are frequently present. In instances of long-continued antidiuretic hormone lack, the rates of growth, sexual maturation and general body metabolism are apt to be reduced.

In addition to the specific symptomatology described above, patients with diabetes insipidus often show signs indicative of intracranial tumor. Headache is frequent. Bitemporal hemianopia may be demonstrated by the confrontation test. Separation of the cranial sutures may be detected by the cracked-pot resonance of the skull. It is of utmost importance to make a detailed neurological examination of any patient having the symptomatology of diabetes insipidus.

LABORATORY STUDIES. Certain of the laboratory findings in diabetes insipidus are specific and, as such, serve as diagnostic tests. The most important are (a) demonstration of a normal response to administration of posterior pituitary extract and (b) demonstration of an inability to maintain hydration under conditions of water deprivation.

Response to administered posterior pituitary extract. Intravenous or subcutaneous administration of 2 units per m^2 of aqueous posterior pituitary extract to patients with diabetes insipidus is regularly followed by a marked reduction

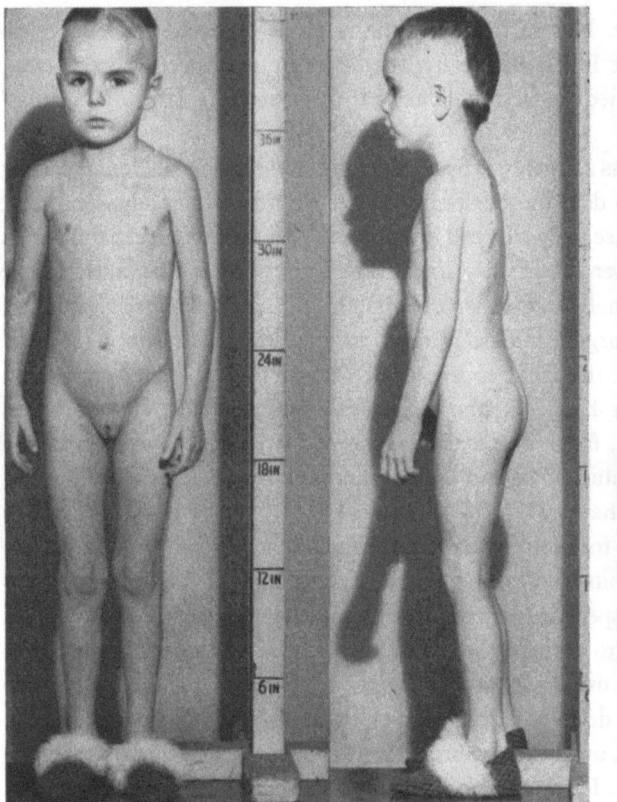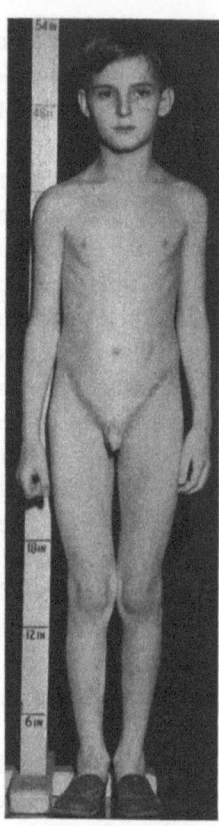

(Left)
FIGURE VIII—11. Diabetes insipidus due to metastatic pinealoma in a girl of six years.

(Right)
FIGURE VIII—12. Idiopathic diabetes insipidus in a boy of 12 years.

CASE HISTORY (FIGURE 11)

The patient was essentially well until the age of four, when she had a sudden generalized convulsion. In the succeeding two years she suffered from progressive weight loss, anorexia, lassitude, easy fatigability and constipation. At five years of age polydipsia and polyuria became noticeable. Initially these complaints were thought to be of emotional origin, but by the time of her admission to the hospital it was clear that she had an organic disease. On physical examination she was found to be completely blind in her left eye and to have temporal hemianopia of the right. There was bilateral optic atrophy. Laboratory studies showed that her urine had a specific gravity of 1.005. The six-hour water deprivation test was positive for diabetes insipidus. Response to pitressin was normal. Urea clearance prior to pitressin therapy was 30 per cent of normal. Following a few months of treatment, it rose to 50 per cent of normal. Spinal fluid contained 12 lymphocytes per mm^3 and 148 mg. per cent of total protein. Roentgenograms indicated that skull and bones were normal.

Exploration of the optic chiasmal region via a left transfrontal craniotomy by Dr. B. Selverstone revealed an ectopic pinealoma anterior to the chiasm. It could not be removed. During this operation and for about 60 hours afterward a team of physicians made half-hourly measurements of hemoglobin and blood specific gravity, of urine volume and specific gravity. Serial determinations of circulating eosinophils were made in anticipation of possible acute adrenocortical insufficiency secondary to anterior pituitary failure. On the basis of these measurements and of the patient's pulse, blood pressure and general condition, the rate of flow of an intravenous infusion of 5 per cent dextrose in water was adjusted at frequent intervals.

The aim was to provide enough water to prevent dehydration, hemoconcentration and cardiovascular failure on the one hand and overhydration, cerebral edema and other manifestations of water intoxication on the other. During and immediately after the operation it was decided not to administer antidiuretic hormone, which would fix urine volume relative to solute output, but to take advantage of the leeway indicated by the discussion on page 505. The patient's water requirements on this regimen varied between 230 and about 350 cc. per m^2 per hour. No overhydration developed until after pitressin therapy was started. She then suffered two brief episodes of hemodilution, bradycardia and loss of mental responsiveness. During one of these she had a convulsion.

The patient's subsequent course has been satisfactory. Following recovery from the operation, a total dose of 3,000 roentgens was administered to the tumor area. The eye changes have not progressed. Symptoms of diabetes insipidus have been controlled by nasal instillations of pitressin. Normal growth has been resumed and the child is able to attend school.

CASE HISTORY (FIGURE 12)

The patient suddenly developed polyuria and polydipsia three months before hospital admission. During this period he lost approximately 3 kg. in weight and became tired, listless and anorexic. Studies of his response to water deprivation and pitressin administration are illustrated in Figures 6, 7 and 9. Since hospital discharge he has been treated with an aqueous solution of posterior pituitary administered in the form of nose drops. Diabetes insipidus has been satisfactorily controlled. He has continued to grow normally, gain in weight and mature sexually. Repeated studies have been unsuccessful in discovering the reason for the failure of the antidiuretic mechanism.

in urine volume and a simultaneous rise in urine concentration (see Figure 6). The aim of administering this relatively large dose is to achieve a rapid and abundant concentration at the kidney. Excess hormone is not harmful if water is withheld until the effect of the drug has been dissipated. A period of two hours should be sufficient. It should be noted that, for reasons not clearly understood, the urine of patients with diabetes insipidus is less concentrated than that of normal persons following administration of posterior pituitary extract. However, if therapy is continued for a period of days or weeks the former may show an increased ability to concentrate urine in response to a given dose of extract.

The water deprivation test. This test should be carried out under careful surveillance. Not only may the result be misleading unless the patient is kept under constant watch, but even during the course of the test water losses may be so rapid as to lead to serious dehydration.

At a time when the patient is well hydrated, he is asked to empty the bladder. He is then weighed and blood is drawn for hemoglobin, hematocrit or serum protein. The volume and concentration of urine passed are noted. Thereafter, all sources of water are withheld for six hours, unless the patient becomes dangerously dehydrated sooner. At hourly intervals until the end of the period he is re-weighed and urine and blood studies are repeated.

During the six-hour test patients with diabetes insipidus show relatively little decrease in urine volume, but some diminution will ordinarily occur, since urinary excretion of solutes becomes smaller in the early hours of fasting. Urine concentration fails to decrease above a specific gravity of approximately 1.005. Weight loss of 1 kg. per m^2 or more occurs. Finally, there is a steep rise in values for serum protein, hemoglobin or hematocrit. These changes reflect a shrinking of intravascular fluid volume and are indicative of depletion in stores of all body water. In Figure 13 the results of water deprivation in the case of a patient with diabetes insipidus are shown graphically. This figure is to be compared with Figure 14, which shows the reactions to a similar test of a patient with normal posterior pituitary function.

Certain other laboratory findings in diabetes insipidus deserve mention. Despite inability of patients with this disease to concentrate urine, other tests of renal function yield essentially normal results. Blood non-protein nitrogen is apt to be low because of the rapid rate of urine excretion as well as the avoidance of protein foods.* Urea clearance may be depressed to 50 or 60 per cent of normal. The reason for this is not entirely clear. A return to normal may be noted after prolonged treatment with posterior pituitary extracts. Values for the

---

* Within certain limits, urea excretion varies directly with the rate of urine flow.

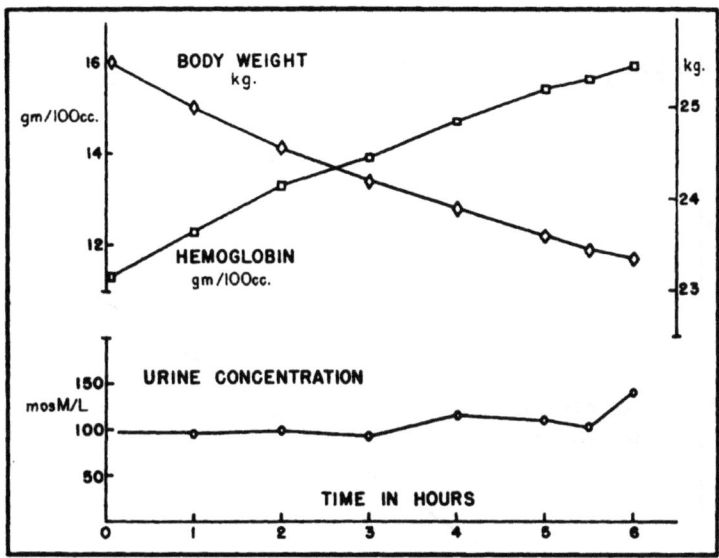

FIGURE VIII—13. Water deprivation test in diabetes insipidus. The subject of this test was a 10-year-old boy with diabetes insipidus. Body weight and hemoglobin concentration are shown on the upper right-hand ordinates. Urine concentration is shown on the lower left-hand ordinate. The abscissa shows time in hours. Note the rapid loss in weight and rise in hemoglobin concentration evidencing rapid dehydration. Little increase in urine concentration was observed as dehydration progressed. Observations of J. D. Crawford, C. U. Lowe and N. B. Talbot as set forth in *Pediatrics* 6:1, 1950.

---

concentration of the various serum electrolytes and for hemoglobin and total protein are generally within the normal range. This is a consequence of the nicety with which the thirst mechanism ordinarily regulates water intake to meet the increased need. Measurements of total serum osmolar concentration usually show values within the normal range.

Finally, certain laboratory data should be obtained in an effort to determine whether a progressive cerebral lesion is present. These studies include visual field perimetry; roentgenographs of the skull, particularly including views of the region of the sella turcica; x-rays of the long bones, if eosinophilic granuloma is suspected; lumbar puncture and electroencephalography. Pneumoencephalography may be a necessary diagnostic step to visualize a lesion in the area of the cisterna chiasmatica. It should be noted in this regard that diabetes insipidus is sometimes the first indication of a progressive cerebral neoplasm. On several occasions exhaustive neurological studies, carried out soon after the onset of this

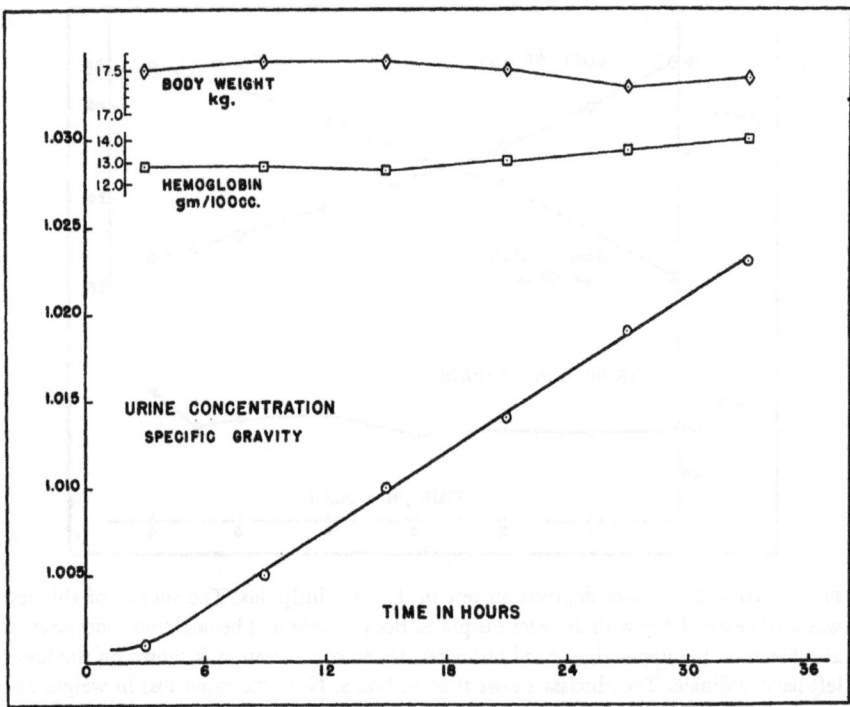

FIGURE VIII—14. Water restriction in psychogenic polydipsia. The subject of this experiment was a 4-year-old girl with psychogenic polydipsia. She was denied water but not food for 36 hours. Note that body weight and hemoglobin concentration remained essentially constant during the 36-hour period. Urine concentration slowly but progressively increased to high normal values. From J. D. Crawford, B. Frame and N. B. Talbot as set forth in *Pediatrics* 6:1, 1950.

disturbance, showed no evidence of a cerebral tumor, and yet in time the lesion became grossly manifest. Hence, studies should be repeated at intervals when the cause is not evident in earlier studies.

DIAGNOSIS AND DIFFERENTIAL DIAGNOSIS. The diagnosis of diabetes insipidus is suspected from the history of polyuria and polydipsia and confirmed by the specific laboratory tests outlined in the previous section.

Table 1 lists the conditions ordinarily to be considered in the differential diagnosis. Note that diabetes insipidus is distinguished from psychogenic polydipsia by the results of the water deprivation test. It differs from nephrogenic diabetes insipidus in that it is responsive to posterior pituitary extract. In pannephritis the serious impairment of several aspects of renal function is usually readily demonstrable, while in the polyuria of the adrenocortical alarm reaction appropriate treatment of the underlying acute disease results in restoration of urine volume and concentration to normal.

It might be anticipated from previous discussion (page 516) that diabetes insipidus sometimes occurs in latent form. On rare occasions a cerebral lesion may initially interrupt the mechanisms of the hypothalamic-neurohypophyseal system, thus producing the clinical manifestations of the disease. When extension of the lesion subsequently results in damage to the anterior pituitary gland, the symptomatology is ameliorated.

In these instances of true panhypopituitarism, demonstration of latent diabetes insipidus has only academic importance. Following replacement therapy with adrenocortical extract or cortisone, the reappearance of marked polyuria with inability to concentrate urine is strongly suggestive of anterior and posterior pituitary failure.

TREATMENT. This will be considered under several headings.

Antidiuretic hormone replacement therapy. Several preparations containing the antidiuretic factor of posterior pituitary are available for use in replacement therapy. Posterior Pituitary Injection (USP) is an aqueous solution with approximately equal antidiuretic and oxytocic activity. Vasopressin Injection (USP), also an aqueous solution, contains 20 units of pressor activity with less than 1.0 units of oxytocic activity per cc. Hence it is preferable to Posterior Pituitary Injection for treatment of diabetes insipidus. Pitressin Tannate Injection (USP) is similar to vasopressin but contains only 5 units of pressor activity per cc. The tannation and oily vehicle provide for relatively slow absorption following intramuscular administration. All three preparations are dispensed in sterile ampules and are intended for parenteral use.

Several preparations are manufactured for topical application. These take advantage of the fact that antidiuretic activity is relatively well absorbed from the surface of several mucous membranes, including the nasal mucosa and the vagina. Posterior Pituitary (USP) is a dry powder containing not less than 1 unit of pressor activity in 1.0 mg. The powder can be used for nasal insufflation but is apt to be irritating. Made up as a 7.5 per cent solution in saline with 0.5 per cent acetic acid added to bring the pH down to 4.5, it is satisfactory for intranasal use as a spray or in drop form. The solution is less irritating than the dry powder.

Vaginal suppositories are manufactured for the control of the disease in females. Incidentally, antidiuretic material is also absorbed from the mucosa of the bladder. In view of the excretion of this substance in urine it is interesting to speculate as to the importance of urinary tract reabsorption in the normal individual. Preparations of posterior pituitary are not useful orally, since absorption is poor and the antidiuretic activity is rapidly destroyed by the gastrointestinal tract.

Control of diabetes insipidus can be obtained by administration of 0.25 to 0.5 cc. per m^2 of pitressin tannate in oil once or twice daily. This is probably the most effective means of treatment. It is often desirable, however, to avoid parenteral injection of medications used by the patient at home. Somewhat less effective but eminently satisfactory control can be achieved by the administration of aqueous solutions of posterior pituitary in doses of one drop in each nostril from three to six times daily. During intranasal administration of aqueous material, the patient should recline on a bed or sofa and let his head hang down over the side at an angle of approximately 30°. A period of one minute or more should be allowed in this position to permit adequate distribution of the solution over the nasal mucosa.

Dietary control of diabetes insipidus. Figure 4 has already demonstrated the remarkable diminution in urine volume which follows reduction of the renal solute load. On the basis of similar observations, the use of dietary measures in place of hormonal therapy has been advocated for control of the polyuria of diabetes insipidus.[17 b] In children, however, this means of control seems less desirable than replacement therapy, in view of the relatively large protein and mineral needs for growth and the emotional disturbances likely to develop when dietary intake is rigidly controlled.

When dietary control of polyuria is employed, foods of high mineral and protein content should be avoided. These include meats, particularly bacon and ham, milk, cheese and fish. In their stead, a diet made up of unsalted cereals, rice, macaroni, potatoes, fresh vegetables and fruits should be taken. As has been mentioned previously, the untreated patient is apt to select for himself a diet which permits increased water economy.

Fluid intake. There is little to be gained from restriction of water intake in patients with diabetes insipidus. When water is readily accessible the thirst mechanism accurately adjusts consumption in proportion to need. Even when the patient is vigorously treated with posterior pituitary extract, there need be no fear of water intoxication from voluntary drinking.

Other aspects of treatment. Several of the lesions which cause diabetes insipidus are highly responsive to medical therapy. Eosinophilic granuloma and pinealoma, for instance, may be held in check for several years by appropriate x-ray treatment. When the cause is infectious, as in syphilis or pyogenic abscess, prompt chemotherapy may prove effective.

When diabetes insipidus results from the impingement of a cerebral tumor on the hypothalamic-neurohypophyseal system neurosurgical advice should be sought. Because of the hazard to life, neurosurgeons are in general agreement that operative intervention is not indicated for the endocrinological disturbance alone. It is imperative, however, when a radio-insensitive lesion begins to jeopardize vision or vital cerebral functions.

PROGNOSIS. The prognosis in diabetes insipidus depends in large measure on the cause. When it is due to non-progressive lesion of the hypothalamic-posterior pituitary system, it is readily controlled by appropriate replacement therapy, but in most instances this must be continued indefinitely. In several instances, when diabetes insipidus has developed as a result of eosinophilic granuloma or syphilis, remissions have been observed after x-ray or antisyphilitic therapy respectively. When it is due to progressive neoplastic lesions, the prognosis depends upon how effectively the lesion can be eradicated. But even after complete eradication of such a lesion, return of normal neurohypophyseal function is not to be expected.

Functional Deficiency of Antidiuretic Hormone (Psychogenic Polydipsia). Pediatricians sometimes encounter patients who have many of the symptoms of true diabetes insipidus, including constant thirst and marked polyuria, but whose histories reveal that the primary disturbance is emotional. Often this disturbance is focused on an abnormal interest in water-drinking and urination.

On physical examination these patients may appear entirely normal. Sometimes there may be evidence of weight loss resulting not only from interruption of normal sleep by the large water exchange but also from emotional turmoil. Evidence of dehydration is regularly absent.

For the most part laboratory determinations give normal results, except for the large volumes of dilute urine which sometimes has a specific gravity below 1.005. Like patients with true diabetes insipidus, these patients show a good response to doses of posterior pituitary extract. They are distinguished from individuals with obligatory diabetes insipidus by the fact that their physiological response to water restriction is fundamentally normal even though their behavior may become hypomanic.

In the course of water restriction, urine volume is rapidly diminished, urine specific gravity rises above 1.015 and weight loss and hemoconcentration of serious proportions are not seen. Figure 14 shows the response of a patient with psychogenic diabetes insipidus to water restriction for a test period of 36 hours' duration.

The disturbances to be considered in the differential diagnosis are outlined in Table 1.

The treatment is psychiatric. An effort should be made to divert the child's morbid interest in fluid intake and excretion to more healthy subjects. As is so often the case in the emotional disturbances of childhood, the physician must include a consideration of all the environmental factors, especially the role of the parents. Therapy should not be directed to the patient alone.

The prognosis is generally excellent. The necessary psychotherapy can usually be given by the pediatrician without recourse to a trained psychiatrist.

Comments on the Water Metabolism of Newborn Infants. The urine passed by the infant immediately after birth usually shows a specific gravity of 1.012 or 1.015. Thereafter, although scant in quantity, it becomes progressively more dilute for a period of five to seven days, until reaching concentrations similar to those seen in diabetes insipidus.[18 a, b] During this period restriction of water is followed by a relatively slight increase in urine concentration.[18 b] These observations suggest that the hypothalamic-neurohypophyseal system, like the parathyroid system, may be functionally immature at this stage (see Chapter II, page 116). Interestingly, this interpretation is supported by the fact that the quantity of antidiuretic material recoverable from the newborn infant's posterior pituitary gland appears to be relatively small compared to that recoverable from the glands of older persons.[18 b]

On the other hand, there are peculiarities of the newborn infant's water metabolism not explained by this concept of simple transient antidiuretic hormone lack. He not only fails to conserve water during deprivation as efficiently as the older infant but shows a relatively poor response to antidiuretic hormone.[18 b] This may be an indication of renal immaturity.[18 c] A further observation is the sluggishness of diuretic response to an administered water load. Possibly this can be correlated with the neonatal tendency to eosinophilia, hypoglycemia and apparently low urinary 11-17-OCS excretion which is indicative of adrenocortical immaturity (see Chapter III, page 154).

Although these peculiarities in water metabolism disappear within two to six weeks after birth, it is interesting to note the appropriateness of breast-feeding during the period when they are present. Breast milk supplies water in relation to solutes in a ratio which permits the metabolic residual to be excreted in a urine of very low specific gravity. With respect to the individual components of the solute load, it has already been stated that breast milk supplies calcium and phosphorus in amounts which satisfy anabolic needs, yet leaves a residual requiring only minimal parathyroid influence for renal elimination (see Chapter II, page 116). It might further be noted that the composition of artificial formulas and intravenous fluids for the newborn should be so modified that they do not put undue demand on immature homeostatic systems. In view of the newborn infant's relative deficiency in antidiuretic hormone, this implies that fluids for maintenance of hydration or correction of dehydration should be hypotonic with respect to plasma.

NON-NEUROHYPOPHYSEAL DISTURBANCES RESEMBLING DIABETES INSIPIDUS

Nephrogenic Diabetes Insipidus (Table 1, Condition 3).[19] This is a rare congenital disease, more frequently seen in males than in females, which is characterized by a failure of end-organ response similar to that seen in pseudohypoparathyroidism (see Chapter II, page 114). It is often hereditary. The cause is unknown.

The symptoms and signs are similar to those of patients with neurohypophyseal diabetes insipidus. But because this disease is present at birth, while true diabetes insipidus is usually acquired after infancy, the symptoms may be modified. Fluid is seldom as readily available to the infant as to the child who is old enough to seek it for himself. Hence, serious dehydration is much more apt to occur. Episodes of dehydration are accompanied by elevations in temperature which rapidly and specifically respond to restoration of normal hydration. Recognition of the large volume of urine is often delayed because of its tendency to be masked in the diapers.

The diagnostic laboratory studies made on patients with nephrogenic diabetes insipidus show not only weight loss, dehydration and inability to concentrate urine on water deprivation, but also unresponsiveness to administered posterior pituitary extract. Measurement of antidiuretic hormone appearing in the urine shows a normal increase during dehydration and diminution following restoration of hydration. Chemical estimations show that serum electrolytes have abnormally elevated concentration values during periods of dehydration but are otherwise usually within normal range. Studies of renal function usually reveal normal values for the glomerular filtration rate, renal blood flow, urea clearance and phenolsulfonphthalein excretion. Seriously impaired renal function is found in some patients. This is probably not a primary characteristic of the disease itself but the result of serious episodes of dehydration which have permanently impaired multiple kidney functions.

The diagnosis of nephrogenic diabetes insipidus depends upon the history of symptoms dating from birth and the demonstration of inability to concentrate urine either on withholding water or on administration of antidiuretic hormone. The differential diagnosis is summarized in Table 1.

Treatment of this disorder of water metabolism consists in dietary measures which provide a large fluid intake but lessen the need for excretion of solutes by the renal route. Although dietary control of urine volumes is considered a less desirable form of treatment than hormonal replacement therapy in true diabetes insipidus, it appears to be the only practicable treatment in nephrogenic diabetes insipidus. During infancy nutritionally adequate formulas can be prepared by diluting 1 part of whole cow's milk with 3 parts of water. The fat content of this material can be brought up to 4 per cent by the addition of 7.5 cc. of 40 per cent cream per 100 cc. The caloric value of the total mixture can then be brought to 0.8 calories per cc. by the addition of 8 gm. of carbohydrate (dextrose or sucrose) per 100 cc. The urinary excretion of solutes by infants on this regimen averages 350 mosM per m^2 per day. As solids are added to the diet, high protein food such as meat purees and cheese should be avoided, and cereals, potatoes, fruit and vegetables, cooked without added salt, used in their stead.[17a] A number of low-sodium foods, including milk substitutes, are prepared commercially for patients with cardiac disease. These can be used advantageously in the case of patients with nephrogenic diabetes.

The prognosis is only fair. As Figure 4 shows, the appropriate dietary measures can be of great aid in reducing the urine volume. Nevertheless, an intercurrent infection may result in mobilization of more solutes from endogenous sources than the kidney can eliminate in water available from glomerular filtrate (see Figure 2). The outcome of this situation may be fatal.

Pannephritis (Table 1, Condition 4). Pannephritis quite commonly results in kidney impairment which is such that the patient is unable to form a urine that is either more dilute or more concentrated than blood plasma. Under such circumstances urine volume is apt to be large in relation to that of the normal individual (see Figure 4) but is seldom as large as that seen in the conditions previously discussed. The specific gravity is fixed at about 1.010 in contrast to the very low specific gravity characteristic of patients with diabetes insipidus of neurohypophyseal origin. As in patients with congenital nephrogenic diabetes insipidus, the neurohypophyseal system is intact, but the ability to respond to administered posterior pituitary extract is lost. Because the excretion of urine isotonic with blood plasma permits a saving of water three times greater than that which can be achieved by the patient with diabetes insipidus, water deprivation is relatively well tolerated.

The diagnosis is suggested by a history of renal disease. Examination of the urine shows not only fixation of the specific gravity but also a nearly neutral pH and the presence of albumin, cellular elements and casts. Additional studies usually show elevation of the non-protein nitrogen and serum phosphorus with depression of values for hemoglobin, serum protein carbon dioxide concentration.

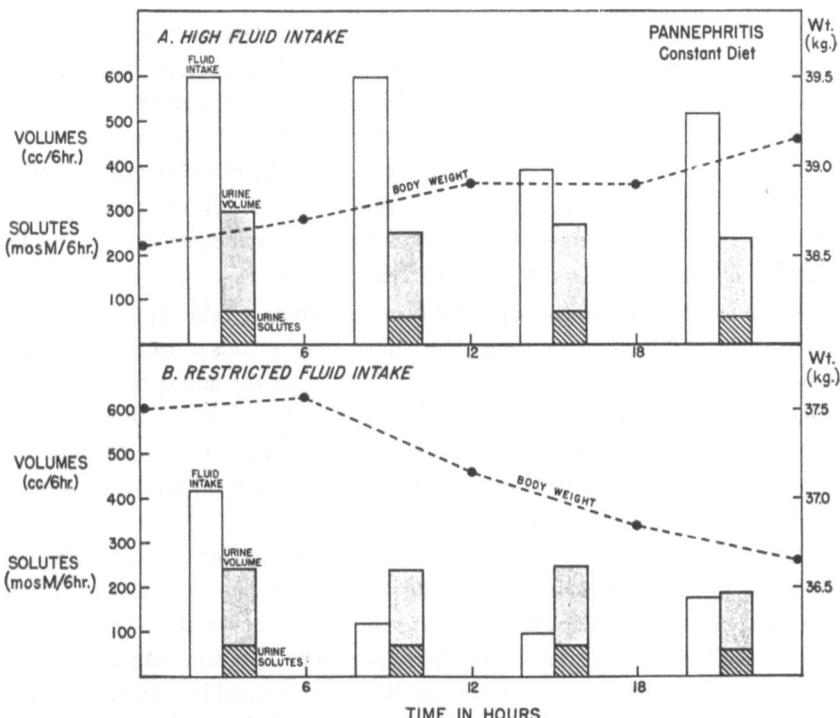

FIGURE VIII—15. Effects of renal tubule disease on water metabolism. The subject of this study was a 10-year-old boy with inability to respond to antidiuretic hormone as a consequence of advanced nephritis. Urine specific gravity was "fixed" at about 1.010.

SECTION A presents data obtained when the patient was given a large fluid intake in conjunction with a constant diet. Under these circumstances the amount of fluid in relation to solutes presenting for renal excretion was greater than that permitted by the damaged kidneys. Urine volume remained essentially constant. Fluid was retained with a resultant gain in weight and fall in hemoglobin concentration.

SECTION B presents data obtained under similar circumstances except for fluid restriction. Note that the diet provided a deficit of water in relation to solutes for renal excretion. As a consequence of the patient's inability to concentrate urine, the excretory volume continued relatively high. Water was withdrawn from body stores (as indicated by weight loss) in order to provide the quantities necessary for urine formation. From J. D. Crawford. Unpublished observations.

Urine volume, as in untreated diabetes insipidus and in cases of congenital unresponsiveness to antidiuretic hormone, is a function of solute excretion. This is demonstrated by the data of Figure 15. In this patient with pannephritis, provision of a constant number of solutes for renal excretion resulted in a constant urine volume. Raising the fluid intake was not effective in increasing water relative to solute output, and hence edema developed (Section A). Conversely, a diminished fluid intake resulted in no decrease in water relative to solute excretion, and dehydration was the obligatory consequence (Section B).

Despite the compromised position of the patient who is unable either to dilute or concentrate urine, water balance is usually successfully maintained by the thirst mechanism. Treatment of the disturbance of water metabolism is far less difficult than the treatment of the underlying disease.

Polyuria and the Adrenocortical Alarm Reaction (Table 1, Condition 5). As has been indicated earlier (page 516) the adrenal glands produce one or more hormones antagonistic in their action to the effect of the antidiuretic hormone. This apparently accounts for the fact that patients who are acutely ill may excrete urine which is far less concentrated than would be expected in view of the degree of dehydration present. Furthermore, these patients are relatively resistant to administered antidiuretic hormone.

This syndrome is seen particularly often among infants with severe diarrhea[20 a, b] and among older children and adults with diabetic acidosis.[21 c] Both of these primary conditions may lead to severe deficiency in intracellular potassium as well as to intracellular migration of sodium. This disturbance of electrolyte metabolism can be reproduced in the laboratory animal by dietary restriction of potassium.[20 d] Here its development is accompanied by enlargement of the zona glomerulosa of the adrenal glands.[20 e] It can also be produced by administration of desoxycorticosterone, particularly if there is excess sodium in the diet.[20 f, g] Inability to concentrate urine normally and resistance to administered antidiuretic hormone are demonstrable in both instances.[20 h] It is not evident, however, whether polyuria develops as a result of direct antagonistic action by the adrenocortical hormone to the antidiuretic influence of the posterior pituitary or whether it is due to loss of ability on the part of the renal tubule cell, when its intracellular constitutents are thus disturbed, to maintain the normal osmotic gradient between urine and cell fluid.

HYPERFUNCTION OF THE POSTERIOR PITUITARY

Although one case of primary pathologic hyperfunction of the posterior pituitary has been postulated and its clinical syndrome described,[21 a, b] no well-documented evidence has yet been reported. Indeed, there is no clear-cut evidence that functional overproduction of posterior pituitary antidiuretic hormone occurs. It is of interest, nevertheless, to note that increases in an antidiuretic substance have been found in the blood and urine of patients with nephrotic and cirrhotic edema, as well as in the blood and urine of patients with the toxemic edema of pregnancy.[7 e, f, 13 d, 15 a, 21 c] It is difficult to reconcile the occurrence of large quantities of antidiuretic hormone in the body fluids of these patients with the fact that the water content of their tissues was increased and solute concentration decreased. In hyperhydremia the stimulus to antidiuretic hormone production, as it is currently conceived, is absent.

The relation of antidiuretic hormone to the occurrence of edema is a subject in need of further investigation.

PHARMACOLOGIC USES OF POSTERIOR PITUITARY EXTRACT OTHER THAN THOSE IN DIABETES INSIPIDUS

Little has been said concerning principles other than the antidiuretic which are contained in posterior pituitary extract. One of these, the oxytocic principle, is frequently used in obstetrics to induce labor or to intensify uterine contractions during the early stages of childbirth. The physiologic importance of the oxytocic hormone has not been clearly established. While normal childbirth has occurred in patients with diabetes insipidus,[22 b, c] marked disturbances of labor have been reported in animal experiments after posterior hypophysectomy.[22 d, e]

Administration of the pressor fraction of posterior pituitary extracts not only results in antidiuresis and frequently in a rise in blood pressure, but also causes an increase in intestinal peristalsis. Advantage is often taken of this action by surgeons in the postoperative treatment of patients with ileus. Roentgenologists favor the use of pitressin to clear the intestine of gas prior to study of the gall bladder or kidneys with radio-opaque dyes. In this connection it is of interest that patients with diabetes insipidus often suffer from constipation.[9 c] It is not entirely clear whether this is a direct manifestation of pressor hormone lack or a result of diet and mild dehydration secondary to antidiuretic hormone deficiency. Clinical use of the pressor fraction in hypotensive states is extremely limited.

Finally, the antidiuretic activity of posterior pituitary extracts may be utilized in performing a rapid test of renal concentrating ability and for inducing temporary states of hyperhydremia as a means of revealing a latent form of epilepsy.[10 b]

REFERENCES

1 (a) VAN DYKE, H. B., CHOW, B. F., GREEP, R. O. and ROTHEN, A. The isolation of a protein from the pars neuralis of the ox pituitary with constant oxytocic, pressor and diuresis-inhibiting activities. *J. Pharmacol. & Exper. Thérap.* 74:190, 1942.
  (b) ROSENFELD, M. The native hormones of the posterior pituitary gland: the pressor and oxytocic principles. *Bull. Johns Hopkins Hosp.* 66:398, 1940.
  (c) HELLER, H. The effect of hydrogen-ion concentration on the stability of the antidiuretic and vasopressor activities of posterior pituitary extracts. *J. Physiol.* 96:337, 1939.
  (d) BUGBEE, E. and KAMM, O. Recent progress in the investigation of the posterior lobe of the pituitary gland. *Endocrinology* 12:671, 1928.

2 HARRIS, G. W. Further evidence regarding the endocrine status of the neurohypophysis. *J. Physiol.* 107:436, 1948.

3 SMITH, H. W. *The Physiology of the Kidney.* New York, Oxford Univ. Press, 1937.

4 (a) GAMBLE, J. L. and BUTLER, A. M. Measurement of the renal water requirement. *Tr. A. Am. Physicians* 58:157, 1944.
  (b) JONES, G. M. Diabetes insipidus; clinical observations in 42 cases. *Arch. Int. Med.* 74:81, 1944.
  (c) LIFSON, N. Note on the total osmotic activity of human plasma or serum. *J. Biol. Chem.* 152:659, 1944.
  (d) OPIE, E. L. The movement of water in tissues removed from the body and its relationship to the movement of water during life. *J. Exper. Med.* 89:185, 1949.

5 GAMBLE, J. L. Physiological information gained from studies on the life raft ration. In *The Harvey Lectures, 1946-47.* Series 42:247. Lancaster, Science Press, 1947.

6 (a) RAPOPORT, S., BRODSKY, W. A. and WEST, C. D. Excretion of solutes and osmotic work of the "resting" kidney of hydropenic man. *Am. J. Physiol.* 157:357, 1949.
  (b) HARE, R. S., HARE, K. and PHILLIPS, D. M. The renal excretion of chloride by the normal and diabetes insipidus dog. *Am. J. Physiol.* 140:334, 1943.
  (c) COREY, E. L. and BRITTON, S. W. The antagonistic action of desoxycorticosterone and posterior pituitary extract on chloride and water balance. *Am. J. Physiol.* 133:511, 1941.

7 (a) LITTLE, J. M., WALLACE, S. L., WHATLEY, E. C. and ANDERSON, G. A. Effect of pitressin on the urinary excretion of chloride and water in the human. *Am. J. Physiol.* 151:174, 1947.
  (b) SILVETTE, H. The influence of posterior pituitary extract on the excretion of water and chlorides by the renal tubules. *Am. J. Physiol.* 128:747, 1940.
  (c) HARRIS, G. W. The excretion of an antidiuretic substance by the kidney after electrical stimulation of the neurohypophysis in the unanaesthetized rabbit. *J. Physiol.* 107:430, 1948.
  (d) SHANNON, J. A. Control of the renal excretion of water; the rate of liberation of the posterior pituitary antidiuretic hormone in the dog. *J. Exper. Med.* 76:387, 1942.
  (e) HAM, G. C. and LANDIS, E. M. A comparison of pituitrin with antidiuretic substance found in human urine and placenta. *J. Clin. Invest.* 21:455, 1942.
  (f) RALLI, E. P., ROBSON, J. S., CLARKE, D. and HOAGLAND, C. L. Factors influencing ascites in patients with cirrhosis of the liver. *J. Clin. Invest.* 24:316, 1945.

8 SHANNON, J. A. Control of the renal excretion of water; the effect of variations in the state of hydration on water excretion in dogs with diabetes insipidus. *J. Exper. Med.* 76:371, 1942.

9 (a) WEIL, A. Uber die hereditäre Form des Diabetes insipidus. *Deutsches Archiv für Klinische Medizin* 93:180, 1908.

- (b) WEIR, J. F., LARSON, E. E. and ROWNTREE, L. G. Studies in diabetes insipidus, water balance and water intoxication. *Arch. Int. Med.* 29:306, 1922.
- (c) CUSHING, H. *Papers Relating to the Pituitary Body, Hypothalamus, and Parasympathetic Nervous System.* Springfield, Ill., C. C. Thomas, 1932.

10. (a) THORN, G. W. and STEIN, K. E. Pitressin tannate therapy in diabetes insipidus. *J. Clin. Endocrinol.* 1:680, 1941.
    (b) MCQUARRIE, I. and PEELER, D. B. Effects of sustained pituitary antidiuresis and forced water drinking in epileptic children; a diagnostic and etiologic study. *J. Clin. Invest.* 10:915, 1931.

11. PICKFORD, M. Control of the secretion of the antidiuretic hormone from the pars nervosa of the pituitary gland. *Physiol. Rev.* 25:573, 1945.

12. (a) VERNEY, E. B. Absorption and excretion of water; the antidiuretic hormone. *Lancet* 251:739, 1946 and *ibid* 781, 1946.
    (b) GAMBLE, J. L. The optimal water requirement in renal function. *Am. J. Physiol.* 88:571, 1929.
    (c) BALDES, E. J. and SMIRK, F. H. The effect of water drinking, mineral starvation and salt administration on the total osmotic pressure of the blood chiefly in relation to the problems of water absorption and water diuresis. *J. Physiol.* 82:62, 1934.

13. (a) GILMAN, A. and GOODMAN, L. S. The secretory response of the posterior pituitary to the need for water conservation. *J. Physiol.* 90:113, 1937.
    (b) BOYLSTON, C. R. and IVY, A. C. An antidiuretic substance present in the urine of dehydrated rats. *Proc. Soc. Exper. Biol. & Med.* 28:644, 1938.
    (c) INGRAM, W. R., LADD, L. and BENBOW, J. T. The excretion of antidiuretic substance and its relation to the hypothalamico-hypophyseal system in cats. *Am. J. Physiol.* 127:544, 1939.
    (d) ROBINSON, F. H., JR. and FARR, L. E. The relation between clinical edema and the excretion of an antidiuretic substance in the urine. *Ann. Int. Med.* 14:42, 1940.
    (e) HARE, K., HICKEY, R. C. and HARE, R. S. The renal excretion of an antidiuretic substance by the dog. *Am. J. Physiol.* 134:240, 1941.
    (f) BIRNIE, J. H., JENKINS, R., EVERSOLE, W. J. and GAUNT, R. An antidiuretic substance in the blood of normal and adrenalectomized rats. *Proc. Soc. Exper. Biol. & Med.* 70:83, 1949.

14. (a) HELLER, H. and URBAN, F. F. The fate of antidiuretic principle of post-pituitary extracts. *J. Physiol.* 85:502, 1935.
    (b) JONES, A. M. and SCHLAPP, W. Actions and fate of injected posterior pituitary extracts in the decapitated cat. *J. Physiol.* 87:144, 1936.
    (c) LESLIE, S. H. and RALLI, E. P. The effect in rats of high fat diets on the renal excretion of water. *Endocrinology* 41:1, 1947.
    (d) GILBERT, A. and LEREBOIULLET, P. Des urines retardies (opsiuric) dans les cirrhoses. *Compt. rend. Soc. de biol.* 11:276, 1901.
    (e) PICK, E. P. The regulation of water metabolism. In *The Harvey Lectures, 1929-30.* Series 25:32. Lancaster, Science Press, 1930.

15. (a) GAUNT, R., BIRNIE, J. H. and EVERSOLE, W. J. Adrenal cortex and water metabolism. *Physiol. Rev.* 29:281, 1949.
    (b) CRAWFORD, J. D. Unpublished observations.

16. SCHOEN, E. J. and CRAWFORD, J. D. Unpublished observations.

17. (a) WARKANY, J. and MITCHELL, A. B. Diabetes insipidus in children. *Am. J. Dis. Child.* 57:603, 1939.
    (b) BEASER, S. B. Renal excretory function and diet in diabetes insipidus. *Am. J. Med.* 213:441, 1947.

18 (a) SMITH, C. A. *The Physiology of the Newborn.* Springfield, Ill., C. C. Thomas, 1945.
   (b) HELLER, H. The renal function of newborn infants. *J. Physiol.* 102:429, 1944.
   (c) MC CANCE, R. A. and YOUNG, W. F. Secretion of urine by newborn infants. *J. Physiol.* 99:265, 1941.
   (d) SMITH, C. A. and ROTH, R. O. Personal communication.

19 (a) DANCIS, J., BIRMINGHAM, J. R. and LESLIE, S. Congenital diabetes insipidus resistant to treatment with pitressin. *Am. J. Dis. Child.* 75:316, 1948.
   (b) WILLIAMS, R. A. Nephrogenic diabetes insipidus occurring in males and transmitted by females. *J. Clin. Invest.* 25:937, 1946.
   (c) WARING, A. J., KAJDI, L. and TAPPAN, V. A congenital defect of water metabolism. *Am. J. Dis. Child.* 69:323, 1945.

20 (a) GAMBLE, J. L., FAHEY, K. R., APPLETON, J. and MAC LACHLAN, E. A. Congenital alkalosis with diarrhea. *J. Pediat.* 26:509, 1945.
   (b) DARROW, D. C. Congenital alkalosis with diarrhea. *J. Pediat.* 26:519, 1945.
   (c) BUTLER, A. M., TALBOT, N. B., BURNETT, C. H., STANBURY, J. B. and MAC LACHLAN, E. A. Metabolic studies in diabetic coma. *Tr. A. Am. Physicians* 60:102, 1947.
   (d) DARROW, D. C., SCHWARTZ, R., IANNUCCI, J. F. and COVILLE, F. The relation of serum bicarbonate concentration to muscle composition. *J. Clin. Invest.* 27:198, 1948.
   (e) DEANE, H. W., SHAW, J. H. and GREEP, R. O. The effect of altered sodium or potassium intake on the width and cytochemistry of the zona glomerulosa of the rat's adrenal cortex. *Endocrinology* 43:133, 1948.
   (f) FERREBEE, J. W., PARKER, D., CARNES, W. H., GERRITY, M. K., ATCHLEY, D. W. and LOEB, R. F. Certain effects of desoxycorticosterone; the development of "diabetes insipidus" and the replacement of muscle potassium by sodium in normal dogs. *Am. J. Physiol.* 135:230, 1941.
   (g) MULINOS, M. G., SPRINGARN, C. L. and LOJKIN, M. E. A diabetes insipidus-like condition produced by small doses of desoxycorticosterone acetate in dogs. *Am. J. Physiol.* 135:102, 1941.
   (h) GARDNER, L. I. and CRAWFORD, J. D. Unpublished observations.

21 (a) JONES, E. I. A new syndrome apparently due to overactivity of the posterior pituitary. *Lancet* 234:11, 1938.
   (b) NOBLE, R. L., RINDERKNECHT, H. and WILLIAMS, P. C. Clinical hyperfunction of the posterior lobe of the pituitary. *Lancet* 234:13, 1938.
   (c) TEEL, H. M. and REID, D. E. Observations upon the occurrence of an antidiuretic substance in the urine of patients with pre-eclampsia and eclampsia. *Endocrinology* 24:297, 1939.

22 (a) GEILING, E. M. K. and OLDHAM, F. K. The neurohypophysis. In *Glandular Physiology and Therapy.* Chicago, A. M. A., 1942.
   (b) HART, S. D. and BREITMAN, H. B. Diabetes insipidus complicating pregnancy. *Am. J. Obst. & Gynec.* 41:527, 1941.
   (c) BLOTNER, H. and KUNKEL, P. Diabetes insipidus and pregnancy. *New Eng. J. Med.* 227:287, 1942.
   (d) DAY, F. L., FISHER, C. and RANSON, S. W. Disturbances in pregnancy and labor in guinea pigs with hypothalamic lesions. *Am. J. Obst. & Gynec.* 42:459, 1941.
   (e) FISHER, C., MAGOUN, H. W. and RANSON, S. W. Dystocia in diabetes insipidus; relation of pituitary oxytocin to parturition. *Am. J. Obst. & Gynec.* 36:1, 1938.

THE PANCREATIC ISLETS

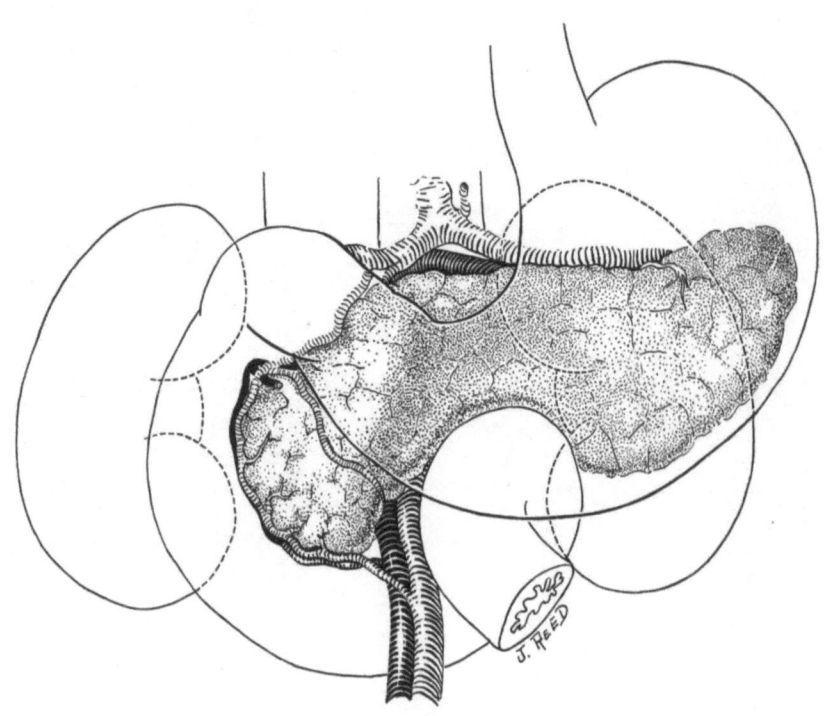

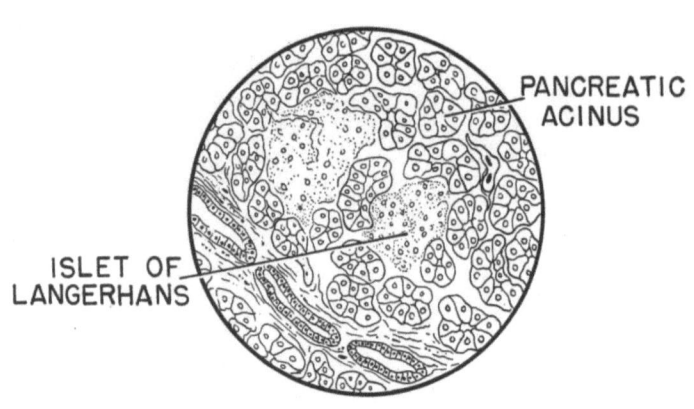

CHAPTER IX

THE PANCREATIC ISLETS

BASIC CONSIDERATIONS

THE HORMONES

Insulin constitutes the best-known and most important endocrine hormone.[1, 2] A protein with a molecular weight of about 35,000, it is standardized by a bioassay procedure. One mg. of pure crystalline insulin contains 22 I.U., each of which is equivalent to the amount required to lower the blood sugar of a normal rabbit (weighing 2 kg. and fasted for 24 hours) to a level of 45 mg. per cent within five hours.

In addition to insulin, it appears that the pancreatic islets produce another hormone, glukagon, which causes a rise rather than a fall in blood sugar values. This substance is absent from insulin preparations made in Denmark but not from those currently being made in this country. It has been postulated that glukagon is produced by the alpha cells of the pancreatic islets. If this is correct, disproportionate production of glukagon in cases of spontaneous diabetes mellitus due to beta cell failure may partly explain why more insulin is required to control this type of diabetes than that following pancreatectomy.

ACTION OF INSULIN

Insulin acts to adjust the rate at which glucose is utilized by body tissues.[2] In the absence of insulin the rate of utilization is slowed, with a resultant tendency for sugar to accumulate in the blood. This is equivalent to saying that insulin deficiency leads to carbohydrate starvation in the tissues, for the first step in glucose utilization, namely formation of glucose-6-phosphate, is markedly slowed when insulin is lacking.

$$\text{Glucose + adenosine triphosphate} \xrightarrow{\text{insulin}} \text{glucose-6-phosphate + adenosine diphosphate}.$$

The chief determinant of this reaction may be the enzyme hexokinase. If so, it may be presumed that insulin acts by modifying the activity of this enzyme.

Once phosphorylation of glucose has occurred, synthesis of glycogen and fatty acids and chain oxidation of carbohydrate are possible even in a diabetic organism. In the absence of insulin this total reaction can therefore occur to a limited extent, for hyperglycemia leads by mass action to some phosphorylation of glucose.

Muscular exercise augments the action of insulin. On the other hand, it does not constitute a substitute for this hormone.[1]

INSULIN ANTAGONISTS

There are several hormones which have an action on carbohydrate metabolism essentially opposite to that of insulin.[2] Among these, the adrenocortical sugar-fat-nitrogen (S-F-N) and anterior pituitary glycotropic* hormones are prominent (see Chapters III and VII). Both substances appear to depress the hypoglycemic effect of insulin by inhibiting its tendency to accelerate the utilization of sugar by peripheral tissues.

Epinephrine (see Chapter IV) and glukagon are also considered antagonistic to insulin in the sense that they tend to prompt a rise rather than a fall in the concentration of blood sugar. Both agents appear to facilitate glycogenolysis, with release of glucose into the circulation.

FACTORS WHICH INFLUENCE THE RATE OF INSULIN PRODUCTION (BLOOD GLUCOSE HOMEOSTASIS BY MEANS OF INSULIN)

It is highly probable that hyperglycemia directly stimulates insulin secretion by the pancreas.[2] The central nervous system, operating through the right vagus nerve, may also stimulate insulin production.[3] It may be presumed that insulin secretion becomes markedly diminished when blood glucose concentration falls below a certain value. Other factors, such as epinephrine, adrenocortical S-F-N hormone, anterior pituitary glycotropic hormone and glukagon have the task of preventing hypoglycemia. Ordinarily this closely knit system operates so well that blood sugar values rarely exceed the limits of approximately 80 to 120 mg. per cent for more than an hour or two (see Chapter III, Figures 11 and 22-26).

In these connections it should be mentioned that chronic treatment with an-

---

* This substance may be identical with the pituitary growth hormone (PGH). On the other hand, it may be a separate substance with very similar physicochemical properties. In this treatise it will arbitrarily be considered as a separate and distinct substance.

terior pituitary extract can prompt degeneration of pancreatic islet tissue and lead to permanent diabetes mellitus.[2c] There is a possibility that this phenomenon is due to a specific pancreatropic hormone. It appears more likely, however, that pituitary glycotropic hormone, by exerting its hyperglycemic (insulin antagonist) effect, causes compensatory islet hyperactivity, with eventual exhaustion and degeneration of beta cells.

The latter hypothesis is supported by observations on partially pancreatectomized dogs, which develop permanent diabetes mellitus and show changes in the beta cells of the pancreas if fed a high carbohydrate diet. On the other hand, if they are fed a high fat, low carbohydrate diet or are subjected to semistarvation, no permanent diabetes develops. Animals of species which fail to develop hyperglycemia in response to anterior pituitary glycotropic hormone therapy do not develop diabetes mellitus.

METABOLIC EFFECTS OF INSULIN LACK

The primary effect of insulin deficiency is decreased utilization of tissue glucose (oxidation, glycogenesis, etc.).[2] As a result of this, numerous secondary phenomena occur. Some of these, such as tendencies to hyperglycemia, glycosuria, polyuria, polydipsia and polyphagia, are both familiar and relatively easy to understand. The glycosuria, for example, simply reflects spillage of glucose into the urine when the glucose content of the glomerular filtrate (serum glucose concentration glomerular filtration rate) exceeds maximum capacity of the tubules for glucose reabsorption (see Chapter II, Figure 2). The increase in urine solutes (osmoles) resulting from this occurrence leads to a proportionate increase in urine water requirements (see Chapter VIII). The increased urine water outgo produces a tendency to dehydration, which is counteracted by the thirst mechanism and polydipsia. The polyphagia reflects carbohydrate starvation in the tissue and loss of calories as glucose in the urine.

As in simple starvation due to dietary restriction, carbohydrate starvation secondary to insulin deficiency prompts a tendency to ketosis and to ketonuria. This tendency is explained as follows[4a]: Persons who are unable to utilize carbohydrate to the full measure of their metabolic need must fall back on fat for their energy requirements. Part of this need is met by the initiation and completion of fat oxidation in the muscles. However, a considerable fraction, estimated as ranging from one-third to one-half of the total caloric need from fat, is obtained by a preliminary oxidation of fats in the liver to ketone bodies. This mobilization of fat for energy purposes apparently is not caused by hepatic glycogen depletion[4b] but may be facilitated by adrenocortical S-F-N hormones (Chapter III).

These ketone bodies are utilized for energy by peripheral tissues without the aid of insulin or simultaneous carbohydrate oxidation. However, the capacity of the tissues to utilize ketone bodies under conditions of normal blood ketone concentration is limited to approximately 100 gm. or 900 calories of fat equivalent per m^2 per day. When larger amounts of fat energy are needed by the organism, blood ketone concentration is increased to supranormal levels. This increase presumably facilitates peripheral ketone utilization by mass action. It also results in the development of clinical ketosis and ketonuria.

As the foregoing effects of insulin lack become extended, other changes may take place. For example, when polydipsia does not completely compensate for polyuria, dehydration ensues. Data concerning this phenomenon are presented in Tables 1 to 3.[5]

Table 1 sets forth information concerning normal body composition for each kilogram of body weight. In addition, it presents calculations based on available evidence of losses incident to dehydration resulting in a 10 per cent body weight (water) loss. This loss is assumed to have an equal effect on extra- and intracellular fluid volumes and to leave the respective electrolyte concentrations unchanged. Note that such a 10 per cent loss of body weight means a 17 per cent loss of total body water, a 25 per cent loss of extracellular water and electrolytes and a 12 per cent loss of intracellular water and electrolytes.

Actual losses sustained by a normal adult during four days of absolute thirsting and fasting are shown in Table 2. The loss of 3 mEq. of potassium as compared with 7 mEq. in Table 1 reflects the concentration of cell potassium which occurs during the dehydration of thirsting. On the other hand, note that the ratio of K to N lost (4.3 mEq. K to 1 gm. N) is greater than that found in normal muscle tissue (2.8 mEq. K to 1 gm. N). This excess loss of potassium in relation to nitrogen is characteristic of starvation and dehydration in persons with intact adrenocortical function.*

Table 3 indicates the actual losses incurred by a diabetic patient during the development of pre-coma dehydration, when insulin was withheld for 3.4 days, plus extrapolated losses of an added theoretical day† of no fluid intake due to nausea and vomiting.[6] Both the actual losses during the first 3.4 days and the total calculated losses for 4.4 days describe tissue losses of potassium (in mEq.)

* As described in Chapter III, this ability to eliminate potassium above nitrogen is impaired in hypoadrenocorticism. The phenomenon appears to be of considerable importance in that it permits the thirsting organism to support extracellular water stores, if need be, at the expense of intracellular water and potassium.

† The losses of this added day were compounded from the losses shown in Table 2 for the fourth day of thirsting plus those calculated to occur as a result of glycosuria and of a 500 cc. vomitus.

TABLE IX—1. Approximate composition of body fluid per kg. of body weight and calculated dehydration losses resulting in a 10 per cent decrease in body weight. Equal losses from extra- and intracellular fluids and maintenance of normal body fluid concentrations are assumed. It should be noted that a 10 per cent loss of body weight due largely to dehydration means a 14 per cent loss of total body water, a 23 per cent loss of extracellular water and electrolytes, and a 10 per cent loss of intracellular water and electrolytes. These are over-all losses including renal and extrarenal losses. Adapted from A. M. Butler, *Acta pædiat.* 38:59, 1949.

	$(H_2O)_T$* ml.	$(H_2O)_E$* ml.	$(H_2O)_I$* cc.	Na_E mEq.	Cl_E mEq.	Na_I mEq.	K_I mEq.
Composition per kg.	600	200	400	30	23	3	60
Dehydration losses per kg.	100	50	50	7	6	0.4	7

*T = total; E = extracellular; I = intracellular.

TABLE IX—2. Losses suffered during four days of complete thirsting and fasting by a normal adult weighing 64 kg. Losses for the fourth day are given separately, since those for the first two days (particularly in Na and Cl) reflect variations dependent on the uncontrolled metabolic state. From A. M. Butler, *Acta pædiat.* 38:59, 1949.

Days	Losses					
	Weight, kg.	Na mEq.	Cl mEq.	K mEq.	P gm.	N gm.
1–3	4.40	247	209	130	2.6	31
4	1.45	45	33	59	1.2	13
Total	5.85	292	242	189	3.8	44
Per kg.	0.09	4.6	3.8	3	0.06	0.7

TABLE IX—3. Losses suffered by a 68-kg. diabetic patient during a 78-hour period of precoma nausea and acidosis following insulin withdrawal plus extrapolated losses for a theoretical day of vomiting and thirsting. From A. M. Butler, *Acta pædiat.* 38:59, 1949.

Days	Losses						
	Weight, kg.	Na mEq.	Cl mEq.	K mEq.	Mg mEq.	P gm.	N gm.
3.4	3.7	217	142	273	41	3	40
1.0 (added)	2.9	105	130	115	12	2	20
Total	6.6	322	272	388	53	5	60
Per kg.	0.1	5	4	6	0.8	0.07	0.9

and nitrogen (in gm.) in a ratio of approximately 7 to 1. This indicates a specific loss of K in excess of N greater than that described for non-diabetic starvation and dehydration.

Figure 1 shows further that the foregoing occurrences can lead to a marked degree of metabolic acidosis.[7] There are two reasons for this. First, certain of the ketone bodies, namely aceto-acetic acid and beta-hydroxy-butyric acid, directly displace plasma bicarbonate. Second, marked dehydration leads to circulatory failure and hence to renal failure. There results a tendency to accumulate such products of tissue catabolism as phosphate and sulfate and to lose such fixed bases as sodium and potassium. These changes add to the previously mentioned tendency to plasma bicarbonate reduction. Another presumably compensatory change is noted in the erythrocytes, which lose a major portion of their organic, acid-soluble phosphorus as diabetic acidosis develops.[8] This phosphorus is replaced by chloride ion.

The foregoing phenomena are accompanied by and in part are occasioned by homeostatic alterations in the activity of certain endocrine systems. For example, it is probable that the tendency toward dehydration elicits increased antidiuretic hormone production by the hypothalamic–posterior pituitary apparatus. This is evidenced by an elevation in urine specific gravity. The tendency to hyperphosphatemia apparently results likewise in a compensatory or functional type of hyperparathyroidism. This is manifested by a tendency to a very low ratio between tubular reabsorption of phosphorus and glomerular filtrate phosphorus (see Chapter II). The combined stress of carbohydrate starvation, dehydration, ketosis and acidosis elicits the anterior pituitary–adrenocortical alarm reaction. This is evidenced by eosinopenia and hyper-11-17-oxycorticosteroiduria (see Figure 2).[9] It probably accounts at least in part for the tissue loss of potassium in excess of nitrogen mentioned above and may in addition explain why diabetic-coma patients show a temporary tendency to resist insulin. Further, it probably contributes to the development of diabetic ketosis by facilitating the mobilization of body depot fat. These changes incident to the alarm reaction are of particular interest, inasmuch as they suggest that homeostatic endocrine reactions, while serving one purpose, may at times aggravate rather than ameliorate the metabolic disturbance in other respects.

METABOLIC EFFECTS OF INSULIN EXCESS

Insulin in excess causes glucose to be utilized by peripheral tissues at such a rapid rate that supply fails to keep pace with demand. Hypoglycemia results. This in turn activates both the sympathetic–adrenomedullary–epinephrine mechanism

Continued on page 550

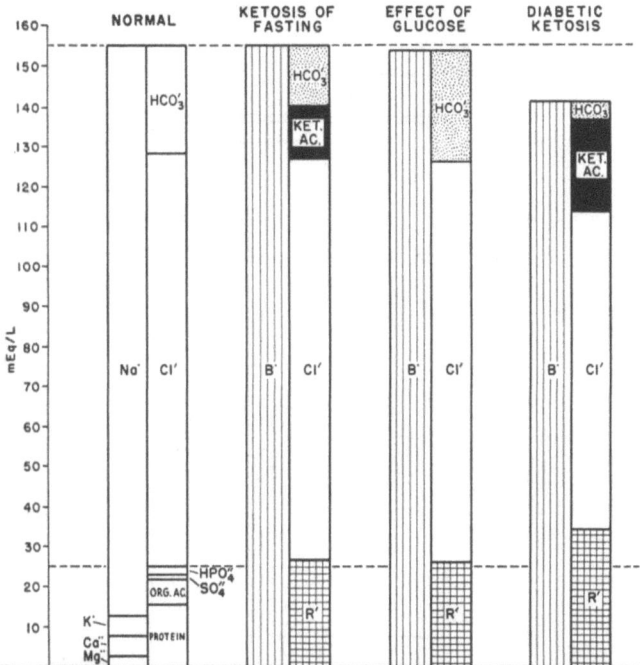

FIGURE IX—1. Effect of fasting ketosis and diabetic ketosis on serum electrolyte composition. In diabetes, ketosis results from a failure of the oxidative processes of carbohydrate metabolism; in many other conditions it may result from a lack or inadequacy of carbohydrate intake. Complete or partial starvation is often an incident of disease processes. Children exhibit ketosis much more frequently than adults. Apparently, during childhood, even very short periods of carbohydrate deprivation may lower the metabolic level to the point where incompletely oxidized fatty acids begin to appear in the extracellular fluid.

Ketone acids must be given space in the electrolyte structure of the plasma, and this space is provided at the expense of the concentration of bicarbonate ion. The measurements used in constructing the diagram which describes the ketosis of fasting were obtained from an epileptic boy who was fasted as a therapeutic measure. R' stands for the residue of anions made up of phosphate, sulfate organic acids and protein; B stands for base. As may be seen, the only change in plasma structure is the reduction of HCO'_3 to the base equivalence of the ketone acids. The next diagram shows the complete removal of the ketone acids and the return of HCO'_3 to its usual value by providing, over a 12-hour period, a small intake of carbohydrate (50 gm. of cane sugar per m^2 per day).

The last diagram in the chart describes the extensive structural changes found in the plasma of a child in diabetic coma, which have together produced an extremely severe acidosis. Besides the very large accumulation of ketone acids, two other changes, a decrease in base (B) and an increase in R', have helped to reduce HCO'_3 to a dangerously small value. These two changes are referable to renal disability caused by the rapid dehydration which is always a prominent feature of diabetic coma. From J. L. Gamble, *Chem. Anat., Physiol. and Pathol. of Extracellular Fluid.* Cambridge, Harvard Univ. Press, 1950.

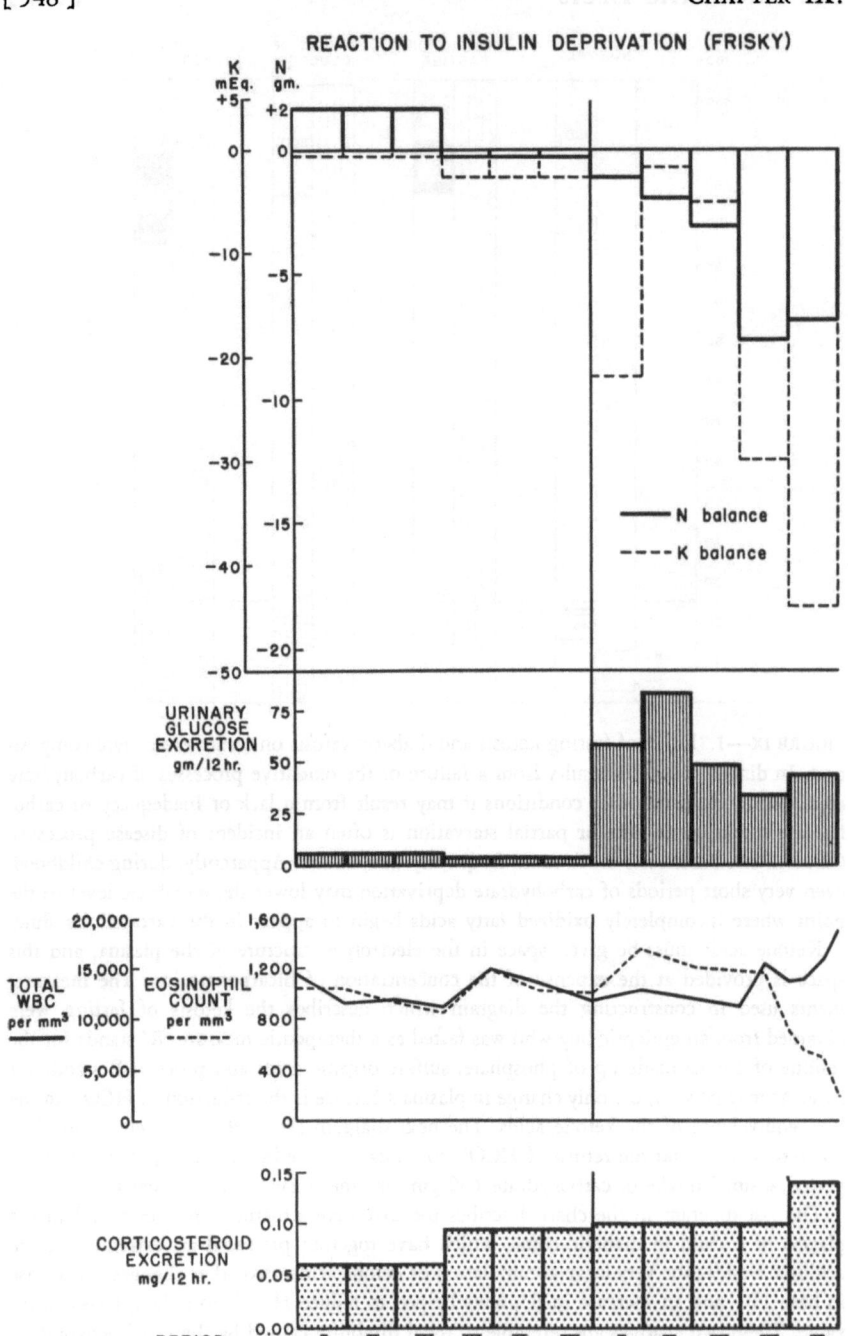

FIGURE IX—2. Effect of sudden insulin deprivation on the nitrogen and potassium balances, the urinary glucose excretion, the eosinophil and total white blood cell counts and the corticosteroid excretion of a depancreatized dog. The vertical line passing through the center of the figure indicates the moment at which insulin was withdrawn and separates the six 24-hour control periods from the five 12-hour experimental periods. At the end of 60 hours the animal had passed into profound diabetic coma and resumption of therapy became mandatory. The ordinate scales in the upper portion of the figure, which is devoted to the presentation of the nitrogen and potassium balances, are so correlated that the length of the column indicating the potassium balance in a given period is identical with that of the column indicating nitrogen balance when these substances are lost or retained in the same proportion that exists in protoplasm (one gram of nitrogen is equivalent to 2.39 mEq. of potassium in dog muscle).

Withdrawal of insulin is followed by: (1) immediate development of a negative nitrogen balance; (2) development of a negative potassium balance, which exceeds the proportionate negative nitrogen balances during two phases—(a) an immediate and transient loss of "excess" potassium, believed to be due to the breakdown of liver glycogen and (b) a progressive terminal loss, believed to be due to the selective loss of potassium from cells; (3) glycosuria, which is maximal during the initial periods after insulin withdrawal, which dwindles when the animal becomes ketotic and anorexic and which increases again when the condition of the animal becomes critical; (4) minimal changes in the eosinophil and total white blood cell counts during the early periods, but marked development of leukocytosis and eosinopenia as keto-acidosis becomes intense; (5) a terminal rise in urinary corticosteroid excretion.

The "alarm reaction," recognizable by the eosinopenia and the increased rate of urinary corticosteroid excretion, is thus seen to be a comparatively late feature of keto-acidosis resulting from insulin omission. It is temporally, and perhaps causally, related to the terminal hyperglycemia (indicated on this chart only by increased glycosuria) and to the loss of potassium from cells. From J. W. McArthur, D. Harting, G. A. Smart, E. A. MacLachlan, M. Terry and A. S. Zygmuntowicz. Unpublished observations.

and the anterior pituitary–adrenocortical alarm reaction mechanism. The epinephrine, by prompting hepatic glycogenolysis, may restore blood sugar concentration to normal at least temporarily. The adrenocortical steroids, produced as a result of the alarm reaction, tend to inhibit insulin action. Hence they may ameliorate if not eliminate the effects of insulin excess.

Under conditions of hyperinsulinism and hypoglycemia the behavior of the central nervous system becomes seriously altered. Since the brain is markedly dependent upon glucose as a source of energy, by prompting hypoglycemia insulin can deprive this organ of this vitally important nutrient. Convulsions, cerebral edema and chromatolysis of cells may follow.[10]

METHODS OF ESTIMATING INSULIN STATUS

At present, although it is technically difficult, it is possible to measure the concentration of insulin in blood by a bio-assay procedure.[2,5] Because this procedure is not suited to general clinical use, insulin status must ordinarily be appraised indirectly with the aid of standardized tests of carbohydrate metabolism. The tests used vary according to whether one suspects (a) insulin deficiency or (b) insulin excess. The general nature of certain of these carbohydrate tolerance tests is illustrated diagrammatically in Figures 22-26 of Chapter III. The information presented there may be extended as follows.

Indications of Insulin Deficiency. These constitute the diagnostic signs of ordinary juvenile diabetes mellitus—chiefly hyperglycemia and glycosuria. The diagnostic significance of these signs depends to a considerable extent upon the factors considered below.

Hyperglycemia. Previous diet, infections and toxemias may exert an appreciable effect on blood sugar values.

Diet. When a normal individual is subjected to a glucose tolerance test (see Chapter III, Table 3) following several days of low carbohydrate intake, he is apt to show a marked reduction in sugar tolerance. This is evidenced by a diabetic type of glucose tolerance curve (capillary, true blood glucose $>$ 120 mg. per cent two hours after 40 gm. of glucose per m^2 have been administered intravenously). Such intolerance for sugar is presumed to be a manifestation of adaptative changes in glucose homeostatic mechanisms. It can be dissipated by providing a relatively high carbohydrate intake (about 180 gm. of CHO per m^2 per day) for three days prior to the glucose tolerance test. Following such preparation, the normal individual has a capillary blood sugar of less than 120 mg. per cent two hours after a standard dose of glucose. Accordingly, it is considered of great importance always to prepare patients for glucose tolerance test by three days of high carbohydrate feeding. There is no evidence that such a regimen seriously harms a patient with diabetes mellitus.

Infections, toxemias and other noxious stimuli. These constitute stress stimuli which may activate the anterior pituitary–adrenocortical alarm reaction. Increased quantities of adrenocortical S-F-N hormones secreted as a result of this reaction may produce a tendency to impaired glucose tolerance as described above (see pages 180 and 546). This phenomenon is sufficiently common and definite to mean that glucose tolerance tests should not be used to appraise pancreatic islet–insulin status while a patient is suffering stress of any significant degree.

Other factors. Diminished glucose tolerance is observed occasionally in patients with hypertension, nephritis, thyrotoxicosis, liver disease, pituitary gigantism (or acromegaly) and Cushing's syndrome. The mechanisms responsible for this change in hypertensive, nephritic and thyrotoxic patients are not known. In severe hepatic disease capacity for glycogenesis is limited. Hence withdrawal of glucose from the circulation under the influence of insulin also is slow. In hyperpituitarism, pituitary glycotropic hormone, and in Cushing's syndrome, adrenocortical S-F-N hormones may explain the tendency to hyperglycemia.

Glycosuria. The quantitative and qualitative aspects of this subject are considered under the following separate subheadings.

Quantitative considerations. When the blood glucose concentration of the normal individual exceeds a critical value, which usually lies between 140 and 180 mg. per cent, the glomerular filtrate contains more glucose than the tubules of the kidney can reabsorb.[11] Glucose not reabsorbed by the tubules appears quantitatively in the urine. Since most diabetic patients develop hyperglycemia in excess of 180 mg. per cent after eating foods containing carbohydrates, they tend to show glycosuria, at least temporarily.

Glycosuria should be considered strongly suggestive of diabetes mellitus until proved otherwise. On the other hand, it is not necessarily diagnostic of this condition. It can occur in persons whose tolerance for sugar in terms of blood glucose values is normal, but whose renal tubule capacity for glucose reabsorption (renal threshold for glucose) is uncommonly low. Such persons may develop glycosuria with blood sugar values between 140 and 100 mg. per cent or even lower. This is called renal glycosuria. It is observed in a few otherwise normal individuals, in patients with nephritis involving the tubules and in patients suffering a stress-induced adrenocortical alarm reaction. It is recognized by making frequent simultaneous blood and urine glucose determinations during the course of a glucose tolerance test or following a meal containing moderate amounts of carbohydrate.

The blood glucose level corresponding to the first appearance of glycosuria approximately indicates the renal glucose threshold.

Qualitative considerations. Glycosuria comprises the commonest of several types of melituria, or sweet urine. Other causes of melituria are galactose,* pentose and levulose (fructose). These substances react like glucose with Benedict's solution and must be distinguished from glucose by means of special tests. Patients having these rare types of melituria do not ordinarily show any impaired tolerance for glucose.

Indications of Insulin Excess. Except in clinics where blood insulin assays can be run, a presumptive metabolic diagnosis of insulin excess can be made only by a process of elimination. This stems from the fact that hypoglycemia, the outstanding manifestation of insulin excess, results from hepatic dysfunction, hypopituitarism and hypoadrenocorticism as well as from hyperinsulinism. Thus, it is necessary to rule out the former conditions before concluding that hyperinsulinism is the probable cause of hypoglycemia.

Hepatic dysfunction as a cause of hypoglycemia can be determined reasonably satisfactorily by applying the epinephrine-glucose tolerance test. The patient is prepared for this test by means of a diet containing 180 gm. of carbohydrate per m^2 per day for three days. On the morning of the fourth day, breakfast is omitted, the fasting blood sugar concentration is determined and a dose of epinephrine (0.3 cc. of 1:1,000 freshly opened epinephrine solution per m^2) is administered subcutaneously. Blood sugar determinations are repeated at 15, 30 and 45 minutes. If liver function is normal, the blood sugar concentration should increase at least 20 mg. per cent during this interval. This increase reflects normal hepatic glycogenolysis under the influence of epinephrine. Failure to show such a rise in blood sugar suggests glycogen storage disease,[13] abnormal hepatic glycogen depletion or other serious disturbance in hepatic function.

Hypopituitarism and hypoadrenocorticism may be recognized as possible causes of hypoglycemia by application of the diagnostic procedures discussed in Chapters III and VII. Of the tests considered in Chapter III, those concerned with

---

* Very occasionally one encounters children with symptoms of hypoglycemia in association with galactosuria and galactosemia. It appears that these patients are unable to metabolize galactose in a normal manner. As a result when foods (such as milk) containing this sugar are eaten, there is a tendency for it to accumulate in the blood stream and to spill over into the urine. The pancreas apparently responds to hypergalactosemia as it does to hyperglycemia. The insulin formed as a result of this stimulus prompts increased utilization of the circulating glucose, but not of the circulating galactose. As a result, though total blood sugar fails to fall promptly to normal levels, blood glucose levels fall to abnormally low levels. Hence, the tendency toward manifestations of hypoglycemia in the presence of high or normal total blood sugar concentration and melituria. The condition is largely prevented by omitting all galactose-containing foods.[12]

carbohydrate metabolism are most pertinent. For practical purposes a normal response to the epinephrine-eosinophil test essentially rules out hypopituitarism and hypoadrenocorticism as likely causes of hypoglycemia.

If the foregoing types of conditions can be ruled out, fasting blood sugar measurements, the glucose tolerance and the 24-hour fast tolerance tests (see Chapter III, Table 3) can be used to separate patients with "functional hyperinsulinism" from patients with "organic hyperinsulinism."[14]

Functional hyperinsulinism is a poorly understood clinical entity which is thought to be due to a disturbance in the nervous and humoral regulation of blood sugar. More specifically, there probably is either (a) hyper-reactiveness to hyperglycemia on the part of the insulin-glucose homeostatic mechanism or (b) failure on the part of this mechanism to discontinue insulin production promptly as blood sugar concentration falls into the normal or hypoglycemic range. Patients with this condition are apt to be high strung and to react excessively to many stimuli. They develop hypoglycemia within a period of two to four hours after meals, but not before breakfast or upon fasting for 24 hours. When subjected to a glucose tolerance test, they may show a sharp drop in blood glucose values to hypoglycemic levels between the second and fourth hours.

Organic hyperinsulinism is characterized by the occurrence of hypoglycemic attacks between midnight and breakfast, two to four hours after meals and after exercise or skipped or late meals. Fasting blood sugars are usually below 50 mg. per cent, and after a 24-hour fast are below 40 mg. per cent. In the glucose tolerance test, they may develop hypoglycemia between the second and fifth hours.

CLINICAL CONSIDERATIONS

JUVENILE "HYPOINSULINISM" OR DIABETES MELLITUS

Despite half a century of investigation, the exact cause and nature of ordinary diabetes mellitus remains obscure. Hence the quotation marks around the term "hypoinsulinism," for it is not known whether ordinary diabetes is due to an absolute lack of insulin, an excess of anti-insulin substances or both. In these connections it is noteworthy that the insulin needs of the patients with spontaneous diabetes usually are considerably larger than those of patients with diabetes secondary to pancreatectomy.*

* The pancreatectomized adult requires from 20 to 60 units of insulin per day.[1]

ETIOLOGY AND INCIDENCE.[1] Certain factors, including heredity, race and obesity appear to bear a relation to the genesis of this condition. With regard to heredity it has been noted that (a) diabetes occurs about 15 times more often in both twins of identical pairs (48.5 per cent incidence) than in both twins of dissimilar pairs (3.2 per cent incidence), and (b) about five times more frequently in blood relatives of diabetics (incidence 6.7 per cent) than in control groups (incidence 1.23 per cent). Mendelian ratios of the recessive type are evident in large series of diabetic cases selected at random. The expected ratios can be demonstrated also in presumably latent cases of diabetes.

Although diabetes is clearly affected by obesity in several important respects, the relation cannot as yet be fully explained. It is almost unknown in persons who are 20 or 30 per cent under weight, but otherwise during childhood it occurs more or less irrespective of weight status. Thus, of 43 diabetic children under 10 years of age,* 44 per cent were below, 37 per cent were within and only 19 per cent were over standard weight. Of 84 diabetics between 10 and 20 years of age, 29 per cent were under, 39 per cent were within and 32 per cent were above standard weight at or prior to the onset of diabetes.

On the other hand, in one large series of successive diabetics, including all ages, maximum body weights were below standard in only 8 per cent, within standard limits in 15 per cent and above standard in 77 per cent. Although obesity tends to precipitate diabetes in predisposed individuals, especially after they pass their twentieth birthday, cases have been observed in which diabetes followed rapid loss of weight by fat persons. Neither the incidence nor the mechanisms of this phenomenon have been thoroughly studied.

Certain other etiologic factors deserve brief mention. As outlined in Chapters III and VII and in the first sections of the present chapter, adrenocortical S-F-N and pituitary glycotropic hormones in excess tend to prompt an insulin-resistant type of glucose intolerance. Thus, by causing an increase in S-F-N hormone production, infection and other forms of stress may aggravate latent diabetes to the point where it becomes manifest. This fits in with the clinical finding that infection can precipitate the onset of diabetes. On the other hand, the data of Figure 27, Chapter III, indicate that S-F-N hormone production by diabetics is normal or low except during periods of stress. This suggests that although S-F-N hormone may accentuate ordinary diabetes, it probably is not an important factor in its etiology. However, chronically excessive S-F-N hormone production is con-

---

* Though diabetes is never apparent as a congenital disturbance, it sometimes develops during the first year of life.

sidered to be responsible for the special type of diabetes seen in patients with Cushing's syndrome.

Glycosuria has been noted in about 35 per cent and diabetes found in about 17 per cent of patients with acromegaly.[15] These observations suggest that clinical diabetes may occasionally be due to hyperpituitarism.

CLINICAL MANIFESTATIONS. In most adults and adolescents, diabetes develops insidiously over a period of months from a latent to a clinically manifest form. In children the syndrome is likely to develop within a period of days or weeks.

In a group of 30 successive diabetic patients who were seen in this clinic and who ranged in age from a few months to 15 years, the commonest presenting symptoms were thirst (89 per cent), polyuria (82 per cent), nocturia or enuresis (52 per cent), loss of or failure to gain weight (48 per cent), increase in appetite (37 per cent), vomiting (33 per cent), easy fatigability or weakness (30 per cent) and constipation (18 per cent). Abdominal pain, irritability and apathy were observed in about 15 per cent of these children. Infection was present in about one-third of the cases at the time of first admission to the hospital.

Except when diabetic acidosis and coma had developed, the signs presented were not striking. Of the patients seen in this clinic, most (90 per cent) were of normal height for age and of normal weight for height. These findings are in apparent contrast to those of others who report a distinct tendency for diabetic children to be from 6 to 8 cm. taller at the onset of the disease than average normal children of the same age and sex.[15 b] The same investigators report that the skeletal and sexual development of the average diabetic child is a year or so in advance of normal for age.

Symptomatically *diabetic acidosis* is characterized by marked thirst and polyuria followed by nausea and vomiting, abdominal pain and general malaise. Prior to the onset of vomiting, dehydration and signs of acidosis may not be very marked. Once vomiting starts, however, dehydration and acidosis develop rapidly. There follows a tendency to labored, long and deep respirations and to drowsiness, stupor and finally coma. Acetone soon becomes detectable in the expired breath and may permeate the atmosphere of the patient's room.

On examination the patient is drowsy or unconscious and presents signs characteristic of dehydration and acidosis (Kussmaul breathing). The face is drawn, the skin cold and dry and subcutaneous tissue elasticity is markedly diminished. The mucous membranes are dry. If ketosis is marked, the lips may be of a reddish blue hue. The eyeballs are soft, the pulse weak and rapid, the blood pressure low. Physical examination may reveal diffuse spasm and tenderness suggestive of an acute abdominal disorder. These signs may be due in part to an accumulation of hard fecal matter in the large bowel or to a lesion requiring surgery. In the latter event there is apt to be an antecedent history of abdominal pain with or without vomiting. In addition there are often definite, localized tenderness and spasm.[16] If diabetes is responsible, the signs usually subside after a few hours of insulin and fluid therapy.

LABORATORY STUDIES. These may be divided into groups relating to (a) impaired glucose tolerance, (b) ketosis, metabolic acidosis, dehydration and renal failure and (c) miscellaneous changes.

Impaired glucose tolerance is reflected by hyperglycemia. The initial blood sugar values obtained on a series of children seen at this clinic ranged between 167 and 1068 mg. per cent. Eighty-five per cent of the values were over 200 mg. per cent. Glycosuria was a universal finding.

Ketonuria (acetonuria) is a variable finding. In mild cases it may be absent. In patients with impending diabetic acidosis or coma it is almost always present. The serum electrolyte changes observed in patients with diabetic acidosis are set forth diagrammatically in Figure 1. The serum carbon dioxide content (serum bicarbonate) is low if the acidosis is pronounced. The acidosis is considered severe when the value obtained is less than 7 mEq. per liter. The serum sodium and chloride values also are somewhat depressed. On the other hand, the concentrations of potassium and inorganic phosphorus may be abnormally elevated, as may the values for total protein, hemoglobin and non-protein nitrogen. The latter changes occur when circulatory failure results in impairment of renal function.

Among the miscellaneous findings, leucocytosis and eosinopenia are of interest. Leukocytosis is the rule in patients in coma. The white cells may total between 15,000 and 50,000 per mm^3, even in the absence of demonstrable infection. In one instance a count of 100,000 was obtained. Eosinophils, on the other hand, may be virtually absent. Such eosinopenia is a relatively late occurrence in the development of diabetic acidosis and indicates that the condition has produced a significant degree of stress. The eosinopenia is due to stress-induced functional hyperadrenocorticism (see above and Chapter III).

DIAGNOSIS AND DIFFERENTIAL DIAGNOSIS. Demonstration of hyperglycemia and glycosuria* in a patient presenting the history, symptoms and signs enumerated above is nearly diagnostic of diabetes mellitus. To be differentiated are patients with (a) transient carbohydrate intolerance secondary to carbo-

---

* These terms must be interpreted strictly to refer to blood and urine glucose content (see pages 550, 551).

hydrate starvation (see page 550), (b) transient tendencies to hyperglycemia and glycosuria secondary to a stress-induced adrenocortical alarm reaction (see page 551), (c) Cushing's syndrome (see Chapter III), (d) pheochromocytoma (see Chapter IV) and (e) salicylate poisoning.

Salicylates in toxic doses produce a picture which can be confused with diabetic coma. They cause hyperpnea by irritating the respiratory center of the brain. In addition, they induce a tendency to diuresis, drowsiness, pseudo-glycosuria and pseudo-ketonuria. If nausea and drowsiness interfere with fluid ingestion, dehydration also results.

A false impression that the patient may have glycosuria arises because salicylates, like glucose, reduce Benedict's qualitative sugar reagent. Similarly, an impression may be gained that the patient has ketonuria because salicylates react in the ferric chloride test for ketones by giving a deep violet color. This error can be avoided by testing samples of urine after boiling. Ketone bodies, being volatile, disappear upon boiling; salicylates, being non-volatile, remain in the urine and continue to give a positive ferric chloride test.

The patient may be thought to have acidosis because of the central hyperpnea. Such centrally induced hyperventilation tends to wash abnormally large amounts of carbon dioxide out of the blood stream. The consequent reduction in the ratio of carbonic acid to base bicarbonate in the plasma causes the plasma pH to rise.* The alkalosis thus produced stimulates a compensatory elimination of sodium with the result that the plasma pH falls toward normal after several hours. Later, when the centrally induced hyperpnea subsides, acidosis may develop on account of this fixed base loss. If the patient also develops starvation ketosis, the tendency to acidosis may increase.

Patients with salicylate poisoning do not have hyperglycemia. They recover from the intoxication within two or three days after salicylates are discontinued, provided that water, calory and electrolyte intake is maintained at reasonable levels. Ordinarily, there is no need for specific acid or alkali therapy. If parenteral fluid therapy is necessary, one-third saline (0.28 gm. per cent NaCl) in 5 or 10 per cent dextrose solution is satisfactory.

* Plasma carbon dioxide values are totally unreliable indices of acidosis versus alkalosis, except when the nature of the primary disturbance is known. In the salicylate-poisoning patient we have an example of lowered plasma carbon dioxide and alkalosis. The same condition can be produced by voluntary hyperventilation. In patients with ammonium chloride intoxication, renal failure or marked ketosis the plasma carbon dioxide undergoes a compensatory depression. Such patients have low carbon dioxide values and metabolic acidosis. Contrariwise, there are patients with metabolic alkalosis and compensatorily increased plasma carbon dioxide values due to alkali (sodium lactate, sodium bicarbonate, etc.) intoxication. Finally, patients with central hyperpnea or with pulmonary obstruction (due to emphysema, fibrosis, edema) tend to accumulate carbon dioxide in the blood stream with resultant elevated plasma carbon dioxide values and acidosis due to carbonic acid retention.

TREATMENT. The treatment of diabetes involves several considerations. For instance, it is well to recognize that one is dealing with a disturbance in homeostasis which is not clearly understood. This means that one is forced for lack of knowledge to undertake alleviative rather than curative therapy. It means also that one is faced with the problem of attempting to serve as a substitute for a homeostatic mechanism. This poses an interesting and important question: Should the physician attempt to keep blood glucose concentration within physiologic limits at all times?

This question has no single anwer. It can only be assumed that perfect control works to the physiologic and physical benefit of a patient with diabetes. Perfect control of blood sugar can usually be attained only by paying detailed attention to diet and exercise, by making numerous blood and urine sugar measurements and by giving insulin several times a day. Such exquisite attention may, however, render the patient an emotional invalid.[17a] This seems a large price to pay for a therapeutic accomplishment of unknown value.

Less than perfect control of blood sugar concentrations means that deviations below or above the normal range must be expected. Errors in the direction of hypoglycemia are encountered most often when attempts are made to keep the patient aglycosuric at all times. To make this error repeatedly is hazardous and undesirable, for pathologic lowering of blood sugar values can cause serious changes in the central nervous system (see Figure 3). Moreover, the stress of hypoglycemia can elicit the adrenocortical alarm reaction. This in turn can cause increased resistance to insulin and hence more severe diabetes.[17b] By contrast, errors in the direction of hyperglycemia do not cause irreversible changes unless the hyperglycemia is of sufficiently marked degree and duration to result in fatal diabetic ketosis and coma.

Concerning the possible deleterious effects of chronic mild-to-moderate hyperglycemia and glycosuria, one can only raise questions. Three come to mind. First, does such hyperglycemia aggravate the diabetic state by prompting degenerative changes in the pancreatic islets? Second, does hyperglycemia or the carbohydrate starvation* primary to it constitute a stress of sufficient magnitude to elicit the adrenocortical alarm reaction? Third, are the vascular and other degenerative changes seen in patients with diabetes of several years' duration due to insulin deficiency, tissue carbohydrate starvation, hyperglycemia and glycosuria or are they due to entirely separate factors? No satisfactory answers to these questions are available today.

* As indicated above, insulin lack leads to loss of ability to utilize glucose. Indirectly, by causing glycosuria there also occurs a loss of calories from the body. Each gram of glucose in the urine indicates a loss of 4 calories.

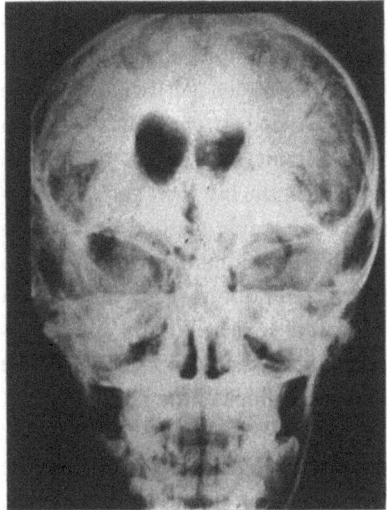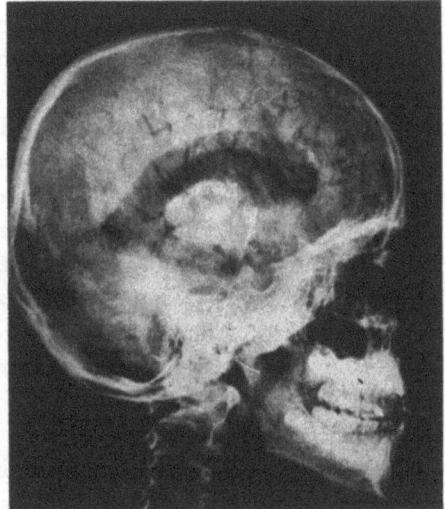

FIGURE IX—3. Dilatation of the ventricles presumably secondary to repeated insulin reactions in a boy of 7½ years.

CASE HISTORY

The patient developed diabetes mellitus at the age of two years. Up to that time his growth, maturation and general health had been satisfactory. During the first two years of his illness he was treated in another clinic with relatively large doses (16 units) of protamine insulin only. Presumably as a consequence of this type of therapy, he suffered numerous severe insulin reactions. At the age of seven years he came to our clinic with the chief complaints of diabetes mellitus and behavior problem. At that time he was receiving 12 units of protamine and 8 units of regular insulin before breakfast and was free from reactions. A complete physical examination revealed no abnormalities. His IQ was 111. While the neurologic examination also failed to reveal definite abnormalities, it was thought that his unusual behavior pattern might be a manifestation of diffuse brain damage secondary to episodes of insulin-induced hypoglycemia. At 7 3/12 years he suffered the first of a series of generalized convulsions. Simultaneously he commenced to show evidences of gradual intellectual deterioration. Three months later enlargement of the lateral and third ventricles was revealed by pneumoencephalography. The left lateral ventricle appeared larger than the right. There was no gross evidence of cortical atrophy or of a causative lesion. A series of electroencephalograms likewise showed increasing abnormalities—most marked over the left occiput. In the three years subsequent to these studies the patient has become aphasic and grossly retarded in mind. From N. B. Talbot, J. D. Crawford and C. C. Bailey, *Pediatrics*, 1:337, 1948.

This lack of information makes it difficult to set forth recommendations concerning the management of diabetes which are not empirical and arbitrary. Because hypoglycemia is definitely harmful, it is recommended that therapy be so directed that the phenomenon is very largely avoided. If one is dealing with an intelligent, stable and cooperative diabetic patient, it may be possible to maintain him in a nearly aglycosuric state without inducing intermittent hypoglycemia. Presumably, this can be considered an acceptable method of management. If, on the other hand, the patient cannot be so maintained without inducing episodes of hypoglycemia, it would appear preferable to gain the margin of safety afforded by intermittent slight-to-moderate hyperglycemia and glycosuria (10 to 30 gm. per m^2 per day). Such deviations should not, however, be permitted to reach the point where the patient develops ketonuria, nocturia, caloric undernutrition or hepatomegaly.

These comments may be extended to include a few remarks concerning the types of diet and types of insulin which may be used in the treatment of diabetes. There is no clear evidence that any one type of dietary regimen is superior to another. It appears reasonable therefore to recommend for the present that dietary advice be kept as simple as possible and that attention be directed chiefly to providing meals that are easy to prepare and appetizing. They also should permit adaptation to daily variations in caloric needs on the one hand and allow reasonable regulation of blood sugar concentrations on the other. Having decided upon some such dietary regimen, insulin is given in accordance with need.

As indicated below, various insulin preparations are available. So far as is known, these differ chiefly with respect to duration of action. Satisfactory results can be obtained by using certain of these preparations in a variety of combinations. One such combination will be outlined below.

Chronic Management of Diabetes

Diet. Diabetic patients under two years of age are fed normal diets for age and weight, the carbohydrate intake being kept at the lower limit of normal. For patients over two years of age, the following instructions are given:

1. Eat no candy, cakes, cookies, jams or sugar, and no desserts to which such ingredients have been added in any considerable amount.
2. Eat only one piece of bread a meal or its equivalent in crackers.
3. Have at any meal only one of the following: rice, macaroni, spaghetti or potatoes, and take only one moderate helping.
4. Eat but half a banana or apple at any one time.
5. In the middle of the morning take some form of food containing between 10 and 20 gm. of carbohydrate. If at any time symptoms of hypoglycemia appear,

FIGURE IX—4. Representation of approximate duration and intensity of action of various types of insulin. Adapted from E. P. Joslin et al., *The Treatment of Diabetes Mellitus*, Philadelphia, Lea & Febiger, 1946.

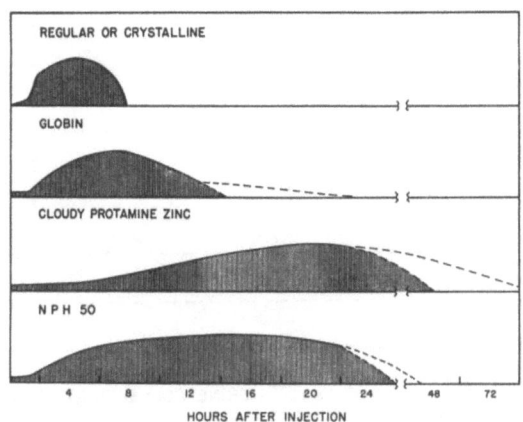

the juice of one orange or some food containing 10 gm. of glucose is to be taken immediately.

6. With the above exceptions, eat as desired at mealtime, provided ordinary common sense is applied in not eating too much of any particular dish.[18a]

Insulin. Figure 4 indicates the approximate time of onset and duration of action of certain available types of insulin.* Of these insulins, crystalline and protamine zinc are most commonly used in this clinic.

It is not possible to indicate any clear quantitative relation between insulin dosage and carbohydrate utilization or intake. This is due to the fact that the various anti-insulin factors greatly modify the action of insulin from time to time. In broad terms, one unit of insulin will permit the body to metabolize somewhere between 1 and 9 gm. of carbohydrate.[1]

Insulin dosage is adjusted to needs as indicated by urine sugar values and sometimes also by blood sugar determinations. Figure 5 may aid in these considerations. Here it is assumed (a) that the patient is following a relatively constant diet of the type suggested above, (b) that hypoglycemia is to be avoided, if need be, at the expense of intermittent mild-to-moderate hyperglycemia and glycosuria and (c) that regular (or crystalline) and protamine zinc insulin are to be

---

* The new Hagedorn protamine insulin preparation, NPH-50, is designed to permit the mixing of crystalline and protamine insulin solutions without alteration in the activity of either type of insulin. The Danish preparation of NPH-50 apparently fulfills this criterion. Accordingly, it is possible to give patients both types of insulin in desired amounts by a single injection. Current reports suggest that great care must be taken in the manufacture of NPH-50 to make sure that there is no excess protamine, since free protamine reacts with regular or crystalline insulin to form protamine insulin. This newly formed protamine insulin has a delayed and prolonged action similar to that shown in Figure 4 for NPH-50.

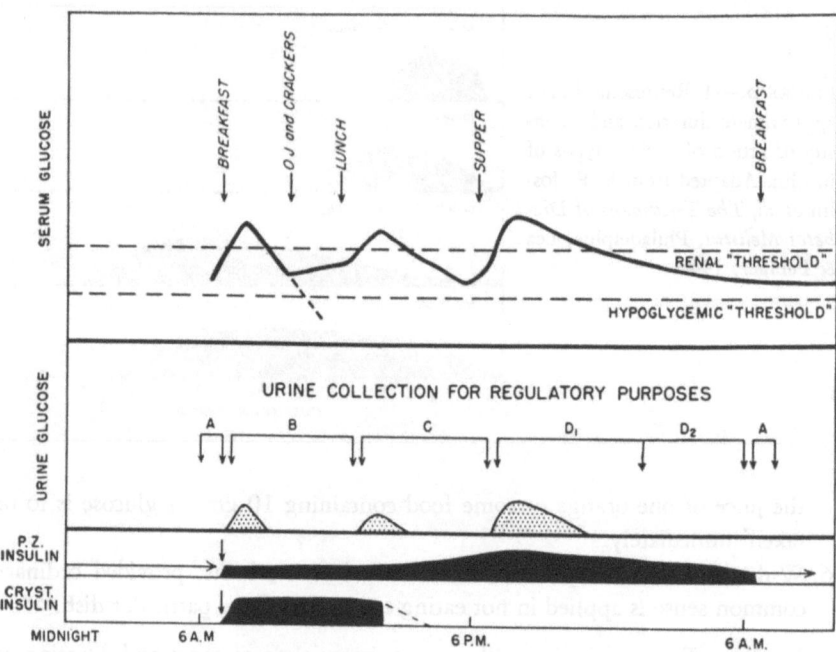

FIGURE IX—5. Diagrammatic representation of certain of the factors to be considered in the management of diabetes mellitus.

TOP DIAGRAM: The interrupted horizontal line labeled "renal threshold" indicates that glycosuria occurs when blood sugar values exceed this level. The lower interrupted horizontal line indicates that clinical symptoms of hypoglycemia develop when the blood sugar falls below this level.

MIDDLE DIAGRAM: The urine collection periods for regulatory purposes are shown by brackets A to D_2. Glycosuria is indicated when blood sugar values exceed the renal threshold.

BOTTOM DIAGRAM: Shows the duration of protamine zinc and crystalline insulin action. The vertical arrows indicate the time of administration of these agents. The horizontal arrows in the protamine zinc area attempt to indicate that this hormone acts more than 24 hours and that it therefore carries over from day to day.

---

given in separate injections by separate syringes and needles a few minutes before breakfast. During periods when the insulin needs of the patient are being determined and insulin dosages are being regulated accordingly, urine may be collected for sugar analysis* in four separate samples, as indicated in the middle section of the figure. Once the needs of the patient are fairly well known, it

* The Somogyi approximate quantitative method (see Appendix, page 590), which is easily performed, serves this purpose satisfactorily.

usually suffices to test urine for sugar by Benedict's test just before breakfast* and before supper and to collect occasional 24-hour urine samples for estimation of total daily glucose losses. Blood sugar determinations are chiefly of value for detecting preprandial hypoglycemia in patients whose preprandial urine sugar tests give negative results.

As the figure indicates, when it is noted that excessive glycosuria occurs before breakfast, the dose of protamine zinc insulin should be increased. If, as sometimes happens in the case of adolescent children, marked glycosuria is noted before and after supper, it may be desirable to administer a small amount† of additional crystalline insulin before supper. This avoids the difficulties incurred by giving such large doses of crystalline insulin before breakfast that hypoglycemia develops in the mid-morning or before lunch and of giving such large doses of protamine zinc insulin that hypoglycemia develops in the hours before breakfast.

A survey of the records of the diabetic children under our care reveals no clear relation between insulin doses and age, weight or surface area. Approximately speaking, the average total daily maintenance dose of insulin is between 20 and 30 units per m^2 (range 8 to 63 units per m^2). Of this insulin about half (range 25 to 67 per cent) is crystalline insulin, the remainder being protamine zinc insulin. There is a tendency for the ratio of crystalline to protamine zinc insulin to be higher (about 1.5 to 1) in young children and lower (about 0.5 to 1) in adolescents. Incidentally, there is an increasing tendency to permit children to give themselves their insulin injections after they reach adolescent age.

The doses of insulin required at the very beginning of diabetic therapy are usually somewhat larger than those needed in the immediately succeeding months.[18 b-d] Moreover, the doses apparently needed during hospitalization may be twice as large as those needed by the patient when he returns home. This is presumed to be due in part to a tendency for the stress of homesickness, needles, finger pricks and so forth to activate the adrenocortical alarm reaction** and in part to the fact that hospitalized patients are unable to get much physical exercise. On account of this phenomenon it is usually advisable to reduce insulin

* Note that collection A of Figure 5 gives information concerning the presence of glycosuria immediately before breakfast. Such information cannot be obtained unless, about 6 a.m., the patient empties his bladder of urine formed during the night and then, approximately one hour later, voids the urine formed during the interval. The same thesis holds with respect to other urine sugar tests designed to indicate preprandial status.

† From 5 to 10 per cent of the pre-breakfast dose.

** Stress of emotional as well as of physical origin can markedly intensify tendencies to ketosis and glycosuria.[18 e]

dosage when a diabetic child is discharged from the hospital. Otherwise, he is apt to have insulin reactions within a few days after returning home.

Infections can lead to increased glycosuria at any time. If the intercurrent condition is severe it may be necessary (a) to place the patient on a diet of simple sweetened fluids, soups and possibly soft solids and (b) to counteract marked glycosuria* by the administration of extra crystalline insulin before lunch or supper or at both times. The occurrence of acetonuria in association with marked glycosuria definitely indicates that more insulin is needed. The occurrence of acetonuria in the absence of glycosuria indicates starvation and need for more carbohydrate.

Parents are instructed always to assume that a disturbance in a diabetic child is an insulin reaction (see below) until proved otherwise. Such a reaction is treated by giving food containing from 10 to 15 gm. of carbohydrate. Alternatively, 2 or 3 teaspoons of sugar in water or Karo syrup may be given in fractional doses. Parents and older children also are taught that exercise augments the action of insulin and that either an increase in food allotments or a decrease in insulin dosages may be necessary on days or during periods (such as weekends and school vacations) when the patient is going to exercise hard. To prevent the disastrous development of an insulin reaction while out of reach of help, diabetic children should never be allowed to go in swimming, ride horseback or go on camping expeditions unless accompanied by a responsible person who is aware of the disease.

Difference between insulin reaction and diabetic coma. This rarely constitutes an urgent problem in the diabetic patient who is receiving insulin. The salient characteristics of these two conditions are summarized in Table 4.

Prevention and treatment of severe insulin reactions. For reasons offered earlier, it is believed that insulin reactions are a very undesirable complication of diabetic therapy. They usually can be avoided if (a) meals are eaten regularly, (b) strenuous exercise is taken after rather than just before meals and (c) the patient and his parents learn the symptoms and signs of hypoglycemia and are prepared to take appropriate corrective measures whenever they appear. Reactions occasionally develop for unexpected reasons, such as changing the site of insulin administration, errors in insulin dosage (due to change in strength of insulin or type of syringe) or sudden upsets with nausea, vomiting or diarrhea.

When the insulin reaction is severe, the patient may be so restless and unreasonable that it is difficult to get him to take sweetened fluids by mouth voluntarily. Under such circumstances and when coma or convulsions have supervened,

---

* Glycosuria may be considered marked if two or more successive samples of preprandial urine cause a red precipitate to be formed when Benedict's qualitative test is applied.

TABLE IX—4. Differential diagnosis of diabetic coma and insulin reaction. Adapted from E. P. Joslin et al., *The Treatment of Diabetes Mellitus*, Philadelphia, Lea & Febiger, 1946.

	Diabetic coma	Insulin reaction*
1. Onset	Slow—days	Sudden—minutes
2. Food	Too much	Too little
3. Insulin	Too little	Too much
4. Presence of infection	Frequent	Rare
5. Thirst	Extreme	Absent
6. Hunger	Absent	Frequent
7. Vomiting	Common	Seldom*
8. Pain in abdomen	Frequent	Absent
9. Fever	Absent except with infection, or marked	Absent
10. Skin	Dry	Moist
11. Tremor	Absent	Frequent
12. Vision	Dim	Double
13. Eyeballs	Soft	Normal
14. Appearance	Florid; extremely ill	Pale; weak; faint; sweating
15. Respiration	Air-hunger	Normal
16. Blood pressure	Tends to fall	Tends to rise
17. Mental state	Restless; distressed	Apathetic or irritable; or hysterical
18. Unconsciousness	Approaches gradually	May intervene suddenly
19. Convulsions	Very rare	Sometimes
20. Urine: sugar	Present	Absent (always in repeat examination)
21. Urine: diacetic acid and acetone	Present	Usually absent
22. Blood sugar	High	Low
23. Specific treatment	Insulin; fluid; salt	Carbohydrate
24. Response to treatment	Gradual—hours	Quick—minutes*

*The features of an insulin reaction listed in this table are those observed after rapidly acting, regular or crystalline insulin. In certain respects reactions due to the slowly acting protamine zinc insulin may differ. Headache (particularly occipital), nausea and even vomiting may occur. These symptoms make the differential diagnosis between reactions from protamine zinc insulin and coma more difficult than that between regular or crystalline insulin and coma. Moreover, response to treatment may be slow in patients suffering hypoglycemia due to one of the slowly acting insulins.

it may be necessary to give glucose intravenously (10 to 20 cc. of 50 per cent glucose). If it is not possible to carry out such treatment promptly, persistent efforts should be made to introduce concentrated sugar solution (table sugar in water or 50 per cent Karo syrup) into the side of the mouth with a teaspoon, a few cubic centimeters at a time. If given in small amounts, such solutions are not apt to choke the patient or be aspirated and at least a portion of the material will find its way into the stomach, whence it is rapidly absorbed into the circulation. When the reaction is due to excess crystalline insulin, recovery is usually rapid and sustained. When the reaction is caused by an excess of one of the longer-acting insulin preparations, it may be necessary to continue sugar therapy for some time before recovery is completed (constant intravenous administration of 10 per cent glucose in ⅓ to ½ isotonic (0.28 to 0.43 gm. per cent) NaCl solution. Other supportive measures, such as oxygen, sedation and suction of airway, are seldom necessary.

Other complications of insulin therapy. Atrophy of subcutaneous fat at sites of insulin injection is seen commonly. The condition may be minimized by using several sites in rotation; however, in time it tends to disappear whether or not the site in question still is being used. Urticaria at the site of injection may occur transiently at the outset of insulin therapy. This is an unimportant phenomenon. Serious allergic reactions to insulin are practically unknown. Infection at one injection site is usually due to contamination of the insulin syringe or needle; multiple abscesses suggest contamination of the insulin solution.

Treatment of Diabetic Coma

Diabetic coma* is the ultimate expression of decreased tissue utilization of glucose resulting from a relative or absolute deficiency of insulin. The progression of metabolic consequence which is initiated by insulin lack has been described on page 543. Successful therapy is founded upon: (a) accurate appraisal of the extent of this progression in the individual patient and (b) recognition of the presence of complicating factors, such as infection, which may modify his response.[19 a, b]

While the gravity of diabetic acidosis demands that treatment be begun with dispatch, the initial study of the patient must be neither cursory nor perfunctory. However, by making the appraisal in a systematic manner one can obtain the necessary information with little loss of time. Specifically, from the history one should seek to determine the precipitating cause of the acidosis and the character and duration of the individual symptoms. The physical examination should be performed with a view to estimating the extent of acidosis, dehydration and shock. A thorough search for infection should be made, particularly if a ready explanation for the occurrence of coma, such as failure of the patient to take insulin, is not apparent. Immediate confirmation of the clinical diagnosis should be obtained by means of laboratory estimations of blood and urine glucose and of urine acetone and diacetic acid. In seriously ill patients additional laboratory examinations may be of material assistance in defining more precisely the therapy required. These include determinations of the serum pH and carbon dioxide content, the serum sodium, chloride, potassium, inorganic phosphorus and protein concentrations and the blood hemoglobin and nonprotein nitrogen levels.

* The demarcation between severe diabetic acidosis and coma is not sharp. Joslin, for example, has suggested that all patients with a plasma CO_2-combining power lower than 20 volumes per cent (9 mEq. per liter) be arbitrarily considered in coma.

The interpretation of the results of these laboratory examinations is deserving of parenthetical comment. The demonstration of hyperglycemia is important from the diagnostic point of view but its degree often correlates poorly with the intensity of acidosis. The serum carbon dioxide content is not an invariably accurate index of the seriousness of the patient's condition or even of the degree of acidosis. A patient so prostrated that he is incapable of responding to acidosis with hyperventilation may have a more severe acidosis with a lower serum pH but a higher carbon dioxide content than a patient whose serum pH level is being defended by hyperpnea. In critical cases serum pH, if obtainable, is thus more informative as to the degree of acidosis than is the carbon dioxide content.

The concentrations of blood hemoglobin and serum protein may not be reliable indices of the degree of dehydration. This is because extracellular fluid and blood volumes are often quite well defended in diabetic acidosis by the marked increases in extracellular osmotic pressure occasioned by hyperglycemia and ketonemia. The extracellular hypertonicity results in movement of fluid from the intracellular to the extracellular compartment and hence in a tendency to severe intracellular dehydration. A useful approximate index of the total extent of dehydration is afforded by body weight measurements. In patients suffering diabetic acidosis of one or two days' duration, the difference between the patient's admission weight and his approximate normal weight is usually due largely to changes in total body water. An acute 10 per cent loss of body weight (water) usually results in marked clinical signs of dehydration. When weight loss spreads gradually over a longer period of time, considerable losses of body solids also occur.

In seriously ill patients the demonstration of high levels of blood non-protein nitrogen or of serum inorganic phosphorus or potassium is of importance because it indicates impairment of renal function as well as increased cellular catabolism.

Once the diagnosis of diabetic acidosis has been established and blood drawn for such chemical examinations as are clinically indicated, therapy must be initiated without delay. The essential features are the administration of insulin in adequate dosage and the restoration of the patient's depleted reserves of water and electrolytes. Each patient in acidosis presents an individual therapeutic problem: his needs must be evaluated from hour to hour by the physician in constant attendance. Many difficulties can be obviated by the preparation of a tabular "coma sheet" on which is entered a running record of the important clinical observations, the results of each laboratory test as it is obtained and a description of all therapy administered.

Insulin. It is our custom to begin treatment by administering crystalline insulin in a dosage of approximately 75 units per m^2. This is given subcutaneously or intramuscularly. An additional dose of about 50 units may be given intravenously if the acidosis is severe. Previously untreated patients are given 25 units of protamine zinc insulin per m^2 in a separate subcutaneous injection. During the first 10 or 12 hours after its administration protamine insulin has little effect and treatment with regular insulin can proceed as if protamine insulin had not been given. At the end of this period the protamine insulin carries on the work of the regular insulin, reducing the number of subsequent insulin injections. Early use of protamine insulin also helps to prevent the escape from control which sometimes occurs late in the course of treatment when the condition of the patient appears so favorable that the physician relaxes his vigilance.[19 c]

Needs for subsequent injections of crystalline insulin are determined from hourly tests of the urine for sugar and acetone and occasional blood sugar measurements. If the urine cannot be collected by spontaneous voidings, an inlying catheter should be introduced promptly. It is usually safe to assume that the blood sugar is abnormally elevated so long as the urine contains appreciable amounts of sugar (red, orange or yellow Benedict's tests). When the urine sugar diminishes below these levels (green or blue Benedict's tests) the possibility of hypoglycemia should be borne in mind. In the first hours of therapy the aim is to reduce glycosuria from very high to moderate levels and to maintain urine sugar at such moderate levels until the urine becomes acetone free. The manner of accomplishing this objective cannot be reduced to a mathematical formula. Generally speaking, one hour after insulin therapy has been begun the urine still gives a red Benedict's test. Under these circumstances we ordinarily give a second dose of about 35 units per m^2 of crystalline insulin. As the urine tests with Benedict's reagent approach yellow to green values, crystalline insulin is administered less and less frequently and the dosage is reduced to 10 or 20 units per m^2.

In severely acidotic patients it may be necessary to repeat the initial 75 units per m^2 dose at hourly intervals for several hours. When this is the case, it is advisable to obtain blood sugar determinations at intervals, as indicated by changes in the patient's condition or the need for information. In this connection the renal threshold for glucose may drop under conditions of severe stress and give a false impression with regard to the height of the blood sugar. We observed appreciable glycosuria with blood sugar values under 100 mg. per cent in a patient with fundamentally normal kidneys. This tendency to lowered renal glucose threshold disappeared after the patient had recovered from the stress of diabetic coma. Such temporary lowering of the renal glucose threshold is probably due to stress-induced hyperadrenocorticism (see Chapter III, page 153).

Following elimination of acetonuria and marked glycosuria, a process which seldom requires more than 12 hours, it is usually possible for the patient to take oral feedings. In addition to one daily dose of protamine zinc insulin, doses of crystalline insulin are given before breakfast, lunch and supper until carbohydrate stores have been replenished. After a few days the total insulin dosage can be administered before breakfast as indicated in Figure 5.

Theoretic considerations of parenteral fluids. [5-9, 19] Since it is imperative to relieve shock, to restore renal function and to terminate hyperpnea, the first objective of parenteral fluid therapy is *reparation of the chemical structure of extracellular fluid.* To accomplish this without further deranging the chemical structure of the intracellular fluid is a minimum goal toward which one should strive. Optimal therapy would promote restoration of the chemical structure of both extra- and intracellular fluids simultaneously. It would be desirable, for instance, to institute prompt replacement of the intracellular deficit of potassium which is known to exist. But since the concentration of serum potassium is sometimes greatly elevated initially, owing to impaired renal function, it is advisable to postpone this replacement until renal function is re-established. Therefore, while present knowledge permits only a distant approximation to the ideal, it suffices to indicate the desirability of modifying the composition of many fluids now in common use.

The administration of isotonic saline solution (i.e., 150 mEq. Na and 150 mEq. Cl per liter), which contains 50 mEq. more chloride ion per liter than plasma and which therefore may result in a chloride acidosis, appears unphysiologic for patients who already are suffering from severe acidosis and exhausting hyperpnea. The custom of some clinics to correct the acidifying effect of isotonic saline by adding molar sodium lactate or bicarbonate until the sodium concentration is elevated to 190 mEq. per liter in order to provide a sodium/chloride ratio similar to that of plasma (i.e., 1.3 to 1) results in a hypertonicity that is not in accord with the need for relatively sodium- and chloride-free water for cellular hydration, renal excretion and extrarenal water loss.

Recognition of the large needs for water in diabetic acidosis has led some authorities to recommend that diluted saline-lactate solutions containing about 100 mEq. of sodium, 65 mEq. of chloride and 35 mEq. of lactate per liter be employed, although such electrolyte dilution renders the fluid hypotonic with respect to red cells. This is an apparently safe change.* Dilution, however, also

---

* Red cells begin to fragment when placed in a solution of about 150 mosM per liter. However, intravenous infusion of solutions, the concentration of which is 150 mosM per liter or less, results in no appreciable hemolysis, because of rapid mixing with large volumes of blood. The above-mentioned diluted saline-lactate solution has an osmotic concentration of about 200 mosM per liter. Thus, it has no tendency to cause hemolysis.

reduces the amount of base available for rapid correction of acidosis, a possibly undesirable change.

At present, we are employing a compromise solution containing 150 mEq. of sodium, 100 mEq. of chloride and 50 mEq. of lactate (Table 8, Solution 1). This solution contributes little to the replacement of intracellular fluid deficits, but, with minimum derangement of intracellular fluid structure, it repairs those extracellular fluid defects whose persistence places the survival of the organism in immediate jeopardy.

Once the pressing extracellular needs have been met, attention must be directed to the *replacement of intracellular deficits*. That sodium salt solutions are inadequate for this purpose is becoming increasingly clear. The intracellular deficits are numerous and their metabolic consequences are only beginning to be understood. Although potassium, phosphorus and magnesium are all known to be lost in large quantities, only with respect to the consequences of potassium loss do we possess even rudimentary information.

Potassium is the chief basic ion of intracellular fluid, and as such it is maintained in ionic and osmotic equilibrium with sodium, the principal cation of extracellular fluid. When, as in diabetic acidosis, potassium is lost from cells,* replacement by sodium occurs, apparently in order that osmotic equilibrium may be preserved. However, this adjustment is effected at the cost of a reduction in the functional efficiency of the cells.

Certain measures necessarily employed in the treatment of diabetic acidosis lead to further distortion of the intracellular environment unless appropriate compensations are introduced. Thus, the prolonged infusion of sodium salts into individuals who are under stress is known to accelerate the depletion of cellular potassium and concomitant sodium replacement (see Figure 6). Moreover, restoration of carbohydrate utilization by means of insulin transfers to the cells from 1 to 1.5 mEq. of potassium per kilogram of body weight, owing to the glycogen stores which are thus replaced.† This process occurs with especial rapidity if glucose is administered with the insulin.

If sufficiently advanced, cellular potassium depletion becomes clinically recognizable. The characteristic signs are peripheral muscle paralysis, respiratory muscle weakness and myocardial failure. The respiratory muscle weakness is manifested by shallow gasping respirations and the myocardial failure by a

* Although the concentration of potassium in the serum is frequently normal or even elevated initially due to shock and renal failure, cellular deficiency in potassium has been demonstrated repeatedly and can be confidently inferred.

† In the presence of severe potassium deficiency, liver glycogen deposition cannot proceed normally, [19 k] for as much potassium is needed to form glycogen as is needed for the formation of an equal amount of muscle protoplasm.

The Pancreatic Islets

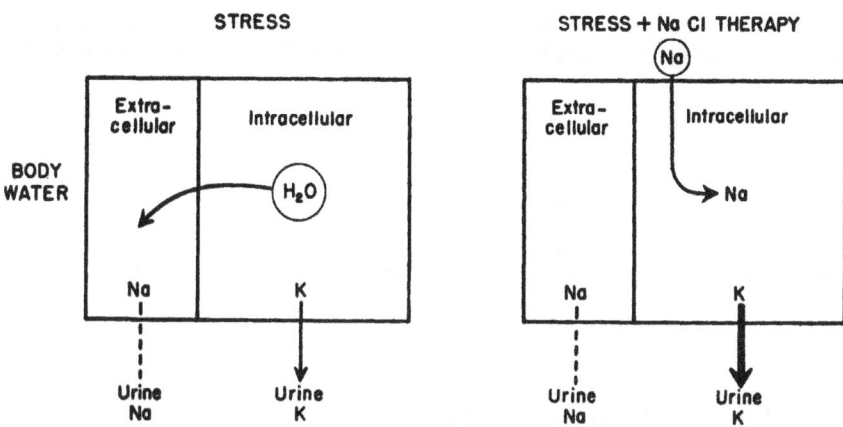

FIGURE IX—6. Schematic diagrams showing how under conditions of stress adrenocortical hormones tend to inhibit renal sodium and to facilitate renal potassium excretion. As shown in the left-hand diagram, the body is thus enabled to sustain extracellular fluid volume for a time at the expense of intracellular water. This is accomplished by osmotic forces as suggested by Chapter III, Figure 10. The right-hand diagram indicates that isotonic sodium chloride therapy may exaggerate the tendency to intracellular potassium loss to a pathologic degree. This is explained by the fact that when excess sodium cannot be eliminated by way of the kidneys, it tends to enter the body cells and to displace the potassium contained therein. When this exchange of sodium for potassium becomes marked, serious degenerative and functional changes develop (see Chapter III, Figures 6 and 35). From N. B. Talbot, *Pediatrics*, 6:1, 1950.

---

weak, rapid pulse and ashen gray pallor.[19 e] After the acidosis has been corrected and the serum sodium, chloride and glucose concentrations restored to normal, the disturbance may still have a fatal termination. Post-mortem examination fails to reveal any anatomic cause for death in such cases. That it results from therapy which is focused on restoration to normal of extracellular fluid concentrations and which neglects intracellular needs seems well substantiated by the fact that the previously mentioned clinical manifestations, which become recognizable before death, can be eliminated promptly by the administration of potassium salts.

The above considerations have stimulated us among others to design solutions which attempt to replace the total electrolyte and water deficits of the acidotic patient rather than to correct isolated abnormalities in plasma electrolyte structure.[5 a, b]

The deficits incurred by the diabetic patient have been discussed on page 544 and are summarized in Table 3. In applying such estimations of losses to replace-

TABLE IX—5. Basic parenteral maintenance requirements of a diabetic patient per m² of body surface during the first 24 hours of therapy. From A. M. Butler, *Acta pædiat.* 38:59, 1949.

Requirement	H$_2$O cc.	Na mEq.	Cl mEq.	K mEq.	Mg mEq.	P gm.	Glucose gm.
Insensible*	500	5	5	2			
Renal:							
normal basic†	250	6	6	10	3	0.2	
added diabetic**	750	12	11	10	4	0.4	50
Caloric							250
Total	1,500	23	22	22	7	0.6	300
Concentration per liter	1,000	15	14	15	5	0.4	200

*Assuming perspiration accounts for 70 per cent of insensible loss and has Na and Cl concentrations of 20 per cent of the extracellular fluid concentration.
†Determined by experimental data on normal subjects.
**Determined by metabolic balance data on diabetic coma patients during therapy.

ment therapy, consideration should be given to the fact that the losses reparable in the first 24 hours of therapy do not include those resulting from tissue catabolism. Such losses can be repaired only by the deposition of new tissue and thus fall outside the scope of rehydration therapy. Moreover, in the case of potassium only that portion of the loss which is in excess of the nitrogen loss (i.e., approximately 3 mEq. K per kg. rather than 6 mEq. as given in Table 3) is immediately replaceable. Extending this method of thinking to other body substances, roughly 80 per cent of the water, sodium and chloride, 50 per cent of the potassium and magnesium and 25 per cent of the phosphorus lost are potentially replaceable in the first 24 to 48 hours of therapy. Restoration of the remaining fractions depends upon regeneration of lost protoplasm. Expressed in other terms, the replacement needs of the first 24 to 48 hours of therapy may be calculated to approximate per kilogram: 80 cc. H$_2$O, 6 mEq. Na, 5 mEq. Cl, 3 mEq. K, 0.4 mEq. Mg and 0.02 gm. P. It is to be noted that the loss and repair values are concerned with changes in body mass and hence are expressed on a per kilogram basis.

During each 24 hours there must be provision for maintenance requirements as well as for repair needs. Maintenance requirements are prescribed by physiologic functions which are proportional to surface area rather than to body mass. Further, they are subject to changes which occur as a result of homeostatic, adaptative alterations in adrenocortical, posterior pituitary and parathyroid activity. Since the latter phenomena have not yet been fully defined and described, it is difficult at present to make dogmatic statements concerning maintenance needs. A rough approximation of the orders of magnitude involved is indicated in Table 5.

TABLE IX—6. Repair and maintenance parenteral therapy during the first 24 hours of treatment for a child of approximately 30 kg., or 1 square meter of body surface. From A. M. Butler, *Acta pædiat.* 38:559, 1949.

	H_2O cc.	Na mEq.	Cl mEq.	K mEq.	Mg mEq.	P gm.	Glucose gm.
Repair (per kg. x 30)	2,400	150	120	90	12	0.6	0
Maintenance (per m² x 1)	1,500	20	20	22	7	0.6	300
Total	3,900	200	170	112	19	1.2	300
Approximate concentrations per liter	1,000	51	44	30	5	0.3	75

From the data of Tables 3 and 5 the total repair and maintenance needs for the first 24 hours of treatment may be estimated. Table 6 gives the approximate therapeutic requirements. To correct such data for a patient of any specific size, multiply the repair data of the table by weight in kilograms divided by 30 and the maintenance data by square meters of body surface (Table 7).

Practical considerations of parenteral fluids. Hydration is begun by intravenous infusion of 500 to 800 cc. per m² at the rate of 8 cc. (about 150 drops) per m² per minute of a solution containing only sodium, chloride and bicarbonate or lactate (Table 8, Solution 1).

As soon as urine flow and circulatory efficiency are satisfactory and signs of hyperpnea have commenced to subside, we ordinarily discontinue the saline-lactate infusion and begin the administration of a glucose containing multiple electrolyte solution (Table 8, Solution 2).* In most instances this solution has given satisfactory results. In a few exceptionally severe instances of diabetic coma, accompanied by profound potassium depletion, it has seemed advisable to modify Solution 2.

---

* A factor of first importance with respect to the administration of potassium is that the cardio-vascular-renal system be functioning efficiently. Under these circumstances potassium is distributed widely, and unneeded surpluses can be eliminated by way of the kidneys. Otherwise it may accumulate within the body in toxic amounts. Hence the clinical recommendation that potassium be withheld until circulation and renal flow have been restored by infusions of sodium salt solutions.

The doses of potassium recommended here are actually very conservative as regards potential toxicity. They are well within maximum limits of tolerance. Thus, it is known that individuals with normal kidneys can eliminate at least as much potassium as is contained in glomerular filtrate (100,000 cc. x 0.05 mEq. or 500 mEq. per m² per 24 hours). In dogs and humans it has been shown that additional potassium can be eliminated by tubular secretion (see Chapter II, Figure 2, Section F).[19 g-1] Humans have been given solutions containing from 40 to 90 mEq. of potassium per liter at rates (250 to 400 cc. per m² per hour) which in 24 hours would total 500 and 900 mEq. of potassium in 6 to 10 liters of water per m² per day.[19 j] Incidentally, for reasons suggested above, the provision of ample water for urine formation probably widens the margin of safety to a considerable extent.

TABLE IX—7. Approximate guide to therapy for diabetic coma patients of various sizes during the first 24 hours. The values given should be considered maximal.

			Parenteral fluid therapy							
			0 to 1 hr. Sol. no. 1†		1 to 6 hr. Sol. no. 2		6 to 8 hr. transfusion**		8 to 24 hr. Sol. no. 2††		Total volume of fluid per 24 hr.
Weight of patient	Surface area	Initial crystalline insulin dose*	Tot. vol. cc.	Infus. rate cc/min.§	Tot. vol. cc.	Infus. rate cc/min.§	Tot. vol. cc.	Infus. rate cc/min.§	Tot. vol. cc.	Infus. rate cc/min.§	
kg.	m²	units	cc.	cc/min.**	cc.	cc/min.**	cc.	cc/min.**	cc.	cc/min.**	cc.
5	0.25	20	125	2.0	200	0.7	75	0.6	575	0.6	975
10	0.5	40	250	4.0	400	1.3	150	1.2	1,150	1.1	1,950
15	0.6	45	300	4.8	500	1.7	180	1.5	1,600	1.6	2,580
20	0.8	60	400	6.5	700	2.3	240	2.0	2,100	2.1	3,440
28	1.0	75	500	8	950	3.2	300	2.5	2,900	2.9	4,650
40	1.3	100	650	10.5	1,300	4.2	390	3.3	3,800	3.8	6,140
50	1.5	110	750	12.0	1,550	5.1	450	3.7	4,700	4.7	7,450
60	1.7	125	850	13.5	1,850	6.2	510	4.2	5,500	5.5	8,710
70	1.8	135	900	14.5	2,100	7.0	540	4.5	6,200	6.2	9,740

*For comments concerning subsequent doses, see text.
†Sometimes it is advisable to extend the first period to 3 or 4 hours before starting to administer Solution 2. In this case, the rate of administering Solution 1 should be reduced after the first hour to the rate indicated in the 1-to-6 hour column.
**Transfusion may not be necessary. If omitted, therapy is continued with Solution 2.
††Usually this infusion may be discontinued and oral feeding instituted between 12 and 18 hours after starting insulin and parenteral therapy.
§The ordinary intravenous drip bulb delivers approximately 1 cc. per 17 or 18 drops.

TABLE IX—8. Composition of solutions suitable for intravenous administration to diabetic coma patients. See text for comments on indications and contraindications for the use of each of these solutions.

	Electrolyte composition per liter					Constituents per liter					
Solution no.	Na mEq.	K mEq.	Cl mEq.	P gm.	Lactate mEq.	NaCl gm.	NaL** gm.	KCl gm.	K₂HPO₄ gm.	KH₂PO₄ gm.	Dextrose gm.
1*	150	—	100	—	50	5.6	4.1	—	—	—	—
2†	30	30	30	0.2	20	0.6	2.2	1.5	0.8	0.2	50

*This solution is easily prepared by adding 40 cc. of molar Na lactate (or NaHCO₃) solution and 210 cc. of water to 500 cc. of 0.85 gm. per cent NaCl solution. If pure distilled water is not available, 5 per cent dextrose solution may be used.
†A 50 cc. ampule containing the salts indicated is made up and sterilized. Just prior to use, the contents of this ampule are added to 1 liter of 5 per cent dextrose solution.
**Sodium lactate.

Potassium depletion is recognized by progressive muscle weakness, electrocardiographic changes (see Chapter III, Figure 35) and falling serum potassium concentration values. Should these signs develop, it may appear advisable to increase the potassium content of Solution 2 by 20 to 40 mEq. per liter. For this purpose it is convenient to have available sterile 20 cc. ampules containing molar potassium acetate or chloride solution.* The former salt appears preferable in patients who are still suffering from severe acidosis. Each cc. of the solution in these ampules contains 1 mEq. of potassium. The amount indicated is added to Solution 2, which, thus fortified, is administered until either the manifestations of potassium insufficiency have disappeared or the patient is able to take potassium-containing fluids (such as orange juice, pineapple juice, milk) by mouth.

Finally, it may be desirable to add magnesium to Solution 2. It is known that this element plays a significant role in carbohydrate utilization. It also has been noted that serum magnesium levels may drop to values as low as 0.5 mEq. per liter during the course of therapy. Magnesium chloride can be infused at a concentration of 5 mEq. (0.3 gm.) per liter with safety. Because it causes clouding of the solution if autoclaved in the presence of phosphate, it should be sterilized separately in a 10 cc. vial, the contents of which can be added to a liter of Solution 2.

The rate of administration of the multiple electrolyte solution should approximate 3 cc. (about 50 drops) per m^2 of body surface per minute. The duration of parenteral therapy varies according to the persistence of the nausea. Usually 70 per cent of the 24-hour requirement given parenterally in 12 hours will result in such improvement that the remainder can be given orally. The fluid may be flavored with ginger ale or orange juice, or it may be diluted with milk.

Supportive measures. A number of additional measures are frequently indicated in the treatment of patients with diabetic acidosis. These include gastric lavage, chemotherapy and blood transfusion.

Since the stomach is likely to be distended with food remnants and with fluid, gastric lavage is usually advisable to reduce the risk of aspiration of regurgitated material and to facilitate subsequent oral feeding.

The importance of detecting the presence of infection in the acidotic patient has already been mentioned. If infection is found, appropriate treatment should be instituted immediately. Sulfonamide therapy should, of course, be postponed until urine flow has become well established.

The transfusion of whole blood frequently appears to be beneficial. Definite anemia (hemoglobin < 9 to 10 gm. per cent) or hypoproteinemia (serum

---

* 2.0 gm. K acetate per 20 cc.; 1.5 gm. KCl per 20 cc.

protein < 5 gm. per cent), appearing as hydration is restored, is an indication for transfusion. Blood should be given somewhat more slowly than the clear parenteral fluids and in an amount not ordinarily exceeding 300 cc. per m². In patients suffering marked potassium deficiency, the relative needs for red blood cells and plasma protein versus readily available potassium ion should be weighed carefully before substituting whole blood for Solution 2 therapy. We have seen the serum potassium and electrocardiographic T waves fall to low levels during the course of a transfusion lasting two hours.

Management of diabetic patients at times of surgery. When it is known in advance that a patient with diabetes is to be subjected to elective surgery, certain preparatory steps should be taken. During the preoperative period enough carbohydrate and insulin should be given to insure satisfactory hepatic glycogen storage. Unless the patient's condition is unsatisfactory, the operation should be performed without delay at the scheduled time, preferably 9 or 10 a.m.

Four hours preoperatively the patient is given some strained orange juice and a piece of toast spread with honey or jelly. At the same time he is given half his regular doses of crystalline and protamine zinc insulin. As soon as he is anæsthetized, an intravenous infusion of Solution 2 in 5 per cent dextrose is started and an inlying catheter is inserted into the bladder. A physician in constant attendance checks the urine for sugar and acetone at half-hourly intervals. In addition, if the patient's status is in question, blood sugar determinations should be made. Crystalline insulin is given intra- and postoperatively at intervals of three to six hours as indicated by these tests. It is better to give too little insulin and to supplement the dose later than to give too much and risk inducing intraoperative hypoglycemia. Ordinarily the individual doses of crystalline insulin given during the intra- and postoperative periods equal approximately one-eighth to one-sixth of the preoperative daily insulin dosage. The aim of this insulin therapy is to maintain slight-to-moderate hyperglycemia and glycosuria and to avoid ketonuria.

When emergency surgery is indicated in the case of a patient suffering diabetic acidosis and dehydration, a difficult problem arises. If circumstances permit, it is very desirable to delay surgery until the patient has been subjected to therapy of the type outlined in Table 7 and its accompanying text for at least an hour and preferably for 6 to 12 hours. Ideally, operation should be postponed until circulatory and renal efficiency are fully restored and ketosis and acidosis have been eliminated.

Postoperatively, if the patient requires continued intravenous fluid infusion, Solution 2 is reasonably satisfactory. Sometimes after prolonged infusions of this solution, a tendency to alkalosis develops. Recent studies suggest that this can be prevented or corrected by fortifying Solution 2 with 15 to 20 mEq. of additional KCl per liter (see page 575). The volume of solution needed for maintenance purposes is determined by the surface area, as indicated in Table 5.

PROGNOSIS. The rate of recovery from diabetic coma by diabetic children is practically 100 per cent. Exceptions are encountered only when coma is accompanied by a condition such as overwhelming sepsis or serious surgical lesion which in itself is potentially lethal.

Provided the diabetes is reasonably well controlled, essentially normal growth and maturation may be anticipated. Like healthy children, diabetic children may show a tendency to retarded growth and development if they suffer from repeated infections or chronic caloric undernutrition.

The really distressing aspect of juvenile diabetes is to be found in the late degenerative sequelæ of the disease. After 15 or 20 years, about 70 per cent of diabetic children develop arteriosclerosis, 65 per cent retinal hemorrhages, 50 per cent retinal exudates, 40 per cent hypertension and 35 per cent albuminuria.[20] As mentioned earlier, the cause of these degenerative changes is not yet known. It is not even known whether they are the result of the disease or of its therapy. This is a sobering fact, which should stimulate much more intensive studies of these problems.

Insulin-reaction hypoglycemia occasionally produces serious degenerative changes (see Figure 3) and occasionally results in death; the commonest cause recorded to date is nephritis (intercapillary glomerulosclerosis[21]). This condition has been listed as responsible for about 50 per cent of the late deaths in a series of 48 diabetic patients who had suffered from the disease for more than 15 years. The other deaths had miscellaneous causes.

HYPERINSULINISM AND RELATED CONDITIONS CAUSING HYPOGLYCEMIA

Introductory Comments. Hypoglycemia can result from a variety of conditions, including hyperinsulinism, hypopituitarism, hypoadrenocorticism, hepatic disease, galactosemia, disorders of the central nervous system, strenuous exercise and starvation. Because methods for appraising insulin status are not generally available, it usually is not possible to determine directly whether a given hypoglycemic patient is suffering from hyperinsulinism. On the contrary, this diagnosis is of necessity made largely by a process of elimination, as discussed above under methods of diagnosis.

The experience of pathologists dealing with pediatric patients indicates that functionally active, pancreatic islet adenomas are probably quite rare. No instances of pancreatic islet adenomas known to have been associated with a tendency toward hypoglycemia during life have been encountered in patients under 16 years of age at the Massachusetts General Hospital or the Children's Medical Center in Boston. On the other hand, the autopsy records of these hospitals do indicate the occasional occurrence of clinically "silent" islet cell adenomas. The significance of the latter is unknown. As might be expected from the foregoing, the literature contains very few records of authentic cases of hypoglycemia due to hyperinsulinism.[22]

Definitions of pathologic hypoglycemia. During approximately the first five days of life, normal infants commonly have true blood sugar values ranging between 20 and 60 mg. per cent.* Thereafter, as in normal older infants, children and adults it is unusual to find blood sugar values of less than 60 mg. per cent. Pre-breakfast blood sugar concentrations of less than 50 mg. per cent with the patient on an ordinary carbohydrate intake and less than 40 mg. per cent with the patient on a low carbohydrate diet are almost always indicative of pathology.[14, 23] The occurrence of similarly low values from three to five hours after meals may also be considered abnormal.

Interpretation of the significance of blood sugar values is enhanced by relating them to clinical symptomatology. The neonatal tendency to low blood sugar is not ordinarily accompanied by definite clinical signs of blood sugar deficiency. Accordingly, the tendency may be considered physiologic and normal for this age group. In older individuals tolerance for lowered blood sugar concentration varies. Most children and adults develop signs of sugar lack when the concentration of glucose in the blood falls below 50 or 40 mg. per cent. Patients with central nervous system defects and patients suffering hypoadrenocorticism[24] may be more sensitive to a lowering of blood sugar concentration and may develop signs of hypoglycemia when blood glucose values fall below 60 or 50 mg. per cent.

In other words, patients are considered to have pathologic hypoglycemia when a decline in blood glucose concentration below a certain value results in symptoms and signs of glucose deficiency. Implicit in this statement is the thought that these symptoms and signs of glucose deficiency disappear promptly when blood glucose concentration is raised above the critical threshold value just mentioned.

* The values obtained for infants born of diabetic mothers fall in approximately the same range.[23]

TABLE IX—9. Summary of certain conditions which may be accompanied by hypoglycemia.

| | | | Approximate characteristics | | | | |
| | | | Blood sugar | | Normal reaction | | |
Condition	Cause	Incidence	Fall on fasting*	Rise post epineph.†	Epineph.-eosino.**	ACTH-eosinophil††	Comments
1. Hyperinsulinism	Pancreatic islet adenoma	Very rare	yes	yes	yes?	yes?	Hypoglycemia apt to occur unpredictably; prolonged
2. Primary hypoadrenocorticism	Destruction of adrenals	Very rare	yes	yes	no	no	See Chapter III
3. Primary hypopituitarism or hypothalamic disturbance with secondary hypoadrenocorticism	Disturbance in anterior pituitary or hypothalamus	?	yes	yes	no	yes	See Chapters III and VII
4. Hepatic disease including von Gierke's disease	Glycogen fixation§ or fatty infiltration with glycogen depletion	Rare	yes	no	yes?	yes?	Hepatomegaly usually present
5. Galactosemia	Disturbance in galactose metabolism	Rare	no	yes	yes?	yes?	Galactosemia, galactosuria, and hypoglycemia occur after eating galactose. See page 552
6. Functional hypoglycemia	Over-reaction to hyperglycemia; mechanism unknown§§	?	no	yes	?	yes?	Hypoglycemia may occur within 3 to 5 hours after meals and be corrected spontaneously within ½ hour

*See Test 5, Table 3, Chapter III. †See page 552, this chapter.
**See Test 2, Table 3, Chapter III. ††See Test 3, Table 3, Chapter III.
§Patients with von Gierke's glycogen-storage disease are apt to show acetonuria, lipemia, and hypercholesterolemia in addition to chronic hypoglycemia.[13] Interestingly, they may not present clinical manifestations of blood sugar lack, even though the blood sugar concentration falls to very low levels.
§§Some of these patients have gross central nervous system defects,[20] of which the functional significance is not clear. In certain cases, it appears that the defect may have been the result rather than the cause of hypoglycemia.[28]

CLINICAL MANIFESTATIONS. The classic manifestations of hypoglycemia are listed above in Table 4. The picture observed in different patients and at different times in a single individual is apt to be moderately variable. Nervousness, trembling, pallor, sweating, weakness, unsteadiness of gait, mental confusion and irritability constitute the common manifestations seen in patients who have retained consciousness. In more severe cases consciousness may be lost and epileptiform convulsions may supervene. These may so dominate the clinical picture that the other manifestations of hypoglycemia are easily overlooked. This error can be avoided by measuring the blood sugar concentration of patients with unexplained convulsions.

DIAGNOSIS. Table 9 presents in outline form information concerning some of the conditions which may be accompanied by pathologic hypoglycemia and indicates some of their distinguishing characteristics.

In dealing with a patient who has been found to have significant hypoglycemia, it is our custom to make the following measurements or tests in the order mentioned: (a) blood sugar determinations in the morning before breakfast after an overnight fast, (b) a combined epinephrine-glucose and epinephrine-eosinophil test, (c) an intravenous glucose tolerance test and (d) a 24-hour fasting tolerance test. These tests are considered above in the section dealing with methods of estimating insulin status.

The occurrence of early morning hypoglycemia is interpreted to mean that the tendency toward low blood sugar does not represent a simple, functional overreaction to the stimulus provided by postprandial hyperglycemia* (Condition 6) or galactosemia (Condition 5, see footnote to page 552). A normal rise in blood sugar following the administration of epinephrine is taken to mean that there is no significant depletion of hepatic glycogen stores or lack of capacity to lyse hepatic glycogen as is noted in patients with certain types of liver disease (Condition 4). A normal drop in eosinophils following the administration of epinephrine is considered valid evidence that there is probably no significant disturbance in the adrenocortical alarm reaction mechanism as may be seen in certain hypopituitary and hypoadrenocortical patients (Conditions 2 and 3).

There now remain two chief possibilities. One is that the patient has a hyperfunctioning pancreatic islet cell tumor, the other and more likely possibility is that he has a tendency to hypoglycemia which cannot be thoroughly explained by the diagnostic procedures available today.† The former can be excluded only

* This is demonstrable by application of the intravenous glucose tolerance test. Transitory hypoglycemia occurs within three to five hours after the hyperglycemic peak is passed. In patients with primary hyperinsulinism, similar post-hyperglycemic hypoglycemia may develop, but it is not so apt to be transitory.

† Some patients have gross evidences of cerebral defects.[29] It is usually not clear whether these defects are the cause or the result of the hypoglycemia.

by meticulous and sometimes repeated surgical exploration of the pancreas. Since this is a major undertaking, one hesitates to recommend it unless there is strong evidence that the patient has a striking tendency to hypoglycemia. To gain such evidence, it may be of value to subject the patient to a carefully planned period of prolonged fasting (but not thirsting).

The fast is performed as outlined in Test 5 of Table 3, Chapter III. The development of acetonuria after 12 to 16 hours of fasting signifies that the patient has depleted his carbohydrate stores and is maintaining blood sugar values by the gluconeogenesis mechanism described in Chapter III. If blood sugar concentrations are still above hypoglycemic levels after 24 hours of fasting, it may be desirable to extend the fast for an additional 12 to 24 hours. If no pathologic hypoglycemia develops after 48 hours of fasting, pancreatic exploration may be postponed. Under the opposite circumstance, where fasting does lead to pathologic hypoglycemia, exploration of the pancreas is usually indicated.

Demonstration of an islet cell adenoma by surgical exploration may be quite difficult. Experience with adult patients indicates that adenomas are located most frequently in the tail of the pancreas. About one-quarter are located in the head or at the junction of the tail and body of the organ. Occasionally multiple small adenomas are encountered. These tumors can vary in size from 0.5 to 15 cm. in diameter. They are slow growing and late to metastasize.[25]

Failure to demonstrate an adenoma at the initial surgical exploration constitutes presumptive rather than positive evidence that no such lesion exists. The literature indicates that tumors which were not discernible at the first operation may be evident at a second exploration.[14, 26]

TREATMENT. Removal of a functioning pancreatic islet cell adenoma usually results in complete cessation of pathologic hypoglycemia. Failure to obtain relief by removal of a single adenoma suggests that other similar tumors may exist.

The therapeutic problem presented by patients with hypoglycemia of unknown cause is a difficult one. Occasionally they suffer only one or two attacks of hypoglycemia, which disappear spontaneously and without explanation. Though the literature describes patients in whom hypoglycemia develops following carbohydrate ingestion (Table 9, Condition 6), we have not encountered them. This condition is said to be controlled by feeding relatively high protein, low carbohydrate meals.[14, 27] Low carbohydrate meals are less apt *per se* to result in postprandial hyperglycemia than high carbohydrate meals. Carbohydrate is formed from protein, but at such a slow rate that it does not cause an elevation in blood sugar.

Recent studies suggest that ACTH therapy may act to correct hypoglycemic tendencies in certain cases.[27c] It remains to be seen whether such therapy is practically satisfactory. Similar results might be expected from the use of cortisone. As discussed in Chapter III, both agents can prompt serious toxic as well as beneficial effects.

In the rare patient who has hypoglycemia which is so severe and protracted that it must be treated by constant carbohydrate feedings, more radical measures may become justified. One such patient was treated with alloxan with apparent success.[28] Others have been treated by subtotal or nearly total pancreatectomy, in many instances with little or no success.

PROGNOSIS. The outlook for patients with repeated hypoglycemia is poor with regard to central nervous system function. Unless the hypoglycemia is brought under control, convulsions and mental deterioration occur.

REFERENCES

1. JOSLIN, E. P., ROOT, H. F., WHITE, P., MARBLE, A. and BAILEY, C. C. *The Treatment of Diabetes Mellitus.* Philadelphia, Lea & Febiger, 1946.

2. (a) SOSKIN, S. and LEVINE, R. *Carbohydrate Metabolism.* Univ. Chicago Press, 1946.
   (b) CORI, C. F. Enzymatic reactions in carbohydrate metabolism. In *The Harvey Lectures, 1945-46.* Series 41:253. Lancaster, Science Press, 1946.
   (c) YOUNG, F. G. The mechanism of action of insulin. *Science Progress* 36:13, 1948.
   (d) HIMSWORTH, H. P. The syndrome of diabetes mellitus and its causes. *Lancet* 1:465, 1949.
   (e) STETTEN, DE W., JR. Carbohydrate metabolism. *Am. J. Med.* 7:571, 1949.
   (f) BORNSTEIN, J. A technique for the assay of small quantities of insulin using alloxan diabetic, hypophysectomized, adrenalectomized rats. *Australian J. Exper. Biol. & M. Sc.* 28:87, 1950.
   (g) BORNSTEIN, J. Normal insulin concentration in man. *Australian J. Exper. Biol. & M. Sc.* 28:93, 1950.

3. LA BARRE, J. The role of the central nervous system in the control of pancreatic secretion. *Am. J. Physiol.* 94:13, 1930.

4. (a) STADIE, W. C. Fat metabolism in diabetes mellitus. *Ann. Int. Med.* 15:783, 1941.
   (b) BONDY, P. K., SHELDON, W. H. and EVANS, L. D. Changes in liver glycogen studied by the needle aspiration technic in patients with diabetic ketosis. *J. Clin. Invest.* 28:1216, 1949.

5. (a) BUTLER, A. M. Parenteral fluid therapy in diabetic coma. *Acta pædiat.* 38:59, 1949.
   (b) BUTLER, A. M. Diabetic coma. *New Eng. J. Med.* 243:648, 1950.

6. (a) ATCHLEY, D. W., LOEB, R. F., RICHARDS, D. W., JR., BENEDICT, E. M. and DRISCOLL, M. E. On diabetic acidosis; a detailed study of electrolyte balances following withdrawal and re-establishment of insulin therapy. *J. Clin. Invest.* 12:297, 1933.
   (b) BUTLER, A. M., TALBOT, N. B., STANBURY, J. B. and MAC LACHLAN, E. A. Metabolic studies in diabetic coma. *Tr. A. Am. Physicians* 60:102, 1947.

7. GAMBLE, J. L. *Chemical Anatomy, Physiology and Pathology of Extracellular Fluid: A Lecture Syllabus.* Cambridge, Harvard Univ. Press, 1947.

8   GUEST, G. M. Organic phosphates of the blood and mineral metabolism in diabetic acidosis. *Am. J. Dis. Child.* 64:401, 1942.

9   MC ARTHUR, J. W., HARTING, D., SMART, G. A. and TALBOT, N. B. Time relations between the metabolic changes of experimental diabetic acidosis and onset of adrenal cortical hyperfunction. *Proc. Am. Soc. Clin. Invest.* 1950. (In press.)

10 (a) GRAYZEL, D. M. Changes in the central nervous system resulting from convulsions due to hyperinsulinism. *Arch. Int. Med.* 54:694, 1934.
   (b) BAKER, A. B. Cerebral lesions in hypoglycemia; some possibilities of irrevocable damage from insulin shock. *Arch. Path.* 26:765, 1938.
   (c) BAKER, A. B. Cerebral damage in hypoglycemia. *Am. J. Psychiat.* 96:109, 1939.

11 (a) SMITH, H. W. *The Kidney: Structure and Function in Health and Disease.* New York, Oxford Univ. Press, 1951.
   (b) BLOTNER, H. and HYDE, R. W. Renal glycosuria in selectees and volunteers. *J. A. M. A.* 122:432, 1943.
   (c) WOLMAN, I. J. Mellituria in healthy American men with special reference to transitory glycosuria. *Am. J. M. Sc.* 212:159, 1946.

12 MASON, H. H. and TURNER, M. E. Chronic galactemia; report of case with studies on carbohydrates. *Am. J. Dis. Child.* 50:359, 1935.

13 MASON, H. H. and ANDERSON, D. H. Glycogen disease. *Am. J. Dis. Child.* 61:795, 1941.

14 CONN, J. W. Diagnosis and management of spontaneous hypoglycemia. *J. A. M. A.* 134:130, 1947.

15 (a) COGGESHALL, C. and ROOT, H. F. Acromegaly and diabetes mellitus. *Endocrinology* 26:1, 1940.
   (b) WHITE, P. Diabetes in childhood. In *The Treatment of Diabetes Mellitus.* By E. P. Joslin, H. F. Root, P. White, A. Marble and C. C. Bailey. Philadelphia, Lea & Febiger, 1946.

16 MC KITTRICK, L. S. Abdominal symptoms with or without abdominal lesions in diabetic acidosis. *New Eng. J. Med.* 209:1033, 1933.

17 (a) BRUCH, H. Physiologic and psychologic interrelationships in diabetes in children. *Psychosom. Med.* 11:200, 1949.
   (b) SOMOGYI, M. Dietary and insulin therapy of diabetics. *Bull. St. Louis Jewish Hosp. Staff* 4:1, 1949.

18 (a) BUTLER, A. M. The dietary management of diabetics at the diabetic clinic of the infants' and children's hospitals, Boston, Mass. *New Eng. J. Med.* 212:760, 1935.
   (b) JACKSON, R. L., BOYD, J. D. and SMITH, T. E. Stabilization of the diabetic child. *Am. J. Dis. Child.* 59:332, 1940.
   (c) BRUSH, J. M. Initial stabilization of the diabetic child. *Am. J. Dis. Child.* 67:429, 1944.
   (d) JOHN, H. J. Diabetes mellitus in children. *J. Pediat.* 35:723, 1949.
   (e) HINKLE, L. E. and WOLF, S. Experimental study of life situations, emotions, and the occurrence of acidosis in a juvenile diabetic. *Am. J. M. Sc.* 217:130, 1949.

19 (a) GUEST, G. M. Diabetic coma; metabolic derangements and principles for corrective therapy. *Am. J. Med.* 7:630, 1949.
   (b) FRANKS, M., BERRIS, R. F., KAPLAN, N. O. and MEYERS, G. B. Metabolic studies in diabetic acidosis: I. The effect of the early administration of dextrose. *Arch. Int. Med.* 80:739, 1948; II. The effect of the administration of sodium phosphate. *ibid* 81:42, 1948.
   (c) KEPLER, E. J., INGHAM, D. W. and CRISLER, J. R. Protamine insulin as an adjunct to the treatment of diabetic acidosis and coma. *Proc. Staff Meet., Mayo Clin.* 12:171, 1937.
   (d) KETY, S. S., POLIS, B. D., NODLER, C. S. and SCHMIDT, C. F. The blood flow and oxygen

consumption of the human brain in diabetic acidosis and coma. *J. Clin. Invest.* 27:500, 1948.
(e) HOLLER, J. W. Potassium deficiency occurring during the treatment of diabetic acidosis. *J. A. M. A.* 131:1186, 1946.
(f) NODLER, C. S., BELLET, S. and LANNING, M. Influence of the serum potassium and other electrolytes on the electrocardiogram in diabetic acidosis. *Am. J. Med.* 5:838, 1948.
(g) BERLINER, R. W. and KENNEDY, T. J., JR. Renal tubular secretion of potassium in the normal dog. *Proc. Soc. Exper. Biol. & Med.* 67:542, 1948.
(h) MUDGE, G. H., FOULKS, J. and GILMAN, A. The renal excretion of potassium. *Proc. Soc. Exper. Biol. & Med.* 67:545, 1948.
(i) LEAF, A. and CAMARA, A. A. Renal tubular secretion of potassium in man. *J. Clin. Invest.* 28:1526, 1949.
(j) HOWARD, J. E. and CAREY, R. A. The use of potassium in therapy. *J. Clin. Endocrinol.* 9:691, 1949.
(k) GARDNER, L. I., TALBOT, N. B., COOK, C. D., BERMAN, H. and URIBE, R. C. The effect of potassium deficiency on carbohydrate metabolism. *J. Lab. & Clin. Med.* 35:592, 1950.

20 ROOT, H. F. Cardio-renal-vascular disease. In *The Treatment of Diabetes Mellitus*. By E. P. Joslin, H. F. Root, P. White, A. Marble and C. C. Bailey. Philadelphia, Lea & Febiger, 1946.

21 KIMMELSTIEL, P. and WILSON, C. Intercapillary lesions in the glomeruli of the kidney. *Am. J. Path.* 12:83, 1936.

22 FRANTZ, V. K. Adenomatosis of islet cells, with hyperinsulinism. *Ann. Surg.* 119:824, 1944.

23 HARTMANN, A. F. and JAUDON, J. C. Hypoglycemia. *J. Pediat.* 11:1, 1937.

24 (a) THORN, G. W., KOEPF, G. F., LEWIS, R. A. and OLSEN, E. F. Carbohydrate metabolism in Addison's disease. *J. Clin. Invest.* 19:813, 1940.
(b) LEWIS, R. A., KUHLMAN, D., DELBUE, C., KOEPF, G. F. and THORN, G. W. The effect of adrenal cortex on carbohydrate metabolism. *Endocrinology* 27:971, 1940.

25 DUFF, G. L. The pathology of islet cell tumors of the pancreas. *Am. J. M. Sc.* 203:437, 1942.

26 MARBLE, A. Hyperinsulinism. In *The Treatment of Diabetes Mellitus*. By E. P. Joslin, H. F. Root, P. White, A. Marble and C. C. Bailey. Philadelphia, Lea & Febiger, 1946.

27 (a) CONN, J. W. Advantage of a high protein diet in the treatment of spontaneous hypoglycemia. *J. Clin. Invest.* 15:673, 1936.
(b) THORN, G. W., QUINBY, J. T. and CLINTON, M., JR. A comparison of the metabolic effects of isocaloric meals of varying composition, with special reference to the prevention of postprandial hypoglycemic symptoms. *Ann. Int. Med.* 18:913, 1943.
(c) MC QUARRIE, I., BAUER, E. G., ZIEGLER, M. R. and WRIGHT, W. S. The metabolic and clinical effects of pituitary adrenocorticotrophic hormone in spontaneous hypoglycemosis. In *Proceedings of the First Clinical ACTH Conference*. Edited by J. R. Mote. Philadelphia, Blakiston, 1950.

28 TALBOT, N. B., CRAWFORD, J. D. and BAILEY, C. C. Use of mesoxalyl urea (alloxan) in treatment of an infant with convulsions due to idiopathic hypoglycemia. *Pediatrics* 1:337, 1948.

29 DARROW, D. C. Mental deterioration associated with convulsions and hypoglycemia. *Am. J. Dis. Child.* 51:575, 1936.

APPENDIX

APPENDIX

BLOOD, PLASMA OR SERUM VALUES

To provide ready reference to the normal values of laboratory procedures referred to in this book and to the methods used, the following tabular summary has been prepared. This summary is based in part on a table published by G. M. Rourke, E. A. MacLachlan and A. M. Butler in *New Eng. J. Med.* 234:24, 1946.

Determination	Material analyzed	Minimum required, cc.	Normal value	Method
Bilirubin (van den Bergh's test)	Serum	2	Direct, 0.4 mg. per 100 cc.; indirect (total) 0.7 mg. per 100 cc.	H. T. Malloy and K. A. Evelyn, *J. Biol. Chem.* 119:481, 1937
Calcium, total	Serum	2	8.5-10.2 mg. per 100 cc.	C. H. Fiske and M. A. Logan, *ibid.* 93:211, 1931
Calcium, ionized	Serum	2	See Figure II-1	See Figure II-1
Carbon dioxide (content)	Serum (obtained without tourniquet)	0.5	Newborn infants 20-26 mEq. per liter, older persons 26-28 mEq. per liter	D. D. Van Slyke and J. M. Neill, *J. Biol. Chem.* 61:523, 1924; J. P. Peters and D. D. Van Slyke, *Quant. Clin. Chem.* II (methods), p. 283, Baltimore, Williams & Wilkins, 1932
Carotenoids: Total	Serum	2	100-300 I. U. per 100 cc.	H. W. Josephs, *Bull. Johns Hopkins Hosp.* 65:112, 1939 (modified for photocolorimeter)
Vitamin A			40-100 I. U. per 100 cc.	
Chloride	Serum	0.5	100-106 mEq. per liter	D. W. Wilson and E. G. Ball, *J. Biol. Chem.* 79:221, 1928
Cholesterol	Serum	0.5	110-280 mg. per 100 cc.	W. R. Bloor, *ibid.* 24:227, 1916
Creatinine (apparent)	Serum	1	0.8-1.5 per 100 cc.	R. W. Bonsnes and H. H. Taussky, *ibid.* 158:581, 1945
Glucose, total	Blood	0.1	70-100 mg. per 100 cc. (fasting)	O. Folin, *Lab. Manual Biol. Chem.*, New York, Appleton, 1934; *New Eng. J. Med.* 206:727, 1932
Hemoglobin	Blood	0.02	Infants and children 10 to 13 gm. per cent; adults 12-16 gm. per cent	K. A. Evelyn, *J. Biol. Chem.* 115:63, 1936
Galactose	Blood	1	<5 mg. per cent	A. M. Basset, T. L. Althausen and G. C. Coltrin, *Am. J. Digest. Dis.* 8:432, 1941

BLOOD, PLASMA OR SERUM VALUES (continued)

Determination	Material analyzed	Minimum required, cc.	Normal value	Method
Iodine, protein-bound (thyroid hormone)	Serum	2	3.5-7 micrograms per cent	S. B. Barker, *J. Biol. Chem.* 173:715, 1948. Values courtesy of Dr. D. Riggs
Magnesium	Serum	2	1.5-2.5 mEq. per liter	R. J. Garner, *Biochem. J.* 40:828, 1946
Non-protein nitrogen	Serum	0.5	15-35 mg. per 100 cc.	O. Folin, *Lab. Manual Biol. Chem.*, p. 265
pH	Serum	0.4	7.35-7.45	A. B. Hastings and J. Sendroy, *J. Biol. Chem.* 61:695, 1924
Phosphatase, alkaline	Serum	0.7	Infants and children 5-12 units per 100 cc.; adults 2.0-4.5 units per 100 cc.	A. Bodansky, *ibid.* 101:93, 1933 (using the method for determining inorganic phosphorus)
Phosphorus, inorganic	Serum (patient fasting)	0.2	Infants 4-5.5 mg. per cent; children 3.5-4.5 mg. per 100 cc.; adults 3.0-4.0 mg. per 100 cc.	C. H. Fiske and Y. Subbarow, *ibid.* 66:375, 1925; O. Folin, *Lab. Manual Biol. Chem.*, p. 341 (modified for photocolorimeter)
Potassium (chemical)	Serum	3-4	4.0-5.5 mEq. per liter	C. H. Fiske and G. Litarczek in O. Folin, *Lab. Manual Biol. Chem.*, p. 353 (chemical)
(Flame photometer)	Serum	0.5	4.0-5.5 mEq. per liter	J. W. Berry, D. G. Chappell and R. B. Barnes: *Indust. & Engin. Chem.* 18:19, 1946 (flame photometry)
Protein, total	Serum	0.5 (macro) 0.05 (micro)	Infants 5.5 to 7.0 gm. per 100 cc.; older persons 6.5-8.0 gm. per 100 cc.	Macro: J. P. Peters and D. D. Van Slyke, *Quant. Clin. Chem.*, II, p. 691 Micro: O. H. Lowry and A. B. Hastings, *J. Biol. Chem.* 143:257, 1942
Prothrombin activity	Plasma	0.3	By control	A. J. Quick, *J.A.M.A.* 110: 1658, 1938; C. A. Tanturi and R. F. Banfi, *J. Lab. & Clin. Med.* 31:703, 1946
Sodium	Serum	0.5	136-145 mEq. per liter	A. M. Butler and E. Tuthill, *J. Biol. Chem.* 93:171, 1931 (chemical). Same as potassium (flame photometer) same as potassium
Urea nitrogen	Serum	1	<28 mg. per 100 cc.	D. D. Van Slyke, *ibid.* 73: 695, 1927; J. P. Peters and D. D. Van Slyke, *Quant. Clin. Chem.*, II, p. 372.

Appendix

URINE VALUES

Determination	Minimum quantity required	Normal value	Method
Ammonia	5 cc.	Variable (see p. 91)	D. D. Van Slyke and G. E. Cullen, *J. Biol. Chem.* 24:117, 1916
Calcium	2 cc.	Variable (see p. 72)	Quantitative: same as serum. Qualitative, Sulkowitch: see Method 1, below
Chloride	0.5 cc.	Varies with intake	Same as serum
Cystine	5 cc. of urine (or 20 mg. of stone)	None	See Method 2, below
Creatinine	0.5 cc.	15-25 mg. per kg. per 24 hr., ± constant per individual, lower in obese, higher in muscular people	O. Folin, *Lab. Manual Biol. Chem.*, p. 159 (modified for photocolorimeter)
Estrogen	1/10 of 24 hr. sample	Not yet available	L. L. Engel, W. R. Slaun-White, P. Carter and I. T. Nathanson, *J. Biol. Chem.* 185:255, 1950
Gonadotropin (FSH)	24-hr. sample (more in small children)	Tables V-1, VI-1	H. F. Klinefelter, F. Albright and G. C. Griswold, *J. Clin. Endocrinol.* 3:529, 1943
17-ketosteroids: (total)	Macro: 24-hr. sample; Micro: 2-hr. sample	See p. 154	A. S. Zygmuntowicz, M. Wood, E. Christo and N. B. Talbot, *J. Clin. Endocrinol.* 11:578, 1951
(3-β-OH fractions)	24-hr. sample	See p. 191	N. B. Talbot, A. M. Butler and E. A. MacLachlan, *J. Biol. Chem.* 132:595, 1940
11-17-oxycorticosteroids (reducing steroids)	24-hr. sample (more in infants)	See p. 154	N. B. Talbot, A. H. Saltzman, R. L. Wixom and J. K. Wolfe, *ibid.* 160:535, 1945
Osmolar concentration	20 cc.	Variable, see Chapter VIII	Bulletin on Hortvet cryoscope (28591/1), Eimer and Amend, 635 Greenwich St., New York 14, N. Y.
Phosphorus		Variable, see p. 65	Same as serum
Potassium		Proportional to intake	Same as serum
Pregnandiol		0 except during progestational phase of menstrual cycle; then from 1 to 6 mg. per day	I. F. Somerville, G. F. Marrian and R. J. Kellar, *Lancet* 2:89, 1948

URINE VALUES (continued)

Determination	Minimum quantity required	Normal value	Method
Sodium		Variable, see Chapter III	Same as serum
Sugar:			
Total (quantitative)	5 cc.	0	S. R. Benedict, *J.A.M.A.* 57:1193, 1911
Total (roughly quantitative)	0.5 cc.	0	M. Somogyi, *J. Lab. & Clin. Med.* 26:1220, 1941
Fermentable	1 cc.	0	P. B. Hawk and O. Bergheim, *Pract. Physiol. Chem.*, p. 750, Philadelphia, Blakiston, 1931
Fructose	1 cc.	0	*Ibid.*, p. 772
Galactose or lactose	6 cc.	0	(Total sugar x 1.24) minus fermentable sugar
Osazone, differentiation of	5 cc.	0	*Ibid.*, p. 50
Titratable acidity	10 cc.	Variable, see p. 95	J. P. Peters and D. D. Van Slyke, *Quant. Clin. Chem.*, II (methods), 0. 825
Urea clearance	Blood and urine (two 1-hr. samples)	75-125 per cent of normal	*Ibid.*, 0. 564

Method 1. *Qualitative determination of urinary calcium (Sulkowitch test).* The test reagent solution is made as follows: Dissolve 2.5 gm. of oxalic acid and 2.5 gm. of $(NH_4)_2 C_2O_4$ in 100 cc. of water. Add 5 cc. of glacial acetic acid and enough water to make a total volume of 150 cc. This is the reagent. In running the test, mix approximately equal volumes of the reagent solution and urine in a test tube. Test the pH of the resultant mixture with nitrazine paper or other standard procedure. The pH for optimal precipitation of calcium oxalate is 5.0. If necessary adjust the pH to this value by the addition of acetic acid or NaOH solution.

Method 2. *Qualitative determination of cystine in urine or renal calculus.* Take 5 cc. of urine (or 20 mg. of calculus) and add concentrated NH_4OH until strongly alkaline. Add 2 cc. of 5 per cent sodium cyanide and let stand 10 minutes. Add a few drops of a freshly prepared, saturated aqueous solution of sodium nitroprusside. In the presence of cystine a deep purple color develops. Acetone reacts to give a red color. The difference in color can be recognized by running an acetone control. We are indebted to Miss E. Dempsey of Dr. F. Albright's laboratory for these directions.

APPENDIX [591]

MISCELLANEOUS TESTS

Determination	Material analyzed	Quantity required	Normal value	Method
Bone age	Roentgenogram of hand and wrist			T. W. Todd, *Atlas of Skeletal Maturation*, St. Louis, Mosby, 1937
Eosinophil count	Blood	0.05 cc.	Fig. III-18	G. G. Randolph, *J. Lab. & Clin. Med.* 34:1696, 1949
Renal calculi				J. F. McIntosh and R. W. Salter, *J. Clin. Invest.* 21:751, 1942
Stool fat	Stool	Representative sample	See p. 86	H. C. Tidwell and L. E. Holt, *J. Biol. Chem.* 112: 605, 1936
Sperm count	Semen	.05 cc.	70-100 million per cc.	E. J. Farris, *J. Urol.* 58:85, 1947
Surface area	Height and weight		See p. 592 and end papers	J. D. Crawford M. E. Terry and G. M. Rourke, *Pediatrics* 5:783, 1950
Vaginal smear	Vaginal secretions	Few drops	See p. 313	E. Shorr, *J. Mt. Sinai Hosp.* 12:667, 1945

UNITS OF MEASUREMENT

In discussing bodily functions, measurements of their components must obviously be expressed in terms of physiologic-chemical equivalents. As Dr. James Gamble has demonstrated so effectively in his *Syllabus on the Chemical Anatomy, Physiology and Pathology of Extracellular Fluid* (Harvard University Press), it is only in this way that their relative magnitudes and inter-relationships can be correctly displayed.

In respect to body electrolytes the suitable term is *equivalent* or *milliequivalent*, which is one-thousandth of an equivalent. In these biochemical connections the term "equivalent" has electrical connotations. This may be illustrated by considering the substance, sodium chloride. Sodium carries a positive charge, chloride a negative charge; it is the mutual attraction of these two charges that holds the two elements together in the form of ordinary dry table salt. When this salt is dissolved in water, however, sodium chloride ceases to exist; it is replaced by exactly equal numbers of positively charged sodium ions (cations) and negatively charged chloride ions (anions), each existing separately in solution.

$$\text{Dry NaCl} \xrightarrow[\text{solution}]{H_2O} Na^+ \text{ and } Cl^-$$

It will be noted that sodium and chloride ions have but one positive or negative electrical charge respectively. This fact is expressed by stating that they are univalent, or that in each case there is a *valence* of one. Another biochemically important univalent substance is potassium. In contrast to these are such other substances as calcium and magnesium which are bivalent cations (two positive charges) and sulfate which is a bivalent anion (two negative charges) under physiologic conditions. As shown below with respect to phosphate, the valence of certain radicles may be variable.

In a stable salt the sum of positive charges must always equal the sum of negative charges. This is true when one bivalent cation is combined with two univalent anions to form a stable salt such as $CaCl_2$ as well as when one univalent cation is combined with one univalent anion as in KCl.

An *equivalent* is a *mole* of any univalent electrolyte, one-half mole of any bivalent electrolyte, one-third mole of any trivalent electrolyte, and so forth. The weight in grams of a mole of any substance is equal numerically to the sum of the atomic weights of its constituents. A milliequivalent is one-thousandth of an equivalent.

On the basis of the foregoing it may be seen that values expressed in terms of milligrams can be converted to milliequivalents by dividing milligrams by total atomic weight and multiplying by valency. To convert values for these substances expressed in terms of milligrams per cent to values expressed in terms of milliequivalents per liter, multiply by the conversion factor indicated in the right-hand column below.

Electrolyte	Atomic Weight	Valence	Conversion Factor
Na^+	23.0	1	.433
K^+	39.1	1	.256
Ca^{++}	40.1	2	.499
Mg^{++}	24.3	2	.823
Cl^-	35.5	1	.282*
P (as $HPO_4^=$)	31.0	1.8	.581
S (as $SO_4^=$)	32.1	2	.624

* It has become the unfortunate custom in some clinics to express serum chloride values as mg. per cent of sodium chloride. As shown above, there is no sodium chloride in serum; there are only sodium ions and chloride ions. Conversion of chloride values thus expressed to milliequivalents per liter is accomplished by application of the multiplication factor .172. Conversion of sodium values similarly expressed is accomplished by use of the same factor.

Note that the valency of $HPO_4^=$ is taken as 1.8. This is because, at the pH of normal extracellular fluid, 20 per cent of the millimoles of this radicle carries one equivalent of univalent base ($B \cdot H_2PO_4$) and 80 per cent carries two equivalents of univalent base ($B_2 \cdot HPO_4$). Base equivalence per unit of phosphate is therefore $(0.2 \times 1) + (0.8 \times 2) = 1.8$.

In the case of carbonic acid ($H \cdot HCO_3$) and of bicarbonate ($B \cdot HCO_3$), which have often been expressed in terms of volumes per cent, conversion to milliequivalents per liter is accomplished by dividing by the factor 2.24. This factor is determined as follows: one mole of a gas under standard conditions of pressure and temperature occupies 22.4 liters. Volumes per cent $\times 10 \div 22.4 =$ volumes per cent $\div 2.24$.

Other commonly used units of measurements are the *osmole* and the *milliosmole*. These units are based on the fact that each millimole of substance in solution exerts an approximately equal amount of osmotic pressure irrespective of its electrical equivalence value. Comparison of milligram, millimole, milliequivalent and milliosmole values for certain representative substances follow:

Substance	Mg.	mM	mEq. +	mEq. −	mosM
Glucose	180	1	0	0	1
Na$^+$—Cl$^-$	58	1	1	1	2
Ca^{++}$\genfrac{}{}{0pt}{}{\diagup \text{Cl}^-}{\diagdown \text{Cl}^-}$	110	1	2	2	3

Note that in the case of glucose, a non-electrolyte, the millimole and milliosmole values are identical but the milliequivalence value is zero. In the case of NaCl, 1 millimole in solution yields 1 cation and 1 anion milliequivalent (2 total) and 2 milliosmoles. By contrast, note that CaCl$_2$ in solution yields 2 cation and 2 anion milliequivalents (4 total), but only 3 milliosmoles.

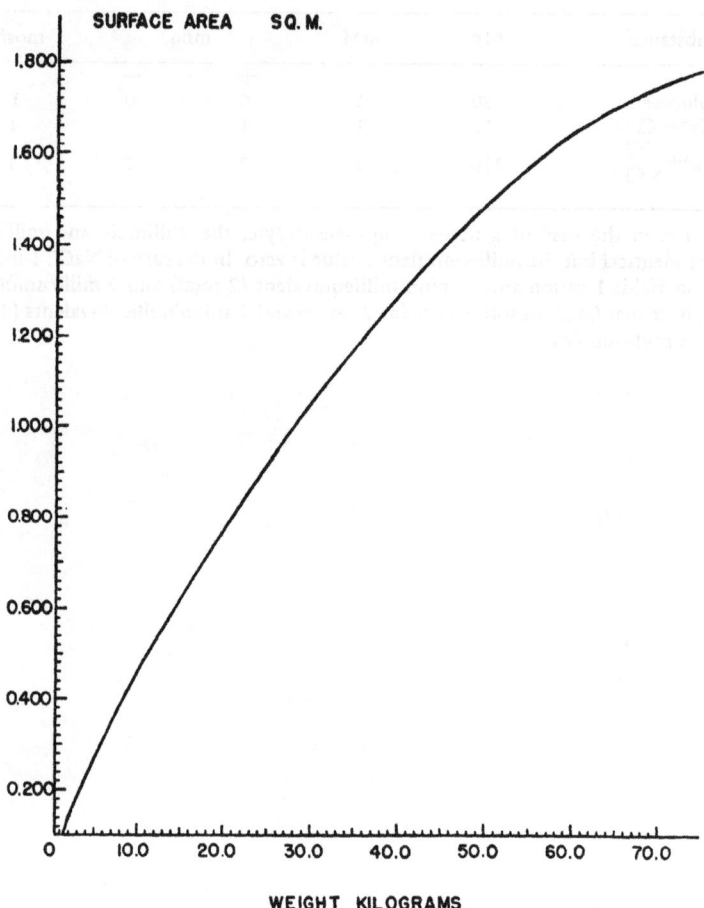

(Left)

FIGURE A-1. Graph estimating surface area from body weight alone. The solid curve running upward from left to right permits an approximate estimation of surface area (ordinate) from body weight (abscissa). The nomograms inside the front and back covers of this book give more accurate information, especially in regard to individuals who are abnormally thin or fat. From J. D. Crawford, M. E. Terry, G. M. Rourke, *Pediatrics* 5:783, 1950.

(Right—opposite page)

FIGURE A-2. Heights and weights of normal boys. The design and origin of these data are the same as for Figure 3.

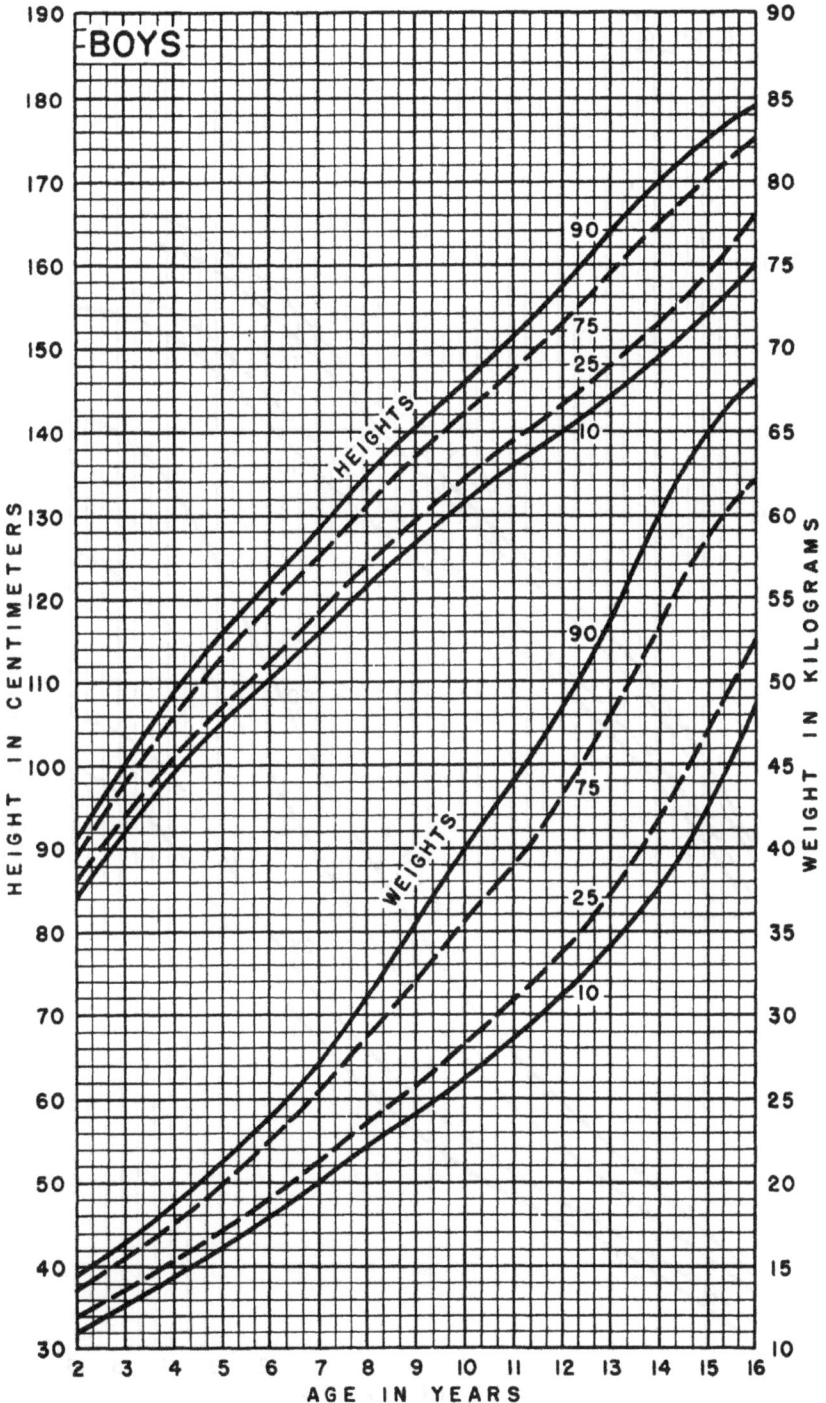

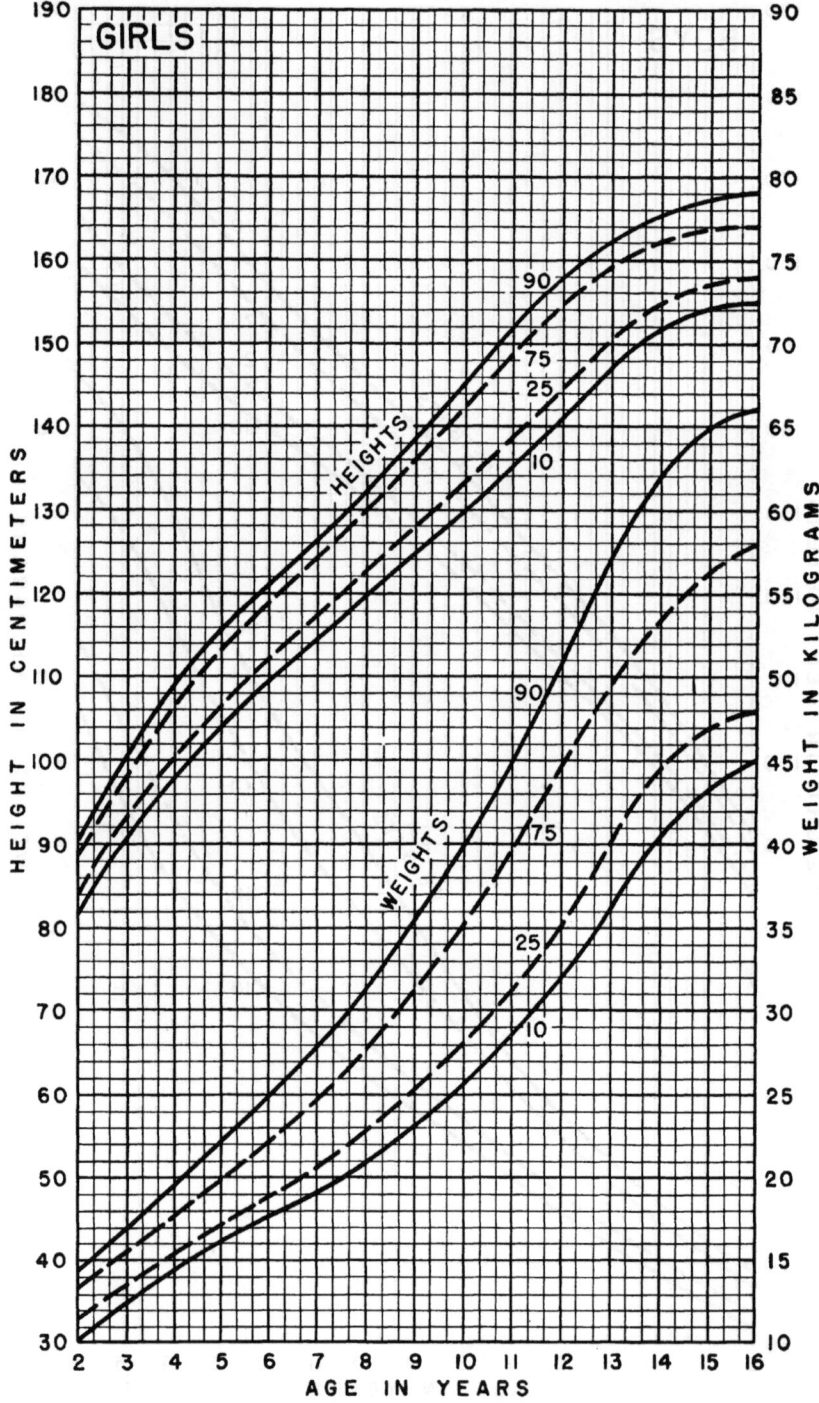

APPENDIX

FIGURE A-3. Heights and weights of normal girls. Normal height ranges are indicated by the uppermost set of curves coursing upward from left to right. The lower set of curves gives corresponding data with relation to weight. The four individual numbers of each set of curves indicate percentile distribution as found in a normal population. Thus with respect to the height curves, 80 per cent of normal girls range in height between the limits of the top and bottom curves—10 per cent being taller and 10 per cent being shorter. Fifty per cent range in height between the limits of the interrupted curves; 15 per cent between the top curve and the first interrupted curve; and 15 per cent between the second interrupted curve and the bottom curve. These curves correspond closely to the data of R. L. Jackson and H. G. Kelley, *J. Pediat.* 27:215,1945.

INDEX

INDEX

INDEX

Abdomen
  calcification in adrenocortical cancer 243
  pain. See Pain, abdominal
Acetylcholine 272, 299
Acholia 82
Acid, lactic 275
  from muscle glycogen 148
Acidosis
  chloride, due to saline therapy 569
  defenses against 91f
  in base-losing nephritis 95
  in diabetes. See under Diabetes mellitus
  in salicylate poisoning 557
  skeletal catabolism in 101
  vs alkalosis 557
Acne
  in adrenocortical virilism 227
  in Cushing's syndrome 237
  iodinization, cause of 39
  testosterone and 381
Acromegaly 481
  diabetes mellitus in 555
  parathyroids in 78
ACTH. See under Anterior pituitary
Addison's disease 195f
Adenoma
  adrenocortical 223
  of anterior pituitary 449f, 481f
  of parathyroids 122
Adenosine triphosphate 541
Adolescence
  definition of 302
  development
    of normal boys 392f
    of normal girls 301f
  goiter in 46f
  gonadotropin production in 3
  hyperthyroidism in 32
  thyroid hormone needs in 47
Adrenal cortices 134f
  activity
    control of 158f
    control of, by ACTH 135, 158
    effect of epinephrine on 160
    effect of hypoglycemia on 550
    Na-K hormone in adrenocortical virilism 228
    physiologic vs pathologic 193f
    S-F-N hormone in adrenocortical virilism 228
  adenoma, in hyperadrenocorticism 223
  adrenalectomy, therapeutic
    in adrenocortical virilism 233
    in Cushing's syndrome 244f
  adrenarche
    in female 308
    precocious, relation to gonadarche 247

Adrenal cortices (cont.)
  adrenosterone, chemistry of 136f
  alarm reaction. See Alarm reaction of Selye
  androgens 156f
    effect on growth and development 226f
  atrophy
    in adrenocortical cancer 219
    unilateral, meaning of 245
  basic considerations 135f
  cancer
    abdominal calcification in 243
    effect on ACTH production 218f
    11-17-OCS output in 185
    in adrenocortical atrophy 219
    in adrenocortical virilism 224
    in hyperadrenocorticism 223
    incidence in Cushing's syndrome 235
    metastases 228
    surgical removal, medical management during 219f
    test for, with cortisone 229
  cell rests
    in congenital adrenocortical virilism 247
    in ovary 227
  clinical considerations 193f
  corticosterone 216
    chemistry of 136
  cortisone
    cause of psychopathic changes 254
    chemistry of 136
  cortisone, effect on
    antidiuretic hormone 152
    diabetes insipidus 527
    electroencephalogram 152
    emotions 254
    erythrocytes 151
    fever 254
    fibroblastic proliferation 150
    immunologic phenomena 152
    macrophages 151
    pain 254
    phagocytes 151
    reticulocytes 151
    serum cholesterol 150
    serum phospholipids 150
    signs of disease 254
    urine 17-KS 229
    water metabolism 152
    wound-healing 150
  cortisone therapy
    dose 210, 255
    general comments 247f, 259f
    in adrenocortical virilism 234
    in hypoadrenocorticism 215

Adrenal cortices, cortisone therapy (cont.)
    in hypoglycemia 582
    in non-endocrine conditions 255f
    theoretical comments 259f
    undesirable effects of 253f
  destruction by DDD 245
  disease, mixed, in infants 245f
  11-desoxycorticosterone
    chemistry of 135
    dosage 205
    effect on breast 440
    effect on sweat chloride–rate index 189
    preparations 205f
    resistance to, in mixed adrenocortical disease 246
    toxicity due to 206f
    use in hypoadrenocorticism 214f
  11-desoxycorticosterone acetate (DOCA) 135f, 206f
  11-17-oxycorticosteroids (OCS). See Adrenal cortices, S-F-N hormones
  estrogens 297
    production in childhood 306
  extract
    aqueous 204f
    lipo 205
  extract, effect on diabetes insipidus 527
  gland zones 135
    zona reticularis in adrenocortical disease 157f, 223
  hemorrhage into 216
  homeostasis
    Na-K hormone 190
    relation to needs 156
    relation to stress 156
    S-F-N hormone 185
  hormones
    actions 137f
    antagonisms 151f
      to antidiuretic hormone 517
    chemistry of 135f
    effect of ACTH production 160
  hormones, need of
    at rest 156
    in hypopituitarism 218
    in hypothyroidism 218
    under stress 156
  hormones, preparations
    aqueous extract 204f
    corticosterone 216
    cortisone 210
    11-desoxycorticosterone acetate (DOCA) 206f
    lipo extract 205
  hormones, types of 135f
    anti-Na-K 246
    11-17-OCS 136
    Na-K 136
    S-F-N 136

Adrenal cortices (cont.)
  hyperadrenocorticism. See Adrenal cortices, hyperadrenocorticism (below)
  hyperplasia 223
    in adrenocortical virilism 224
  hypoadrenocorticism. See Adrenal cortices, hypoadrenocorticism (below)
  Na-K hormone 136, 137f
    activity, index of 138
    deficiency, effects of 142f
    excess, effects of 139f
    production determinants 147
    production of, by man 190
  Na-K hormone, effects of
    on kidney 137f
    on salivary gland 139
    on sweat gland 138
  reciprocal relations with posterior pituitary 534
  response to ACTH
    age variations in 172f
    time required for 173
  role in water metabolism 516f
  17-ketosteroid precursors (17-KS-Gens) 156f
    effects of abnormal 157f
    effects of normal 157f
  S-F-N hormones 136, 148f
    insulin relations 542
    production rate in normal 154f
    production rate under stress 156
  S-F-N hormones, effects on
    brain metabolism 152
    electrolyte metabolism 151
    fat metabolism 149f
    glycogenesis 275
    histamine metabolism 153
    immunologic phenomena 152
    muscle fatigue 151
    nitrogen metabolism 150
    renal function 152
    sugar metabolism 148f
    water metabolism 152
  sodium-potassium homeostasis 146f
  status, indices of 163f
    ACTH–11-17-OCS test 170f
    ACTH-eosinophil test 170f
    ACTH–17-KS test 170f
    ACTH–urinary uric acid test 170f
    electrolyte measurements 185f
    eosinophil count 173f
    epinephrine-eosinophil test 168f
    glucose tolerance test 175f
    insulin tolerance test 175f
    sodium deprivation test 186f
    sweat test 189f
    24-hour fast 174f
    urinary 11-17-OCS 180f
    urinary 17-KS 190f
    water diuresis test 163

INDEX

Adrenal cortices (cont.)
  sugar homeostasis in infancy 154
  tumor, local signs of 228
  virilism 224f
    clinical manifestations 225f
    diagnosis 228
    11-17-OCS output in 185
    prognosis 234f
    pseudo-hermaphroditism and 365
    treatment 229f
    urine 17-KS in 157
  zona reticularis
    in adrenocortical virilism 157f
    in hyperadrenocorticism 223
Adrenal cortices, hyperadrenocorticism 223f
  adrenocortical feminization in 247
  adrenocortical virilism and pseudo-
    hermaphroditism 365
  amenorrhea and 354
  congenital 245f
  gynecomastia and 440
  mixed types 229, 244
  pathologic 223f
    adrenocortical virilism 224f, 245, 343
    Cushing's syndrome. See Cushing's syndrome
    diabetes mellitus and 224
    due to DOCA intoxication 206f
    manifestations 224
    primary due to cancer or hyper-
      plasia 223, 235
    secondary due to hyperpituitarism 223
  physiologic
    in diabetic acidosis 546
    in stress 156, 158f, 571
    vs pathologic 185
  polyuria and 526, 534
  relative to needs 193
  sexual infantilism in girls and 343
  sexual precocity in girls and 334f
  therapy 247f
  types of 223f
Adrenal cortices, hypoadrenocorticism 194f
  absolute vs relative 193
  acute, due to infection 216f
  adrenocortical surgery and 229f
  amenorrhea and 354
  crisis
    due to sodium salt deprivation 186, 197
    prevention of 215
  11-17-OCS output in 181
  epinephrine-eosinophil test in 169
  hypoglycemic threshold in 178
  pathologic
    ACTH-eosinophil test in 168
    and adrenocortical cancer removal 219

Adrenal cortices, hypoadrenocorticism, pathologic (cont.)
    and hypopituitarism 218f
    clinical manifestations 195f
    diagnosis 203f
    prevention of 218f
    primary vs secondary 194f
    prognosis 215f
  physiologic vs pathologic 190
  reactions to
    ACTH 168
    glucose infusion 177, 180
    insulin 177f
    stress 168
  renal, Na and Cl clearances in 188
  secondary to
    ACTH withdrawal 252
    cortisone withdrawal 252f
  surgical stress, effect of 215
  sweat chloride–rate index in 189
  treatment 204f
    with parenteral fluids 210f
  water metabolism in 516
  water test in 163
Adrenal medullæ 270f
  activity 272
    effect of hypoglycemia on 546f
  anti-epinephrine substances 275
  basic considerations 271f
  clinical considerations 275f
  control of
    by histamine 272
    by potassium 272
    by sympathetic system 272
  epinephrine 271f
    dose 287
    in normal adrenal medullæ 276
    preparations 287
    therapy 287f
  epinephrine, effect on
    ACTH production 155, 167
    antidiuretic hormone production 511
    hepatic glycogenolysis 149, 179
    tumors 276
  epinephrine-glucose tolerance test 552
  hormones
    actions 272f
    epinephrine 271f
    nor-epinephrine 271f
  hormones, effect on
    ACTH 275
    cardiovascular system 275
    metabolism 273f
    TSH 275
  hyperepinephrinism, pathologic 276f
    clinical manifestations 276f
    diagnosis 281
    diagnostic procedures 284f
    differential diagnosis 36, 281f

Adrenal medullæ, hyperepinephrinism, pathologic (cont.)
      due to pheochromocytoma and related tumors 276
      prognosis 286f
      treatment 286
  hypoepinephrinism 275
  nor-epinephrine 271f
      in pheochromocytoma 276
      preparation 286
      origin 271
Adrenalectomy, therapeutic. See under Adrenal cortices
Adrenarche, precocious 247
Adrenocorticotropic hormone. See Anterior pituitary, ACTH
Adrenosterone, chemistry of 136f
Age
  height age, defined 441
  physiologic vs chronologic 191
Age at onset of hypothyroidism, relation to intelligence quotient 20
  prognosis 29
Age, relation to
  adrenocortical responsiveness to ACTH 172f
  adrenocortical virilism 225
  appearance, in sexually precocious boys 413f
  blood sugar 578
  breast development in girls 305
  cortisone tolerance 255
  11-17-OCS output 181
  FSH production 385f
  gonadotropin production in male castrate 431f
  incidence of hyperthyroidism 32
  kidney function 530
  manifestations of hypothyroidism 15
  nodules in chronic goiter 20
  normal serum phosphatase 8f
  normal serum protein-bound iodine 14
  normal skeletal maturation 12
  ovarian development 303f
  parathyroid histology 53
  posterior pituitary maturation 530
  sexual development
    of boys 385f, 392f
    of girls 301f, 308f
  spermatogenesis 386
  testicular development 386, 391f
  urine estrogens 306f
  urine gonadotropins, in ovarian insufficiency 320
  urine pregnandiol 308
  urine 17-KS output 191
  water metabolism 530
Alarm reaction of Selye 156
  effect of stress on
    adrenocortical activity 147, 158,

Alarm reaction of Selye, effect of stress on, adrenocortical activity (cont.)
    167, 173, 184, 193, 259, 571
  adrenocortical hormone needs 156, 193, 247
Alkalosis
  due to parenteral fluid therapy 576f
  due to salicylate poisoning 557
  in central hyperpnea 557
  in Cushing's syndrome 243
  in hyperadrenocorticism 141
  vs acidosis 557
Allergic conditions, treatment with adrenocortical hormones 257f
Alloxan therapy for hypoglycemia 582
Aluminum hydroxide
  added to milk 120
  dose 91
  inhibits phosphorus assimilation 91
Amenorrhea. See under Menstruation
Ammonium
  chloride, tolerance test 95f
  production
    by renal tubules 91
    mechanism impaired in base-losing nephritis 93
Anaphylaxis, effect of adrenocortical hormones on 153
Androgens. See under Adrenal cortices; Testes
Anemia
  erythroblastic 128
  in hypothyroidism 20
  in pathologic hyperparathyroidism 126
Anorexia. See under Appetite
Anorexia nervosa 5, 473f
  and central nervous system disease 475
  treatment with adrenocortical hormones 258
Anterior pituitary 448f
  ACTH characteristics 158
  ACTH control, homeostatic 160f
  ACTH deficiency in hypoadrenocorticism 218f
  ACTH dose 254f
  ACTH effect on
    adrenal cortices of infant 155
    adrenocortical activity 135, 158, 250f
    blood ketones 149f
    blood sugar 153
    emotions 254
    fever 254
    glucose excretion 153
    glutathione 153
    insulin action 153
    kidney function 153
    pain 254
    phosphorus excretion 153
    signs of disease 254
    skin tests 152

Index

Anterior pituitary, ACTH effect on (cont.)
    sodium metabolism 246
    sweat chloride–rate index 190
    urine histamine 153
    urine histidine 153
    wound-healing 150
  ACTH-eosinophil test 168, 170f
  ACTH in adrenocortical surgery 223
  ACTH in detection of diabetes mellitus 253
  ACTH production
    effect of estrogens on 299, 345
    effect of thyroid on 2f
    hyperadrenocorticism caused by rise in 223
    inhibited by adrenocortical hormones 160
    suppressed by ACTH therapy 250f
  ACTH standardization 254
  ACTH therapy 247f, 259f
    in hyperthyroidism 36
    in hypoadrenocorticism 216
    in hypoglycemia 582
    in non-endocrine conditions 255f
    undesirable effects of 253f
  ACTH, types of 158
  activity, indices of 455f
  adenoma
    basophilic 235, 449, 481
    eosinophilic 449, 481f
  adrenocortical mechanism, maturation of 155
  basic considerations 449f
  basophiles
    adenoma of, in Cushing's syndrome 235, 481
    hyaline changes in Cushing's syndrome 235
  blood supply 497
  cells, types of 449
  craniopharyngioma, and sexual infantilism in girls 340
  disturbances
    outline of 460
    physiologic vs pathologic 460
  extract, effect on parathyroids 78
  FSH, effect on
    ovary 295
    testes 385f
  FSH therapy 428
  gigantism. *See* Gigantism
  glycotropic hormone
    and diabetes mellitus 543
    insulin relations 542
  gonadotropins
    in body fluids 295
    in fetal pituitary 302f
  gonadotropins, effect on ovaries 294f
  gonadotropins, production
    age relation 307

Anterior pituitary, gonadotropins, production (cont.)
    cyclic 295
    in boys 345
    in girls 345f
    in sexual precocity in boys 408
    indices of, urine gonadotropin 319f
    neurologic control of 295f, 303, 348, 385
    sporadic, in adolescence 308
  gonadotropins, types of 295
    FSH 295
    ICSH 295
    lactogenic 295
    LH 295
    luteotropin 295
  growth hormone (PGH) 451f
    actions 451f
    clinical considerations 460f
    effect on body composition 452
    excess, effects of 482
    hormone interrelations 454
    insulin relations 542
    nature of 451
    production, effect on
      of caloric balance 455
      of estrogen 454
      of thyroid 2f, 454f
  homeostasis 162, 451, 481, 486
  hormones
    actions of 450
    effect on water metabolism 516
    relation to antidiuretic hormone 516
    therapy 468
    types of 450f
  hyperpituitarism. *See* Anterior pituitary, hyperpituitarism (*below*)
  hypophysectomy, effects of
    on growth 452
    on parathyroids 78
  hypopituitarism. *See* Anterior pituitary, hypopituitarism (*below*)
  ICSH 295, 451
    effect on testes 385, 391f
    relation to chorionic gonadotropin 385
    therapy 428
  lactogenic hormone production, effect of estrogen on 295, 299
  LH
    effect of progesterone on production of 301
    effect on ovary 295
    index of, endometrial biopsy 317
  luteotropin, effect on ovary 295
  origin of 449
  PGH. *See* growth hormone (*above*)
  position in body economy 450
  radiation of, in Cushing's syndrome 245

Anterior pituitary (cont.)
   reciprocal relations with
      ovary 295
      thyroid 3
   relation to hypothalamus 450
   sex differences 345f
   tall stature and 492
   target-gland relations 450, 481
   TSH
      control of thyroid activity by iodine block 37
      production
         effect of thyroid on 3
         influence of thyroid hormone on 5
Anterior pituitary, hyperpituitarism 481f
   fractional 413, 481
   pathologic 481f
   pathologic, primary organic 481f
      clinical manifestations 482
      diagnosis 483f
      treatment 484f
   pathologic, secondary functional 484
   physiologic 486f
   physiologic, functional, with tall stature 492f
   physiologic, secondary to caloric hypernutrition 486f
      clinical manifestations 488f
      differential diagnosis 489
      etiology 486f
      laboratory studies 489
      prognosis 492
      treatment 490f
Anterior pituitary, hypopituitarism 461f
   acute, due to sepsis 216
   adrenocortical responsiveness in 173
   amenorrhea and 350f
   cause of hypoadrenocorticism 218f
   effect of thyroid in 469
   effect on diabetes insipidus 527
   11-17-OCS output in 181
   epinephrine-eosinophil test in 169
   fractional 480f
      and sexual infantilism in boys 429f
      etiology 429
      treatment 429f
   fractional, hypogonadotropic in girls 342
   Froehlich's syndrome and 462
   functional
      due to athyrosis 430
      due to caloric undernutrition 430
      sexual infantilism and 342, 430
   generalized
      clinical manifestations 423f
      diagnosis 428
      prognosis 428f
      treatment 428f
   generalized, and sexual infantilism in boys 423f

Anterior pituitary, hypopituitarism, generalized, and sexual infantilism (cont.)
      in girls 342
   growth promotion in 472
   hypoadrenocorticism in 469
   inability to react to stress 167
   need for adrenocortical hormones 469
   organic, primary pathologic 461f
      clinical manifestations 461f
   pathologic, primary idiopathic 462f
      differential diagnosis 468
      laboratory studies 465f
      physical examination 464f
      prognosis 472
      treatment 468f
   pathologic, secondary functional 472
   physiologic 472f
   physiologic, secondary to primary athyrosis 473
   physiologic, secondary to starvation 473f
      clinical manifestations 473
      diagnosis 474f
      laboratory tests 473f
      prognosis 476f
      treatment 476
   sensitivity to insulin in 177f
   sexual infantilism in girls and 341f
   spontaneous remission 428
   testes development in 391
   tests for 466f
   vs hypothyroidism 469
   with hypothyroidism 30f
"Anterior-pituitary-like" hormone 385
Antibodies, effect of adrenocortical hormone on 152
Antidiuretic hormone 498f
Antidiuretic hormone serum, increased in edema 534f
Anxiety
   in hyperthyroidism 35
   in hypothyroidism 35
Appetite
   anorexia
      in base-losing nephritis 93
      in diabetes insipidus 521
      in hypoadrenocorticism 197
   diminished, in diabetes insipidus 510
   effect on
      of adrenocortical hormones 258
      of thyroid 2
   in hypothyroidism 21
   increased in
      craniopharyngioma 459
      diabetes mellitus 555
      hyperepinephrinism 280
      insulin lack 543
   large, causes of 486f
Apprehension, feeling of, in hyperepinephrinism 280
Arteriosclerosis 287, 577

INDEX

Arthritis, rheumatoid
    treatment with adrenocortical hormone 256
    water test in 163
Asthma
    effect of epinephrine on 288
    treatment with adrenocortical hormones 257
A.T.-10. See Dihydrotachysterol
Athetoid motions and hypocalcemia 104
Athyrosis. See Thyroid, hypothyroidism

Backache in Cushing's syndrome 272
Bartholin's gland 304
Basal energy metabolism
    in hyperepinephrinism 280
    in normal persons 6
    in obesity 6, 487
    in thyroid disease 7
    influence on
        of caloric balance 5
        of thyroid 2, 6f
        of "X" factors 6
    response to iodinization 39
Base, fixed
    body stores of 92
    conservation by kidney 91
    therapy with 97f
Base, urine excretion, parathyroid hormone and 123
Behavior
    effect of testosterone on 384
    emotional, in sexual precocity 412f
    manic
        in diabetes insipidus 521
        in psychogenic polydipsia 529
Benedict's test 563
Benzodioxane
    actions 285f
    adrenolytic 275
    test 285f
Bile estrogens 298
Blood
    amino acid, effect of pituitary growth hormone on 452
    anemia. See Anemia
    bleeding, control with epinephrine 288
    circulation
        collapse, and acute hypoadrenocorticism 216
        disturbances of, in mixed adrenocortical disease 246
    concentration, effect on antidiuretic hormone production 511
    dyscrasias and menorrhagia 358f
    11-17-OCS increased during stress 162
    eosinopenia
        due to adrenocortical hormones 150
        in Cushing's syndrome 243

Blood, eosinopenia (cont.)
        in diabetic acidosis 556
        of non-endocrine origin 173
    eosinophils, count
        as index of 11-17-OCS activity 167, 168
        in abnormal 173
        in acute hypoadrenocorticism 218
        in normal 168
    erythrocytes
        chloride of, in diabetic acidosis 546
        hemolysis, osmotic 569
        organic phosphorus of, in diabetic acidosis 546
        polycythemia in Cushing's syndrome 243
        sedimentation rate, effect of adrenocortical hormones on 256
    glucose. See Serum glucose
    ketones, effect of adrenocortical hormones on 149f
    leukocytes
        increased in diabetic acidosis 556
        leukopenia in pathologic hyperparathyroidism 126
    pressure. See Blood pressure (below)
    purpura in pathologic hyperparathyroidism 125
    sugar. See Serum glucose
    transfusion
        indication for, in diabetic acidosis 575f
        size of 576
    vessels. See Blood vessels (below)
    volume, decrease in hypoadrenocorticism 143
    See also Serum
Blood pressure
    decreased in hypoadrenocorticism 143
    effect on
        of epinephrine 273
        of posterior pituitary extract 535f
        of posterior pituitary hormones 498
    hypertension
        in Cushing's syndrome 237
        in diabetes mellitus 577
        in hyperadrenocorticism 139, 224
        in hyperepinephrinism 280
        in obesity 489, 492
        in ovarian agenesis 344
    hypotension
        in acute hypoadrenocorticism 216
        in diabetic acidosis 555
        in hypothyroidism 21
Blood vessels
    anomalies, in ovarian agenesis 344
    arteriosclerosis
        in diabetes mellitus 577
        in hyperepinephrinism 287
    constriction by epinephrine 288

Blood vessels (cont.)
    effect on
        of epinephrine 273
        of estrogen 300
        of nor-epinephrine 273
        of testosterone 383
Body
    composition, effect of pituitary growth hormone on 452
    electrolytes 544
    fat. *See* Fat
    growth. *See* Growth
    height. *See* Height
    proportions. *See* Body proportions (*below*)
    stature. *See* Height
    surface area. *See* Surface area
    temperature. *See* Fever; Temperature of body
    water 544
        homeostasis 518
        relation to solutes 503
    weight. *See* Weight
Body proportions
    eunuchoid
        in female castrate 345
        in fractional hypopituitarism 342
        in male castrate 431
    in hypothyroidism 20
    relation to menarche 337
    See also Growth; Height; Weight
Bone age. *See* Skeleton, maturation rate
Brain. *See under* Central nervous system
Breast
    atrophy in menopause præcox 351
    budding, normal age of 337
    development
        in adrenocortical virilism 226
        in girls, during adolescence 305
        precocious, as isolated change 335
        transient 335
    effect of estrogen therapy on 341
    fat in obesity 488
    gynecomastia
        adolescent 440
        adolescent, in boys 392
        causes of 440
        in newborn 302
        with testis tubular disease 437f
    in hypothalamic infantilism 340
    lobules, effect of progesterone on 301

Cachexia in primary organic hypopituitarism 462
Calcium
    assimilation, by intestines 77
    bound 54
    calcification
        metastatic 79
        of renal tubules 72

Calcium (cont.)
    chloride
        dose 110, 111
        in treatment of hypoparathyroidism 110f
    content, in milk 117
    deficiency 82f
        causes 82
        clinical manifestations 84f
        diagnosis 86
        differential diagnosis 87
        effect on skeleton 84
        prognosis 88
        treatment 87f, 97
    excretion, by kidneys 72
    gluconate
        added to milk 120
        calcium content 102
        dose 102
        effects 107
    hypocalcemia
        activates parathyroids 74
        and pannephritis 100
        and renal failure 119
        and tetany 77f
    in glomerular filtrate 54f
    intake, effect on
        parathyroids 79f
        phosphorus assimilation 79
    ionized, determination 54
    lactate, dose 87
    metabolism
        effect of estrogen on 300
        parathyroids and 72f
    output in pathologic hyperparathyroidism 126
    oxalate stones 123
    phosphate stones 123
    phosphorus-calcium ratio in milk 117
    requirements 87
    salt, therapy 87f
    serum. *See* Serum calcium
Caloric balance. *See* Diet; Milk; Nutrition; Vitamins
Cancer
    adrenal cortices. *See under* Adrenal cortices
    cervix of the uterus and menorrhagia 359
    interstitial cell 418f
    parathyroids 122
    renal, hypercalcemia in 128
    thyroid 20, 39, 48
Carbohydrate
    metabolism, effect on
        of adrenocortical hormone 148f, 150
        of testosterone 374
    See also Glucose
Carbon dioxide serum. *See* Serum carbon dioxide

INDEX [609]

Carotene serum. *See* Serum carotene
Carpopedal spasm
  in hypocalcemia 103
  in meningitis 119
Cartilage, calcification failure in osteomalacia and rickets 84
Castration
  ovaries 345
  testes 431
Celiac syndrome 82
Cells
  metabolism and thyroid 2
  organization and thyroid 2
Central nervous system
  brain damage due to hypocalcemia 121
  brain edema due to
    hypocalcemia 114
    hypoglycemia 550
  brain, effect on
    of adrenocortical hormone 152
    of insulin reactions 559
  damage to, by hypoglycemia 558
  defects, and hypoglycemia 580
  disease, and
    anorexia 475
    hypopituitarism 472
  effect on
    insulin production 542
    of hypoglycemia 550
  hydrocephalus due to craniopharyngioma 458
  hypothalamus
    amenorrhea and 349, 350
    in polyostotic fibrous dysplasia 327
    maturation of sex center 325
    morbid hunger and 487
  hypothalamus, effect on
    anterior pituitary 3, 450
    of various stimuli 511f
    posterior pituitary 511, 514
  hypothalamus, lesions of
    diagnosis 325
    sexual precocity in boys and 408, 409
    sexual precocity in girls and 323f
  hypothalamus, relation to
    gonadotropin production 385
    hyperadrenocorticism 223
    posterior pituitary structure 497
    sexual development 385
    sexual infantilism in boys 422f
    sexual infantilism in girls 337, 338, 340f
    sexual precocity 323f
  irritability. *See under* Emotional disturbances
  lesions, manifestations of, in diabetes insipidus 520f, 525f
  relation to gonadotropin secretion 302f
  tumors, cause of diabetes insipidus 520

Chloride
  extracellular, deficiency in hyperadrenocorticism 141, 142
  metabolism, effect on
    of progesterone 301
    of testosterone 375
  serum. *See* Serum chloride
Cholesterol, serum. *See* Serum cholesterol
Chondrodystrophy 11
Chvostek test 104
Climate, relation to menarche 337
Clitoris, hypertrophy
  congenital 228
  in adrenocortical virilism 226
  in hermaphroditism 365
Colitis, ulcerative
  treatment with adrenocortical hormone 259
  water test in 163
Colloid goiter 47
Coma
  diabetic. *See under* Diabetes mellitus
  in hypercalcemia 122
  in hypoadrenocorticism 196
  in hypoglycemia 580
  in thyroid storm 35
Conception, effect on ovary 293
Congenital goiter 46
Congenital malformations in cystinosis 99
Constipation
  in diabetes insipidus 535
  in diabetes mellitus 555
  in hypercalcemia 122
  in hypoadrenocorticism 197
  in hypothyroidism 21
  in undernutrition 373
Convulsions
  due to
    craniopharyngioma 458
    hypoadrenocorticism 196, 216
    hypoglycemia 550, 580
    posterior pituitary extract 535
    water intoxication 505
  epileptiform 103, 196, 535, 580
Corpus albicans 293
Corpus luteum. *See under* Ovaries
Corticosterone. *See under* Adrenal cortices; Adrenal cortices, hormones, preparations
Cortisone. *See under* Adrenal cortices; Adrenal cortices, hormones, preparations
Cortisone test for adrenocortical cancer 229
Coxa vara 10
Cramps, uterine. *See* Menstruation, dysmenorrhea
Craniopharyngioma
  cause of diabetes insipidus 520
  origin of 449
  symptoms and signs 456f
Cretinism. *See* Thyroid, hypothyroidism
Cryptorchidism 442f

Cushing's syndrome 235f
    anterior pituitary in 481
    cancer incidence in 235
    clinical manifestations 235f
    diagnosis 244
    differential diagnosis 244
    11-17-OCS output in 185
    emaciation in 235
    forms of 224
    prognosis 244f
    therapy 244f
    tongue in 25
Cyanosis and acute hypoadrenocorticism 216
Cystine stones 123
Cystinosis 99
    and stunted growth 476

Deafness
    in osteogenesis imperfecta 128
    in ovarian agenesis 344
Debility, effect of testosterone on 441f
Dehydration. See under Water
Delirium in thyroid storm 35
Depression, mental
    in Cushing's syndrome 237
    in hypercalcemia 122
Dermatomyositis, treatment with
    adrenocortical hormones 256
    testosterone 257
Diabetes insipidus 520f
    anorexia in 510
    clinical manifestations 521
    diagnosis and differential diagnosis 526f
    etiology 520f
    in craniopharyngioma 459
    in Froehlich's syndrome 340
    laboratory studies 521f
    latent form 527
    maximum and minimum urine volumes
        in 505
    nephrogenic 531f
    prognosis 529
    treatment 527f
Diabetes mellitus 553f
    acidosis 555f
        endocrine homeostasis in 546
        hyperadrenocorticism and, effect on
            glucose excretion 154
        losses due to 544f
        metabolic 546
        polyuria in 534
        treatment 566f
        treatment with parenteral fluids
            569f
    amenorrhea and 354
    clinical manifestations 555f
    coma
        due to acidosis 555
        treatment 566f
        vs insulin reaction 564

Diabetes mellitus (cont.)
    degenerative changes in 577
    detection with ACTH 253
    diagnosis and differential diagnosis 556f
    etiology 554f
    in Cushing's syndrome 237
    in glycotropic hormone treatment 543
    in hyperadrenocorticism 224
    in hypopituitarism 343
    in sexual infantilism 343
    incidence 554f
    laboratory studies 556
    obesity and 492
    prognosis 577
    surgery and 576f
    treatment 558f
    vs hyperepinephrinism 284
Diarrhea
    due to thyroid dose 25
    effect of adrenocortical hormones on 259
    in acute hypoadrenocorticism 216
Dibenamine vs epinephrine 275
Diet
    effect on glucose tolerance 550f
    for diabetes mellitus 560f
    for nephrogenic diabetes insipidus 532
    high caloric regimen 478
    high mineral content 528
    high protein content 528
    history of obese children 486f
    low caloric regimen 490f
    low mineral content 510
    low sodium content 186
        in hyperadrenocorticism 245
    protein in, effect on serum glucose 581
    therapy for diabetes insipidus 528
    See also Milk; Nutrition; Vitamins
Diethylstilbestrol. See Stilbestrol
Dihydrotachysterol
    dose equivalents 110
    effects 77f
    resistance to 110
Dinitrophenol, effects on metabolic rate 2
Dizziness
    due to hypercalcemia 122
    in hypoadrenocorticism 196
DOCA (11-desoxycorticosterone acetate)
    135f, 206f
Drowsiness due to salicylate poisoning 557
Dwarfism. See under Growth, stunted
Dysmenorrhea. See under Menstruation
Dysplasia, polyostotic fibrous 127f
    and sexual precocity 325, 327f

Ears. See Deafness
Eczema, treatment with adrenocortical hormones 258f
Edema
    antidiuretic hormone production in 534f

INDEX [611]

Edema (cont.)
  cerebral, due to
    hypocalcemia 114
    hypoglycemia 550
  due to antidiuretic hormone excess 511
  endometrial, during menstrual cycle 311
  in hyperadrenocorticism 139
  in hypoadrenocorticism 145, 211
  in pannephritis 534
  nephrotic, effect of adrenocortical hormones on 258f
  premenstrual 301
Electrocardiogram. See under Heart
Electroencephalogram, effect of adrenocortical hormone on 152
Electrolytes
  losses in dehydration 513, 544f
  losses, repair of
    in diabetic acidosis 572f
    in hypoadrenocorticism 210f
  maintenance needs 210
    in diabetic acidosis 573
    in hypoadrenocorticism 210f
  serum composition in ketosis 547
11-desoxycorticosterone. See under Adrenal cortices
11-desoxycorticosterone acetate (DOCA) 135f, 206f
11-17-oxycorticosteroids (11-17-OCS). See Adrenal cortices, S-F-N hormones; Urine, 11-17-OCS
Emotional disturbances
  amenorrhea and 350
  anorexia and 473
  anxiety in hyperthyroidism 35
  apprehension due to hyperepinephrinism 280
  behavior of sexually precocious boys 412f
  cause of polydipsia 529
  depression
    due to hypercalcemia 122
    in Cushing's syndrome 237
  due to ACTH 254
  effect on adrenomedullary activity 272
  hyperexia and 486f
  instability 35
  invalidism, emotional, due to therapy 558
  irritability
    due to hypoglycemia 580
    due to thyroid dose 25
    in diabetes insipidus 521
    in diabetes mellitus 555
    in hyperthyroidism 35
    in hypothyroidism 22
  placidity in hypothyroidism 22
  polydipsia, psychogenic 529f
  reaction to tall stature 492
  stress
    effect on antidiuretic production 511

Emotional disturbances, stress (cont.)
    effect on basal body temperatures 319
    fingernails and 489
  stress, relation to
    glycosuria 563
    insulin needs 563
    ketosis 563
Endometrium. See under Uterus
Epilepsy. See Convulsions, epileptiform
Epinephrine. See under Adrenal medullæ
Epinephrine-eosinophil test of adrenocortical status 168f
Epinephrine-glucose tolerance test 552
Epiphyses. See under Skeleton
Equivalent, definition of 595
Ergotamine vs epinephrine 275
Ergotoxine vs epinephrine 275
Estradiol, chemistry of 296f
Estriol, chemistry of 296f
Estrogens. See under Ovaries
Estrone, chemistry of 296f
Eunuchoidism 431
  pseudo- 393
Exercise and insulin 564
Extremities
  abnormalities in mongolism 23
  athetoid motions and hypocalcemia 104
  metacarpals, early fusion in 114
  See also Feet; Fingers and toes
Eyes
  buphthalmos in cystinosis 99
  cataracts in cystinosis 99
  exophthalmos 34
  fundus, abnormal due to hyperepinephrinism 280
  lid lag 33
  pathology in ovarian agenesis 344
  proptosis in polyostotic fibrous dysplasia 327
  retinal changes in diabetes mellitus 577
  retinitis pigmentosa in Laurence-Moon-Biedl syndrome 341
  scleræ, blue, in osteogenesis imperfecta 128
  soft
    in diabetic acidosis 555
    in hypoadrenocorticism 197
  strabismus in pseudo-hypoparathyroidism 114
  vision loss due to craniopharyngioma 458
Face
  effect of testosterone on development of 381
  moon-shaped
    in Cushing's syndrome 236
    in pseudo-hypoparathyroidism 114
  spasm in hypothyroidism 22

Faintness in hypoadrenocorticism 196
Fallopian tubes 292
   development of
      during adolescence 304
      during childhood 304
   effect of estrogen on 298f
   origin 292
Familial adrenocortical virilism 224
Fanconi's syndrome 99
Fasting
   effect of
      in hypoadrenocorticism 175
      in normal 175
   losses incident to 544
   metabolism, effect of testosterone on 374
Fat
   body, distribution in obesity 488
   fatty acids, formation from glucose 542
   hip, in adolescence 306
   in blood. See Serum lipids
   metabolism, effect on
      of adrenocortical hormones 148, 150
      of pituitary growth hormone 452
      of testosterone 374
   metabolism in diabetes mellitus 543
   pads in hypothyroidism 22
   stores, effect of protein anabolic hormone on 480
   subcutaneous, atrophy due to insulin 566
Fatigue
   effect on
      of adrenocortical hormones 151
      of blood glucose 151
   in diabetes insipidus 521
   in hypercalcemia 122
   in hypoadrenocorticism 195f
   in hypothyroidism 21
   See also Weakness
Feces. See Stool
Feet, abnormalities of, in mongolism 23
   See also Carpopedal spasm
Feminization, abnormal, due to adrenocortical cancer 247
Ferric chloride test 557
Fetus
   adrenocortical activity in 154
   parathyroid activity in 116
Fever
   due to
      craniopharyngioma 459
      glucose infusion in hypoadrenocorticism 177
      hyperepinephrinism 281
      hyperthyroidism 34
      thyroid storm 35
   lysis by cortisone 254
   metabolic origin in hypoadrenocorticism 215

Fever (cont.)
   septic, and acute hypoadrenocorticism 216f
Fibroblastic proliferation, inhibited by adrenocortical hormone 150
Fingers and toes
   abnormalities in mongolism 23
   fingers, short in pseudo-hypoparathyroidism 114
   nails
      in hypothyroidism 20
      monilia infection in hypoparathyroidism 105
   polydactylism in Laurence-Moon-Biedl syndrome 341
Fluids, parenteral, treatment
   for diabetic acidosis 569f
   for hypoadrenocorticism 210f
Follicle-stimulating hormone (FSH). See under Anterior pituitary
Fontanelles in hypothyroidism 21
Food. See Diet; Nutrition; Milk; Vitamins
Fractures 86
   in base-losing nephritis 93
   in osteogenesis imperfecta 128
   in pathologic hyperparathyroidism 125
   in polyostotic fibrous dysplasia 327
Francis test 152
Froehlich's syndrome 462
   and amenorrhea 350
   in girls 340f
FSH. See under Anterior pituitary

Galactosemia 552
Gastrointestinal tract
   insufficiency 82
   obstruction in hypoadrenocorticism 197
   perforation masked by cortisone 254
   peristalsis, effect of posterior pituitary extract on 535
   See also Constipation; Diarrhea; Stool; Vomiting
Genetic factors
   familial adrenocortical virilism 224
   in diabetes mellitus 554
   in sex determination 291
   relation to
      growth and maturation 345, 475
      retarded adolescence in boys 429
      sexual precocity in boys 408
      sexual precocity in girls 325
   relation to genital development
      in boys 392
      in girls 337
Genital tract
   effect of adrenocortical androgens on 226f
   malformations
      amenorrhea and 348f

INDEX

Genital tract, malformations (cont.)
    in adrenocortical virilism 225
    in mixed adrenocortical disease 246
Genitalia
    female, development during adolescence 304
    male, development during adolescence 392
    male, development in adrenocortical virilism 227
    See also under names of individual organs
Gigantism 481f
    clinical manifestations 482
    diagnosis 483
    treatment 484
    See also under Growth, increased
Glucose
    gluconeogenesis, effect of adrenocortical hormone on 148
    homeostasis 550
    in blood. See Serum glucose
    in urine. See Urine, glucose
    infusion, effect in hypoadrenocorticism 180
    metabolism, effect on
        of adrenocortical hormones 148
        of insulin 149, 178f, 541
        of insulin deficiency 543
        serum phosphorus 125
    oxidation, effect of epinephrine on 275
    phosphorylation 541
    renal tubule reabsorption 60
    tolerance
        decreased in Cushing's syndrome 244
        effect of diet on 550f
        epinephrine-glucose test 552
    tolerance test 175f
        meaning of 550f
    See also Carbohydrate
Glukagon hormone 541
Glutathione
    effect of adrenocortical hormone on 152
    relation to blood sugar 153
Glycogen
    glycogenesis and need for potassium 570
    glycogenesis, effect on
        of epinephrine 275
        of insulin 542
    glycogenolysis due to
        epinephrine 179, 273
        glukagon 542
    in vaginal cells, due to estrogen 299
    metabolism 148
    muscle, effect of epinephrine on 275
    storage disease
        hypoglycemia in 175
        test for 552

Glycosuria. See under Urine, glucose
Glycotropic hormone 542f
Goiter 44f
    adolescent 46f
    colloid, involution 47
    congenital 46
    due to thiouracil 40
    in hyperthyroidism 33
    in hypothyroidism 20
    in polyostotic fibrous dysplasia 328
    neonatal 44f
Gonadotropins. See under Anterior pituitary; Urine
Gonadotropins, chorionic
    dosage 402
    effect on
        male sex development 391
        pseudo-cryptorchidism 443
        test for testes activity 402
        testes 385
        true cryptorchidism 442
    in urine. See under Urine
    therapy
        for hypopituitarism in boys 428f
        sexual precocity and 419, 422
Graafian follicles. See Ovaries, follicles
Graves' disease. See Thyroid, hyperthyroidism
Growth
    accelerated, in obesity 486
    disturbances in hypothyroidism 20
    effect on, of
        adrenocortical androgens 226f
        adrenocortical hormones 454
        estrogen 300
        gonadal hormones 454
        pituitary growth hormone 454
        testosterone 436, 440f
        thyroid 454
    genetic factors and 345, 475
    gigantism 481f
    hormone. See Anterior pituitary, growth hormone (PGH)
    in diabetic children 577
    in fractional hypopituitarism 342, 480f
    in hypoadrenocorticism 216
    increased
        causes of 471
        hereditary tall stature 492
        in anterior pituitary adenoma 481f
        in sexual precocity in boys 224, 409, 418
        in sexual precocity in girls 224, 321, 330
    normal
        in anovarianism 345
        in male castrate 431
    rate, effect of thyroid on 26f
    stunted
        calcium deficiency and 86

Growth, stunted (cont.)
  causes of 468
  chondrodystrophy 11
  in adrenocortical virilism 227
  in base-losing nephritis 93
  in caloric undernutrition 473
  in Cushing's syndrome 237
  in cystinosis 476
  in diabetes mellitus 555
  in functional hyperpituitarism 492f
  in hypopituitarism 31
  in hypothalamic sexual infantilism 340
  in hypothyroidism 20
  in kidney disease 476
  in ovarian agenesis 344
  in pathologic hyperparathyroidism 125
  in primary idiopathic hypopituitarism 462, 464
  in primary organic hypopituitarism 462
  in pseudo-hypoparathyroidism 114
  in sexual precocity 325, 413
  serum phosphatase in 9
  See also Height
Gynecomastia. See under Breast

Hair
  axillary
    and adrenarche 247
    and masculinity 383f
    and menarche 306
    in hypoadrenocorticism 202
  axillary, development
    in adolescence 305
    in male castrate 431
  axillary, diminished in ovarian agenesis 344
  axillary, effect on
    of estrogen 345
    of genetic factors 383
    of testosterone 383
  axillary, lack of
    due to hypopituitarism 218
    in hypothalamic infantilism 340
    in primary idiopathic hypopituitarism 464
    in primary organic hypopituitarism 462
  axillary, normal in fractional hypopituitarism 342
  baldness, in adrenocortical virilism 227
  body, unresponsive to androgens, in pseudo-eunuchoidism 393
  hirsutism in
    adrenocortical virilism 227
    Cushing's syndrome 237
    ovarian fibrocystic disease 351
    testes cancer 419

Hair (cont.)
  in hypothyroidism 20
  loss in pathologic hyperparathyroidism 125
  pubic
    and adrenarche 247
    and masculinity 384
    in hypoadrenocorticism 202
    in hypopituitarism 428
    in sexual precocity in boys 409
  pubic, development of
    in adolescence 305
    in male castrate 431
  pubic, diminished in ovarian agenesis 344
  pubic, effect on
    of estrogen 345
    of genetic factors 383
    of testosterone 383
  pubic, lack of
    due to hypopituitarism 218
    in hypothalamic infantilism 340
    in primary idiopathic hypopituitarism 464
    in primary organic hypopituitarism 462
  pubic, normal
    in fractional hypopituitarism 342
Hashimoto thyroiditis 48
Headache
  due to
    craniopharyngioma 458
    hyperepinephrinism 280
  in hypoadrenocorticism 196
Heart
  action, effect of epinephrine on 273
  decompensation in hyperthyroidism 35
  disease, congenital
    and adrenocortical disease 246
    and mongolism 23
  electrocardiogram
    abnormal, due to hyperepinephrinism 280
    in hypothyroidism 21
    Q-T interval in hypocalcemia 119
  enlargement, pseudo-, in hyperthyroidism 34
  failure, effect of epinephrine on 288
  fibrillation due to epinephrine 288
  murmur in hyperthyroidism 34
  myocarditis in hyperthyroidism 35
  rate
    bradycardia due to undernutrition 473
    bradycardia in hypercalcemia 102
    irregular due to hypercalcemia 122
  size decreased
    causes of 202
    due to hypoadrenocorticism 143, 197f

INDEX [615]

Heart, size decreased (cont.)
    sign of dehydration 197f
    x-ray 202
  size increased
    due to hyperepinephrinism 280
    in hypothyroidism 21
    in neonatal goiter 44
Height
  age, definition of 441
  decreased 468
  increased 471
  normal 592f
  relation to
    general health 484
    sexual maturation 484
  ultimate, prediction of 492f
  See also under Growth
Hemorrhage, epinephrine in 288
Heredity. See Genetic factors
Hermaphroditism 365f
  causes 365
  classification 365
  diagnosis 366
  pseudo-hermaphroditism
    due to hyperadrenocorticism 225
    non-endocrine 228
    treatment 366
Hernia, umbilical, in hypothyroidism 21
Hexestrol, chemistry of 296f
Hexokinase 541
Hip, coxa vara 10
Hirsutism. See under Hair
Histaminase, effect of adrenocortical hormone on 153
Histamine
  actions 285
  metabolism, effect of adrenocortical hormone on 153
  test for pheochromocytoma 284f
  vs epinephrine 275
Homeostasis
  adrenal medullæ 272
  adrenocortical Na-K hormone 190
  adrenocortical S-F-N hormone 156, 185
  anterior pituitary 451, 486
  blood sugar 175, 273, 542f
    during fasting 175
  caloric undernutrition and 476
  glucose 550
  in newborn, and breast milk 530
  insulin 542f
  paradoxical 546
  parathyroid 64f
  phosphorus 64f
  posterior pituitary 517f
  potassium, and adrenal cortices 146f
  sodium, and adrenal cortices 146f
  substitution for 558
  thyroid 5
  water 517

Hormones
  acetylcholine 272, 299
  ACTH. See under Adrenal cortices
  adrenocortical amorphous fraction 137
  "anterior-pituitary-like" 385
  antidiuretic 498f
  11-17-OCS. See under Adrenal cortices
  epinephrine. See under Adrenal medullæ
  estradiol, chemistry of 296f
  estriol, chemistry of 296f
  estrogens. See under Ovaries
  estrone, chemistry of 296f
  follicle-stimulating (FSH). See under Anterior pituitary
  glukagon 541
  glycotropic 542f
  gonadotropins. See Anterior pituitary, gonadotropins; Gonadotropins, chorionic; Urine, gonadotropins
  growth. See under Anterior pituitary
  inhibin 373
  insulin. See under Pancreatic islets
  interstitial-cell-stimulating (ICSH). See under Anterior pituitary
  lactogenic 295, 451
  luteinizing (LH) 295, 451
  luteotropin 295, 451
  Na-K. See under Adrenal cortices
  nor-epinephrine. See under Adrenal medullæ
  oxytocin 498
  parathyroid. See under Parathyroids
  pituitary growth (PGH). See under Anterior pituitary
  progesterone. See under Ovaries
  progestins. See under Ovaries
  protein anabolic 480
  17-ketosteroid-precursors (17-KS-Gens). See under Adrenal cortices
  S-F-N. See under Adrenal cortices
  steroid
    adrenocortical, chemistry 135f
    metabolism, possible changes with age 173
    ovarian 296f, 300f
    testicular, chemistry 136
    testosterone 373
    urinary 17-KS chemistry and origin 137
  sympathin 272
  thyroid-stimulating (TSH; thyrotropin). See under Anterior pituitary
  vasopressin 498
Hot flashes in menopause præcox 351
Hunger, effect on adrenomedullary activity 272
Hyaluronidase activity, effect of adrenocortical hormone on 153
Hymen, imperforate and amenorrhea 349

Hyperadrenocorticism. *See* Adrenal cortices, hyperadrenocorticism
Hyperaminoaciduria 99
Hypercalcemia. *See under* Serum calcium
Hypercalcuria. *See under* Urine, calcium
Hypercarotenemia. *See* Serum carotene
Hyperchloremia. *See under* Serum chloride
Hyperepinephrinism. *See under* Adrenal medullæ
Hyperglycemia. *See under* Serum glucose
Hyperinsulinism. *See under* Pancreatic islets
Hyperkalemia. *See under* Serum potassium
Hypernatremia. *See under* Serum sodium
Hyperparathyroidism. *See* Parathyroids, hyperparathyroidism
Hyperphosphatasemia. *See under* Serum alkaline phosphatase
Hyperphosphatemia. *See under* Serum phosphorus
Hyperpituitarism. *See* Anterior pituitary, hyperpituitarism
Hyperproteinemia. *See under* Serum protein
Hyperthermia. *See* Fever
Hyperthyroidism. *See* Thyroid, hyperthyroidism
Hypoadrenocorticism. *See* Adrenal cortices, hypoadrenocorticism
Hypocalcemia. *See under* Serum calcium
Hypocalcuria. *See under* Urine, calcium
Hypochloremia. *See under* Serum chloride
Hypoepinephrinism. *See under* Adrenal medullæ
Hypoglycemia. *See under* Serum glucose
Hypogonadism. *See under* Testes
Hypoinsulinism. *See* Diabetes mellitus
Hypokalemia. *See under* Serum potassium
Hyponatremia. *See under* Serum sodium
Hypoparathyroidism. *See* Parathyroids, hypoparathyroidism
Hypophosphatasemia. *See under* Serum alkaline phosphatase
Hypophosphatemia. *See under* Serum phosphorus
Hypopituitarism. *See* Anterior pituitary, hypopituitarism; Posterior pituitary, deficiency; Posterior pituitary, hypopituitarism
Hypothalamus. *See under* Central nervous system
Hypothyroidism. *See* Thyroid, hypothyroidism

ICSH. *See under* Anterior pituitary
Idiocy, mongolian 23f
Illness, chronic, and skeletal maturation 12
Immunologic phenomena, effect of adrenocortical hormones on 152
Infantilism, sexual. *See* Sexual infantilism
Infants
 adrenocortical activity in 154
 adrenocortical responsiveness in 154
 newborn, endocrine function in 530

Infants (cont.)
 parathyroid activity in 117
Infection
 chronic
  and amenorrhea 354
  effect on pituitary function 343
 diabetic coma and 566f
 effect on glucose tolerance 551
 overwhelming, hypoadrenocorticism in 216f
 spread, increased by ACTH 254
Inhibin 373
Instability, emotional 35
Insulin. *See under* Pancreatic islets
Intelligence. *See* Mental development
Interstitial-cell-stimulating hormone (ICSH). *See under* Anterior pituitary
Interstitial cells. *See under* Testes
Intestines. *See* Gastrointestinal tract
Invalidism, emotional, due to therapy 558
Iodine
 deficiency
  cause of hypothyroidism 14f
  in congenital goiter 46
 effect on goiter 47
 in neonatal goiter 44f
 in thyroid hormone, daily requirement 1
 radio-active
  treatment in hyperthyroidism 36, 39
  uptake by thyroid 39
 salt, prophylaxis 46
 serum, protein-bound. *See* Serum iodine, protein-bound
 treatment
  dose iodide 37
  in hyperthyroidism 36, 37f
  mode of action 37
  preparation for thyroidectomy 42, 43
  toxic reactions 39
  use with propyl thiouracil 42
 treatment, response to
  in hyperthyroidism 38f
  in normal 37
 uptake by thyroid
  in normal 12
  in thyroid disease 13
  inhibited by certain foods 46
IQ. *See* Mental development
Irritability. *See under* Emotional disturbances

Jaw development, effect of testosterone on 381

Ketone bodies
 metabolism of 543f
 See also under Blood; Urine
Ketosis
 effect on serum electrolytes 547
 See also Diabetes mellitus, acidosis

Ketosteroids. *See* Adrenal cortices, hormones; Urine, 11-17-OCS; Urine, 17-KS
Kidney
    anomalies, in ovarian agenesis 344
    base economy, test for 94f
    calcification 88
        due to pathologic hyperparathyroidism 123
        in base-losing nephritis 95
        in Cushing's syndrome 237
        in pathologic hyperparathyroidism 123
        types of 123
        x-ray appearance 123
    carcinoma, serum calcium in 128
    clearance of uric acid and adrenocortical hormone 152
    colic in pathologic hyperparathyroidism 123
    disease
        and stunted growth 476
        effect on parathyroids 88f
    effect of testosterone on 381
    function 54f
        in diabetes insipidus 524
        in nephrogenic diabetes insipidus 531
    function, effect on
        of ACTH 153
        of adrenocortical hormone 137f, 153
        of dehydration 531
        of parathyroid extract 53f, 66
    function failure, due to
        atresia 119
        circulatory failure 556
        dehydration 119
        polycystic disease 119
    function impaired, due to hypoadrenocorticism 143
    function, osmotic and antidiuretic hormone 508
    glomerular filtration
        of calcium 54f
        of phosphorus 54f
    glomerular filtration rate 54f
        in newborn 117
        urea clearance 90
    infection
        in Cushing's syndrome 237
        in pathologic hyperparathyroidism 123
    nephritis. *See* Nephritis
    nephrosis
        serum cholesterol, effect of cortisone on 150
        serum phospholipids, effect of cortisone on 150
        treatment, with adrenocortical hormones 258f

Kidney (cont.)
    perirenal air insufflation 228
    phosphorus excretion and parathyroid hormone 62f
    refractoriness to parathyroid hormone in pseudo-hypoparathyroidism 114
    response to antidiuretic hormone, in newborn 530
    Tm, endocrine influence on 62
    tubular excretion
        of calcium 55
        of phosphorus 55
        of water 533
    tubular reabsorption
        of calcium 55, 72
        of glucose 551
        of phosphorus 55, 72
    tubular reabsorption mechanisms 60f
        endocrine influence on 60f
        fractional 60f
        threshold 60
    tubules
        calcification 72
        disease 533
        effect of antidiuretic hormone on 499f
        function, in potassium deficiency 534
    tubules, base economy
        by ammonia production 91f
        by excretion of acid urine 91
Klinefelter's syndrome 437f

Lactation 299
    in newborn 302
Lactogenic hormone 295, 451
Larynx
    development, effect of testosterone on 381
    spasm in hypothyroidism 23
    stridor, causes of 119
    unresponsive to androgens 393
Laurence-Moon-Biedl syndrome
    hypothalamic-pituitary relations in 385
    in girls 341
Leydig cells. *See* Testes, interstitial cells
LH (luteinizing hormone) 295, 451
Lipids serum in hypothyroidism 8
Liver
    cirrhosis and gynecomastia 440
    disease
        hypoglycemia in 175
        menorrhagia and 359
    effect of pituitary growth hormone on 452
    extract, effect on water metabolism 515
    glycogen
        metabolism 148
        stock of 177
        storage disease 552

Liver (cont.)
    glycogenolysis
        epinephrine and 273
        test for 552
    insufficiency, effect on antidiuretic hormone metabolism 515
    role in
        metabolism of antidiuretic hormone 515
        steroid metabolism 298, 300
Lupus erythematosus, treatment with adrenocortical hormone 150, 257
Luteinizing hormone (LH) 295, 451
Luteotropic hormone 295, 451
Luteotropin 295, 451
Lymph nodes
    Delphian
        in Hashimoto thyroiditis 48
        in thyroid carcinoma 20
        in thyroiditis 20
    involution due to adrenocortical hormone 150
    lymphadenopathy, effect of adrenocortical hormone on 256
Lysozyme activity, effect of adrenocortical hormone on 153

Macroglossia. *See under* Tongue
Magnesium
    intracellular, loss in diabetic acidosis 570
    salt, preparations 575
    serum, in diabetic acidosis 575
Malnutrition. *See* Nutrition, undernutrition
Marine cycle 47
"Medical" dilatation and curettage
    in postmenarcheal amenorrhea 350
    index of estrogen production 316
    progesterone in 316
Menarche. *See under* Menstruation
Menopause præcox 351
Menorrhagia. *See under* Menstruation
Menstruation 309f
    amenorrhea
        diagnosis 351f
        postmenarcheal 349f
        treatment 355
        types of 348f
        vaginal smear in 314f
    amenorrhea due to
        adrenocortical virilism 226, 235
        Cushing's syndrome 237
        hyperparathyroidism 125
        hyperthyroidism 35
        ovarian disease 351
        pregnancy 351
    anovulatory
        in pseudo-precocious puberty 330
        pregnandiol excretion in 318
    bleeding during 312
    calendar of 353

Menstruation (cont.)
    cycles 294
        anovulatory 312
        ovulatory 312
    disorders of
        during adolescence, physiologic considerations 345f
        obesity and 492
    due to adrenocortical cancer 334
    dysmenorrhea 361f
        absence of, in metropathia hemorrhagica 356
        causes 361
        in ovulatory cycle 319
        manifestations 361f
        prognosis 364
        treatment 364
        types of 361
    estrogen-withdrawal 341
    evolution 309
    induced by
        progesterone treatment 316
        stilbestrol treatment 341
    menarche
        definition 302
        delayed, due to genital tract defects 348f
        in adrenocortical virilism 235
        mothers vs daughters 337
    menarche, relation to
        age 348
        axillary hair 306
        body build 337
        climate 337
        hormone production 308
        ultimate stature 492f
        urine gonadotropins 308
    menopause
        in "constitutional" precocity 327
        præcox 351
    menorrhagia
        definition 355
        endometrial biopsy in 317
        ovarian 356f
        ovarian, differential diagnosis 358
        treatment 359f
        types of 355f
    metropathia hemorrhagica 356f
    neonatal 302
    oligomenorrhea 350
        due to hyperthyroidism 35
        due to hypothyroidism 342
        due to ovarian fibrocystic disease 351
    ovulatory, in true precocious puberty 323
    pregnandiol excretion and 318
    proliferative phase 311
    regressive phase 312
    secretory phase 311f

INDEX

Mental confusion
  due to hypoglycemia 580
  in hypoadrenocorticism 196
Mental deficiency
  in cystinosis 99
  in Laurence-Moon-Biedl syndrome 341
  in ovarian agenesis 344
  thyroid dose in 25f
Mental development
  effect of thyroid hormone on 28f
  in hypopituitarism 472
  in hypothyroidism 20
  of sexually precocious child 412
  relation to age at onset of hypothyroidism 29f
  retarded, in pseudo-hypoparathyroidism 114
Mental disturbances. *See* Emotional disturbances; Mental confusion; Psychic pathology
Metabolism, basal energy. *See* Basal energy metabolism
Metropathia hemorrhagica 356f
Milk
  cow's
    comparison with human milk 530
    composition 117
  human
    composition 117
    virtues of 530
  intake, effect on serum calcium 79
  "witch's" 302
Milliequivalent (mEq.), definition of 595
Milliosmole (mosM), definition of 596
Mongolian idiocy 23f
Monilia albicans
  hypoadrenocorticism and 195
  hypoparathyroidism and 103, 105
Morphine intolerance in
  hypoadrenocorticism 214
  hypothyroidism 23
Mouth, monilia infection in hypoparathyroidism 105
Mucoprotein secretion, effect of adrenocortical hormone on 153
Mucoproteose secretion, effect of adrenocortical hormone on 153
Mucous membranes
  effect of estrogen on 299
  pigmentation
    in hypoadrenocorticism 202
    in polyostotic fibrous dysplasia 128
Müllerian ducts, effect of estrogen on 298f
Muscles
  development, effect on
    of adrenocortical 17-KS-Gens 157
    of pituitary growth hormone 452
    of testosterone 381
  diastasis of rectus in hypothyroidism 21
  fatigue. *See* Fatigue
  glycogen, metabolism 148

Muscles (cont.)
  glycogenolysis, effect of epinephrine on 275
  hypertrophy in adrenocortical virilism 227
  irritability, and hypocalcemia 105
  myositis, effect of adrenocortical hormone on 257
  paralysis 141
  spasms in hypothyroidism 22, 23
  tone, hypotonia due to hypercalcemia 122
  weakness due to
    potassium deficiency 141
    potassium excess 142
  weakness in
    Cushing's syndrome 237
    hyperthyroidism 35
    hypoadrenocorticism 195f
Myeloma, multiple 128
Myocarditis 35
Myositis, effect of adrenocortical hormone on 257
Myotonia congenita 23
Myxedema. *See* Thyroid, hypothyroidism
Myxedema, pituitary type 30f, 342f

Na-K hormone. *See under* Adrenal cortices
Nasal obstruction in polyostotic fibrous dysplasia 327
Nausea in diabetes insipidus 521
  See also Vomiting
Neck, webbing of, in ovarian agenesis 344
Neonatal goiter 44f
Nephritis
  base-losing 91f
    diagnosis 93f
    Fanconi's syndrome 99
    parathyroid histology and 53
    prognosis 99
    test for 95f
    treatment 97f
  cause of diabetes insipidus 531
  glomerular
    and parathyroid histology 53
  glomerular plus tubular. *See* pannephritis (*below*)
  glomerular without tubular insufficiency 89f
    diagnosis and differential diagnosis 90
    prognosis 91
    treatment 90f
  intercapillary glomerulosclerosis in diabetes mellitus 577
  pannephritis 100f
    diagnosis 101
    due to pathologic hyperparathyroidism 123
    prognosis 102

Nephritis, pannephritis (cont.)
    treatment 101f
    urine volume in 532f
    tubular without glomerular. See base-
        losing (above)
Nervous system. See Central nervous system;
    Sympathetic nervous system
Neuroblastoma 276
Nipple pigmentation due to stilbestrol 335
Nitrogen
    balance vs caloric balance 452
    losses relative to potassium in acute de-
        hydration 510
    metabolism, effect on
        of adrenocortical hormone 150
        of caloric intake 455
        of estrogen 300
        of nitrogen intake 454
        of pituitary growth hormone 452
        of testosterone 374
        of thyroid 2
    non-protein, serum. See Serum non-pro-
        tein nitrogen
Nodules, subcutaneous, effect of adrenocortical
    hormones on 256
Non-protein nitrogen serum. See Serum non-
    protein nitrogen
Nor-epinephrine. See under Adrenal medullæ
Nutrition
    caloric balance
        relation to obesity 487
        vs nitrogen balance 452
    caloric balance, effect on
        nitrogen balance 455
        pituitary growth hormone produc-
            tion 455
    caloric content of foods 492
    caloric stores and survival 480
    disturbances and amenorrhea 354
    overnutrition, effect on anterior pituitary
        function 486f
    relation to
        pituitary growth hormone action
            452
        wound-healing 478f
    undernutrition and sexual infantilism
        in boys 430
        in girls 343
    undernutrition, effect on
        anterior pituitary function 473f
        growth and maturation 473
        ovaries 478
        pituitary function 343
        skeletal maturation 12
        thyroid function 5
    See also Diet; Milk; Vitamins

Obesity
    amenorrhea and 354
    basal metabolic rate in 6

Obesity (cont.)
    "buffalo type" 236
    causes 489
    diabetes mellitus and 554
    relation to
        craniopharyngioma 459
        Cushing's syndrome 235f
        hypothyroidism 21
        Laurence-Moon-Biedl syndrome
            341
        primary idiopathic hypopituitarism
            464
        primary organic hypopituitarism
            462
        pseudo-hypoparathyroidism 114
    simple dietary 486f
        clinical manifestations 488f
        differential diagnosis 489
        etiology 486f
        laboratory studies 489
        prognosis 490
        treatment 490f
Oligomenorrhea. See under Menstruation
Osmole
    concentrations, relation to body water
        distribution 144f
    definition 498, 596
    serum. See Serum osmole
    water relations, and antidiuretic hor-
        mone 498
Osmoreceptors 514
Osmotic equilibrium 503
    in diabetic acidosis 570
Osteoblasts and osteoid formation 84
Osteochondritis deformans 10f
Osteogenesis. See Skeleton, growth
    imperfecta 128
Osteomalacia. See under Skeleton
Osteoporosis. See under Skeleton
Ovaries 290f
    activity
        control of, by anterior pituitary
            294f
        cycles 295
    agenesis 344f
    anatomy and general physiology 292f
    androgens 296
    arrhenoblastoma and
        amenorrhea 351
        pseudo-hermaphroditism 365
    basic considerations 291f
    castration 345
    changes during menstrual cycle 311
    chorionepithelioma 330, 334
    clinical considerations 320f
    corpus luteum
        evolution 348
        formation 292f
        lack of, in metropathia hemor-
            rhagica 356

Ovaries (cont.)
    deficiency
        cause of amenorrhea 351
        urine gonadotropins in 320
    development
        during adolescence 303
        during childhood 303f
    disease, and menorrhagia 356f
    ectopic 365
    embryology 291f
    estrogens 296f
        actions 298f
        definition 296
        dosage 341
        inactivation 298
        maternal, effect on newborn 302
        metabolism 298
        role in menstruation 312
        source of, extra-ovarian 297f
        source of, ovarian 292
        stilbestrol. See Stilbestrol
        use of, in adrenocortical virilism 233
    estrogens, chemistry of
        diethylstilbestrol 296f
        estradiol 296f
        estriol 296f
        estrone 296f
        hexestrol 296f
        triphenylchlorethylene 296f
    estrogens, deficiency 316
        effect on skeleton 341
        effect on skin 341
    estrogens, effect on
        ACTH production 299
        blood vessels 300
        body growth 494
        breast 299
        electrolyte metabolism 300
        epiphyseal closure 484
        genital organs 298f
        gonadotropin production 295, 348
        lactogenic hormone production 299
        mucous membranes 299
        pituitary growth hormone production 300, 454
        17-KS production 345
        skeleton 300
        skin 299
        testes 412
        urine citric acid 300
    estrogens, production
        decreased, in menopause præcox 351
        sporadic, during adolescence 308
    estrogens, production indices 312f
        endometrial biopsy 316
        "medical" dilatation and curettage 316
        urine estrogen 313

Ovaries, estrogens, production indices (cont.)
        urine sediment 313
        vaginal pH 313
        vaginal smear 313f
    estrus cycle 294
    failure, relation to nutrition 478
    fibrocystic disease 351
        and menorrhagia 358
    follicles
        atresia 293
        cyst 330, 334
        growth 292
        in metropathia hemorrhagica 356
    gonadarche, precocious 247
        relation to adrenarche 247
    granulosa cell tumor 330f
        and menorrhagia 358
    hermaphroditism and 365
    hormones 296f
    hypoovarianism. See Sexual infantilism, in girls
    in adrenocortical virilism 226f
    infantile, in hypopituitarism 342
    menopause præcox 351
    menses. See Menstruation
    oogenesis 292
    ovotestes 366
    ovulation 292f
        basal body temperature and 318f
        dysmenorrhea and 319, 361
        effect on ovary 304
        failure of, in fibrocystic disease 351
        inception of 309
        inhibition of, with stilbestrol 364
        urine pregnandiol and 318
    progesterone
        chemistry 300
        conversion to pregnandiol 300
        cyclic therapy with 359f
        "medical" dilatation and curettage and 316
        role in menstruation 312
        sources 293, 300
    progesterone, effect on
        electrolyte metabolism 301
        estrogen metabolism 301
        genital organs 301
        gonadotropin production 295, 301
    progesterone, production indices 317f
        basal body temperature 318f
        endometrial biopsy 317
        urine pregnandiol 317f
    progestins
        chemistry 300
        definition 296
        dosages 300
        dysmenorrhea and 361
        lack of, in metropathia hemorrhagica 356

Ovaries (cont.)
   teratoma 330, 334
Overnutrition. *See under* Nutrition
Oxygen consumption, effect of epinephrine on 275
Oxytocin hormone 498

Pain
   abdominal
      due to dysmenorrhea 361
      in acute hypoadrenocorticism 216
      in diabetes mellitus 555
      in hypoadrenocorticism 197
   analgesia by cortisone 254
   effect on adrenomedullary activity 272
   in back, in Cushing's syndrome 237
Pancreas
   cystic fibrosis 82
   pancreatectomy, needs of insulin after 553
Pancreatic islets 540f
   adenoma 578
      surgical excision 581
   basic considerations 541f
   cell degeneration due to glycotropic hormone treatment 543
   clinical considerations 553f
   glukagon 541
   homeostasis 542f
   hormones 541
   hyperinsulinism 577f
      hypoglycemia in 175
      types of 553
   "hypoinsulinism." *See* Diabetes mellitus
   insulin
      actions 541f
      antagonists 542
      deficiency, effects of 543f
         See also Diabetes mellitus
      dosage 561f
      dosage for diabetic coma 567f
      excess, effects of 546f
      exercise and 542, 564
      indices of 550f
      needs after pancreatectomy 553
      preparations 561
      production, control of 542f
      therapy, complications of 566
      tolerance test 175f
      tolerance test in hypopituitarism 467
      unit of 541
      withdrawal, effects of 549
   insulin, effect on
      glucose metabolism 149, 178
      glycogenesis 275
      serum glucose 561f
   insulin reactions
      causes 564
      effect on brain 559

Pancreatic islets, insulin reactions (cont.)
      manifestations 564
      on leaving hospital 564
      prevention 564f
      treatment 564f
   insulin, resistance to
      in Cushing's syndrome 237
      in diabetic acidosis 546
      relation to glutathione 153
Panhypogonadism. *See* Testes, hypogonadism, primary complete
Panhypopituitarism. *See* Anterior pituitary, hypopituitarism, generalized
Pannephritis. *See under* Nephritis
Parathyroidectomy. *See under* Parathyroids
Parathyroids 52f
   activity
      at birth 117
      control of 74f
      in fetus 116
      index of 64
   activity, relation to
      calcium intake 79f
      calcium metabolism 72f
      kidney diseases 88f
      needs 73
      phosphorus intake 66
      renal tubule calcium and phosphorus reabsorption 72f
      serum calcium 74
      serum phosphorus 66
   adenoma 122
   aphasia 103
   basic considerations 53f
   carcinoma 122
   clinical considerations 78f
   extract, effects 77f
      in newborn 117
      on kidney function 53f, 66, 72, 74
      on skeleton 53f
      on urine phosphorus 66
   extract, hormone types in 73
   extract therapy, intoxication due to 111
   fibrosis 103
   histology of
      abnormal 53
      normal 53
   homeostasis 64f
      abnormal 102f
      in newborn 118
      temporal aspects 70f
   hormones
      inactivation 53
      molecular weight 53
      placenta, barrier to 116
      sites of action 53
      test for responsiveness to 107f
      types of 53, 73
   hormones, effect on
      bones 75f

INDEX

Parathyroids, hormones, effect on (cont.)
    phosphorus excretion 62f
    phosphorus metabolism 62f
    renal base excretion 123
    renal chloride excretion 123
    renal water excretion 123
  hyperparathyroidism. See Parathyroids, hyperparathyroidism (below)
  hyperplasia, primary 122
  hypoparathyroidism. See Parathyroids, hypoparathyroidism (below)
  hypoplasia 103
  in pseudo-hypoparathyroidism 114
  parathyroidectomy and
    hypocalcemia 74
    tetany 129
    tumor in pathologic hyperparathyroidism 125
    urine phosphorus 66
  reciprocal relations with other endocrines 78
  size of
    activity and 73f
    at birth 117
    fetal 116
    increased in pannephritis 100
    phosphorus intake and 66
Parathyroids, hyperparathyroidism
  and osteoclastic activity 82
  pathologic 122f
    calcium Tm in 72
    clinical manifestations 122f
    diagnosis 126f
    differential diagnosis 127f
    etiology 122
    laboratory studies 125f
    prognosis 129
    roentgenography in 125
    treatment 128f
  physiologic 66, 82
    in base-losing nephritis 92
    in kidney insufficiency 90
    in pannephritis 100
    lack of effect on bones 90
Parathyroids, hypoparathyroidism
  pathologic
    calcium Tm in 72
    clinical manifestations 103f
    diagnosis 105f
    differential diagnosis 107f
    maternal 116
    prognosis 111
    response to A.T.-10 and vitamin D 77f
    treatment 110f
  physiologic 66
    in newborn 117
  pseudo-hypoparathyroidism 111f
Pelvis, female, development during adolescence 305

Penis
  development
    effect of testosterone on 384
    in hypopituitarism 428
    in sexual precocity 409
    precocious in adrenocortical virilism 227
  size
    in obesity 489
    index of androgens 393f
Pepsin secretion, effect of adrenocortical hormones on 153
Periarteritis nodosa
  serum cholesterol, effect of cortisone on 150
  serum phospholipids, effect of cortisone on 150
  treatment with adrenocortical hormone 257
PGH. See Anterior pituitary, growth hormone
pH plasma. See Serum pH
Pheochromoblastoma 276
Pheochromocytoma. See *under* Adrenal medullæ, hyperepinephrinism
Phosphatase serum. See Serum alkaline phosphatase
Phospholipids serum, effect of cortisone on 150
Phosphorus
  assimilation reduced by
    aluminum hydroxide 91
    calcium lactate 91
  balance 70
  content of
    food 90
    milk 117
  excretion
    capacity for, in newborn 117
    effect of ACTH on 153
    mechanism 55
    parathyroid hormone and 62f
  homeostasis 64f
    limits of 70f
    temporal aspects 70f
  in glomerular filtrate 54f
  intake
    and parathyroid gland histology 53
    and parathyroid gland size 66
    and serum phosphorus 66
  intracellular, losses in diabetic acidosis 570
  metabolism
    effect of estrogen on 300
    effect of testosterone on 375
    parathyroids and 62f
  nitrogen ratio in muscle 375
  organic, acid-soluble loss of, in diabetic acidosis 546
  serum. See Serum phosphorus

Pinealoma
    cause of diabetes insipidus 520
    sexual precocity and 408
Pituitary growth hormone (PGH). *See*
    Anterior pituitary, growth hormone
Planned Parenthood Federation of America,
    temperature reading charts 318
Pneumonia masked by cortisone 254
Polydactylism in Laurence-Moon-Biedl syndrome 341
Polydipsia
    in base-losing nephritis 95
    in diabetes insipidus 521
    in pathologic hyperparathyroidism 123
    psychogenic 529f
Polyuria. *See under* Urine
Posterior pituitary 496f
    activity
        control of 498, 518
        control of, by hypothalamus 511
        excess 534f
        reserve 518
    antidiuretic hormone
        actions 505f
        deficiency, effects of 510f
        excess, effects of 511
        metabolism 514f, 516f, 527
        production, control of 498f
    antidiuretic hormone, effect of
        "all-or-none effect" 505
        on body metabolism 510f
        on kidneys 499f
    antidiuretic hormone, relation to
        adrenocortical hormone 152, 516, 534
        anterior pituitary hormone 516
        solute load 503f
        urine volume 503f
        water load 505
    antidiuretic hormone, resistance to
        in adrenocortical alarm reaction 534
        in nephrogenic diabetes insipidus 531
        in pathologic hyperparathyroidism 123
        in potassium deficiency 534
    basic considerations 497f
    clinical considerations 518f
    deficiency 518f
        causes of 519
        pathologic 520f
    disease, extent of, and diabetes insipidus 518
    homeostasis 517f
        in edema 535
    hormones 497f
        oxytocin 498
        preparations 527f

Posterior pituitary, hormones (cont.)
        vasopressin 498
    hypopituitarism, physiologic 529f
    innervation of 497
    maturation during infancy 530
    origin 497
    preparations 527f
        doses 528
        effect on urine chloride 509
        impurities in 509
        miscellaneous uses 535
        test for response to 521f
Potassium
    citrate
        dose 207
        therapy in base-losing nephritis 97f
    content of muscle 375
    deficiency
        cause of death 571
        effect on glycogenesis 570
        repair of 572f
        signs of 570f
    dosage 573
    gains after adrenocortical hormone withdrawal 143f
    gains, excessive
        in hypoadrenocorticism 186
        serum K in 186
    homeostasis
        and the adrenal cortices 146f
        disturbed by stress 147
    intake, relation to adrenocortical hormone 143
    intracellular, deficiency
        adrenocortical histology in 534
        antidiuretic hormone resistance in 534
        cell changes in 141
        due to diarrhea 142
        due to diet 142
        due to hyperadrenocorticism 139
        due to nephritis 142
        due to stress 148
        due to stress plus saline 571
        in diabetic acidosis 570f
        prevention by sodium restriction 141f
        production of 534
        weakness in 141
    intracellular, depletion due to sodium therapy 97f
    intracellular, excess
        cause of death 142
        weakness in 142
    intracellular, normal content 140
    losses due to thirsting 143
    losses relative to nitrogen
        in acute dehydration 510
        in dehydration 544, 546

INDEX

Potassium (cont.)
   metabolism, effect on
      of adrenocortical hormones 137f, 151f
      of progesterone 301
      of testosterone 375
   need of, for glycogenesis 570
   nitrogen ratio, in muscle 375
   retention, in excess of nitrogen 375
   salt
      preparations 575
      solutions for intravenous therapy 571
   serum. *See* Serum potassium
   therapy in DOCA intoxication 207
   toxicity
      avoidance of 573
      due to orange juice 102
      in pannephritis 102
Precocity, sexual. *See* Sexual precocity
Pregnancy
   cause of amenorrhea 351
   complications of, and menorrhagia 359
   parathyroids in 78
   risk of, in "constitutional" sexual precocity 325f
Pregnandiol
   metabolism 300
   relation to ovulation 318
Pregneninolone 300
Progeria, effect of testosterone on 374
Progesterone. *See under* Ovaries
Progestins. *See under* Ovaries
Promizole, cause of sexual precocity 335
Propyl thiouracil
   action, mode of 39f
   dose 42
   use with iodide 42
Prostate
   development
      effect of testosterone on 384
      index of androgen production 384
   size, index of androgens 393f
Protein anabolic hormone 480
Protein-bound iodine, serum. *See* Serum iodine, protein-bound
Protein, serum. *See* Serum protein
Protoplasm growth, effect on
   of pituitary growth hormone 452
   of testosterone 374
Pseudo-cryptorchidism 443
Pseudo-eunuchoidism 393
Pseudo-hermaphroditism. *See under* Hermaphroditism
Pseudo-hypoparathyroidism 111f
   clinical manifestations 114
   diagnosis 114f
   prognosis 116
   treatment 116

Pseudo-precocious puberty. *See under* Puberty, precocious
Psychic pathology due to cortisone 254
Psychogenic polydipsia 529f
Puberty
   definition of 302
   delayed. *See under* Sexual infantilism
Puberty, precocious
   definition of 321f
   pseudo-, in boys 418f
   pseudo-, in girls 321, 329f
   true precocious, in boys
      complete 408f
      incomplete 413f
   true precocious, in girls 321f
   See also Sexual precocity
Pulse
   rate, rapid in
      hyperthyroidism 34
      thyroid storm 35
   rate, slow in
      anorexia nervosa 5
      hypothyroidism 21
   weak in
      acute hypoadrenocorticism 216
      diabetic acidosis 555
      hypoadrenocorticism 197
Pyloric stenosis and adrenocortical disease 246

Rathke's pouch 449
Reflexes, nervous, in hyperthyroidism 35
Respirations
   increased in
      central hyperpnea 557
      diabetic acidosis 555
      salicylate poisoning 557
   Kussmaul 555
   rapid, and acute hypoadrenocorticism 216
   rate, vs pH and CO_2 567
Respiratory tract
   laryngeal stridor, causes 119
   obstruction
      due to hypocalcemia, in pseudo-hypoparathyroidism 116
      in hypocalcemia 103, 105
      in hypothyroidism 22
      in neonatal goiter 44
Rheumatic fever
   treatment with adrenocortical hormones 256f
   vs hyperepinephrinism 281f
Rheumatoid arthritis. *See* Arthritis, rheumatoid
Rhinitis, vasomotor, effect of adrenocortical hormone on 258
Rickets
   base-losing nephritis and 95

Rickets (cont.)
    due to vitamin D lack
        growth rate and 84
        nutritional state in 84
        parathyroid histology in 53
    healing, due to vitamin D lack, and tetany 120
    hyperaminoaciduria and 100
    in pannephritis 101
    vs osteoporosis 84
    vs scurvy 84f
    x-rays in 84

Salicylate poisoning 557
Salivary gland, effect of adrenocortical hormone on 139
Sarcoidosis, serum calcium in 128
Sarcoma botryoides and menorrhagia 359
Scrotum development
    effect of testosterone on 384
    index of androgen production 384
Scurvy and rickets 84f
Sella turcica
    calcification due to craniopharyngioma, x-ray of 459
    lesions of, in hypothalamic infantilism 340
Seminal vesicles development
    effect of testosterone on 384
    index of androgen production 384
Serum
    concentration, effect on antidiuretic hormone production 511
    water-solute ratio in relation to urine water-solute ratio 503, 511f
Serum alkaline phosphatase
    calcium deficiency and 82
    effect on
        of pituitary growth hormone 452
        of thyroid 26
    hyperphosphatasemia in
        base-losing nephritis 92
        healing rickets 121
        pathologic hyperparathyroidism 126
    hypophosphatasemia in hypoparathyroidism 105
    in achondroplasia 9
    in anemia 9
    in arthritis 9
    in Cushing's syndrome 237
    in dwarfism 9
    in hypothyroidism 8f
    in malnutrition 9
    in mongolism 9
    in polyostotic fibrous dysplasia 328
    in rickets 9
    in scurvy 9
    osteoblastic activity and 9

Serum calcium
    concentration, in fetus 116
    effect on parathyroid activity 75
    ionization, in acidosis 101
    ionized, determination 54
    hypercalcemia
        causes 79
        clinical manifestations 122
        death due to 111, 122
        in acute osteoporosis 128
        in multiple myeloma 128
        in neuroblastoma 128
        in pathologic hyperparathyroidism 126
        in renal carcinoma 128
        in sarcoidosis 128
        in vitamin D intoxication 88
    hypocalcemia
        causes 82
        Chvostek test for 104
        clinical manifestations 103
        despite hyperparathyroidism 84
        differential diagnosis 107
        in base-losing nephritis 92
        in healing rickets 120f
        in neonatal period 116
        in pseudo-hypoparathyroidism 111f
        reflexes and 105
        skeletal anabolism and 84
        Trousseau test for 103
Serum carbon dioxide
    decreased
        in diabetic acidosis 556
        in hypoadrenocorticism 185
    significance of 557
Serum carotene, hypercarotenemia
    in Cushing's syndrome 8
    in hypothyroidism 8
    in liver disease 8
    in primary idiopathic hypopituitarism 465
Serum chloride
    hyperchloremia in Fanconi's syndrome 99
    hypochloremia
        in Cushing's syndrome 243
        in diabetic acidosis 556
        in hypoadrenocorticism 185, 203
Serum cholesterol
    effect on
        of cortisone 150
        of thyroid 8, 26
    in diabetes mellitus 8
    in hepatic disease 8
    in hypopituitarism 31
    in malnutrition 8
    in renal disease 8
    in thyroid disease 8

Serum cholesterol (cont.)
    in xanthomatosis 8
    normal range 7f
Serum electrolytes, composition in ketosis 547
Serum glucose
    effect on
        of anterior pituitary extract 455
        of testosterone 374
    homeostasis 175, 273, 542f
        in fasting 175
    hyperglycemia
        and epinephrine 273
        and nor-epinephrine 273
        due to hyperadrenocorticism 149, 180
        due to insulin lack 543
        effect on insulin production 180, 542
        in diabetes mellitus 556
        in diabetic coma 567
        significance of 550f
        unresponsiveness 177, 180
    hyperglycemia, chronic, effects 558
        on pancreatic islets 543
    hypoglycemia
        and epinephrine production 273f
        causes 275, 552f, 577f
        definition 578
        diagnosis 580f
        due to galactosemia 552
        due to hypoadrenocorticism 149
        effects 550
            on adrenomedullary activity 179, 272
            on central nervous system 558
        functional 580
        idiopathic 580
        in hepatic disease 175
        in hyperinsulinism 175, 546
        in hypoadrenocorticism 175
            prevention by lipo-adrenal cortex extract 205
        in newborn 578
        in regulation of diabetes mellitus 558
        manifestations 578f
        prognosis 582
        treatment 258, 581f
        unresponsiveness 175, 177f
    in hyperepinephrinism 280
    in hypoadrenocorticism 203
    metabolism 148f
    osmotic effect in diabetic coma 567
    relation to
        glukagon 541
        glutathione 153
    testing, in diabetes mellitus 563
Serum iodine, protein-bound
    effect of thyroid therapy on 4

Serum iodine, protein-bound (cont.)
    in adolescent goiter 47
    in anorexia nervosa 5
    in hypopituitarism 31
    in hypothyroidism 23
    in normal 14
    in thyroid disease 14
    in undernutrition 473
    thyroid dose and 25
Serum ketones
    increased due to insulin lack 543f
    osmotic effects of 567
Serum lipids, in hypothyroidism 8
Serum magnesium, in diabetic acidosis 575
Serum non-protein nitrogen
    in base-losing nephritis 95
    in diabetic coma 567
    increased in
        hypoadrenocorticism 143
        pannephritis 101
        renal failure 119
Serum osmole
    concentration
        decreased in edema 535
        rate of change and antidiuretic hormone production 514
    effect on antidiuretic hormone production 511f
Serum pH 557
    in diabetic coma 567
Serum phospholipids, effect of cortisone on 150
Serum phosphorus
    determination, collection of blood for 125
    effect on
        of pituitary-growth hormone 452
        parathyroid activity 66, 75
    hyperphosphatemia
        effect of diet on 126
        in diabetic acidosis 556
        in diabetic coma 567
        in healing rickets 120f
        in hypoparathyroidism 66, 105
        in multiple myeloma 128
        in neonatal period 116
        in pannephritis 100
        in pseudo-hypoparathyroidism 111
        in renal failure 119
        in renal glomerular insufficiency 89
        in sarcoidosis 128
        with high phosphorus intake 70f
    hypophosphatemia
        due to glucose metabolism 125
        in base-losing nephritis 92
        in pathologic hypoparathyroidism 125
        with low phosphorus intake 70f
    normal range 64

Serum phosphorus (cont.)
    skeletal anabolism and 84
Serum potassium
    hyperkalemia
        and epinephrine 273
        in diabetic acidosis 556
        in hypoadrenocorticism 185
        in pannephritis 102
    hypokalemia
        due to testosterone 375
        in Cushing's syndrome 243
        in hyperadrenocorticism 139
        in hypoadrenocorticism 187
Serum protein
    as dehydration index in diabetic coma 567
    hyperproteinemia
        in multiple myeloma 128
        in sarcoidosis 128
    relation to calcium 54
Serum sickness, treatment with adrenocortical hormones 258
Serum sodium
    hypernatremia in hyperadrenocorticism 139
    hyponatremia
        in diabetic acidosis 556
        in hypoadrenocorticism 185f
        significance of urine sodium in 188
    in hypoadrenocortical patients 203
Serum urea, variability of 60
17-hydroxy-11-dehydrocorticosterone 136
    See also Adrenal cortices, cortisone
17-ketosteroid-precursors (17-KS-Gens).
    See under Adrenal cortices
Sex
    determination by
        chromosomes 291
        hormones 291
    incidence, in
        hyperparathyroidism 122
        hyperthyroidism 32
        nephrogenic diabetes insipidus 531
Sex characters. See under Sexual development
Sexual development
    characteristics, order of appearance
        in female 308f
        in male 392f
    effect on
        of adrenocortical 17-KS-Gens 157
        of testosterone 157, 384
    female 301f
        during adolescence 304f
        in adrenocortical virilism 235
        relation to hormone production 308f
    in Cushing's syndrome 237
    in hypothyroidism 21
    male, effect of chorionic gonadotropin on 391

Sexual development (cont.)
    maturation
        in hypoadrenocorticism 216
        in relation to stature 484, 492
    maturation, accelerated in obesity 486
    maturation, retarded
        due to caloric undernutrition 473
        due to diabetes insipidus 521
    retarded, in hypopituitarism 31
    See also Sexual infantilism; Sexual precocity; and under names of organs
Sexual infantilism
    in boys 422f
        causes 422
        definition 422
        hypothalamic types 422f
        pituitary types 423f
        testicular types 431f
    in girls 337f
        causes 337f
        definition 337
        functional types 342f
        hypothalamic types 337, 338, 340f
        incidence 338
        manifestations 338
        ovarian types 343
        pituitary types 341f
        vaginal smear in 315
    in primary idiopathic hypopituitarism 464
    in primary organic hypopituitarism 462
Sexual maturation. See under Sexual development
Sexual precocity
    in boys
        age of occurrence 325
        constitutional 325f
        due to hypothalamic lesions 323f
        idiopathic 325f
        types of 408f
    in girls
        age of occurrence 325
        constitutional 325f, 334
        definition of 320
        due to adrenocortical cancer 334f
        due to hypothalamic lesions 323f
        due to medication 335
        due to polyostotic fibrous dysplasia 127f, 325, 327f
        end organ type 335
        idiopathic 325f
        incidence 321
        manifestations 321
        physiologic 247
        true precocious puberty 321f
        types of 320f
    mixed iso- plus heterosexual 334f
    neonatal 301f
    See also Puberty, precocious
S-F-N hormone. See under Adrenal cortices

INDEX [629]

Shock, effect of epinephrine on 288
Simmonds' disease 461f
Skeleton
    arthritis. *See* Arthritis, rheumatoid
    atrophy of disuse 79, 87
    cartilage, calcification failure in osteomalacia and rickets 84
    catabolism
        in acidosis 101
        in calcium deficiency 82
    chondrodystrophy 11
    contractures, due to DOCA intoxication 206
    costochondral junctions 86
    coxa vara 10
    cranial fontanelles in hypothyroidism 21
    craniotabes 86
    cysts
        dysplasia, polyostotic fibrous 127f, 325, 327f
        multiple 127
        solitary 127
        solitary, giant cell 128
    deformities
        in ovarian agenesis 344
        in pathologic hyperparathyroidism 123
        osteomalacia and 86
    demineralization
        in hyperparathyroidism 75f
        in pseudo-hypoparathyroidism 114
    effect of parathyroid extract on 53f
    epiphyses, closure of
        and stilbestrol 484
        and testosterone 484
    epiphyses, cupping of, in rickets 84
    epiphyses, dysgenesis
        in hypopituitarism 31, 466
        in hypothyroidism 9f
    fractures. *See* Fractures
    growth, effect on
        of estrogen 300
        of pituitary growth hormone 452
        of testosterone 381, 436, 440f
    hyperossification, in hypoparathyroidism 107
    insulation, by osteoid tissue 84
    maturation, accelerated in
        adrenocortical virilism 227
        obesity 486
        sexual precocity 325, 408
    maturation rate, effect on
        of estrogen 300
        of testosterone 381, 436, 440f
        of thyroid 27
    maturation, relation to ultimate stature 440f, 492f
    maturation, retarded in
        hypopituitarism 31, 342, 462
        hypothyroidism 12

Skeleton, maturation, retarded in (cont.)
        sexual infantilism 337, 422
        undernutrition 12, 473
    metacarpals, early fusion in pseudo-hypoparathyroidism 114
    metastases in 128
    osteoblasts and osteoid formation 84
    osteochondritis deformans 10f
    osteoclastic activity in calcium deficiency 82
    osteogenesis imperfecta 128
    osteoid formation 84
        in scurvy 86
    osteomalacia 76, 84
        effects of 86
        in base-losing nephritis 92
        in pannephritis 100f
    osteoporosis 84
        local, in polyostotic fibrous dysplasia 328
    osteoporosis, due to
        estrogen lack 341
        immobilization 128
    osteoporosis in
        Cushing's syndrome 237
        menopause præcox 351
        ovarian agenesis 344
    polydactylism in Laurence-Moon-Biedl syndrome 341
    protein matrix 84
    refractoriness to parathyroid hormone, in pseudo-hypoparathyroidism 114
    rickets. *See* Rickets
    sodium in 140
        increase, in hypoadrenocorticism 143
    tenderness, in pathologic hyperparathyroidism 123
    tumors, in pathologic hyperparathyroidism 125
Skin
    atrophy, due to estrogen lack 341
    bluish, due to hyperepinephrinism 280
    coarseness, in hypothyroidism 22
    cold, due to hyperepinephrinism 280
    dry
        in diabetes insipidus 521
        in hypothyroidism 22
    ecchymoses, in Cushing's syndrome 236
    effect of estrogen on 299
    elasticity loss, in hypoadrenocorticism 197
    petechiæ, in Cushing's syndrome 236
    pigmentation
        in hypoadrenocorticism 202
        in hypothyroidism 22
        in polyostotic fibrous dysplasia 128
        sexual precocity and 327
        vitiligo, in base-losing nephritis 95
    senile, in menopause præcox 351

INDEX

Skin (cont.)
  sensitivity to
    Francis test and adrenocortical hormones 152
    tuberculin test and adrenocortical hormones 152
  striæ
    in Cushing's syndrome 236
    in obesity 489
  subcutaneous plaques, in pseudo-hypoparathyroidism 114
  texture, effect of testosterone on 381
  yellowish
    in hypopituitarism 465
    in hypothyroidism 22
  See also Acne

Sodium
  bicarbonate, effect on serum calcium 79
  bicarbonate, therapy
    comments on 569
    in base-losing nephritis 97f
  chloride, therapy
    comments on 569
    in hypoadrenocorticism 209
  citrate, therapy in base-losing nephritis 97f
  extracellular, deficiency due to hypoadrenocorticism 142
  homeostasis
    and the adrenal cortices 146f
    disturbed by stress 147
  intake, adjustment to, time for 188
  intake, effect on
    adrenocortical activity 143, 190
    sweat chloride–rate index 190
  intracellular, increase due to
    diabetic acidosis 570
    hyperadrenocorticism 139
  intracellular, normal content in body 140
  lactate, therapy, comments on 569
  loss, due to
    adrenocortical hormone withdrawal 143f
    thirsting 143
  loss, excessive
    due to hypoadrenocorticism 186
    effect of DOCA on 189
  metabolism, effect on
    of adrenocortical hormone 137f
    of estrogen 300
    of progesterone 301
    of testosterone 375
  movement into bones, in hypoadrenocorticism 143
  needs, in hypoadrenocorticism 211
  salt, administration, effect on posterior pituitary activity 498, 514
  salt, craving for, by individual with hypoadrenocorticism 197

Sodium (cont.)
  salt, therapy
    for intravenous use 569f
    hyperadrenocorticism and 571
    in diabetic acidosis 570
    in hypoadrenocorticism 214
    in stressed individual 148
  serum. *See* Serum sodium
  therapy and intracellular potassium deficiency 97f
  total, normal content in body 140

Solute load
  effect on urine volume 503f
  relation to antidiuretic hormone effect 498, 507f
  relation to diet 503f
  tolerance for 505

Solutions
  multiple electrolyte 573f
  parenteral 573f

Somogyi test 562
Spermatogenesis. *See under* Testes
Splenomegaly, effect of adrenocortical hormone on 256
Sprue, water test in 163

Starvation
  carbohydrate, due to insulin lack 543
  effect on gonadotropin production 296
  losses incident to 544

Steatorrhea. *See under* Stool
Stein-Leventhal syndrome 351, 355
Steroid hormones. *See under* Hormones

Stilbestrol
  chemistry 296f
  dosage 341, 343
  effect on ovulation 364
  therapy in menorrhagia 360
  See also Ovaries, estrogens

Stool
  fat content, normal 86
  fatty. *See* steatorrhea (*below*)
  lysozyme, effect of adrenocortical hormone on 153
  steatorrhea
    and calcium deficiency 82
    characteristics 86
    diagnosis 86f
  water content
    decreased in diabetes insipidus 511
    increased due to posterior pituitary extract 511

Stress
  adaptation to, effect of adrenocortical hormones on 151
  cause of death, in hypoadrenocorticism 203
  determinant in adrenocortical Na-K hormone production 147f
  effect on
    ACTH production 163f

Stress, effect on (cont.)
    adrenocortical activity 147, 156, 158, 167, 173, 184, 193, 259, 571
    adrenocortical hormone needs 156f, 193, 247
    11-17-OCS output 185
    glucose tolerance 551
    plus saline, cause of intracellular potassium deficiency 571
    See also under Emotional disturbances
Stupor and acute hypoadrenocorticism 216
Sulfhydryl groups. *See* Glutathione
Sulkowitch test 88, 590
Surface area, calculation
    from weight 592
    from weight and height. *See* end papers
Sweat
    chloride, relation to rate of sweating 189
    decreased in diabetes insipidus 510
    electrolyte content, effect of adrenocortical hormone on 138
    electrolyte test for adrenocortical status 189
    glands, effect of adrenocortical hormone on 138
    increased due to
        hyperepinephrinism 280
        hypoglycemia 580
        posterior pituitary extract 511
Sympathetic nervous system
    hormones
        acetylcholine 272, 299
        sympathin 272
    role in ACTH production 162
Sympathin 272
Sympathogonioma 276
Syndromes
    celiac 82
    Cushing's. *See* Cushing's syndrome
    Fanconi's 99
    Froehlich's. *See* Froehlich's syndrome
    Klinefelter's 437f
    Laurence-Moon-Biedl 341
        hypothalamic-pituitary relations in 385
    Stein-Leventhal 351, 355
    Turner's 344f
    Waterhouse-Friderichsen 216f

Teeth, in hypothyroidism 21
Temperature of body
    decreased in
        anorexia nervosa 5
        hypothalamic infantilism 340
        hypothyroidism 21f
        in undernutrition 473
    relation to ovulation 318
    See also Fever

Tendons
    calcification, in pseudo-hypoparathyroidism 116
    reflexes in hypocalcemia 105
Testes 372f
    adrenocortical cell rests in 373
    androgens
        actions of 374f
        source of urinary 17-KS 191
    androgens, production
        chorionic gonadotropin test for capacity of 402
        cryptorchidism and 442
        indices of 393f
    anorchia, congenital 431
    basic considerations 373f
    biopsy 402
        in adrenocortical virilism 227, 246
        in hypopituitarism 428
        in incomplete true precocity 413
        in interstitial cell cancer 419
        in normal person 388
        in sexual precocity 409
        tubule hyalinization in 438f
    cancer of interstitial cells and sexual precocity 418f
    castration 431
    clinical considerations 408f
    components 373
    cryptorchidism
        pseudo- 443
        true 442f
    development
        in normal persons 392
        in sexual precocity 409
    disease, cause of sexual infantilism 431f
    estrogens 298
        effect on testes 412
    eunuchoidism 431f
        pseudo- 393
    hermaphroditism and 365
    hormones
        chemistry 373f
        metabolism 373
    hypogonadism 422f
    hypogonadism, primary complete 431f
        clinical manifestations 431f
        prognosis 436f
        treatment 436
    hypogonadism, primary incomplete 437f
        clinical manifestations 437f
        diagnosis and differential diagnosis 439f
        etiology 437
        treatment 440
    interstitial cells
        cancer and sexual precocity 418f
        development in sexual precocity 409

Testes, interstitial cells (cont.)
    development, normal, relation to age 388
    pseudo-hyperplasia of 418
    pseudo-hyperplasia of, in Klinefelter's syndrome 439
  interstitial cells, effect on
    ICSH relations 391f
    of chorionic gonadotropin 391
  ovotestes 366
  size
    in adrenocortical virilism 227, 235
    in hypopituitarism 423f
    in incomplete true precocity 413
    normal 392
    significance of 395
    small 438
  spermatogenesis
    aspermatogenesis 422f
    in adrenocortical virilism 235
    in sexual precocity 409
  spermatogenesis, effect on
    of cryptorchidism 442
    of follicle-stimulating hormone 385
    of testosterone 386
  testosterone 373
    dosage in male hypogonadism 436
    metabolism to estrogens 391
    methyl 436
    pellets 436
    propionate 436
    use of, as growth hormone 440f
  testosterone, effect on
    ACTH production 245, 392
    body growth 436
    body structure 375f
    cryptorchidism, pseudo- 443
    cryptorchidism, true 442
    debilitated patient 441f, 480
    epiphyseal closure 484
    general metabolism 374f
    gonadotropin production 386
    gynecomastia 440
    interstitial cells 392
    nitrogen anabolism 436
    spermatogenesis 386
  testosterone, therapy
    for hypopituitarism in boys 429
    intermittent 429
    sexual precocity in boys and 419f
  tubules
    activity, index of 402f
    damage, and gonadotropin production 386
    deficiency 437f
    degeneration 402
    development, normal 386
    effect of FSH on 385
    hyalinization 402

Testes, tubules (cont.)
    immaturity 402
    tumor, in congenital adrenocortical virilism 247
Testosterone. *See under* Testes
Tests
  ACTH-eosinophil 170f
  ACTH-11-17-OCS 170f
  ACTH-17-KS 170f
  ACTH status 467
  ACTH-urinary uric acid 170f
  ammonium chloride tolerance 95f
  antidiuretic hormone response 521f
  Benedict's 563
  benzodioxane 285f
  chorionic gonadotropin 402
  Chvostek 104
  cortisone 229
  endometrium adequacy 355
  eosinophil count 173f
  epinephrine-eosinophil 168
  epinephrine-glucose tolerance 552
  ferric chloride 557
  Francis 152
  glucose tolerance 175f
    meaning of 550f
  gonadotropins, status 467f
  histamine 284f
  insulin tolerance 175f
  parathyroid hormone 107f
  pituitary growth hormone status 466f
  serum electrolyte measurements 185f
  sodium deprivation plus potassium feeding 186f
  Somogyi 562, 590
  Sulkowitch 88, 590
  sweat 189
  thyroid therapeutic 28f
  Trousseau 103
  TSH status 467
  24-hour fast 174f
  urinary 11-17-OCS 180f
  urinary 17-KS 190f
  vitamin A tolerance 86
  water deprivation 524f
  water test 163
Tetany
  diagnosis, by response to calcium 119
  due to
    hyperventilation 107
    hypocalcemia in hypoparathyroidism 103, 116
  following parathyroidectomy 129
  in pannephritis 101f
  in the spring 77f
  neonatal 116f
    clinical manifestations 118f
    diagnosis 118f
    differential diagnosis 119
    etiology 116f

INDEX   [633]

Tetany, neonatal (cont.)
    prognosis 120
    treatment 119f
  neonatal, relation to
    feeding 118
    maternal hyperparathyroidism 118
  of healing rickets 120f
Thiocyanate, cause of hypothyroidism 14
Thiouracil
  action
    effect of iodinization on 40
    mode of 39f
  cause of hypothyroidism 14
  dose 41
  metabolism 40
  response to 40f
  toxic reactions 41f
  use in
    preparation for thyroidectomy 40
    treatment of hyperthyroidism 36
Thiourea, cause of hypothyroidism 14
Thirst
  homeostatic factor 528
  in diabetes mellitus 555
  losses incident to thirsting 544
  See also Polydipsia
Thymus
  effect of pituitary growth hormone on 452
  involution, due to adrenocortical hormone 150
Thyroglobulin 1
Thyroid 1f
  activity, control of
    by caloric balance 5
    by environmental temperature 5
    by TSH 3
  activity, in obesity 489
  basic considerations 1f
  bruit 33
  carcinoma 20, 39, 48
  clinical considerations 14f
  enlargement. *See* Goiter
  exhaustion 47
  goiter. *See* Goiter
  homeostasis 5
  hormone 1
    inactivation 5
    needs during adolescence 47
    synthesis 1, 46
  hormone actions 2f
    on body growth and maturation 2f
    on cell organisms 2
    on energy metabolism 2
  hormone dose 25f
    in goiter 47
  hormone effects on
    constipation 26
    goiter 47
    gonadotropin production 296

Thyroid, hormone effects on (cont.)
    growth 26f
    hair 27
    mental development 28f
    nails 28
    pituitary growth hormone production 454f
    skeletal maturation 27
    skin 27
    TSH 47
  hormone therapy
    cause of hypoadrenocorticism 32
    dose 4
    dose in hypopituitarism 32
    effect of withdrawal 30
    in anorexia nervosa 5
    in hypopituitarism 31, 468f
    in obesity 492
    in thyroiditis 48
    intolerance for 469
    need for, in hypothyroidism 30
    rate response 4
  hormone therapy, effect on
    athyrotic 4
    body fat stores 480
    functional hypopituitarism 476
    normal 4f
  hyperplasia 47
  hyperthyroidism. *See* Thyroid, hyperthyroidism (*below*)
  hypothyroidism. *See* Thyroid, hypothyroidism (*below*)
  in hypothyroidism 20
  inflammation. *See* thyroiditis (*below*)
  nodules 33
    in adolescent goiter 47
  reciprocal relations with anterior pituitary 3
  size, effect of TSH on 3
  status, methods of appraising 6f
    alkaline phosphatase 8f
    basal metabolic rate 6f
    carotene 8
    cholesterol 7f
    epiphyseal dysgenesis 9f
    lipids 8
    radio-active iodine uptake 12f
    rate of skeletal maturation 11f
    serum protein-bound iodine 13f
    urine creatine 12
  storm 35, 43
  tenderness 48
  thrills 33
  thyroidectomy
    hypoparathyroidism after 103
    in hyperthyroidism 36f
    in thyroiditis 48
    preparation for 42f
  thyroiditis
    cause of hypothyroidism 15

Thyroid, thyroiditis (cont.)
    Hashimoto type 48
    thiouracil, cause of 42
    treatment 48
Thyroid, hyperthyroidism 32f
  after adolescent goiter 47
  amenorrhea and 354
  clinical manifestations 32f
  diagnosis 35f
  etiology 32
  gynecomastia and 440
  hypopituitarism in 342f
  in polyostotic fibrous dysplasia 328
  incidence 32
  medicational 4f
  medicational, effect on
    growth 26
    maturation 26
    mental development 26
  nutritional needs in 37
  recurrence 37
  sexual infantilism and 342f
  toxic effects 42
  treatment 36f
    goal of 43
    initial 37
    iodinization 36, 37f
    post-operative care 43
    propyl thiouracil 39f
    radio-active iodine 39
    surgical 42f
    thiouracil 39f
Thyroid, hypothyroidism 14f
  amenorrhea and 354
  clinical manifestations 15f
  congenital 15
  diagnosis 23
  differential diagnosis 23f
  due to hypopituitarism 30f, 342f
  due to thiouracil 39
  due to thyroidectomy 43
  due to thyroiditis 15, 48
  11-17-OCS output in 181
  etiology 15f
  goiter. See Goiter
  menorrhagia and 358
  prognosis 29f
  sexual infantilism and
    in boys 430
    in girls 342f
  treatment 25f
    test for 28f
    thyroid dose 25f
    thyroid dose, response to 25, 26f
  vs hypopituitarism 469
Thyroid-stimulating hormone. See Anterior pituitary, TSH
Thyroidectomy. See under Thyroid
Thyroiditis. See under Thyroid
Thyrotoxicosis. See Thyroid, hyperthyroidism

Thyrotropin (TSH). See Anterior pituitary, TSH
Tm glucose 60
Toes. See Fingers and toes
Tongue
  macroglossia 24f
  protuberant
    in hypothyroidism 22
    in mongolism 23
Toxemia, effect on glucose tolerance 551
Trauma, cause of hyperthyroidism 32
Triphenylchlorethylene, chemistry of 296f
Trousseau test 103
TSH. See under Anterior pituitary
Tuberculin test 152
Tuberculosis
  cause of hypoadrenocorticism 195
  water test in 163
Turner's syndrome 344f
24-hour-fast test 174f
Tyrosine, precursor of epinephrine 271

Undernutrition. See under Nutrition
Urea
  effect on osmoreceptors 514
  in blood, variability of 60
  in urine. See under Urine
Urethral cells, effect of estrogen on 313
Uric acid. See under Urine
Uric acid stones 123
Urinary tract, reabsorption of antidiuretic hormone 527
Urine
  abnormalities, in pathologic hyperparathyroidism 126
  aceto-acetic acid in 99
  acetone. See below, ketones
  albuminuria, in diabetes mellitus 577
  aminoaciduria 99
  ammonium
    content 95
    in pannephritis 101
  antidiuretic hormone 514f
    decreased, in newborn 530
    in nephrogenic diabetes mellitus 531
    increased, in edema 534f
    osmotic load, and 508
  calcium
    effect of adrenocortical hormone on 150
    excretion mechanism 55
    hypercalcuria 88
    hypercalcuria, idiopathic 99f
    hypocalcuria 82
    in base-losing nephritis 97
    in hypoparathyroidism 105
    relation to serum calcium 111
    Sulkowitch test 88, 590

Urine (cont.)
  calcium, increased in
    Cushing's syndrome 235
    polyostotic fibrous dysplasia 328
  chloride, effect on
    of posterior pituitary extract 509
    of urinary antidiuretic hormone 509
  citric acid, effect of estrogen on 300
  concentration 93
    control of 499
    in adrenocortical alarm reaction 534
    in diabetes insipidus 524
  corticoids. See below, 11-17-OCS
  creatine, in hypothyroidism 12, 23
  cystinuria 99
    and stunted growth 476
  11-OCS. See 11-17-OCS
  11-17-OCS output
    by normal 181
    in various diseases 181
    measurement of, specificity 180f
    relation to production 155f
  11-17-OCS output, effect on
    of ACTH 172
    of testosterone 392
  11-17-OCS output, increased
    in diabetic acidosis 546
    meaning of 185
  estrogens 298
    assay 313
    derived from testosterone 391
    in chorionepithelioma 334
    in constitutional precocity 325
    in female 297, 306f
    in male 297, 306
    in newborn 302
    in true precocious puberty 323
  estrogens, decreased in
    female castrate 345
    ovarian agenesis 344
    postmenarcheal amenorrhea 350
  estrogens, increased in
    chorionepithelioma 440
    pseudo-precocious puberty 330
  formaldehydogenic substances. See 11-17-OCS (above)
  fructose 552
  FSH. See gonadotropins (below)
  galactose 552
  glucose
    in acromegaly 555
    in diabetes mellitus 556, 562f
    in diabetic coma 568
    in functional hyperadrenocorticism 568
    in insulin deficiency 543
    pseudo-glycosuria in salicylate poisoning 557

Urine, glucose (cont.)
    qualitative considerations 552
    quantitative considerations 551f
    renal 551f
  glucose, relation to
    emotional stress 563
    infection 564
  glucuronides 298, 300
  glycogen and fat metabolism 543
  gonadotropins
    in chorionepithelioma 334
    chorionic, in pregnancy 316, 351
    during menstrual cycle 320
    effect of testosterone on 386
    in children 320
    in constitutional precocity 325
    in female castrate 345
    in idiopathic true precocity in boys 408
    in incomplete true precocity in boys 413
    in normal boys 386
    in normal girls 307f
    in postmenarcheal amenorrhea 350
    in pseudo-precocious puberty in girls 330
    in true precocious puberty in girls 323
  gonadotropins, absent in
    hypopituitarism 342
    hypothalamic infantilism 340
    hypothyroidism 342
    interstitial cell cancer 418
  gonadotropins, decreased in
    hypopituitarism 428
    undernutrition 474
  gonadotropins, increased
    despite hypopituitarism 468
    in chorionepithelioma 440
    in male castrate 431f
    in menopause præcox 351
    in ovarian agenesis 344
    in sexual precocity in boys 409
    in testicular tubule disease 386, 402, 437f
  gonadotropins, normal in
    ovarian fibrocystic disease 351
    testicular tubule failure 402
  histidine, effect of adrenocortical hormone on 153
  infection 93
  ketones
    during fasting 175
    in diabetes mellitus 556
    increased, due to insulin lack 543f
    output, effect of testosterone on 374
    relation to emotional stress 563
    significance of 564
  ketonuria, pseudo-, in salicylate poisoning 557

Urine (cont.)
    magnesium in base-losing nephritis 97
    nocturia in diabetes mellitus 555
    organic acids 99
    pentose 552
    pH 93
        in pannephritis 101
    phosphorus output
        effect of adrenocortical hormone on 150
        effect of parathyroid hormone on 62
        in hypoparathyroidism 105
        mechanism 55f
    phosphorus output, increased
        by parathyroid extract 66
        in pathologic hyperparathyroidism 126
    phosphorus output, relation to
        intake 65f, 71
        serum phosphorus 89f
    polyuria
        causes 518
        control by diet 528
        in adrenocortical alarm reaction 534
        in base-losing nephritis 95
        in diabetes insipidus 521
        in diabetes mellitus 555
        in diabetic acidosis 534
        in infantile diarrhea 534
        in pathologic hyperparathyroidism 123
        in salicylate poisoning 557
    potassium output
        effect of adrenocortical hormone on 137f
        in base-losing nephritis 97
    pregnandiol 300
        during menstrual cycle 318
        in children 318
        in constitutional precocity 325
    prolactin, in newborn 302
    salicylates, test for 557
    sediment, effect of estrogen on cytology of 313
    17-KS
        origin of 156, 191
        3-beta-17-KS 191
    17-KS output
        in hyperadrenocorticism 224
        in hypopituitarism 342, 428
        in obesity 486
        in ovarian agenesis 344
        in sexual precocity in boys 409
        in testis cancer 419
        in undernutrition 473
        in various conditions 191f
        meaning of 190f, 397f

Urine, 17-KS output (cont.)
        prognostic value, in adrenocortical cancer 234f
        qualitative aspects 157
        relation to age 156
    17-KS output, effect on
        of ACTH 172
        of cortisone 229
        of estrogen 345
        of testosterone 392
    sodium output
        effect of adrenocortical hormone on 137f
        in base-losing nephritis 97
    sodium output, increased
        by ACTH 246
        by adrenocortical 11-17-OCS 151
    solute output
        composition, and antidiuretic hormone 508f
        minimum 503
    solute output, relation to
        diet 503f
        fasting 524
        infection 532
        urine volume 503f, 533f
    specific gravity, fixed in
        base-losing nephritis 95
        pannephritis 101, 532
    specific gravity in diabetes insipidus 524
    sulfates 298
    titratable acidity 95f, 99
    urea clearance, decreased
        in diabetes insipidus 524
        in pannephritis 101
    urea clearance in nephrogenic diabetes insipidus 531
    urea excretion mechanism 60, 514
    uric acid-creatinine ratio, as index of adrenocortical activity 172
    uric acid, effect of adrenocortical hormone on 150
    volume
        control of 499
        effect of diet on 528
        relation to solute output 503f, 533f
    volume increased
        in hyperadrenocorticism 527
        in pannephritis 532, 533
    volume, maximum 502f, 505
        in diabetes insipidus 505
    volume, minimum 502f
        and antidiuretic hormone lack 510
        in diabetes insipidus 505
    water-solute ratio, effect of antidiuretic hormone on 502f
Urogenital sinus 365
Uterus
    cervix, cancer of, and menorrhagia 359

INDEX

[637]

Uterus (cont.)
  changes, during menstrual cycle 309f
  congenital absence 349
  contractions 299
    effect of posterior pituitary extract on 535
    in diabetes insipidus 535
  cramps, relation to ovulation 301
  development, during adolescence 304
  diseases of, and dysmenorrhea 361
  effect on
    of estrogen 298f
    of estrogen therapy 341
    of oxytocin 498
    of progesterone 301
  endometrium
    adequacy test 355
    biopsy 316f
    biopsy in "constitutional precocity" 325
    congenital absence of 355
    destruction by tuberculosis 349
    in metropathica hemorrhagica 356
    zones of 311f
  hypoplastic, in hermaphroditism 365
  in newborn 302
  malformation 349
    in ovarian agenesis 344
  origin of 292
  sarcoma botryoides of, and menorrhagia 359
  shrinkage in menopause præcox 351

Vagina
  absent in hermaphroditism 365
  development during adolescence 304
  effect on
    of estrogen 298f
    of estrogen therapy 341
  in newborn 301f
  mucosa, atrophy in menopause præcox 351
  origin of 292
  pH, effect of estrogen on 313
Vaginal smear
  atrophic type 315
  effect of estrogen on 313f
  in postmenarcheal amenorrhea 350
Vasopressin 498
Virilism, adrenocortical. *See under* Adrenal cortices
Vision loss due to craniopharyngioma 458
Vitamins
  need for, in hyperthyroidism 37
  vitamin A tolerance test 86
  vitamin D
    deficiency and steatorrhea 82
    dose equivalents 110
    dose in D deficiency rickets 122

Vitamins, vitamin D (cont.)
  effects 77f
  intoxication 79, 88
  requirements, normal 87f
  resistance to 82
Voice
  effect of testosterone on 381
  genetic factors and 381
  hoarse, in hypothyroidism 22
  puerile, in pseudo-eunuchoidism 393
  See also Larynx
Vomiting
  due to craniopharyngioma 458
  due to hypercalcemia 122
  due to hyperepinephrinism 280
  in diabetes mellitus 555
  in hypoadrenocorticism 197
  See also Nausea

Water
  balance, and obesity 487
  dehydration
    acute, nature of 513
    body weight as index of 567
    in infants, and diabetes insipidus 531
    losses in 544
  dehydration due to
    adrenocortical hormone withdrawal 143f
    antidiuretic hormone deficiency 510
    diabetes insipidus 521
    diabetic acidosis 555
    hypoadrenocorticism 143, 197
      treatment of 210f
    insulin lack 544f
    pannephritis 534
    salicylate poisoning 557
    thirsting 143f
  dehydration, effect on
    antidiuretic hormone production 498f
    kidney function 531
    thirst 510
  dehydration, repair of
    comments 569
    in diabetic acidosis 569f
    relation to losses 572
  deprivation
    and survival 145
    test for diabetes insipidus 524
  diuresis test for hypoadrenocorticism 163
  edema. *See* Edema
  excretion, and nephritis 533
  extracellular
    decrease due to hypoadrenocorticism 143

Water, extracellular (cont.)
    in diabetic coma 567
  extracellular, dehydration
    due to hypoadrenocorticism 145f, 211
    repair of 569f
  extracellular, edema due to hyperadrenocorticism 139
  extracellular, losses in dehydration 544
  homeostasis 517f
  hyperhydremia, production of, by post-pituitary extract 535
  insensible loss 2, 572
  intake
    in base-losing nephritis 95
    in diabetes insipidus 521
    in pathologic hyperparathyroidism 123
    psychogenic 529f
    relation to antidiuretic hormone production 515
  intoxication 505
  intracellular, dehydration
    in diabetic coma 567
    repair of 570
  intracellular, edema due to hypoadrenocorticism 145, 211
  intracellular, losses in dehydration 544
  metabolism
    in liver disease 515
    in newborn 530
  metabolism, effect on
    of adrenocortical hormone 152, 516f
    of anterior pituitary 516f
    of antidiuretic hormone 498f
    of testosterone 375

Water (cont.)
  needs for electrolyte-free water 569
  needs for maintenance
    in diabetic acidosis 573
    in hypoadrenocorticism 210
    in normal 210
  needs for repair
    in diabetic acidosis 573
    in hypoadrenocorticism 211f
  reabsorption by renal tubules 499
  serum water–solutes ratio in relation to urine water–solutes ratio 503, 511f
  shifts, due to osmotic forces 144f, 567
  solute relations
    and antidiuretic hormone 498f
    in renal glomerular filtrate 499f
Waterhouse-Friderichsen syndrome 216f
Weakness
  due to hypoglycemia 580
  in base-losing nephritis 95
  in diabetes mellitus 555
  See also Fatigue
Weight
  index of dehydration 567
  loss in
    diabetes mellitus 555
    hyperepinephrinism 280
    hyperthyroidism 34
    hypoadrenocorticism 197
  normal 592f
  See also Obesity
Wound-healing
  effect on
    of ACTH 150
    of adrenocortical hormone 150
  relation to caloric intake 478f

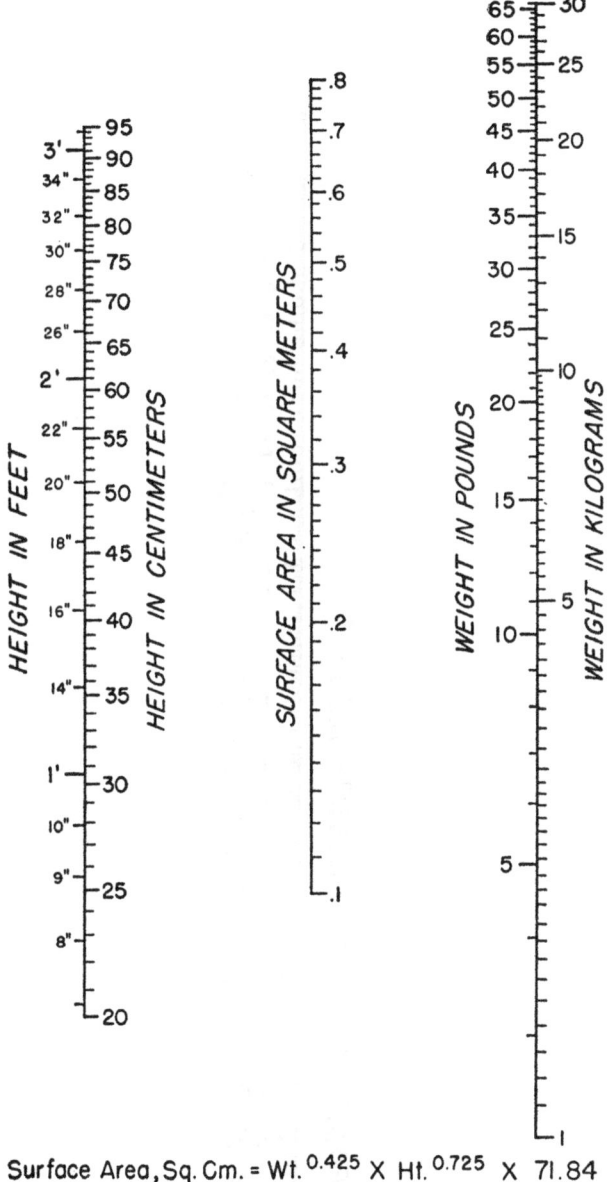

Surface Area, Sq. Cm. = Wt.$^{0.425}$ × Ht.$^{0.725}$ × 71.84

Nomograms estimating surface area from height and body weight. The patient's surface area is found by drawing a straight line between the point representing his weight and the point representing his height. From J. D. Crawford, M. E. Terry, G. M. Rourke, *Pediatrics* 5:783, 1950. See also Figure 1, page 594.

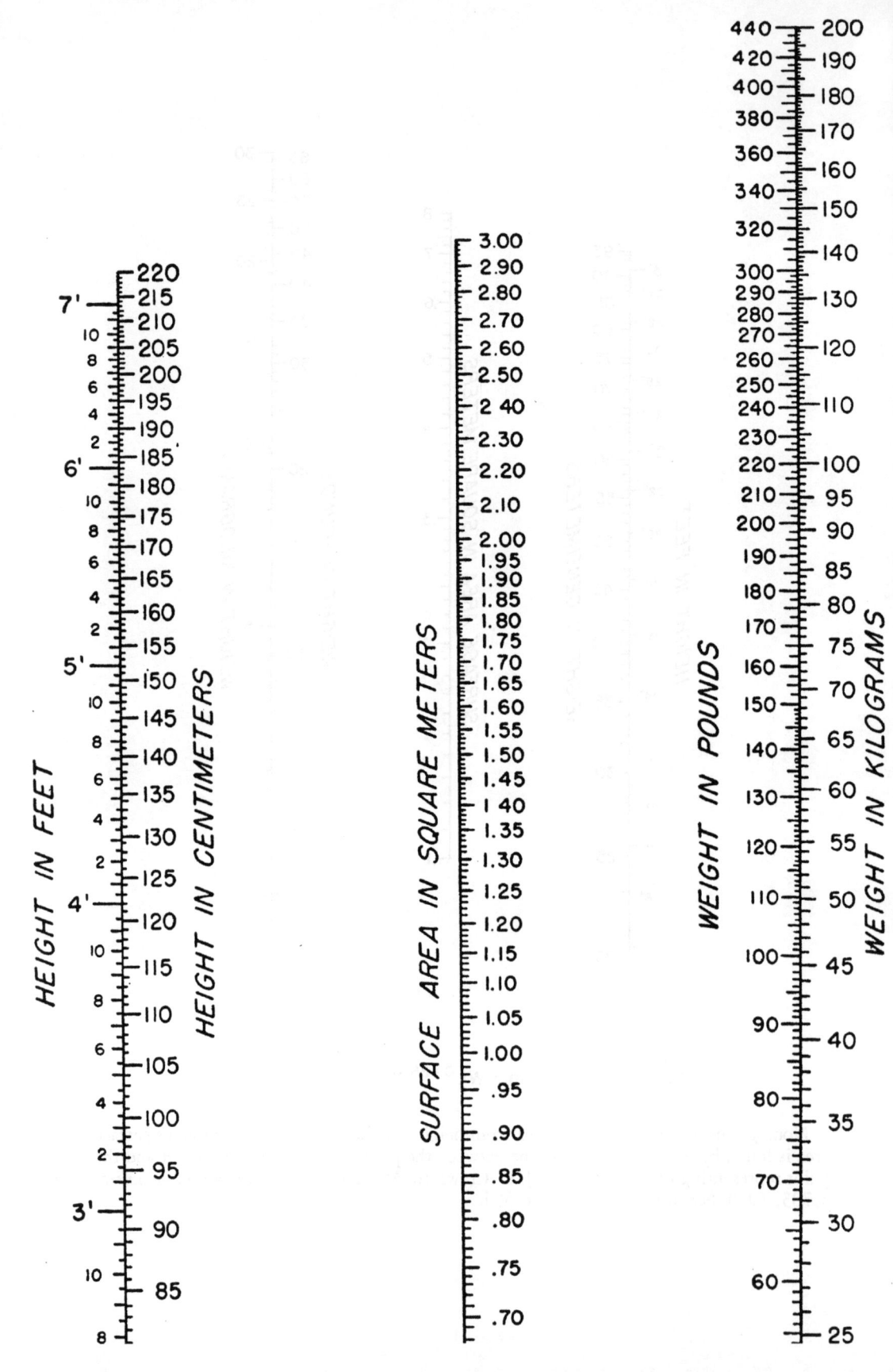

Bei Fragen zur Produktsicherheit wenden Sie sich bitte an:
If you have any questions regarding product safety,
please contact:

Walter de Gruyter GmbH
Genthiner Straße 13
10785 Berlin
productsafety@degruyterbrill.com